NASM ESSENTIALS OF
CORRECTIVE EXERCISE TRAINING

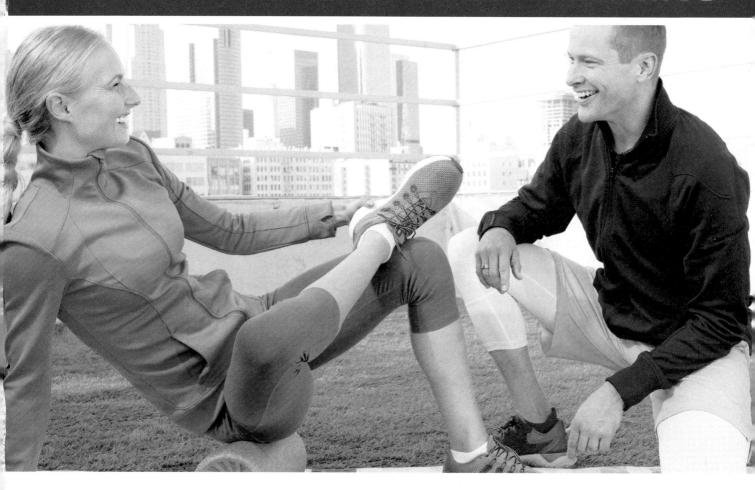

EDITOR

Rich Fahmy, MS, NASM-CPT, CES, PES

Content Development and Production Manager

National Academy of Sports Medicine

Gilbert, Arizona

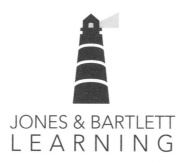

JONES & BARTLETT
LEARNING

Jones & Bartlett Learning
5 Wall Street
Burlington, MA 01803
978-443-5000
info@jblearning.com
www.jblearning.com

National Academy of Sports Medicine
355 E. Germann Road
Suite 201
Gilbert, AZ 85297
800-460-6276
www.nasm.org

Jones & Bartlett Learning books and products are available through most bookstores and online booksellers. To contact Jones & Bartlett Learning directly, call 800-832-0034, fax 978-443-8000, or visit our website, www.jblearning.com.

Substantial discounts on bulk quantities of Jones & Bartlett Learning publications are available to corporations, professional associations, and other qualified organizations. For details and specific discount information, contact the special sales department at Jones & Bartlett Learning via the above contact information or send an email to specialsales@jblearning.com.

Copyright © 2022 by the National Academy of Sports Medicine, an Ascend Learning Company

All rights reserved. No part of the material protected by this copyright may be reproduced or utilized in any form, electronic or mechanical, including photocopying, recording, or by any information storage and retrieval system, without written permission from the copyright owner.

The content, statements, views, and opinions herein are the sole expression of the respective authors and not that of NASM or Jones & Bartlett Learning, LLC. Reference herein to any specific commercial product, process, or service by trade name, trademark, manufacturer, or otherwise does not constitute or imply its endorsement or recommendation by NASM or Jones & Bartlett Learning, LLC and such reference shall not be used for advertising or product endorsement purposes. All trademarks displayed are the trademarks of the parties noted herein. *NASM Essentials of Corrective Exercise Training, Second Edition* is an independent publication and has not been authorized, sponsored, or otherwise approved by the owners of the trademarks or service marks referenced in this product.

You should always review the instructions and recommendations of the manufacturer of any exercise equipment before use, even equipment that appears in any NASM product, as the manufacturer's instructions and recommendations may have changed since the publication of the NASM product. NASM is not responsible for harm that may arise from the misuse of any exercise equipment.

There may be images in this book that feature models; these models do not necessarily endorse, represent, or participate in the activities represented in the images. Any screenshots in this product are for educational and instructive purposes only. Any individuals and scenarios featured in the case studies throughout this product may be real or fictitious, but are used for instructional purposes only.

20089-8

Production Credits
Director of Product Management: Cathy L. Esperti
Product Manager, Whitney Fekete
Manager, Project Management: Kristen Rogers
Project Specialist: Jennifer Risden
Director of Marketing: Andrea DeFronzo
Production Services Manager: Colleen Lamy
Product Fulfillment Manager: Wendy Kilborn

Composition: S4Carlisle Publishing Services
Text and Cover Design: NASM
Senior Media Development Editor: Troy Liston
Rights Specialist: Benjamin Roy
Cover Image: © National Academy of Sports Medicine
Printing and Binding: LSC Communications

Library of Congress Cataloging-in-Publication Data
Names: Fahmy, Rich, editor. | National Academy of Sports Medicine, issuing
  body.
Title: NASM essentials of corrective exercise training / editor, Rich
  Fahmy.
Other titles: Essentials of corrective exercise training
Description: Second edition. | Burlington, Massachusetts : Jones & Bartlett
  Learning, 2020. | Includes bibliographical references and index. |
Identifiers: LCCN 2020022136 | ISBN 9781284200898 (hardcover)
Subjects: MESH: Athletic Injuries--rehabilitation | Athletic
  Injuries--diagnosis | Athletic Injuries--prevention & control | Exercise
  Movement Techniques | Exercise Therapy--methods | Sports Medicine
Classification: LCC RD97 | NLM QT 261 | DDC 617.1/027--dc23
LC record available at https://lccn.loc.gov/2020022136

6048

Printed in the United States of America
24 23 22 21 20   10 9 8 7 6 5 4 3 2 1

YOUR TEXT

The following is the framework for the Corrective Exercise Specialist learning experience. This edition has been updated with the latest evidence and techniques, all with the goal of helping the reader apply them throughout the assessment and exercise program design processes. The text is divided into four sections.

Section 1 provides the rationale for and purpose of corrective exercise, along with the underpinning applied sciences.

Section 2 reviews the scientific rationale for and application variables of the exercise techniques used by the professional to optimize movement.

Section 3 outlines the assessment process that will be carried out by the professional to observe an individual's preferred movement strategies. The results of that assessment process will inform the individual's program design.

Section 4 focuses on putting it all together with programming detail for multiple kinetic chain regions. Section 4 also discusses effective recovery and application strategies necessary to promote client success.

CONTENTS

FOREWORD

Congratulations on taking this step in your health and fitness career! Thank you for entrusting us to provide the education and tools to improve your skill sets and enhance the services you provide to your clients and athletes.

Now more than ever, we are witnessing an increased reliance on technology and the prevalence of sedentary lifestyles. On the other end of the movement spectrum are overuse patterns and overtraining, which also lead to suboptimal movement strategies and musculoskeletal dysfunction. Focusing on quality of movement, movement efficiency, injury resistance, and recovery is vital to your clients' success and to you as a professional.

NASM is the world leader in fitness certification, continuing education, and professional development for health and fitness and sports performance professionals. Our evidence-based approach to creating applicable strategies has created what many consider to be the current standard in professional education in the health and fitness industry.

The backbone of the corrective exercise process is the NASM Corrective Exercise Continuum. The continuum was created by Dr. Mike Clark, DPT, PT, MS, in his work with elite athletes and has since become the standard in corrective exercise programming in the health and fitness industry. It has been applied successfully with clients and athletes of all backgrounds, abilities, and goals. The NASM Corrective Exercise Continuum is a simple, straightforward approach to designing customized programs that will enhance and improve the ability of your clients to move freely and move well.

This new edition of *NASM Essentials of Corrective Exercise Training* has been updated with the current evidence, strategies, and training techniques designed to equip health and fitness professionals with the necessary skills to optimize the movement performance of their clients and athletes.

Welcome to a select group of professionals; we wish you much success in your professional pursuits.

Sincerely,
Rich Fahmy, MS, NASM-CPT, CES, PES
Content Development and Production Manager
Managing Editor, *NASM Essentials of Corrective Exercise Training*

PROGRAM LEARNING OBJECTIVES

- **Relate** fundamental concepts of human movement and anatomy and physiology to corrective exercise.
- **Identify** attributes of and rationale for corrective exercise programming.
- **Identify** scope of practice and referral strategies for allied health professionals.
- **Evaluate** proficiency of movement using various assessment methodologies.
- **Design** individualized movement and exercise programs.
- **Apply** a spectrum of corrective tools, protocols, and modalities aligned to client needs and goals.
- **Demonstrate** effective coaching and communication techniques to maximize adherence and engagement.
- **Communicate** effective recovery strategies for a client's overall wellness.

CONTRIBUTORS

MANAGING EDITOR

Rich Fahmy

LEAD REVIEWERS

Kyle Stull, Scott W. Cheatham

AUTHORS

Tony Ambler-Wright
MS, CSCS, NASM-CPT, CES, PES, NASM Master Instructor

Adam Annaccone
EdD, LAT, ATC, NASM-CES, PES

David G. Behm
PhD

Allison Brager
PhD

Scott W. Cheatham
PhD, DPT, PT, OCS, ATC, CSCS

Mike Clark
DPT, PT, MS, NASM-CES, PES

Rich Fahmy
MS, NASM-CPT, CES, PES, NASM Master Instructor

Chris Frederick
PT, NASM-CPT

Ed Le Cara
DC, PhD, MBA, ATC, CSCS, NASM-CES

Ken Miller
MS, NASM-CPT, CES, PES, NASM Master Instructor

Rick Richey
DHSc, NASM Faculty Instructor

Eric Sorenson
PhD, ATC

Emily Splichal
DPM, MS, NSCA-CPT, NASM-CES, PES

Kyle Stull
DHSc, MS, LMT, CSCS, NASM-CPT, CES, PES, NASM
Faculty Instructor

David A. Titcomb
DPT, PT, EP-C, NASM-CES

PRODUCT TEAM

Jeri Dow
Senior Instructional Designer

Rich Fahmy
Content Development and Production Manager

Andrew Payne
Instructional Designer

Prentiss Rhodes
Product Manager

SPECIAL THANKS

Special thanks to the professionals who provided consumer and technical reviews of our previous and current editions. Your insight was very beneficial to our process of creating a relevant and applicable course for today's professional.

Technical Review: Adam Annaccone, Dave Behm, Robert Lardner, Ed Le Cara, Eric Sorenson, and Emily Splichal

Consumer Review: Georgia Fischer, Adam Ortman, and Theresa Peasley

An additional thanks is owed to Dr. Mike Clark, whose work in creating the NASM Optimum Performance Training Model and Corrective Exercise Continuum have laid the foundation for NASM's legacy of excellence in education and practical application.

USER'S GUIDE

Please take a few moments to look through this User's Guide, which will introduce you to the tools and features that will enhance your learning experience.

Learning Objectives open each chapter and present learning goals to help you focus and retain the crucial information discussed.

Key terms will appear bold within the text and be defined in the margin.

Extensive full-color art and photographs illustrate numerous exercise techniques, anatomy and physiology, professional forms, and important concepts.

Key term sidebars

Key term sidebars provide the definitions of key terms presented in the chapter. The key terms are bolded throughout the chapter for easy reference and for stronger comprehension of the material presented. Definitions are also presented in the glossary.

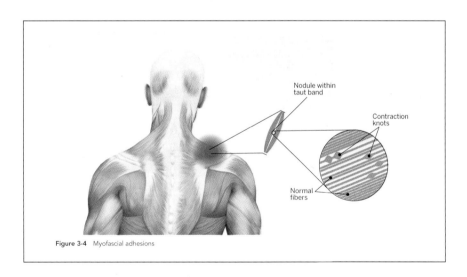

Figure 3-4 Myofascial adhesions

The **Corrective Exercise Assessment Flow** outlines the client intake process, static postural assessment, movement assessment, and mobility assessment.

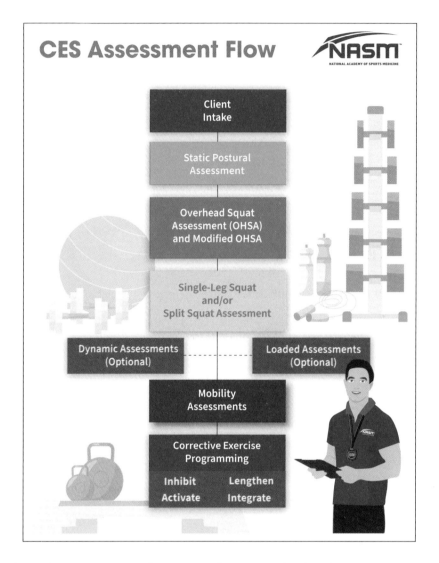

Call-out boxes draw attention to information and activities related to the text content.

Check It Out boxes provide you with fun or interesting information as a sidebar to the discussed content.

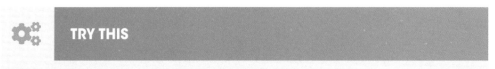

Try This boxes provide activities you can practice on your own.

CRITICAL

Critical boxes supply key information that you need to know before moving on to the next section.

TRAINING TIP

Training Tip boxes provide practical applications of the concepts being discussed.

HELPFUL HINT

Helpful Hint boxes help you retain information by providing analogies or memory tips.

GETTING TECHNICAL

Getting Technical callout boxes emphasize key concepts and findings from current research.

The appendix contains the full CES Assessment Flow and assessment forms for reference.

Introduction to Corrective Exercise Training

CHAPTER 1

Rationale for Corrective Exercise

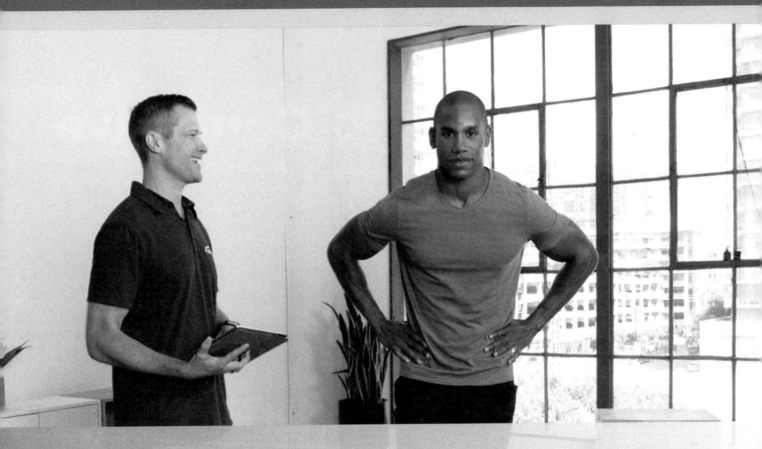

Learning Objectives

After reading this content, students should be able to demonstrate the following objectives:

- **Describe** the rationale for corrective exercise.
- **Define** *corrective exercise.*
- **Identify** the results of common physical conditions and lifestyle factors on the kinetic chain.
- **Identify** scope of practice parameters through the continuum of client care and performance.
- **Summarize** the phases of the Corrective Exercise Continuum.

Introduction

From the mid-1980s to the present, the wealth of technology and automation in the United States has taken a toll on public health. Work and home environments are inundated with automation, computers, mobile devices, and other technology that are more prevalent today than ever before. With the rise of technology, people are likely to be less active and spend less time engaged in physical activity outside of their occupation. As many as a quarter of Americans engage in no leisure-time activity at all (U.S. Department of Health and Human Services, 2020). Sedentary behavior increases all-cause mortality (U.S. Department of Health and Human Services, 2018). Additionally, lack of regular physical activity creates a kinetic chain that is less prepared to adapt and recover from activity, leading to increased injury rates (U.S. Department of Health and Human Services, 2008).

Rationale for Corrective Exercise

Research suggests that musculoskeletal pain is more common now than it was 50 years ago (Harkness et al., 2005). Poor movement quality may also adversely affect injury rate, biomechanical stress (e.g., ground reaction forces), and even physiological stress (e.g., increased cortisol) (Frank et al., 2019; Powers, 2010). Conversely, the application of an appropriate movement preparation technique, utilizing an integrated approach combining flexibility, core, balance, targeted strength, and dynamic warm-up exercises, may improve force absorption and reduce the incidence of injury (Al Attar & Alshehri, 2019; Pollard et al., 2017). This lends support to the concept that decreased activity and poor movement quality may lead to muscular dysfunction and, ultimately, injury. Corrective exercise and the optimization of movement quality have applications across populations and environments. All clients and athletes, regardless of current activity level, can benefit from the skills of a Corrective Exercise Specialist.

Corrective Exercise Philosophy

The primary objective of the Corrective Exercise Specialist is to optimize movement quality. This enhances performance, results, injury resistance, movement efficiency, and recovery. Optimization of movement quality is accomplished by minimizing less-than-ideal motor recruitment strategies that result in observable postural distortion and movement impairment. The Corrective Exercise Specialist's role is not to treat musculoskeletal injury after it has occurred but to reduce its likelihood in a currently healthy client or athlete. Corrective exercise strategies may also be applied post-injury after the athlete or client has received treatment and clearance from a healthcare provider to return to normal activity.

The Corrective Exercise Continuum

Corrective exercise is a term used to describe the systematic process of identifying a neuromusculoskeletal dysfunction, developing a plan of action, and implementing an integrated corrective strategy (**Figure 1-1**). It is a sophisticated and straightforward implementation of assessment and exercise program design processes. This implementation requires knowledge and application of an integrated assessment process, corrective exercise program design, and exercise technique. Collectively, the three-step process is as follows:

1. Identify the problem.
2. Solve the problem.
3. Implement the solution.

> **Corrective exercise**
>
> The systematic process of identifying a neuromusculoskeletal dysfunction, developing a plan of action, and implementing an integrated corrective strategy.

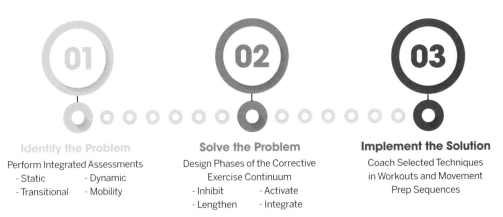

Figure 1-1 Corrective exercise process

01 — **Identify the Problem**
Perform Integrated Assessments
- Static
- Transitional
- Dynamic
- Mobility

02 — **Solve the Problem**
Design Phases of the Corrective Exercise Continuum
- Inhibit
- Lengthen
- Activate
- Integrate

03 — **Implement the Solution**
Coach Selected Techniques in Workouts and Movement Prep Sequences

Corrective Exercise Continuum

The systematic programming process used to address neuromusculoskeletal dysfunction using inhibitory, lengthening, activation, and integration techniques.

Inhibitory techniques

Corrective exercise techniques used to reduce tension or decrease activity of overactive neuromyofascial tissues in the body.

Solving the identified neuromusculoskeletal problems will require a systematic plan. This plan is known as the **Corrective Exercise Continuum** and will specifically outline the necessary steps needed to properly structure a corrective exercise program.

The Corrective Exercise Continuum includes four primary phases (**Figure 1-2**). The first phase is the Inhibit phase using **inhibitory techniques**. Inhibitory techniques are used to reduce tension or decrease activity of overactive neuromyofascial tissues in the body. This can

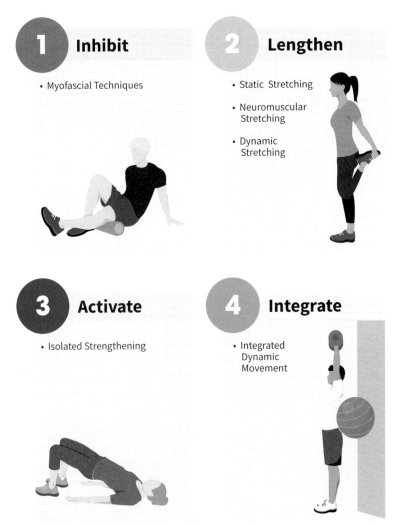

1 Inhibit
• Myofascial Techniques

2 Lengthen
• Static Stretching
• Neuromuscular Stretching
• Dynamic Stretching

3 Activate
• Isolated Strengthening

4 Integrate
• Integrated Dynamic Movement

Figure 1-2 NASM Corrective Exercise Continuum

be accomplished with self-myofascial techniques (e.g., foam rolling). The second phase is the Lengthen phase using **lengthening techniques**. Lengthening techniques are used to increase the extensibility and range of motion (ROM) of neuromyofascial tissues in the body. This can be accomplished using static stretching, dynamic stretching, and neuromuscular stretching. The third phase is the Activate phase using **activation techniques**. Activation techniques are used to reeducate or increase activation of underactive tissues as identified during the assessment process. This can be accomplished using isolated strengthening exercises. The fourth and final phase is the Integrate phase using **integration techniques**. Integration techniques are used to retrain the collective synergistic function of all muscles through functionally progressive exercise using integrated dynamic movements. Before implementing the Corrective Exercise Continuum, an integrated assessment process must be done to determine dysfunction and, ultimately, the design of the corrective exercise program. This assessment process should include (but not be limited to) postural assessments, movement assessments, and mobility assessments. This integrated assessment process will help in determining which tissues need to be inhibited and lengthened and which tissues need to be activated and strengthened through the use of the continuum. At its simplest form, the Corrective Exercise Continuum is a sequence of targeted flexibility and strengthening exercises tailored to an individual's posture and movement quality.

The Regional Interdependence Model

The concept of the **Regional Interdependence (RI) model** will be woven throughout the content. Regional interdependence is a relatively new concept posed by physical therapists and rehabilitation professionals to describe how the region of a patient's primary musculoskeletal complaint is affected by remote sites or factors. For example, a patient may complain of knee pain, but the pain is affected by dysfunction or impairment at the hip, ankle, or both. The patient's experience of symptoms may also be influenced by multiple physiological and psychological systems beyond the musculoskeletal (Sueki et al., 2013). The RI model provides an additional framework used by clinicians to expand their treatment strategies beyond local biomedical intervention at the site.

Although Corrective Exercise Specialists are not clinicians, the RI model provides a useful paradigm from which to assess and improve movement dysfunction; that is, impairments in one musculoskeletal region will influence the movement quality and functional capacity of others. With this understanding, it is imperative that the health and fitness professional take a global as well as a local perspective when assessing their clients' and athletes' movement and designing exercise strategies.

Professional Scope of the Corrective Exercise Specialist

Those who work in the health and fitness profession are fortunate to work in a field that can positively affect the lives of many. A variety of factors contribute to a sound mind and body, and, for all clients, optimized movement quality will have a significant effect on the achievement of their fitness goals. A Corrective Exercise Specialist plays an integral part in the health and fitness industry, and understanding the professional scope of practice is critical.

Lengthening techniques

Corrective exercise techniques used to increase the extensibility, length, and range of motion of neuromyofascial tissues in the body.

Activation techniques

Corrective exercise techniques used to reeducate or increase activation of underactive muscle tissues.

Integration techniques

Corrective exercise techniques used to retrain the collective synergistic function of all muscles through functionally progressive movements.

Regional Interdependence (RI) model

Assessment and intervention model used by clinicians based on the concept that the site of a patient's primary complaint or symptoms is affected by dysfunction in remote musculoskeletal regions.

Health Care and Fitness

The healthcare system is composed of various overlapping and complementary disciplines. For example, the physical therapist will work in conjunction with the orthopedic surgeon to facilitate maximum recovery of their shared patient with boundaries that must be acknowledged and adhered to for ethical and legal reasons. The **scope of practice** defines the limitations and boundaries of certain medical interventions that a person can and cannot perform. This applies to clinical, licensed professionals and those who are not licensed. Licensed healthcare providers have a range of responsibilities and licensing requirements established by their governing bodies (e.g., specific state professional board). Scope of practice can also include acceptable caseloads, practice guidelines, and recommendations for referral to another professional.

Much debate has taken place within the fitness industry regarding a distinct scope of practice for all fitness professionals. Scope of practice serves to define how services should be delivered, the minimum responsibilities of those providing the services, who can receive such services, and, in some instances, the setting in which the services are delivered. In general, the scope of practice for a professional describes the actions, procedures, and processes that they are permitted to undertake in meeting the set terms of the professional's license or credential.

Procedures that fall outside of the fitness professional's scope should be avoided, and the client should be referred to the appropriate healthcare professional. Unlike healthcare professionals, Corrective Exercise Specialists do not currently occupy a role that requires registry of state licensure. However, because they interact with apparently healthy individuals and offer a pay-for-service relationship, it has become essential to create a set level of standards to help ensure the safety of the public. In general, and except where the professional is a currently licensed healthcare provider, Corrective Exercise Specialists and other fitness professionals share an identical scope of practice.

The Continuum of Client Care and Performance

As healthcare costs escalate, emphasis on preventive care has become a priority. Certified Personal Trainers, Corrective Exercise Specialists, and other fitness professionals are being welcomed into the healthcare system and are becoming an asset in the Care and Performance Continuum (**Figure 1-3**).

It is vitally important for Corrective Exercise Specialists to understand their role along the continuum and to refer to other disciplines whenever a situation arises that is out of their scope of practice.

The Care and Performance Continuum incorporates the following disciplines:

- Hospitals, including emergency clinics and trauma centers
- Ambulatory care centers, including personal physicians and specialists
- Therapists, including physical therapists, cardiac rehabilitation professionals, massage therapists, and athletic trainers
- Ancillary facilities, including dentists and optometrists
- Behavioral health specialties, including psychiatrists and psychologists
- Alternative medicine practitioners (licensed), including chiropractors and acupuncture physicians
- Long-term care, including home health and hospice

CARE AND PERFORMANCE CONTINUUM

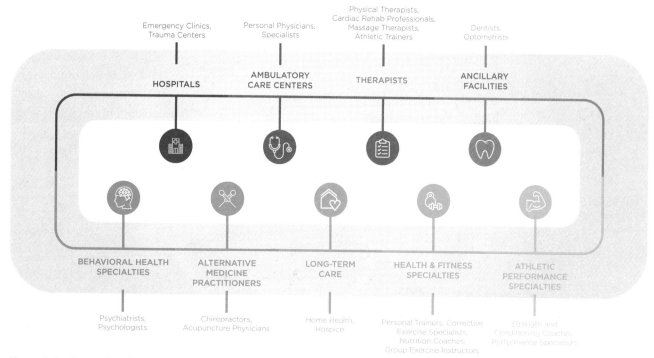

Figure 1-3 Care and Performance Continuum

- Health and fitness specialties, including Certified Personal Trainers, Corrective Exercise Specialists, nutrition coaches, and group exercise instructors
- Athletic performance specialties, including strength and conditioning coaches and performance specialists

Professional Responsibilities

A Corrective Exercise Specialist is a health and fitness professional who performs individualized assessments and designs safe, effective, and individualized exercise programs that are scientifically valid and based on evidence. They serve clients who have no medical or special needs or collaborate with the licensed healthcare professionals of clients currently undergoing treatment or who are post-rehabilitative treatment. The objective of the exercise program is to optimize the movement quality of the participants to enable them to perform at a level consistent with their desired fitness or performance outcome.

Goals

Corrective Exercise Specialists focus on optimizing an individual's movement quality to maximize performance and resistance to injury. When working with allied health professionals, it is the Corrective Exercise Specialist's role to take clients along the continuum of post-rehabilitative treatment to optimal performance. While one cannot claim that corrective exercise programming definitively prevents injury, optimized movement quality may increase a client's resistance to muscle and tendon injury due to the improved neuromuscular efficiency and control, kinetic chain management of force, and mobility achieved. Programs targeting specific movement compensations (e.g., knee valgus) related to particular injuries (e.g., anterior cruciate ligament tear) have been shown to be successful at reducing occurrence rates (Al Attar & Alshehri, 2019; Padua & Marshall, 2006).

Populations

Populations appropriate for the Corrective Exercise Specialist include clients who are post-rehabilitative treatment, fitness clients with no medical or special needs, and recreational and competitive athletes. History of relevant injury requires a medical release from the client's healthcare provider. If a client is currently under the care of a licensed healthcare provider (e.g., physical therapist, certified athletic trainer, or chiropractor) the Corrective Exercise Specialist is obligated to regularly consult with and obtain clearance from that professional (**Figure 1-4**).

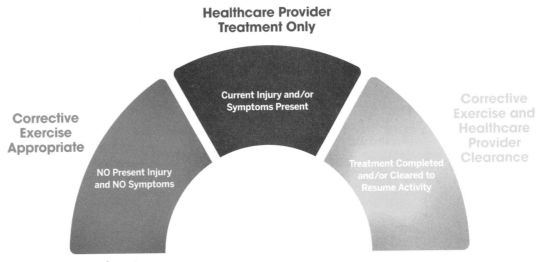

Figure 1-4 Scope of practice

Professional Settings

Common settings for Corrective Exercise Specialists include, but are not limited to, fitness facilities, private studios, independent service providers, and healthcare offices providing exercise services.

Techniques and Skills

Corrective Exercise Specialists are skilled in two primary domains: assessment and program design. Relative to Certified Personal Trainers, Corrective Exercise Specialists implement a more detailed and individualized level of assessment to create a comprehensive profile of a client's movement quality. The specialist interprets the results to design and implement an individualized and effective program to improve the client's movement performance. A specialist is also proficient in interfacing with other members of the Care and Performance Continuum to create a support team around a client. In addition, fitness professionals are required to hold current cardiopulmonary resuscitation (CPR) and automated external defibrillator (AED) certifications in order to be able to respond appropriately in emergency situations.

Diagnosis and Treatment

Diagnosis involves a comprehensive review and understanding of an individual's health history, current medical conditions, current symptoms, and then—after a complete review—determining a specific condition or disease. Treatment involves providing specific plans, including but not limited to therapeutic exercise programs, dietary counseling, nutritional supplementation, home remedies, therapeutic aids, medical intervention, or prescription drugs in order to treat certain conditions or diseases. Because they often work in fitness-related settings, Corrective Exercise Specialists will receive many questions from customers and clients, such as the following:

- "I'm experiencing knee pain. Can you tell me what it is?"
- "I have high blood pressure and high cholesterol. What's the best workout program for me?"

The professional must refer the client to the appropriate licensed provider when the client reports symptoms or conditions that fall outside their professional skill set.

Pain

Pain can be acute or chronic in duration and can originate from multiple systems (e.g., musculoskeletal or neuropathic). Pain is a complex multifactorial and personal experience influenced by biological, psychological, and social variables (i.e., the **biopsychosocial model of pain**). While many individuals may share a similar pain or dysfunction, each person's thoughts, previous experiences, behaviors, and expectations will influence their response to exercise or treatment differently. This understanding should factor into the practitioner's assessment and technique approaches (Booth et al., 2017). As such, the origin of pain requires a proper diagnosis from a licensed healthcare provider. It is irresponsible, and potentially dangerous, for Corrective Exercise Specialists to assume that pain reported by their clients is rooted in musculoskeletal dysfunction and that they are sufficiently equipped to address it. It is not appropriate to diagnose or treat areas of pain or disease. Instead, clients must be referred to other healthcare professionals or practitioners every time pain is reported that is outside of the usual workout soreness, particularly if it is acute and localized.

> **Biopsychosocial model of pain**
>
> Treatment paradigm for chronic musculoskeletal pain that accounts for the role of biological, psychological, and social factors in an individual's experience of pain.

 CRITICAL

Pain is a complex multifactorial and personal experience influenced by biological, psychological, and social variables. Corrective Exercise Specialists should not assume client pain originates in musculoskeletal dysfunction and should refer their client to the appropriate licensed healthcare provider when necessary.

The Future

A specific and sophisticated skill set is required to meet the needs of today's client and athlete. The health and fitness industry has recognized the trend toward nonfunctional living. Health and fitness professionals are witnessing a decrease in the physical functionality of their clients and athletes and are striving to address it.

This is a new state of training in which the client has been physically molded by furniture, gravity, and inactivity; and the athlete injured by overuse patterns (Patel et al., 2017). Today's client is not ready to begin physical activity at the same level that a typical client could 20 to 30 years ago. Therefore, current training programs cannot stay the same as programs of the past.

The advanced mindset in fitness should cater to creating programs that address functional capacity as part of a safe program designed particularly for each individual. In other words, training programs must consider each person, that person's environment and goals, and the tasks that will be performed. It will also be important to address any potential muscle imbalances and movement deficiencies to improve function and decrease the risk of injury. This is best achieved by introducing an integrated approach to program design. It is on this premise that the National Academy of Sports Medicine (NASM) presents the rationale for the Corrective Exercise Continuum and the importance of its integration into current exercise programs.

SUMMARY

Today, more people work in offices, have longer work hours, use more advanced technology and automation, and are required to move less on a daily basis. This environment produces more people who are inactive and have impaired function and leads to dysfunction and increased rates of musculoskeletal pain and injury.

In working with today's typical client and athlete, who more than likely possesses muscle imbalances, health and fitness professionals must take special consideration when designing programs. An integrated approach should be used to create safe programs that consider the functional capacity for each individual. They must address factors such as appropriate forms of flexibility, increasing strength and neuromuscular control, working in different types of environments, and training in different planes of motion. These are the basis for the use of corrective exercise and NASM's Corrective Exercise Continuum model. All the phases included in the model have been specifically designed to follow biomechanical, physiological, and functional principles of the human movement system (HMS). The Corrective Exercise Continuum is an easy-to-follow systematic process that will help address muscle imbalances, improve resistance to injury, optimize movement quality, and maximize results.

REFERENCES

Al Attar, W. S. A., & Alshehri, M. A. (2019). A meta-analysis of meta-analyses of the effectiveness of FIFA injury prevention programs in soccer. *Scandinavian Journal of Medicine & Science in Sports, 29*(12), 1846–1855. https://doi.org/10.1111/sms.13535

Booth, J., Moseley, G. L., Schiltenwolf, M., Cashin, A., Davies, M., & Hübscher, M. (2017). Exercise for chronic musculoskeletal pain: A biopsychosocial approach. *Musculoskeletal Care, 15*(4), 413–421. https://doi.org/10.1002/msc.1191

Frank, B. S., Hackney, A. C., Battaglini, C. L., Blackburn, T., Marshall, S. W., Clark, M., & Padua, D. A. (2019). Movement profile influences systemic stress and biomechanical resilience to high training load exposure. *Journal of Science and Medicine in Sport, 22*(1), 35–41. https://doi.org/10.1016/j.jsams.2018.05.017

Harkness, E. F., Macfarlane, G. J., Silman, A. J., & McBeth, J. (2005). Is musculoskeletal pain more common now than 40 years ago? Two population-based cross-sectional studies. *Rheumatology (Oxford, England), 44*(7), 890–895. https://doi.org/10.1093/rheumatology/keh599

Padua, D. A., & Marshall, S. W. (2006). Evidence supporting ACL-injury-prevention exercise programs: A review of the literature. *Athletic Therapy Today, 11*(2), 11–23. https://doi.org/10.1123/att.11.2.11

Patel, D. R., Yamasaki, A., & Brown, K. (2017). Epidemiology of sports-related musculoskeletal injuries in young athletes in United States. *Translational Pediatrics, 6*(3), 160–166. https://doi.org/10.21037/tp.2017.04.08

Pollard, C. D., Sigward, S. M., & Powers, C. M. (2017). ACL injury prevention training results in modification of hip and knee mechanics during a drop-landing task. *Orthopaedic Journal of Sports Medicine, 5*(9), 1–7. https://doi.org/10.1177/2325967117726267

Powers, C. M. (2010). The influence of abnormal hip mechanics on knee injury: A biomechanical perspective. *The Journal of*

Orthopaedic & Sports Physical Therapy, 40(2), 42–51. https://doi.org/10.2519/jospt.2010.3337

Sueki, D. G., Cleland, J. A., & Wainner, R. S. (2013, May). A regional interdependence model of musculoskeletal dysfunction: research, mechanisms, and clinical implications. *Journal of Manual & Manipulative Therapy, 21*(2), 90–102. https://doi.org/10.1179/2042618612Y.0000000027

U.S. Department of Health and Human Services. (2008). *Physical activity guidelines advisory committee report.* https://health.gov/paguidelines/2008/report/

U.S. Department of Health and Human Services. (2018). *Physical activity guidelines advisory committee scientific report to the Secretary of Health and Human Services.* https://health.gov/paguidelines/second-edition/report/

U.S. Department of Health and Human Services. (2020). Physical activity. Healthy People 2020 objective. https://www.healthypeople.gov/2020/topics-objectives/topic/physical-activity

CHAPTER 2

Human Movement Science and Corrective Exercise

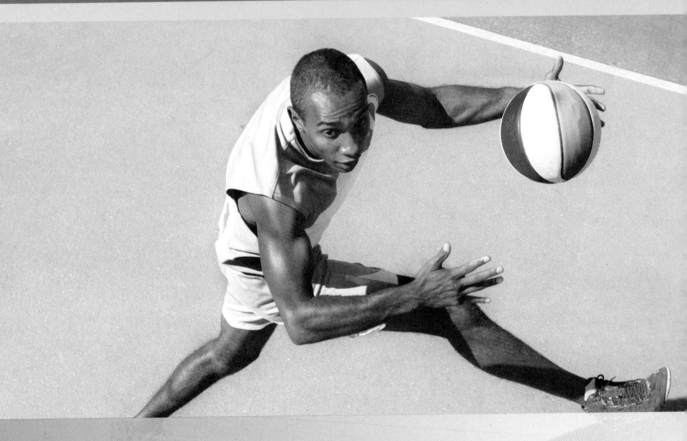

Learning Objectives

After reading this content, students should be able to demonstrate the following objectives:

- **Explain** functional anatomy as it relates to movement.
- **Explain** the effect that posture has on movement and performance.
- **Describe** the influence of optimal neuromuscular efficiency on human movement.
- **Explain** potential causes for common altered movement patterns.
- **Relate** altered movement patterns to muscle imbalance.
- **Explain** the influence altered movement patterns will have on client programming.
- **Explain** the relationship between pain and corrective exercise.

Introduction

Human movement science is the study of how the human movement system (HMS) functions in an interdependent, interrelated scheme. The HMS consists of the muscular system, the skeletal system, and the nervous system (**Figure 2-1**) (Byström et al., 2013; Neumann, 2016; Sahrmann et al., 2017). Although they appear separate, each system and its components must collaborate to form interdependent links. In turn, this entire interdependent system must be aware of its relationship to internal and external environments while gathering the necessary information to produce the appropriate **movement patterns**. This process ensures optimal functioning of the HMS and optimal human movement.

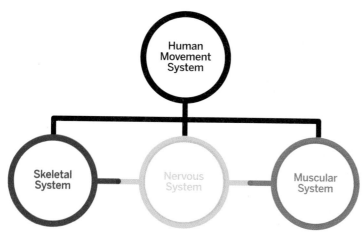

Figure 2-1   Components of the human movement system

Functional Anatomy

Traditional training has focused on training specific body parts, often in single, fixed planes of motion. In turn, anatomy has been traditionally taught in similarly isolated, fragmented components. That approach mapped the body, provided simplistic answers about the structures, and categorized each component. However, the everyday functioning of the human body is an integrated and multidimensional system, not a series of isolated, independent pieces. The new paradigm is to present anatomy from a functional, integrated perspective.

Although muscles have the ability to dominate a certain plane of motion, the central nervous system (CNS) optimizes the selection of muscle synergies, not simply the selection of individual muscles. The CNS coordinates deceleration, stabilization, and acceleration for all muscles of the body in all three planes of motion. Muscles must also react to external stimuli such as gravity, momentum, ground reaction forces, and forces created by other functioning muscles. So, with so many factors involved in the functioning of the HMS, muscles, like actors in a movie, can switch up the role they play depending on what is required of them. Based on the load, the direction of resistance, body position, and the movement pattern being performed, muscles can dynamically take on one of four movement production roles. Those roles include the following:

- **Agonist**: A muscle is an agonist when it acts as the prime mover for a given movement pattern. This muscle provides a majority of force generation. For example, the gluteus maximus is the agonist for hip extension, the pectoralis major is the agonist for pressing movements, and the biceps brachii is the agonist for elbow flexion.

- **Antagonist**: A muscle is an antagonist when it acts in direct opposition of the agonist. When the agonist contracts, the antagonist must relax to allow the joint to move—a neuromuscular interaction known as **reciprocal inhibition**. For example, both the psoas and the rectus femoris (hip flexors) are antagonistic to the gluteus maximus.
- **Synergist**: Muscles in the synergist role are meant to assist the agonist but are not supposed to be the primary source of force production. For example, the triceps brachii are synergistic to the pectoralis major for pressing movements, whereas the hamstrings assist the gluteus maximus during hip extension.
- **Stabilizer**: Muscles in the role of stabilizer help support associated joints while the prime movers and the synergists contract to create movement. For example, the muscles of the rotator cuff support the glenohumeral joint, whereas muscles such as the deltoids and latissimus dorsi create movement at the shoulder.

Although they may have different characteristics, shapes, and sizes, all muscles work in concert to produce efficient motion. For some movements, a muscle should be the agonist, whereas for others it may be an antagonist or a synergist. It all has to do with the movement pattern that needs to be accomplished. For example, muscles that are agonists for flexion are antagonists when the respective joint needs to extend. This realization allows one to view the function of a muscle in all planes of motion throughout the full **muscle action spectrum** (**eccentric**, **concentric**, and **isometric**) (Page et al., 2010; Sahrmann et al., 2017; Thomeé et al., 1995).

Skeletal Muscles

The traditional, simplistic explanation of skeletal muscles is that they work concentrically and predominantly in one plane of motion. However, muscles should be viewed as functioning in all planes of motion, throughout the full muscle action spectrum. Corrective exercise programs become more specific when there is a broader understanding of functional anatomy. The following section lists the **origins** (i.e., the beginning attachment point of the muscle) and **insertions** (i.e., where it connects back to the skeleton), the **isolated** (concentric) and **integrated** (eccentric and isometric) functions, and the **innervations** of the major muscles of the HMS (Neumann, 2016; Seeley et al., 2004; Watkins, 2010).

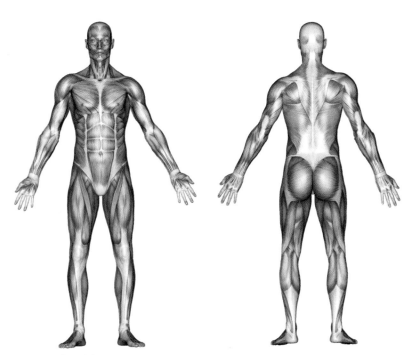

© Ecliptic blue/Shutterstock

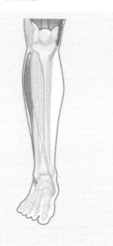

ANTERIOR TIBIALIS

ORIGIN
- Lateral condyle and proximal two-thirds of the lateral surface of the tibia

INSERTION
- Medial and plantar aspects of the medial cuneiform and the base of the first metatarsal

ISOLATED FUNCTION
Concentric Action
- Ankle dorsiflexion and inversion

INTEGRATED FUNCTION
Eccentric Action
- Ankle plantar flexion and eversion

Isometric Action
- Stabilizes the arch of the foot

INNERVATION
- Deep fibular (peroneal) nerve

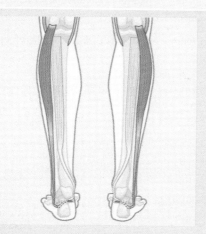

POSTERIOR TIBIALIS

ORIGIN
- Proximal two-thirds of posterior surface of the tibia and fibula

INSERTION
- Every tarsal bone (navicular, cuneiform, and cuboid) but the talus plus the bases of the second through the fourth metatarsal bones—the main insertion is on the navicular tuberosity and the medial cuneiform bone.

ISOLATED FUNCTION
Concentric Action
- Ankle plantar flexion and inversion of the foot

INTEGRATED FUNCTION
Eccentric Action
- Ankle dorsiflexion and eversion

Isometric Action
- Stabilizes the arch of the foot

INNERVATION
- Tibial nerve

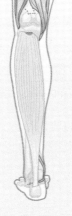

SOLEUS

ORIGIN
- Posterior surface of the fibular head and proximal one-third of its shaft and from the posterior side of the tibia

INSERTION
- Calcaneus via the Achilles tendon

ISOLATED FUNCTION
Concentric Action
- Accelerates plantar flexion

INTEGRATED FUNCTION
Eccentric Action
- Decelerates ankle dorsiflexion

Isometric Action
- Stabilizes the foot and ankle complex

INNERVATION
- Tibial nerve

Concentric muscle action

Occurs when a muscle generates force while shortening to accelerate an external load.

Isometric muscle action

Occurs when a muscle generates force equal to an external load to hold it in place.

Muscle origin

The beginning attachment point of a muscle.

Muscle insertion

Where the end point of a muscle connects back to the skeleton.

Isolated muscle function

The joint motion created when a muscle contracts concentrically.

Integrated muscle function

The joint motion(s) created when a muscle contracts eccentrically or isometrically.

Muscle innervation

A muscle's point of connection to the nervous system.

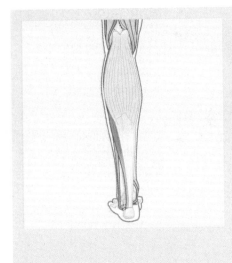

GASTROCNEMIUS

ORIGIN
- Posterior aspect of the lateral and medial femoral condyles

INSERTION
- Calcaneus via the Achilles tendon

ISOLATED FUNCTION
Concentric Action
- Accelerates plantar flexion

INTEGRATED FUNCTION
Eccentric Action
- Decelerates ankle dorsiflexion

Isometric Action
- Isometrically stabilizes the foot and ankle complex

INNERVATION
- Tibial nerve

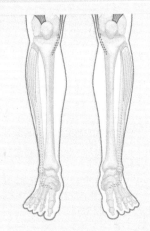

FIBULARIS (PERONEUS) LONGUS

ORIGIN
- Lateral condyle of tibia, head and proximal two-thirds of the lateral surface of the fibula

INSERTION
- Lateral surface of the medial cuneiform and lateral side of the base of the first metatarsal

ISOLATED FUNCTION
Concentric Action
- Plantar flexes and everts the foot

INTEGRATED FUNCTION
Eccentric Action
- Decelerates ankle dorsiflexion and inversion

Isometric Action
- Stabilizes the foot and ankle complex

INNERVATION
- Superficial fibular (peroneal) nerve

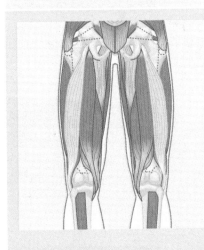

BICEPS FEMORIS, LONG HEAD

ORIGIN
- Ischial tuberosity of the pelvis, part of the sacrotuberous ligament

INSERTION
- Head of the fibula

ISOLATED FUNCTION
Concentric Action
- Accelerates knee flexion, hip extension, and tibial external rotation

INTEGRATED FUNCTION
Eccentric Action
- Decelerates knee extension, hip flexion, and tibial internal rotation

Isometric Action
- Stabilizes the lumbo-pelvic-hip complex and knee

INNERVATION
- Tibial nerve

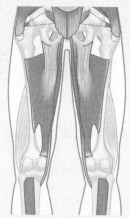

BICEPS FEMORIS, SHORT HEAD

ORIGIN
- Lower one-third of the posterior aspect of the femur

INSERTION
- Head of the fibula

ISOLATED FUNCTION
Concentric Action
- Accelerates knee flexion and tibial external rotation

INTEGRATED FUNCTION
Eccentric Action
- Decelerates knee extension and tibial internal rotation

Isometric Action
- Stabilizes the knee

INNERVATION
- Common fibular (peroneal) nerve

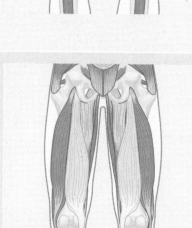

SEMIMEMBRANOSUS

ORIGIN
- Ischial tuberosity of the pelvis

INSERTION
- Posterior aspect of the medial tibial condyle of the tibia

ISOLATED FUNCTION
Concentric Action
- Accelerates knee flexion, hip extension, and tibial internal rotation

INTEGRATED FUNCTION
Eccentric Action
- Decelerates knee extension, hip flexion, and tibial external rotation

Isometric Action
- Stabilizes the lumbo-pelvic-hip complex and knee

INNERVATION
- Tibial nerve

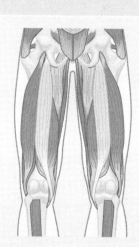

SEMITENDINOSUS

ORIGIN
- Ischial tuberosity of the pelvis and part of the sacrotuberous ligament

INSERTION
- Proximal aspect of the medial tibial condyle of the tibia (pes anserine)

ISOLATED FUNCTION
Concentric Action
- Accelerates knee flexion, hip extension, and tibial internal rotation

INTEGRATED FUNCTION
Eccentric Action
- Decelerates knee extension, hip flexion, and tibial external rotation

Isometric Action
- Stabilizes the lumbo-pelvic-hip complex and knee

INNERVATION
- Tibial nerve

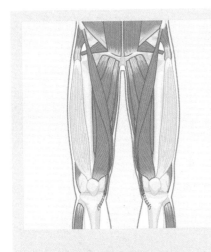

VASTUS LATERALIS

ORIGIN
- Anterior and inferior border of the greater trochanter, lateral region of the gluteal tuberosity, and lateral lip of the linea aspera of the femur

INSERTION
- Base of patella and tibial tuberosity of the tibia

ISOLATED FUNCTION
Concentric Action
- Accelerates knee extension

INTEGRATED FUNCTION
Eccentric Action
- Decelerates knee flexion

Isometric Action
- Stabilizes the knee

INNERVATION
- Femoral nerve

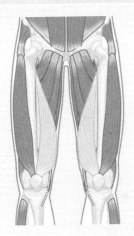

VASTUS MEDIALIS

ORIGIN
- Lower region of intertrochanteric line, medial lip of linea aspera, and proximal medial supracondylar line of the femur

INSERTION
- Base of patella and tibial tuberosity of the tibia

ISOLATED FUNCTION
Concentric Action
- Accelerates knee extension

INTEGRATED FUNCTION
Eccentric Action
- Decelerates knee flexion

Isometric Action
- Stabilizes the knee

INNERVATION
- Femoral nerve

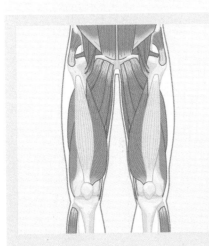

VASTUS INTERMEDIUS

ORIGIN
- Anterior-lateral regions of the upper two-thirds of the femur

INSERTION
- Base of patella and tibial tuberosity of the tibia

ISOLATED FUNCTION
Concentric Action
- Accelerates knee extension

INTEGRATED FUNCTION
Eccentric Action
- Decelerates knee flexion

Isometric Action
- Stabilizes the knee

INNERVATION
- Femoral nerve

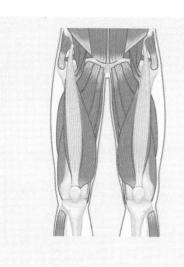

RECTUS FEMORIS
ORIGIN
- Anterior-inferior iliac spine of the pelvis

INSERTION
- Base of patella and tibial tuberosity of the tibia

ISOLATED FUNCTION
Concentric Action
- Accelerates knee extension and hip flexion

INTEGRATED FUNCTION
Eccentric Action
- Decelerates knee flexion and hip extension

Isometric Action
- Stabilizes the lumbo-pelvic-hip complex and knee

INNERVATION
- Femoral nerve

HIP MUSCLES

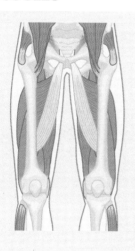

ADDUCTOR LONGUS
ORIGIN
- Anterior surface of the inferior pubic ramus of the pelvis

INSERTION
- Linea aspera of the femur

ISOLATED FUNCTION
Concentric Action
- Accelerates hip adduction, flexion, and internal rotation

INTEGRATED FUNCTION
Eccentric Action
- Decelerates hip abduction, extension, and external rotation

Isometric Action
- Stabilizes the lumbo-pelvic-hip complex

INNERVATION
- Obturator nerve

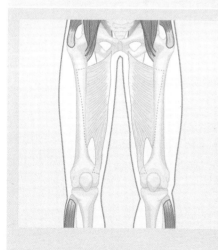

ADDUCTOR MAGNUS, ANTERIOR FIBERS
ORIGIN
- Ischial ramus of the pelvis

INSERTION
- Linea aspera of the femur

ISOLATED FUNCTION
Concentric Action
- Accelerates hip adduction, flexion, and internal rotation

INTEGRATED FUNCTION
Eccentric Action
- Decelerates hip abduction, extension, and external rotation

Isometric Action
- Stabilizes the lumbo-pelvic-hip complex

INNERVATION
- Obturator nerve

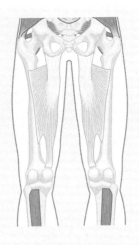

ADDUCTOR MAGNUS, POSTERIOR FIBERS

ORIGIN
- Ischial tuberosity of the pelvis

INSERTION
- Adductor tubercle on femur

ISOLATED FUNCTION

Concentric Action
- Accelerates hip adduction, extension, and external rotation

INTEGRATED FUNCTION

Eccentric Action
- Decelerates hip abduction, flexion, and internal rotation

Isometric Action
- Stabilizes the lumbo-pelvic-hip complex

INNERVATION
- Sciatic nerve

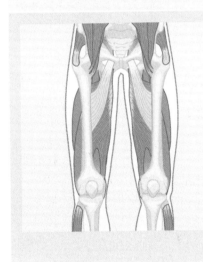

ADDUCTOR BREVIS

ORIGIN
- Anterior surface of the inferior pubic ramus of the pelvis

INSERTION
- Proximal one-third of the linea aspera of the femur

ISOLATED FUNCTION

Concentric Action
- Accelerates hip adduction, flexion, and internal rotation

INTEGRATED FUNCTION

Eccentric Action
- Decelerates hip abduction, extension, and external rotation

Isometric Action
- Stabilizes the lumbo-pelvic-hip complex

INNERVATION
- Obturator nerve

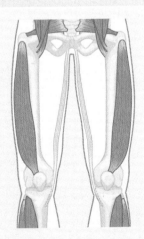

GRACILIS

ORIGIN
- Anterior aspect of lower body of pubis

INSERTION
- Proximal medial surface of the tibia (pes anserine)

ISOLATED FUNCTION

Concentric Action
- Accelerates hip adduction, flexion, and internal rotation and assists in tibial internal rotation

INTEGRATED FUNCTION

Eccentric Action
- Decelerates hip abduction, extension, and external rotation

Isometric Action
- Stabilizes the lumbo-pelvic-hip complex and knee

INNERVATION
- Obturator nerve

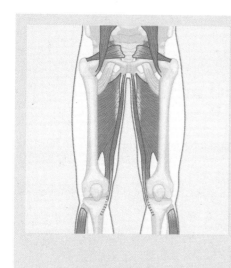

PECTINEUS

ORIGIN
- Pectineal line on the superior pubic ramus of the pelvis

INSERTION
- Pectineal line on the posterior surface of the upper femur

ISOLATED FUNCTION

Concentric Action
- Accelerates hip adduction, flexion, and internal rotation

INTEGRATED FUNCTION

Eccentric Action
- Decelerates hip abduction, extension, and external rotation

Isometric Action
- Stabilizes the lumbo-pelvic-hip complex

INNERVATION
- Obturator nerve

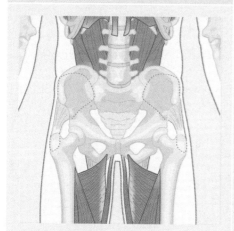

GLUTEUS MEDIUS, ANTERIOR FIBERS

ORIGIN
- Outer surface of the ilium

INSERTION
- Lateral surface of the greater trochanter of the femur

ISOLATED FUNCTION

Concentric Action
- Accelerates hip abduction and internal rotation

INTEGRATED FUNCTION

Eccentric Action
- Decelerates hip adduction and external rotation

Isometric Action
- Dynamically stabilizes the lumbo-pelvic-hip complex

INNERVATION
- Superior gluteal nerve

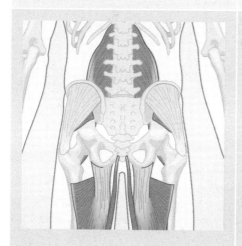

GLUTEUS MEDIUS, POSTERIOR FIBERS

ORIGIN
- Outer surface of the ilium

INSERTION
- Lateral surface of the greater trochanter of the femur

ISOLATED FUNCTION

Concentric Action
- Accelerates hip abduction and external rotation

INTEGRATED FUNCTION

Eccentric Action
- Decelerates hip adduction and internal rotation

Isometric Action
- Stabilizes the lumbo-pelvic-hip complex

INNERVATION
- Superior gluteal nerve

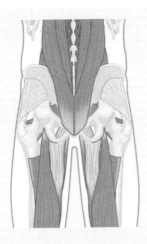

GLUTEUS MINIMUS
ORIGIN
- Ilium between the anterior and inferior gluteal line

INSERTION
- Greater trochanter of the femur

ISOLATED FUNCTION
Concentric Action
- Accelerates hip abduction, flexion, and internal rotation

INTEGRATED FUNCTION
Eccentric Action
- Decelerates frontal plane hip adduction, extension, and external rotation

Isometric Action
- Stabilizes the lumbo-pelvic-hip complex

INNERVATION
- Superior gluteal nerve

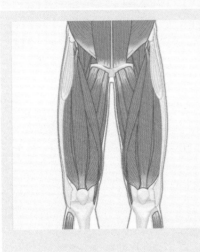

TENSOR FASCIA LATAE
ORIGIN
- Outer surface of the iliac crest just posterior to the anterior superior iliac spine of the pelvis

INSERTION
- Proximal one-third of the iliotibial band

ISOLATED FUNCTION
Concentric Action
- Accelerates hip flexion, abduction, and internal rotation

INTEGRATED FUNCTION
Eccentric Action
- Decelerates hip extension, adduction, and external rotation

Isometric Action
- Stabilizes the lumbo-pelvic-hip complex

INNERVATION
- Superior gluteal nerve

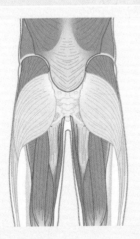

GLUTEUS MAXIMUS
ORIGIN
- Outer ilium, posterior side of sacrum and coccyx, and part of the sacrotuberous and posterior sacroiliac ligament

INSERTION
- Gluteal tuberosity of the femur and iliotibial tract

ISOLATED FUNCTION
Concentric Action
- Accelerates hip extension and external rotation

INTEGRATED FUNCTION
Eccentric Action
- Decelerates hip flexion, internal rotation, and tibial internal rotation via the iliotibial band

Isometric Action
- Stabilizes the lumbo-pelvic-hip complex

INNERVATION
- Inferior gluteal nerve

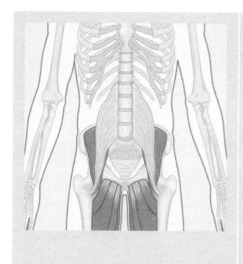

PSOAS MAJOR

ORIGIN
- Transverse processes and lateral bodies of the last thoracic and all lumbar vertebrae, including intervertebral discs

INSERTION
- Lesser trochanter of the femur as the iliopsoas tendon

ISOLATED FUNCTION

Concentric Action
- Accelerates hip flexion and external rotation and extends and rotates lumbar spine

INTEGRATED FUNCTION

Eccentric Action
- Decelerates hip internal rotation and decelerates hip extension

Isometric Action
- Stabilizes the lumbo-pelvic-hip complex

INNERVATION
- Spinal nerve branches of L1–L3

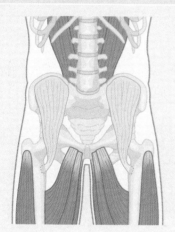

ILIACUS

ORIGIN
- Iliac fossa

INSERTION
- Lesser trochanter of the femur as the iliopsoas tendon

ISOLATED FUNCTION

Concentric Action
- Accelerates hip flexion and external rotation and extends and rotates lumbar spine

INTEGRATED FUNCTION

Eccentric Action
- Decelerates hip internal rotation and decelerates hip extension

Isometric Action
- Stabilizes the lumbo-pelvic-hip complex

INNERVATION
- Spinal nerve branches of L2–L4

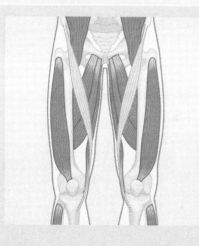

SARTORIUS

ORIGIN
- Anterior superior iliac spine of the pelvis

INSERTION
- Proximal medial surface of the tibia

ISOLATED FUNCTION

Concentric Action
- Accelerates hip flexion, external rotation, and abduction and accelerates knee flexion and internal rotation

INTEGRATED FUNCTION

Eccentric Action
- Decelerates hip extension and external rotation and knee extension and external rotation

Isometric Action
- Stabilizes the lumbo-pelvic-hip complex and knee

INNERVATION
- Femoral nerve

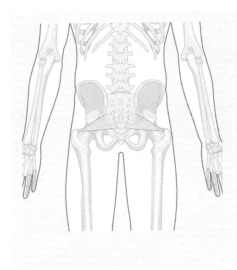

PIRIFORMIS
ORIGIN
- Anterior surface of the sacrum

INSERTION
- The greater trochanter of the femur

ISOLATED FUNCTION
Concentric Action
- Accelerates hip external rotation, abduction, and extension

INTEGRATED FUNCTION
Eccentric Action
- Decelerates hip internal rotation, adduction, and flexion

Isometric Action
- Stabilizes the hip and sacroiliac joints

INNERVATION
- Sciatic nerve

ABDOMINAL MUSCLES

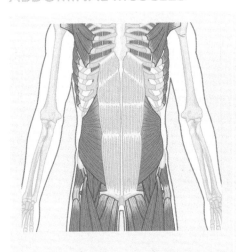

RECTUS ABDOMINIS
ORIGIN
- Pubic symphysis of the pelvis

INSERTION
- Ribs 5–7

ISOLATED FUNCTION
Concentric Action
- Spinal flexion, lateral flexion, and rotation

INTEGRATED FUNCTION
Eccentric Action
- Spinal extension, lateral flexion, and rotation

Isometric Action
- Stabilizes the lumbo-pelvic-hip complex

INNERVATION
- Intercostal nerve T7–T12

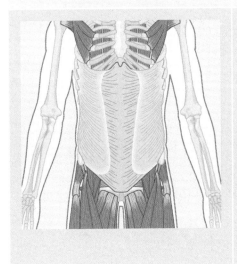

EXTERNAL OBLIQUE
ORIGIN
- External surface of ribs 4–12

INSERTION
- Anterior iliac crest of the pelvis, linea alba, and contralateral rectus sheaths

ISOLATED FUNCTION
Concentric Action
- Spinal flexion, lateral flexion, and contralateral rotation

INTEGRATED FUNCTION
Eccentric Action
- Spinal extension, lateral flexion, and rotation

Isometric Action
- Stabilizes the lumbo-pelvic-hip complex

INNERVATION
- Intercostal nerves (T8–T12), iliohypogastric (L1), and ilioinguinal (L1)

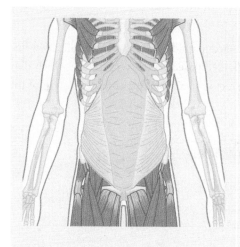

INTERNAL OBLIQUE
ORIGIN
- Anterior two-thirds of the iliac crest of the pelvis and thoracolumbar fascia

INSERTION
- Ribs 9–12, linea alba, and contralateral rectus sheaths

ISOLATED FUNCTION
Concentric Action
- Spinal flexion (bilateral), lateral flexion, and ipsilateral rotation

INTEGRATED FUNCTION
Eccentric Action
- Spinal extension, rotation, and lateral flexion

Isometric Action
- Stabilizes the lumbo-pelvic-hip complex

INNERVATION
- Intercostal nerves (T8–T12), iliohypogastric (L1), and ilioinguinal (L1)

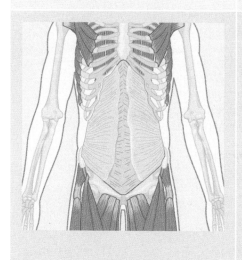

TRANSVERSE ABDOMINIS
ORIGIN
- Ribs 7–12, anterior two-thirds of the iliac crest of the pelvis, and thoracolumbar fascia

INSERTION
- Linea alba and contralateral rectus sheaths

ISOLATED FUNCTION
Concentric Action
- Increases intra-abdominal pressure and supports the abdominal viscera

INTEGRATED FUNCTION
Isometric Action
- Synergistically with the internal oblique, multifidus, and deep erector spinae to stabilize the lumbo-pelvic-hip complex

INNERVATION
- Intercostal nerves (T7–T12), iliohypogastric (L1), and ilioinguinal (L1)

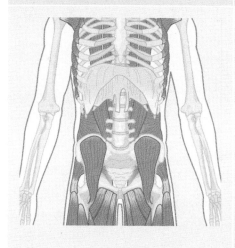

DIAPHRAGM
ORIGIN
- Costal part: Inner surfaces of the cartilages and adjacent bony regions of ribs 6–12
- Sternal part: Posterior side of the xiphoid process
- Crural (lumbar) part: (1) Two aponeurotic arches covering the external surfaces of the quadratus lumborum and psoas major and (2) right and left crus, originating from the bodies of L1–L3 and their intervertebral discs

INSERTION
- Central tendon

ISOLATED FUNCTION
Concentric Action
- Pulls the central tendon inferiorly, increasing the volume in the thoracic cavity

INTEGRATED FUNCTION
Isometric Action
- Stabilization of the lumbo-pelvic-hip complex

INNERVATION
- Phrenic nerve (C3–C5)

SUPERFICIAL ERECTOR SPINAE

The superficial erector spinae are a complex muscle group made up of the iliocostalis, longissimus, and spinalis muscles, each of which are subdivided based on the vertebrae at which they insert, respectively. All muscles of the superficial erector spinae share a common origin of the iliac crest of the pelvis, sacrum, and spinous and transverse processes of T1–L5.

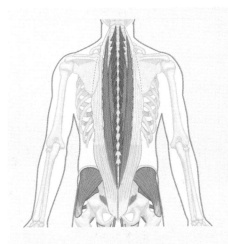

ILIOCOSTALIS: LUMBORUM DIVISION
ORIGIN
- Common origin

INSERTION
- Inferior border of ribs 7–12

ISOLATED FUNCTION
Concentric Action
- Spinal extension, rotation, and lateral flexion

INTEGRATED FUNCTION
Eccentric Action
- Spinal flexion, rotation, and lateral flexion

Isometric Action
- Stabilizes the spine during functional movements

INNERVATION
- Dorsal rami of thoracic and lumbar nerves

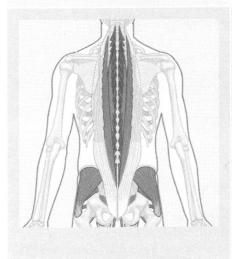

ILIOCOSTALIS: THORACIS DIVISION
ORIGIN
- Common origin

INSERTION
- Superior border of ribs 1–6

ISOLATED FUNCTION
Concentric Action
- Spinal extension, rotation, and lateral flexion

INTEGRATED FUNCTION
Eccentric Action
- Spinal flexion, rotation, and lateral flexion

Isometric Action
- Stabilizes the spine during functional movements

INNERVATION
- Dorsal rami of thoracic nerves

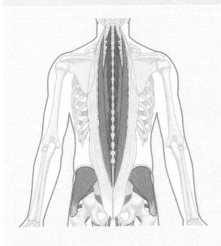

ILIOCOSTALIS: CERVICUS DIVISION
ORIGIN
- Common origin

INSERTION
- Transverse processes of C4–C6

ISOLATED FUNCTION
Concentric Action
- Spinal extension, rotation, and lateral flexion

INTEGRATED FUNCTION
Eccentric Action
- Spinal flexion, rotation, and lateral flexion

Isometric Action
- Stabilizes the spine during functional movements

INNERVATION
- Dorsal rami of thoracic nerves

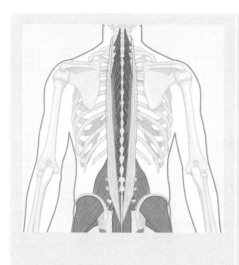

LONGISSIMUS: THORACIS DIVISION
ORIGIN
- Common origin

INSERTION
- Transverse processes of T1–T12 and ribs 2–12

ISOLATED FUNCTION
Concentric Action
- Spinal extension, rotation, and lateral flexion

INTEGRATED FUNCTION
Eccentric Action
- Spinal flexion, rotation, and lateral flexion

Isometric Action
- Stabilizes the spine during functional movements

INNERVATION
- Dorsal rami of thoracic and lumbar nerves

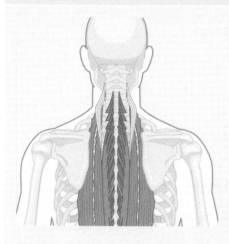

LONGISSIMUS: CERVICUS DIVISION
ORIGIN
- Common origin

INSERTION
- Transverse processes of C6–C2

ISOLATED FUNCTION
Concentric Action
- Spinal extension, rotation, and lateral flexion

INTEGRATED FUNCTION
Eccentric Action
- Spinal flexion, rotation, and lateral flexion

Isometric Action
- Stabilizes the spine during functional movements

INNERVATION
- Dorsal rami of cervical nerves

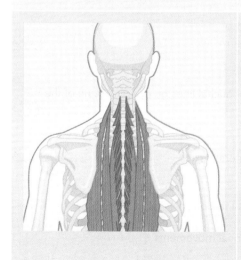

LONGISSIMUS: CAPITIS DIVISION
ORIGIN
- Common origin

INSERTION
- Mastoid process of the skull

ISOLATED FUNCTION
Concentric Action
- Spinal extension, rotation, and lateral flexion

INTEGRATED FUNCTION
Eccentric Action
- Spinal flexion, rotation, and lateral flexion

Isometric Action
- Stabilizes the spine during functional movements

INNERVATION
- Dorsal rami of cervical nerves

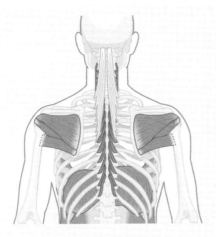

TRANSVERSOSPINALIS: CAPITUS DIVISION

ORIGIN
- Transverse processes of T6–C7
- Articular processes of C6–C4

INSERTION
- Nuchal line of occipital bone of the skull

ISOLATED FUNCTION
Concentric Action
- Produces spinal extension and lateral flexion and extension and contralateral rotation of the head

INTEGRATED FUNCTION
Eccentric Action
- Decelerates lateral flexion of the spine, and flexion and contralateral rotation of the head

Isometric Action
- Stabilizes the spine

INNERVATION
- Dorsal rami C1–T6 spinal nerves

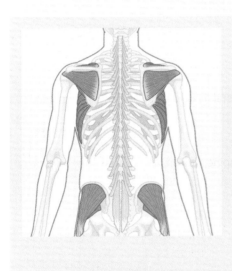

MULTIFIDUS

ORIGIN
- Posterior aspect of the sacrum and processes of the lumbar, thoracic, and cervical spine

INSERTION
- Spinous processes 1 to 4 segments above the origin

ISOLATED FUNCTION
Concentric Action
- Spinal extension and contralateral rotation

INTEGRATED FUNCTION
Eccentric Action
- Spinal flexion and rotation

Isometric Action
- Stabilizes the spine

INNERVATION
- Corresponding spinal nerves

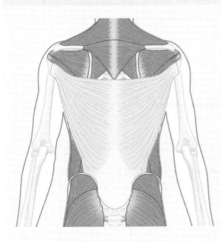

LATISSIMUS DORSI

ORIGIN
- Spinous processes of T7–T12, iliac crest of the pelvis, thoracolumbar fascia, and ribs 9–12

INSERTION
- Inferior angle of the scapula and intertubercular groove of the humerus

ISOLATED FUNCTION
Concentric Action
- Shoulder extension, adduction, and internal rotation

INTEGRATED FUNCTION
Eccentric Action
- Shoulder flexion, abduction, external rotation, and spinal flexion

Isometric Action
- Stabilizes the lumbo-pelvic-hip complex and shoulder

INNERVATION
- Thoracodorsal nerve (C6–C8)

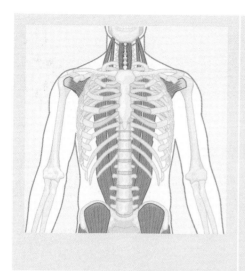

SERRATUS ANTERIOR
ORIGIN
- Ribs 4–12

INSERTION
- Medial border of the scapula

ISOLATED FUNCTION
Concentric Action
- Scapular protraction

INTEGRATED FUNCTION
Eccentric Action
- Scapular retraction

Isometric Action
- Stabilizes the scapula

INNERVATION
- Long thoracic nerve (C5–C7)

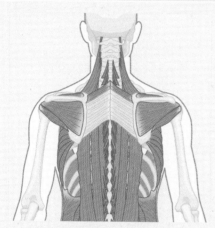

RHOMBOIDS
ORIGIN
- Spinous processes of C7–T5

INSERTION
- Medial border of the scapula

ISOLATED FUNCTION
Concentric Action
- Produces scapular retraction and downward rotation

INTEGRATED FUNCTION
Eccentric Action
- Scapular protraction and upward rotation

Isometric Action
- Stabilizes the scapula

INNERVATION
- Dorsal scapular nerve (C4–C5)

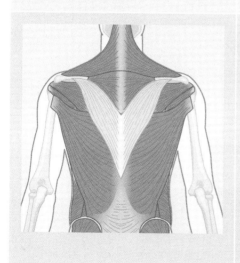

LOWER TRAPEZIUS
ORIGIN
- Spinous processes of T6–T12

INSERTION
- Spine of the scapula

ISOLATED FUNCTION
Concentric Action
- Scapular depression

INTEGRATED FUNCTION
Eccentric Action
- Scapular elevation

Isometric Action
- Stabilizes the scapula

INNERVATION
- Cranial nerve XI and ventral rami C2–C4

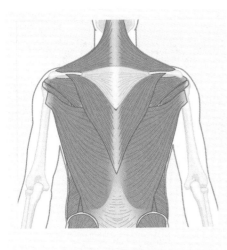

MIDDLE TRAPEZIUS

ORIGIN
- Spinous processes of T1–T5

INSERTION
- Acromion process of the scapula and superior aspect of the spine of the scapula

ISOLATED FUNCTION
Concentric Action
- Scapular retraction

INTEGRATED FUNCTION
Eccentric Action
- Scapular protraction and elevation

Isometric Action
- Stabilizes scapula

INNERVATION
- Cranial nerve XI and ventral rami C2–C4

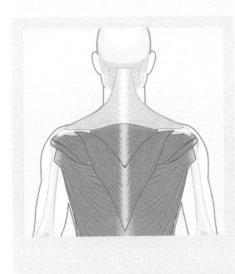

UPPER TRAPEZIUS

ORIGIN
- External occipital protuberance of the skull and spinous process of C7

INSERTION
- Lateral third of the clavicle and acromion process of the scapula

ISOLATED FUNCTION
Concentric Action
- Cervical extension, lateral flexion, and rotation and scapular elevation

INTEGRATED FUNCTION
Eccentric Action
- Cervical flexion, lateral flexion, rotation, and scapular depression

Isometric Action
- Stabilizes the cervical spine and scapula and stabilizes the medial border of the scapula creating a stable base for the prime movers during scapular abduction and upward rotation

INNERVATION
- Cranial nerve XI and ventral rami C2–C4

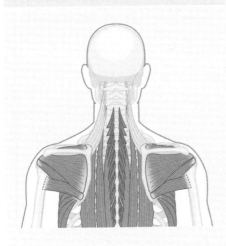

LEVATOR SCAPULA

ORIGIN
- Transverse processes of C1–C4

INSERTION
- Superior vertebral border of the scapula

ISOLATED FUNCTION
Concentric Action
- Cervical extension, lateral flexion, and ipsilateral rotation when the scapula is anchored and assists in elevation and downward rotation of the scapula

INTEGRATED FUNCTION
Eccentric Action
- Cervical flexion, contralateral cervical rotation, lateral flexion, scapular depression, and upward rotation when the neck is stabilized

Isometric Action
- Stabilizes the cervical spine and scapula

INNERVATION
- Ventral rami C3–C4 and dorsal scapular nerve

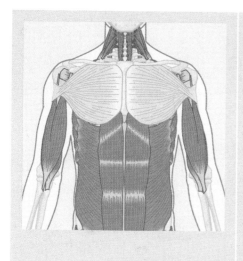

PECTORALIS MAJOR
ORIGIN
- Anterior surface of the clavicle, anterior surface of the sternum, and cartilage of ribs 1–7

INSERTION
- Greater tubercle of the humerus

ISOLATED FUNCTION
Concentric Action
- Shoulder flexion (clavicular fibers), horizontal adduction, and internal rotation

INTEGRATED FUNCTION
Eccentric Action
- Shoulder extension, horizontal abduction, and external rotation

Isometric Action
- Stabilizes the shoulder girdle

INNERVATION
- Medial and lateral pectoral nerves (C5–C7)

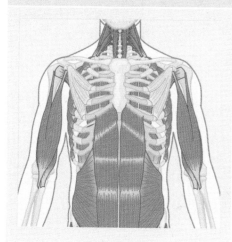

PECTORALIS MINOR
ORIGIN
- Ribs 3–5

INSERTION
- Coracoid process of the scapula

ISOLATED FUNCTION
Concentric Action
- Protracts the scapula

INTEGRATED FUNCTION
Eccentric Action
- Scapular retraction

Isometric Action
- Stabilizes the shoulder girdle

INNERVATION
- Medial pectoral nerve (C6–T1)

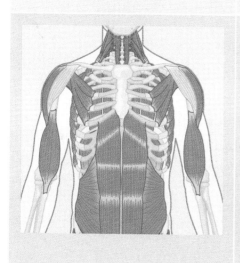

ANTERIOR DELTOID
ORIGIN
- Lateral third of the clavicle

INSERTION
- Deltoid tuberosity of the humerus

ISOLATED FUNCTION
Concentric Action
- Shoulder flexion and internal rotation

INTEGRATED FUNCTION
Eccentric Action
- Shoulder extension and external rotation

Isometric Action
- Stabilizes the shoulder girdle

INNERVATION
- Axillary nerve (C5–C6)

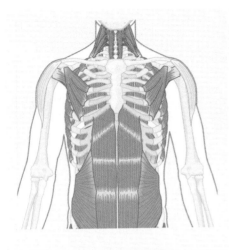

MEDIAL DELTOID

ORIGIN
- Acromion process of the scapula

INSERTION
- Deltoid tuberosity of the humerus

ISOLATED FUNCTION

Concentric Action
- Shoulder abduction

INTEGRATED FUNCTION

Eccentric Action
- Shoulder adduction

Isometric Action
- Stabilizes the shoulder girdle

INNERVATION
- Axillary nerve (C5–C6)

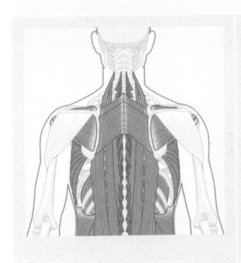

POSTERIOR DELTOID

ORIGIN
- Spine of the scapula

INSERTION
- Deltoid tuberosity of the humerus

ISOLATED FUNCTION

Concentric Action
- Shoulder extension and external rotation

INTEGRATED FUNCTION

Eccentric Action
- Shoulder flexion and internal rotation

Isometric Action
- Stabilizes the shoulder girdle

INNERVATION
- Axillary nerve (C5–C6)

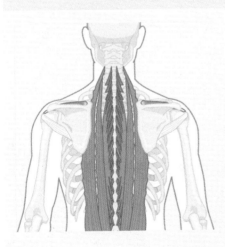

TERES MINOR

ORIGIN
- Lateral border of the scapula

INSERTION
- Greater tubercle of the humerus

ISOLATED FUNCTION

Concentric Action
- Shoulder external rotation

INTEGRATED FUNCTION

Eccentric Action
- Shoulder internal rotation

Isometric Action
- Stabilizes the shoulder girdle

INNERVATION
- Axillary nerve (C5–C6)

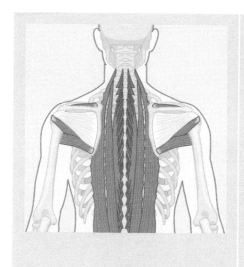

INFRASPINATUS
ORIGIN
- Infraspinous fossa of the scapula

INSERTION
- Middle facet of the greater tubercle of the humerus

ISOLATED FUNCTION
Concentric Action
- Shoulder external rotation

INTEGRATED FUNCTION
Eccentric Action
- Shoulder internal rotation

Isometric Action
- Stabilizes the shoulder girdle

INNERVATION
- Suprascapular nerve (C5–C6)

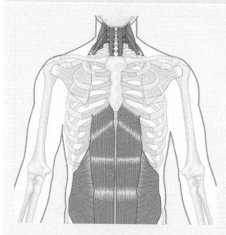

SUBSCAPULARIS
ORIGIN
- Subscapular fossa of the scapula

INSERTION
- Lesser tubercle of the humerus

ISOLATED FUNCTION
Concentric Action
- Shoulder internal rotation

INTEGRATED FUNCTION
Eccentric Action
- Shoulder external rotation

Isometric Action
- Stabilizes the shoulder girdle

INNERVATION
- Upper and lower subscapular nerves (C5–C6)

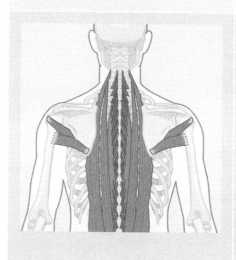

SUPRASPINATUS
ORIGIN
- Supraspinous fossa of the scapula

INSERTION
- Superior facet of the greater tubercle of the humerus

ISOLATED FUNCTION
Concentric Action
- Abduction of the arm

INTEGRATED FUNCTION
Eccentric Action
- Adduction of the arm

Isometric Action
- Stabilizes the shoulder girdle

INNERVATION
- Suprascapular nerve (C5–C6)

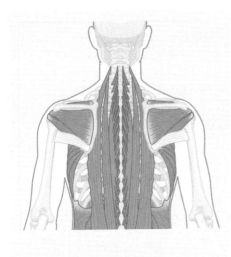

TERES MAJOR
ORIGIN
- Inferior angle of the scapula

INSERTION
- Lesser tubercle of the humerus

ISOLATED FUNCTION
Concentric Action
- Shoulder internal rotation, adduction, and extension

INTEGRATED FUNCTION
Eccentric Action
- Shoulder external rotation, abduction, and flexion

Isometric Action
- Stabilizes the shoulder girdle

INNERVATION
- Lower subscapular nerve

ARM MUSCLES

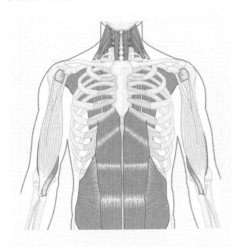

BICEPS BRACHII
ORIGIN
- Short head: Coracoid process
- Long head: Tubercle above glenoid cavity on the humerus

INSERTION
- Radial tuberosity of the radius

ISOLATED FUNCTION
Concentric Action
- Elbow flexion, supination of the radioulnar joint, and shoulder flexion

INTEGRATED FUNCTION
Eccentric Action
- Elbow extension, pronation of the radioulnar joint, and shoulder extension

Isometric Action
- Stabilizes the elbow and shoulder girdle

INNERVATION
- Musculocutaneous nerve

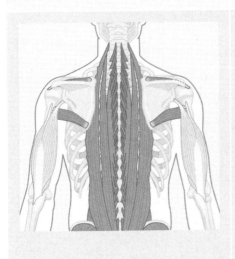

TRICEPS BRACHII
ORIGIN
- Long head: Infraglenoid tubercle of the scapula
- Short head: Posterior humerus
- Medial head: Posterior humerus

INSERTION
- Olecranon process of the ulna

ISOLATED FUNCTION
Concentric Action
- Elbow extension and shoulder extension

INTEGRATED FUNCTION
Eccentric Action
- Elbow flexion and shoulder flexion

Isometric Action
- Stabilizes the elbow and shoulder girdle

INNERVATION
- Radial nerve

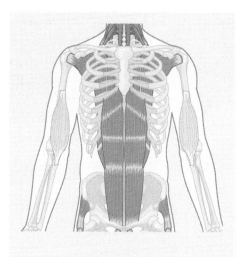

BRACHIALIS

ORIGIN

- Humerus

INSERTION

- Coronoid process of the ulna

ISOLATED FUNCTION

Concentric Action

- Flexes elbow

INTEGRATED FUNCTION

Eccentric Action

- Elbow extension

Isometric Action

- Stabilizes the elbow

INNERVATION

- Musculocutaneous and radial nerve

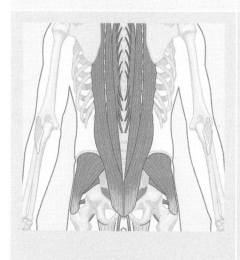

ANCONEUS

ORIGIN

- Lateral epicondyle of humerus

INSERTION

- Olecranon process and posterior ulna

ISOLATED FUNCTION

Concentric Action

- Extends elbow

INTEGRATED FUNCTION

Eccentric Action

- Elbow flexion

Isometric Action

- Stabilizes the elbow

INNERVATION

- Radial nerve

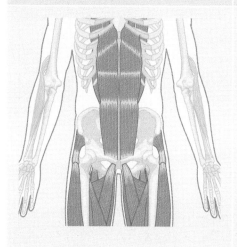

BRACHIORADIALIS

ORIGIN

- Lateral supracondylar ridge of humerus

INSERTION

- Styloid process of radius

ISOLATED FUNCTION

Concentric Action

- Flexes elbow

INTEGRATED FUNCTION

Eccentric Action

- Elbow extension

Isometric Action

- Stabilizes the elbow

INNERVATION

- Radial nerve

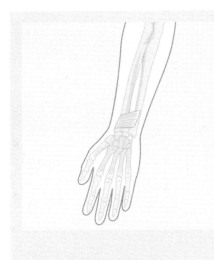

PRONATOR QUADRATUS

ORIGIN
- Distal ulna

INSERTION
- Distal radius

ISOLATED FUNCTION

Concentric Action
- Pronates forearm

INTEGRATED FUNCTION

Eccentric Action
- Forearm supination

Isometric Action
- Stabilizes distal radioulnar joint

INNERVATION
- Anterior interosseous nerve

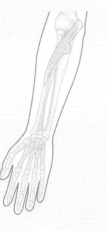

PRONATOR TERES

ORIGIN
- Medial epicondyle of humerus and coronoid process of ulna

INSERTION
- Radius

ISOLATED FUNCTION

Concentric Action
- Pronates forearm

INTEGRATED FUNCTION

Eccentric Action
- Forearm supination

Isometric Action
- Stabilizes proximal radioulnar joint and elbow

INNERVATION
- Median nerve

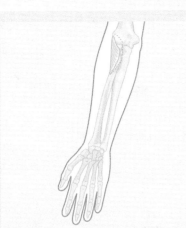

SUPINATOR

ORIGIN
- Lateral epicondyle of humerus

INSERTION
- Radius

ISOLATED FUNCTION

Concentric Action
- Supinates forearm

INTEGRATED FUNCTION

Eccentric Action
- Forearm pronation

Isometric Action
- Stabilizes proximal radioulnar joint and elbow

INNERVATION
- Radial nerve

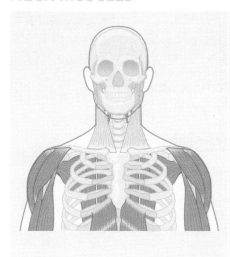

STERNOCLEIDOMASTOID
ORIGIN
- Sternal head: Top of manubrium of the sternum
- Clavicular head: Medial one-third of the clavicle

INSERTION
- Mastoid process and lateral superior nuchal line of the occiput of the skull

ISOLATED FUNCTION
Concentric Action
- Cervical flexion, rotation, and lateral flexion

INTEGRATED FUNCTION
Eccentric Action
- Cervical extension, rotation, and lateral flexion

Isometric Action
- Stabilizes the cervical spine and acromioclavicular joint

INNERVATION
- Cranial nerve XI

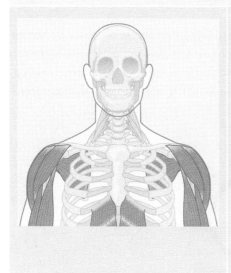

SCALENES
ORIGIN
- Transverse processes of C3–C7

INSERTION
- First and second ribs

ISOLATED FUNCTION
Concentric Action
- Cervical flexion, rotation, and lateral flexion and assists rib elevation during inhalation

INTEGRATED FUNCTION
Eccentric Action
- Cervical extension, rotation, and lateral flexion

Isometric Action
- Stabilizes the cervical spine

INNERVATION
- Ventral rami (C3–C7)

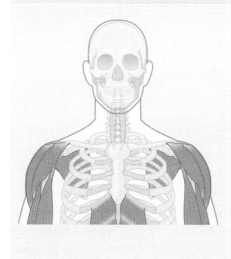

LONGUS COLLI
ORIGIN
- Anterior portion of T1–T3

INSERTION
- Anterior and lateral C1

ISOLATED FUNCTION
Concentric Action
- Cervical flexion, lateral flexion, and ipsilateral rotation

INTEGRATED FUNCTION
Eccentric Action
- Cervical extension, lateral flexion, and contralateral rotation

Isometric Action
- Stabilizes the cervical spine

INNERVATION
- Ventral rami (C2–C8)

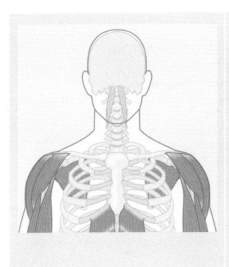

LONGUS CAPITIS
ORIGIN
- Transverse processes of C3–C6
INSERTION
- Inferior occipital bone
ISOLATED FUNCTION
Concentric Action
- Cervical flexion and lateral flexion
INTEGRATED FUNCTION
Eccentric Action
- Cervical extension
Isometric Action
- Stabilizes the cervical spine
INNERVATION
- Ventral rami (C1–C3)

Motor Behavior

Functional movement is learned, applied, and retained using the concept of **motor behavior**. The study of motor behavior examines how the nervous, skeletal, and muscular systems interact to produce skilled movement using **sensory information** from internal and external environments. Collectively, motor behavior represents the combination of motor control, motor learning, and motor development (**Figure 2-2**).

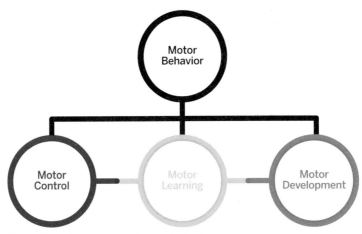

Figure 2-2 Components of motor behavior

Motor control is the study of posture and movements with the involved structures and mechanisms used by the CNS to assimilate and integrate sensory information with previous experiences. Motor control is concerned with what CNS structures are involved with motor behavior to produce movement. **Motor learning** is the utilization of motor control processes through practice and experience, leading to a relatively permanent change in capacity to produce skilled movement. Finally, **motor development** is defined as the cumulative change in motor behavior over time throughout the entire life span.

Motor Control

To move in an organized and efficient manner, the HMS must exhibit precise control over its collective segments. This segmental control is an integrated process involving neural, skeletal, and muscular components working together to produce appropriate motor responses. This process is known as motor control and focuses on the involved structures and mechanisms used by the CNS to integrate internal and external sensory information with previous experiences to produce a skilled motor response. One of the most important concepts in motor control and motor learning is how the CNS incorporates the information it receives to produce, refine, manipulate, and remember a movement pattern.

SENSORY INFORMATION

Sensory information is the data that the CNS receives from sensory receptors to determine things such as the body's position in space and limb orientation as well as information about the external environment such as temperature, sights, sounds, and textures. This information allows the CNS to monitor the internal and external environments to modify motor behavior using adjustments ranging from simple reflexes to intricate movement patterns.

Sensory information is essential in protecting the body from harm. It also provides feedback about movement to acquire and refine new skills through sensory **sensations** and **perceptions**. A sensation is a process by which sensory information is received by the receptor (afferent) and transferred either to the spinal cord for reflexive motor behavior, to higher cortical areas for processing, or both. This sensory pathway is supported by **afferent** neurons, whereas the motor response utilizes **efferent** neurons. Perception is the integration of sensory information with past experiences or memories (Fulkerson, 2002; Irving et al., 2007; Leetun et al., 2004). The body uses sensory information in three ways (Fulkerson, 2002; Ireland et al., 2003; Irving et al., 2007):

- Sensory information provides information about the body's spatial orientation to the environment and itself before, during, and after movement.
- It assists in planning and manipulating movement action plans. This may occur at the spinal level in the form of a reflex or at the cerebellum, where actual performance is compared.
- Sensory information facilitates learning new skills as well as relearning existing movement patterns that may have become dysfunctional.

PROPRIOCEPTION

Proprioception is one form of sensory (afferent) information that uses mechanoreceptors (from cutaneous, fascia, muscle, tendon, and joint receptors) to provide information about static and dynamic positions, movements, and sensations related to muscle force and movement (Kopeinig et al., 2015). It is the cumulative neural input from sensory afferents to the CNS that allows for the perception and awareness of the body's relative position in space. This vital information ensures optimal motor behavior and **neuromuscular efficiency**. This afferent information is delivered to different levels of motor control within the CNS to use in monitoring and manipulating movement.

As many of the receptors are located in and around joints, any joint injury will likely also damage proprioceptive components that could be compromised for some time after an injury. When one considers the 80% of our population that experiences low back pain (LBP) (National Institute of Neurological Disorders and Stroke, 2014), or the estimated 100,000 to 200,000 anterior cruciate ligament (ACL) injuries annually (Friedberg et al., 2017), or the

Sensations

A process by which sensory information is received by the receptor and transferred either to the spinal cord for reflexive motor behavior, to higher cortical areas for processing, or both.

Perceptions

The integration of sensory information with past experiences or memories.

Afferent

Sensory neurons that carry signals from sensory stimuli toward the central nervous system.

Efferent

Motor neurons that carry signals from the central nervous system toward muscles to create movement.

Proprioception

The cumulative neural input from sensory afferents to the central nervous system.

Neuromuscular efficiency

The ability of the neuromuscular system to allow agonists, antagonists, synergists, and stabilizers to work synergistically to produce, reduce, and dynamically stabilize the human movement system in all three planes of motion.

more than 2 million ankle sprains (Waterman et al., 2010), these individuals may have altered proprioception as a result of past injuries (Herzog et al., 2019). A thorough rehabilitation program after a musculoskeletal injury normally will contain a proprioceptive component. Thus, there is a need for core and balance training to enhance proprioceptive capabilities and increase postural control.

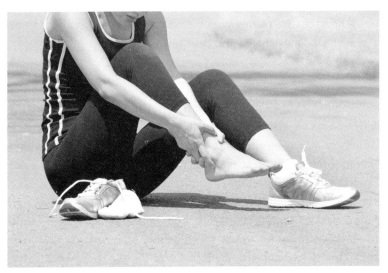

Ankle sprain
© Sawaddeebenz/Shutterstock

SENSORIMOTOR INTEGRATION

Sensorimotor integration

The ability of the central nervous system to gather and interpret sensory information to execute the proper motor response.

Sensorimotor integration is the ability of the CNS to gather and interpret sensory information to execute the proper motor response (Coker, 2018; Magill & Anderson, 2016). Sensorimotor integration is only as effective as the quality of the incoming sensory information (Biedert, 2000; Schmidt & Lee, 2014). An individual who trains with improper form delivers improper sensory information to the CNS, which can lead to **movement compensation** and potential injury. Thus, programs need to be designed to train and to reinforce correct technique. For example, the individual who consistently performs a squat with an arched lower back and adducted femur will alter the length-tension relationships of muscles, force-couple relationships, and arthrokinematics. This can ultimately lead to back, knee, and hamstring problems (Kaya et al., 2018; Sahrmann et al., 2017; Thomeé et al., 1995).

MUSCLE SYNERGIES

Movement compensation

When the body moves in a suboptimal way in response to kinetic chain dysfunction.

As previously mentioned, muscles take on changing roles as they work together to produce movement. One of the most important concepts in motor control is that the CNS recruits muscles in groups, or synergies. This simplifies movement by allowing muscles to operate as a functional unit. For example, during a pushing movement, forces are produced by the pectoralis major as the agonist (prime mover), with the anterior deltoids and triceps brachii assisting synergistically; for pull-type movements, the agonist is the latissimus dorsi, with the posterior deltoids and biceps brachii synergistically assisting (**Figure 2-3**). Through practice of proper movement patterns and technique, muscle synergies become more fluent and automated (Fulkerson, 2002; Irving et al., 2007; Payne & Berg, 1997). This practicing of proper movement patterns and techniques is the focus of the fourth phase in the Corrective Exercise Continuum, integration.

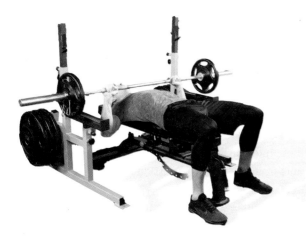

Figure 2-3A Pushing movements

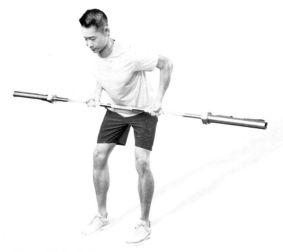

Figure 2-3B Pulling movements

Motor Learning and Development

Motor learning is the integration of motor control processes through practice and experience, leading to a relatively permanent change in the capacity to produce skilled movements. At its most basic, the study of motor learning looks at how movements are learned and retained for future use. For this to occur, feedback is necessary to ensure optimal learning of skilled movements (Fulkerson, 2002; Ireland et al., 2003; Irving et al., 2007).

Motor development then represents the accumulation of all motor learning that happens throughout an entire lifetime. Motor development begins in infancy with the development of gross and fine motor skills. Those skills are also considered developmental milestones and include grasping objects, rolling, sitting, standing, and walking. Motor development continues as we age from infancy to adolescence to adulthood, with humans developing the ability to do more comprehensive and complicated tasks as they get older.

Proper practice and experience will lead to motor learning, which, over time, leads to a permanent change in an individual's ability to perform skilled movements effectively. The fitness professional should consider that motor development occurs throughout the life span and becomes refined as individuals are exposed to new environments, movements, and tasks (Leversen et al., 2012).

FEEDBACK

Feedback is the utilization of sensory information and sensorimotor integration to aid in the development of permanent neural representations of motor patterns for efficient movement. This is achieved through internal (or sensory) feedback and external (or augmented) feedback. **Internal (sensory) feedback** is the process by which sensory information is used by the body to monitor movement and the environment. Internal feedback acts as a guide, steering the HMS to create the proper force, speed, and amplitude of movement required for any given situation. Proper form during movement ensures that the incoming internal (sensory) feedback is the correct information, allowing for optimal sensorimotor integration.

External (augmented) feedback is information provided by some external source. Examples of external feedback include cues from a fitness professional, reviewing performance videos, performing exercises in front of a mirror, or wearing a heart rate monitor. This information is used to supplement internal feedback. External feedback provides another source of information that allows the individual to associate the outcome of the achieved movement pattern (*good* or *bad*) with what is felt internally.

Feedback

The utilization of sensory information and sensorimotor integration to aid in the development of permanent neural representations of motor patterns for efficient movement.

Internal (sensory) feedback

The process by which sensory information is used by the body via length-tension relationships, force-couple relationships, and arthrokinematics to monitor movement and the environment.

External (augmented) feedback

Information provided by some external source, for example, a health and fitness professional, video, mirror, or heart rate monitor.

Knowledge of results

Used after the completion of a movement to inform individuals about the outcome of their performance.

Knowledge of performance

Provides information about the quality of the movement.

Sarcomere

The functional unit of a muscle made up of overlapping actin and myosin filaments.

Cross-bridge mechanism

The collective physiological processes that cause actin and myosin filaments to slide across each other, functionally shortening the muscle as it develops tension.

Length-tension relationship

The resting length of a muscle and the tension the muscle can produce at this resting length.

Resting length

A muscle's state when the body is standing still; not contracting or stretching.

Two major forms of external feedback are **knowledge of results** and **knowledge of performance**. Knowledge of results is used after the completion of a movement to inform individuals about the outcome of their performance. This can come from the fitness professional, the client, or some technological means. The fitness professional might inform individuals that their squats were "good" and ask clients whether they could "feel" or "see" their form. By getting clients involved with knowledge of results, they increase their own awareness and augment their impressions with multiple forms of feedback. This can be done after each repetition, after a few repetitions, or once the set is completed. As individuals become more familiar with a desired movement technique, knowledge of results from the fitness professional should be given less frequently, helping to improve neuromuscular efficiency.

Knowledge of performance provides information about the quality of the movement. An example would be noticing that, during a squat, the individual's feet were externally rotated and the femurs were excessively adducting and then asking whether the individual felt or saw anything different about those repetitions. Or, to get individuals to absorb the shock of landing from a jump (and not landing with extended knees, which places the ACL in a precarious position), tell them to listen to the impact and land quietly, effectively teaching the individual to absorb the shock of landing. These examples get the client involved in his or her own sensory process. Such feedback will be given less frequently as the client becomes more proficient.

These forms of external feedback identify performance errors. It is also an important component in motivation. Furthermore, feedback gives the client supplemental sensory input to help create an awareness of the desired action. It is important to state, however, that a client must not become too dependent on external feedback, especially from the fitness professional, as this may detract from the individual's own responsiveness to internal sensory input. This could alter sensorimotor integration and may affect clients' learning and their ultimate performance of new movements (Fulkerson, 2002; Ireland et al., 2003; Irving et al., 2007).

Muscular Force

In order to correctly produce movement, muscles must work together in synergies. However, changes in both the length of and tension within individual muscles surrounding a joint can alter the joint's resting position, increase stresses placed on the joint, impair how forces are produced, and lead to compensations in posture and movement that increase the risk of injury.

Length-Tension Relationships

The functional unit of muscle is the **sarcomere** (**Figure 2-4**), which is made up of overlapping filaments known as actin and myosin. When a muscle contracts, small, teethlike structures on each of the filaments grab hold and cause the actin and myosin to slide across each other, functionally shortening the muscle as it develops tension. This is known as the **cross-bridge mechanism**. When a muscle relaxes, the filaments let go and slide back to a neutral position.

A **length-tension relationship** refers to the resting length of a muscle and the tension the muscle can produce at that resting length (Feher, 2017) (**Figure 2-5**). The **resting length** of a muscle is its state when the body is standing still and the muscle is neither contracting nor being stretched. If the resting length of a muscle is shorter than it should be, the amount of available actin–myosin cross-bridging becomes limited and reduces available force output. Muscles with resting lengths that are longer than they should be will also have limited force generation capabilities.

The resting length of a muscle and its ability to contract (shorten) and relax (lengthen) are a consequence of the **neural drive** it is receiving. Neural drive represents the effective amount

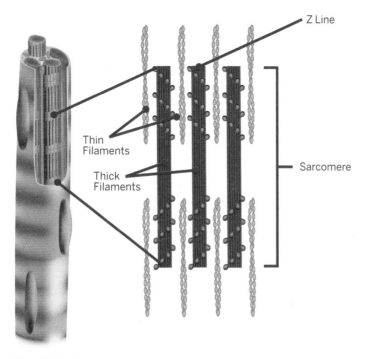

Figure 2-4 Sarcomere

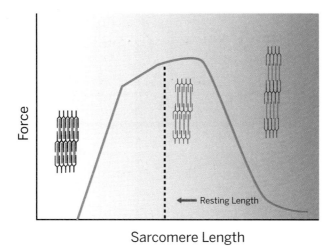

Figure 2-5 Length-tension relationship

of signaling to contract that a muscle receives from the CNS. Even when standing still, muscles surrounding the joints are all in a subconscious state of activation, receiving signals from the CNS to apply tension and keep the skeleton held upright. If muscles completely relaxed, the body would simply fall limp to the ground.

If a muscle is identified as **overactive/shortened**, it does not mean that the protein structures that make it up are physically being made shorter; rather, it means that excessive neural drive is causing the muscle to be held in a partial contraction when at rest, effectively shortening the resting length of that muscle. When it comes time for that muscle to activate and generate force, the amount of total available muscle contraction is reduced due to the muscle's actin and myosin filaments already being in a more overlapped position. Conversely, a lengthened resting state means that actin and myosin filaments have less overlap than they should, reducing a muscle's ability to generate force opposite to how excessive overlap reduces shortened muscles' force production. In this scenario, the muscle's actin and myosin filaments do not have enough resting overlap to optimally generate or control force.

Neural drive

The rate and volume of activation signals a muscle receives from the central nervous system.

Overactive/ shortened

Occurs when elevated neural drive causes a muscle to be held in a chronic state of contraction.

Titin: The Third Filament

Established evidence has shown that the unit for muscle contraction is the sarcomere, which has two sliding filaments (actin and myosin) that follow what is called the cross-bridge mechanism of function in muscle contraction. However, the two-filament model does not quite account for what happens during eccentric muscle contractions when the muscle is in a fully lengthened state. When sarcomeres are stretched to a point beyond functional overlap of the actin and myosin filaments, the two-filament model makes it impossible for cross bridges to contribute directly to active force.

This is where the third filament comes in. Titin is a protein that runs the entire length of the sarcomere and is thought to be responsible for muscle elasticity, preventing the actin and myosin filaments from being pulled apart and assisting the muscle to return to its resting length after being stretched (**Figure 2-6**). Since 1949, research has firmly established the presence of titin, but its function in the role of force production has not yet been fully confirmed (Dos Remedios & Gilmour, 2017). However, increasingly compelling evidence has yielded outcomes for sound theories that explain what the two-filament model cannot.

Given the apparent inability of cross bridges alone to account for the increased force enhancement proven with eccentric contractions, the likelihood that titin plays a significant role has become evident. Leading hypotheses include a winding–unwinding effect of the titin protein structure as well as a dynamic spring theory that may explain how the sarcomere filaments perform lengthening contractions at a length-tension position that does not require maximal overlap of cross bridges for optimal force to occur (Nishikawa et al., 2018). This has resulted in growing support for a three-filament model for sarcomere functioning.

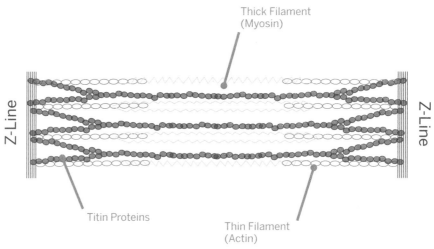

Figure 2-6   Titin proteins

Underactive/ lengthened

Occurs when inhibited neural drive allows a muscle's functional antagonist to pull it into a chronically elongated state.

Muscle imbalance

Alteration of muscle length surrounding a joint.

Additionally, when a muscle on one side of a joint is overactive/shortened, a state of reduced neural drive is created in muscles on the other side of the joint. Recall the natural effects of reciprocal inhibition—when a movement needs to be performed, a signal from the CNS to activate a muscle on one side of a joint causes the inhibition of CNS signals to its functional antagonist, causing it to relax and lengthen to allow the desired movement to occur. If a muscle is chronically overactive and receiving elevated contraction signals in its resting position, then reciprocal inhibition dictates that its functional antagonist will have its neural drive chronically inhibited, in turn. When that inhibited muscle needs to be an agonist for a movement, the chronic inhibition prevents it from correctly doing its job, reducing the amount of force it can produce. Muscles in this situation are referred to as **underactive/lengthened**.

When a situation of overactivity/underactivity exists between muscles on two sides of a joint (e.g., the agonist is overactive/shortened and the antagonist is underactive/lengthened), a **muscle imbalance** is said to exist. This concept is paramount to the corrective exercise process because it directly coincides with the concept of joint alignment. If muscle lengths and

Overactive: Chronically elevated neural drive to a muscle, which puts the muscle in a chronically contracted, shortened state.

Underactive: Chronically inhibited neural drive to a muscle, which allows the overactive muscle on the opposing side of the joint to pull it into a lengthened state.

tensions surrounding a joint are not balanced, joints will be pulled into suboptimal positions. With movement at one joint being interdependent on movement of other joints, any dysfunction in the chain of events producing movement will have direct effects elsewhere (Thomeé et al., 1995). It is for this reason that the interworking segments that move the human body are referred to as the **kinetic chain**; disruption at just one link can alter the functionality of the whole. Essentially, a person with optimal posture has proper length-tension relationships throughout the entire musculature, which allows for proper joint alignment.

Kinetic chain

The combination and interrelation of the nervous, muscular, and skeletal systems.

CHECK IT OUT

What came first, the chicken or the egg? This classic dilemma closely relates to the relationship between muscle imbalances and joint positioning. Did excessive or reduced neural drive (overactivity/underactivity) cause the joint to be pulled into a position where muscles on one side are shortened with the other side lengthened? Or, is a joint chronically held in a position that makes the muscles around it adapt to shortened/lengthened states, causing disruptions to their neural drive?

The comprehensive assessment process with clients will help to uncover the answer. Sometimes, daily life causes the body to be kept in compromising positions that the body adapts to. In these cases, chronic alterations in muscle length come first and lead to states of overactivity/underactivity. In other situations, repetitive activity or an injury can cause a muscle to become overactive first. In this case, the effects of reciprocal inhibition reduce neural drive to its antagonist, and the overactivity/underactivity is what leads to the muscles being shortened/lengthened.

Either way, it is a vicious cycle that the fitness professional will work to end by inhibiting and lengthening overactive/shortened muscles in phases 1 and 2 of the Corrective Exercise Continuum, activating and strengthening underactive/lengthened muscles in phase 3, and then integrating those corrected length-tension relationships into functional movement patterns in phase 4.

Force-Couple Relationships

Muscles produce a force that is transmitted to bones through group connections and by individual muscle attachments to tendons. Because muscles are recruited as groups, many muscles at a time will transmit force onto their respective bones, creating movement at the joints. This synergistic action of muscles to produce movement around a joint is also known as a **force-couple**. Muscles in a force-couple provide divergent (i.e., multidirectional) tension to the bone or bones as well as to the adjacent muscles to which they attach (**Figure 2-7**).

Proper force-couple relationships are needed so that the HMS moves in the desired manner. This can only happen if the muscles have optimal length-tension relationships that let the joints have proper kinematics (i.e., joint motion). One common example is the force-couple created by the hip flexors (e.g., rectus femoris and psoas) and the hip extensors (e.g., gluteus maximus). When each muscle on each side of the hip has an optimal length-tension relationship (not too

Force-couple relationship

The synergistic action of muscles to produce movement around a joint.

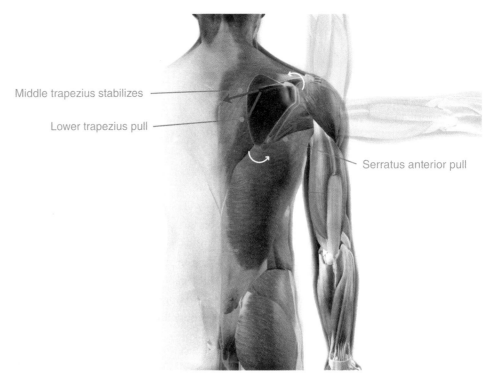

Middle trapezius stabilizes

Lower trapezius pull

Serratus anterior pull

Figure 2-7 Example force-couple relationships

long or too short), the lumbo-pelvic-hip complex (LPHC) is maintained in the ideal neutral position. However, if the hip flexors are in a chronically overactive/shortened state with the extensors in an underactive/lengthened state, the hip will be pulled into a chronic state of flexion, altering the force-couple and creating a scenario where forces are not distributed evenly around the hip. Collectively, optimal length-tension relationships within individual muscles help create optimal, balanced force-couple relationships surrounding joints; when the muscles are all balanced around a joint, optimal and efficient movement is produced (Neumann, 2016; Vleeming et al., 2007) (**Figure 2-8**).

The Regional Interdependence Model

The regional interdependence (RI) model came into being after physical therapists concluded that the traditional biomedical model of treatment for common musculoskeletal conditions had poor outcomes. Oftentimes, it was noticed that when patients were treated at areas far from where they complained of pain, they had better, faster outcomes. For example, in many cases, when the hip was treated, LBP was improved or even eliminated (Wainner et al., 2007).

As more studies into the concepts of RI came out, it became apparent that systems beyond just the musculoskeletal respond when a dysfunction disrupts homeostasis. Those systems include the neurophysiological and somatovisceral. Psychological and social factors also have been shown to affect patient treatment responses (Sueki et al., 2013). Because the medical literature has established the importance of incorporating the RI model into clinical practice, it is crucial that other members of the allied health industry (e.g., fitness professionals) become familiar with and implement this model in their practice as well. In fitness, the RI model can be used to better assess and design corrective exercise programs for more rapid, accurate, and complete results.

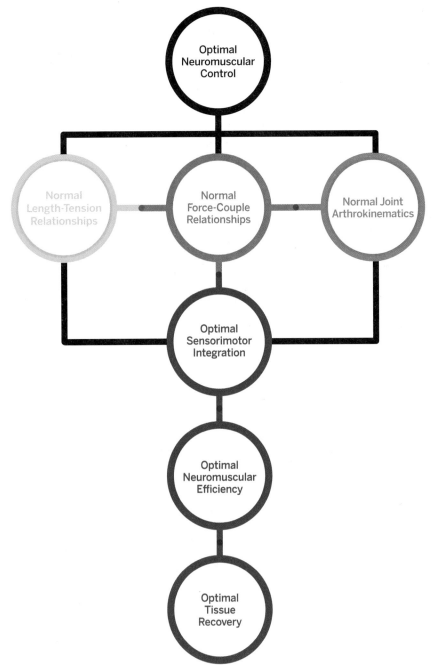

Figure 2-8 Efficient human movement

 CRITICAL

The RI model should simply be used to strengthen one's understanding of the interconnected nature of the HMS. It is outside a fitness professional's scope of practice to address issues beyond correcting posture and improving mobility. If a medical condition is suspected at any time, that client needs to be referred to a qualified medical professional.

The HMS is a very complex, well-orchestrated system of interrelated and interdependent myofascial (muscle and fascia), neuromuscular (neural and muscle), and articular (bone, cartilage, and ligament) components. The functional integration of each system allows for optimal neuromuscular efficiency during functional activities (**Figure 2-9**). Optimal alignment and functioning of all components (and segments of each component) result in optimal length-tension relationships, force-couple relationships, precise arthrokinematics (movement of joint surfaces), and neuromuscular control (Hamill et al., 2014; Neumann, 2016). Optimal alignment and functioning of each component of the HMS depends on the structural and functional integrity of each of its interdependent systems. This structural alignment of the skeleton—as it is held in place by muscles, ligaments, and tendons—is known as posture. **Posture** is the independent and interdependent alignment and function of all components of the HMS at any given moment and is controlled by the CNS (Schmidt et al., 2019).

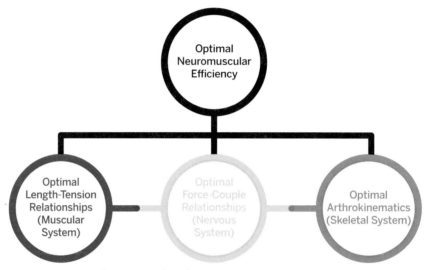

Figure 2-9   Optimal neuromuscular efficiency

Efficiency and longevity of the HMS requires integration of all systems. **Structural efficiency** is the alignment of each segment of the HMS, which allows posture to be balanced in relation to one's center of gravity. This enables individuals to maintain their center of gravity over their constantly changing base of support during functional movements. **Functional efficiency** is the ability of the neuromuscular system to recruit correct muscle synergies, at the right time, with the appropriate amount of force to perform functional tasks with the least amount of energy and stress on the HMS.

Using the RI Model for Corrective Exercise

The RI model, as it pertains to human movement, recognizes that, for a person to function optimally and successfully perform tasks in life and exercise, coordinated and integrated action of all systems of the body is required. If this does not happen, then dysfunction in one region can cause impairment in another more distant region or regions (Buckland et al., 2017; Sueki et al., 2013). For example, during training, a person may experience LBP, not because of issues with the lumbar spine, but rather due to a lack of mobility in the hips (Buckland et al., 2017).

Corrective Exercise Specialists should use the RI model as a foundation to assess the posture and functional movement of the HMS. Clients commonly exhibit poor movement patterns due to musculoskeletal issues far from the observable movement itself.

One example is when the ankle lacks dorsiflexion and the individual leans excessively forward into hip flexion during a squat as a compensation. At first glance, both of these movement compensations (excessive forward lean/hip flexion) seem to indicate impairment at the hip where the movement compensation is directly observed. However, using the RI model reminds

Corrective Exercise Specialists that limited mobility at the ankles can easily create a cascade of effects up the legs that lead to movement compensations at or even above the hip (Byström et al., 2013).

Another common example of RI is when the foot and ankle excessively pronate and turn out during movement. When the foot turns out, the knee usually compensates by collapsing into the valgus position, thereby straining the medial knee (and ankle) ligaments, compressing lateral knee joint structures, and causing dynamic malalignment of the patella. This may result in knee joint discomfort, excessive movement, weakness, and lack of stability in the muscles surrounding the knee. The hips then compensate for the altered ankle and knee mobility, which may result in an excessive anterior pelvic tilt and resultant low back tightness (Kosashvili et al., 2008).

Alterations from optimal movement patterns may occur together or separately in different degrees depending on the individual. By always keeping the concepts of RI in mind, the fitness professional is prepared to optimally assess the entire HMS to identify and correct clients' posture and movement with confidence and accuracy.

Muscular Movement and Stabilization Systems

It has been proposed that muscles can be categorized into two distinct, yet inter-reliant, systems that enable our bodies to maintain proper stabilization and ensure efficient distribution of forces for the production of movement. Muscles that are located centrally to the spine provide intersegmental stability (support from vertebra to vertebra), whereas the more superficial muscles support the spine as a whole and also help generate forces for movement. Bergmark categorized these different groups of muscles in relation to the trunk (LPHC) and termed them the local and global muscular systems (Petersen et al., 2014).

These systems represent many of the most common, interworking force-couples that all human bodies call on to create movement and deal with forces from the external environment and are a clear example of how the RI model applies to the kinetic chain. Understanding the paths that forces commonly take through the body sheds light on why dysfunction at one place of the body can lead to detrimental effects elsewhere.

The Local Muscular System (Stabilization System)

The **local musculature system** consists of muscles that attach directly to the spine and are predominantly involved in stabilization (**Figure 2-10**). These muscles are primarily type 1, or slow-twitch, muscle fibers. They are most suitable for endurance, balance, and slow movement training with parameters of long duration, light resistance, low load, and slow velocity (Wilson et al., 2012). The joint support system of the LPHC includes muscles that either originate in or insert into, or both, the lumbar spine, including the transversus abdominis, multifidus, internal oblique, psoas, diaphragm, and the muscles of the pelvic floor (Crossley et al., 2001; Regev et al., 2011; Thomeé et al., 1995). One of the best examples of local musculature working synergistically is the drawing-in maneuver that is used during virtually every resistance training exercise to protect and stabilize the spine.

> **Local musculature system**
>
> Muscles that connect directly to the spine and are predominantly involved in LPHC stabilization.

JOINT SUPPORT SYSTEMS

Although local muscles are primarily responsible for joint support throughout the LPHC, joint support systems are not confined to just the spine and are evident in the peripheral joints as well.

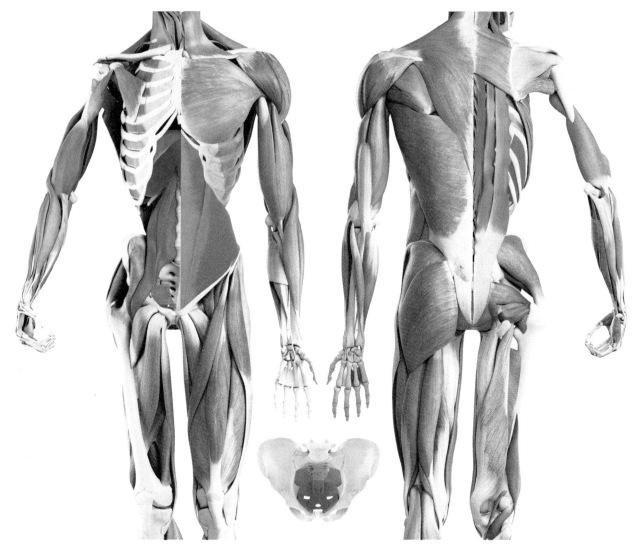

Figure 2-10 Local muscular system

Joint support systems consist of muscles that are not movement specific; rather, they provide stability to allow movement of a joint. They usually are located in close proximity to the joint with a broad spectrum of attachments to the joint's passive elements (ligaments), which makes them ideal for increasing joint stiffness and stability. A common example of a peripheral joint support system is the rotator cuff, which provides dynamic stabilization for the humeral head in relation to the glenoid fossa. Other joint support systems include the posterior fibers of the gluteus medius and the external rotators of the hip, which provide pelvo-femoral stabilization, and the oblique fibers of the vastus medialis, which provide patellar stabilization at the knee (Neumann, 2016; Richardson et al., 2004; Vleeming et al., 2007).

The Global Muscular Systems (Movement Systems)

The **global muscular system** is predominantly responsible for movement and consists of more superficial tissues that originate from the pelvis to the rib cage, the lower extremities, or both (**Figure 2-11**). These muscles are primarily type 2, or *fast-twitch*, muscle fibers. They are most suitable for strength, coordination, agility, and fast velocity training with a large variety of

Global muscular system

Muscles responsible predominantly for movement and consisting of more superficial musculature that originates from the pelvis to the rib cage, the lower extremities, or both.

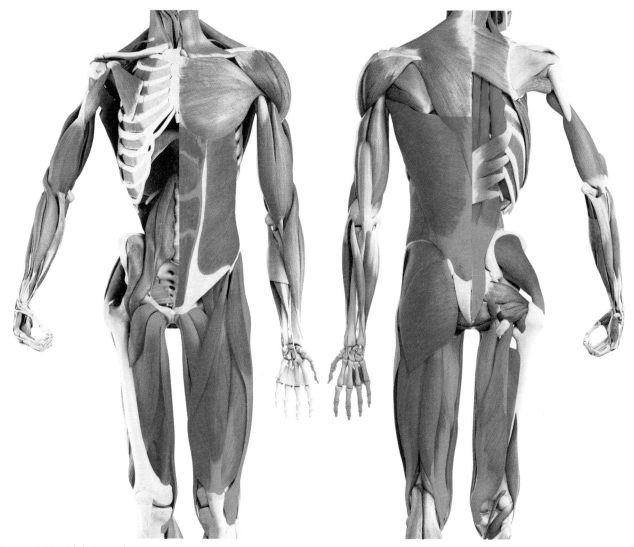

Figure 2-11 Global muscles

movement patterns and parameters of short duration across a spectrum of light to heavy resistance and loads (Wilson et al., 2012). Some of these major muscles include the rectus abdominis, external obliques, erector spinae, hamstring complex, gluteus maximus, latissimus dorsi, adductors, quadriceps, and gastrocnemius. The movement system muscles are predominantly larger and associated with movements of the trunk and limbs that equalize external loads placed on the body. These muscles also are important in transferring and absorbing forces from the upper and lower extremities through the LPHC.

Due to common muscle synergies we all exhibit during functional movement, global muscles can be categorized as working in four distinct (yet interdependent) subsystems: the deep longitudinal, posterior oblique, anterior oblique, and lateral subsystems. This distinction not only allows for an easier description and review of functional anatomy, it also helps the Corrective Exercise Specialist better understand the paths that forces take as they move through the body. This provides a clear picture of RI at work, showing, for example, how forces of a load held overhead move down through the trunk, cross the hip, and can ultimately affect the ankles.

Subsystems are also referred to in the science literature as myofascial slings, chains, or meridians (Wilke et al., 2016). It is crucial for fitness professionals to think of these subsystems operating as an integrated functional unit. Remember, the CNS optimizes the selection of muscle synergies, not just isolated muscles (Page et al., 2010; Richardson et al., 2004; Vleeming et al., 2007).

This concept is especially important for the fourth phase of the Corrective Exercise Continuum—integration. Phases 1 through 3 are concerned with specific muscles—inhibiting and lengthening ones identified as overactive/shortened and activating ones identified as underactive/lengthened—in order to bring force-couple relationships back into balance. Then, phase 4 uses big functional movements that integrate the now-efficient force-couples (optimized in corrective exercise phases 1 through 3) into the working relationships outlined by the global muscular subsystems.

THE DEEP LONGITUDINAL SUBSYSTEM (DLS)

The major soft tissue contributors to the deep longitudinal subsystem (DLS) are the erector spinae, thoracolumbar fascia, sacrotuberous ligament, biceps femoris, tibialis anterior, and fibularis (peroneus) longus. The DLS may provide a longitudinal means of reciprocal force transmission from the trunk to the ground. As illustrated in **Figure 2-12**, the long head of the biceps femoris attaches, in part, to the sacrotuberous ligament at the ischium. The sacrotuberous ligament, in turn, attaches from the ischium to the sacrum. The erector spinae attach from the sacrum and ilium up the ribs to the cervical spine. Thus, activation of the biceps femoris increases tension in the sacrotuberous ligament, which, in turn, transmits force across the sacrum, stabilizing the sacroiliac joint (SIJ), and then up the trunk through the erector spinae. One example of a basic exercise to activate the DLS unilaterally is starting from the quadruped position and then first positioning the head to neutral while also extending the hip and knee of one leg, then lifting the straight leg against gravity toward the ceiling, and then lowering. This exercise would provide concentric and eccentric exercise of the DLS.

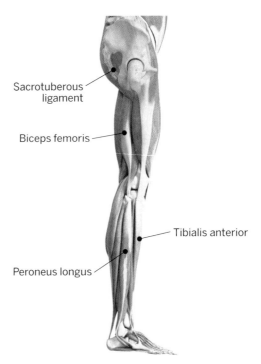

Figure 2-12 Deep longitudinal subsystem

This transference of force is apparent during normal gait. Before heel strike, the biceps femoris activates to eccentrically decelerate hip flexion and knee extension. Simultaneously, the anterior tibialis activates to concentrically dorsiflex and invert the ankle and foot. Just after heel strike, the anterior tibialis eccentrically decelerates to lower the foot as the biceps femoris is further loaded through the lower leg via posterior movement of the fibula. This tension from the lower leg up through the biceps femoris into the sacrotuberous ligament and up the erector spinae creates a force that assists in stabilizing the SIJ. An example of training DLS activation for gait would be in standing and performing a repetitive gait phase interval pattern of midstance to swing phase and heel strike and then retract to repeat with or without resistance bands for concentric and eccentric training.

Another force-couple not often mentioned in this subsystem consists of the superficial erector spinae, the psoas, and the intrinsic core stabilizers (transverse abdominis and multifidus). Although the erector spinae and psoas create lumbar extension and an anterior shear force at L4 through S1, during functional movements, the local muscular system provides intersegmental stabilization and a posterior shear force. Dysfunction in any of these structures can lead to SIJ instability and LBP (Vleeming et al., 2007).

THE POSTERIOR OBLIQUE SUBSYSTEM (POS)

The posterior oblique subsystem (POS) works synergistically with the DLS. As illustrated in **Figure 2-13**, both the gluteus maximus and latissimus dorsi have attachments to the thoracolumbar fascia, which connects to the sacrum, whose fibers run perpendicular to the SIJ. Thus, when the contralateral gluteus maximus and latissimus dorsi contract, a stabilizing force is transmitted across the SIJ (force closure). Just before heel strike, the latissimus dorsi and the contralateral gluteus maximus are eccentrically loaded, which adds pretension to the entire subsystem before weight bearing. At heel strike, each muscle accelerates its respective limb (through its concentric action) and creates tension across the thoracolumbar fascia. This tension also assists in stabilizing the SIJ. Thus, when an individual walks or runs, the POS transfers forces that are summated from the muscle's transverse plane orientation to propulsion in the sagittal plane.

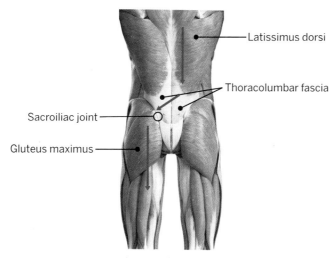

Figure 2-13 Posterior oblique subsystem

The POS is also of prime importance for rotational activities such as swinging a golf club or a baseball bat or throwing a ball. Dysfunction of any structure in the POS can lead to SIJ instability and LBP. The weakening of the gluteus maximus, the latissimus dorsi, or both, can lead to increased tension in the hamstring complex—a factor in recurrent hamstring strains. If performed in isolation, squats for the gluteus maximus and pulldowns/pull-ups for the latissimus dorsi will not adequately prepare the POS to perform optimally during functional activities. In contrast, prone flat or quadruped contralateral arm and leg lift exercises will activate the POS. Another example in standing is to perform simultaneous combination movements of shoulder internal rotation–adduction–extension with contralateral hip external rotation–extension with or without resistance bands (Steele, 2012; Thomeé et al., 1995).

The anterior oblique subsystem (AOS) (**Figure 2-14**) is similar to the POS in that it also functions in a transverse plane orientation, mostly in the anterior portion of the body. The prime contributors are the internal and external oblique muscles, the adductor complex, and the hip external rotators. Electromyography of these AOS muscles shows that they aid in pelvic stability and rotation as well as contributing to leg swing. The AOS is also a factor in the stabilization of the SIJ.

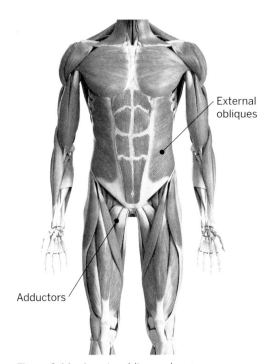

External obliques

Adductors

Figure 2-14   Anterior oblique subsystem

When people walk, their pelvis rotates in the transverse plane to create a swinging motion for the legs. The POS (posteriorly) and the AOS (anteriorly) contribute to this rotation. Knowing the fiber arrangements of the muscles involved (latissimus dorsi, gluteus maximus, internal and external obliques, adductors, and hip rotators) emphasizes this point. The AOS is also necessary for functional activities involving the trunk and upper and lower extremities. The obliques, in concert with the adductor complex, not only produce rotational and flexion movements but are also instrumental in stabilizing the LPHC. A basic exercise example for the AOS is performing supine oblique core activation while reaching a hand to touch the flexed knee of a contralateral flexed and adducted hip. Another example would be while standing to perform a cross-body kicking motion using the contralateral arm to counter the motion with or without resistance bands (Steele, 2012; Thomeé et al., 1995).

THE LATERAL SUBSYSTEM (LS)

The lateral subsystem (LS) is composed of the gluteus medius, tensor fascia latae, adductor complex, and the quadratus lumborum, all of which participate in frontal plane and pelvo-femoral stability. **Figure 2-15** shows how the ipsilateral gluteus medius, tensor fascia latae, and adductors combine with the contralateral quadratus lumborum to control the pelvis and femur in the frontal plane during single-leg functional movements such as in gait, lunges, or stair climbing. RI is demonstrated here by assessing how a client's foot with excessive pronation will result in decreased stability and control of the LPHC.

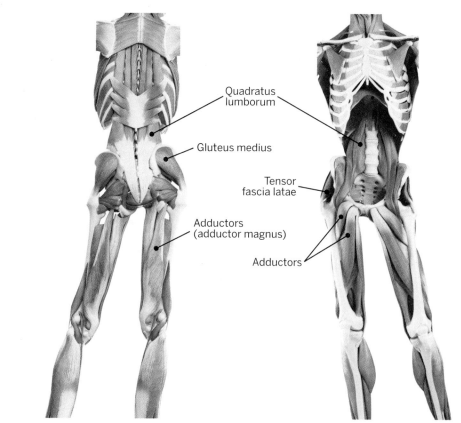

Figure 2-15 Lateral subsystem

Quadratus lumborum

Gluteus medius

Tensor fascia latae

Adductors (adductor magnus)

Adductors

Dysfunction in the LS starts on the ground during increased subtalar joint pronation and moves up the leg with increased tibial and femoral adduction and internal rotation during functional activities. At the top of this kinetic chain of RI, the low back follows the rest of the leg with unwanted frontal plane movement, all characterized by decreased strength and decreased neuromuscular control in the LS. An example of activating the LS and correcting RI dysfunction is side stepping in a knee extended or flexed position progressed with a resistance band placed just above knee joint (easier) or ankle joint (more challenging). Corrective Exercise Specialists would observe and correct any faulty movement patterns, including excessive foot pronation, tibio-femoral internal rotation and adduction, or a laterally tilted pelvis.

The descriptions of these four systems have been simplified; however, realize that the human body simultaneously coordinates these subsystems during activity. Each system individually and collectively contributes to the production of efficient movement by accelerating, decelerating, and dynamically stabilizing the HMS during motion (Michaud, 2011; Thomeé et al., 1995).

Introduction to Movement Impairment

Impairment or injury to the HMS rarely involves just one structure. Because the HMS is an integrated system, impairment in one system leads to compensations and adaptations in other systems. As outlined in **Figure 2-16**, if one component in the HMS is out of alignment (muscle tightness, muscle weakness, or altered joint arthrokinematics), it creates predictable patterns of tissue overload and dysfunction, which leads to decreased neuromuscular control and

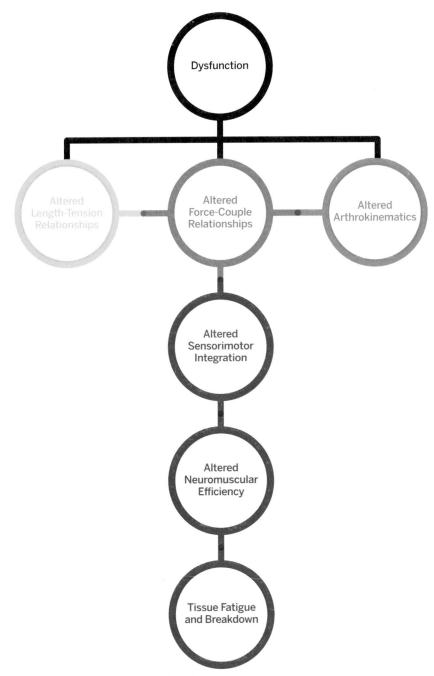

Figure 2-16   Human movement impairment

microtrauma and initiates the cumulative injury cycle (**Figure 2-17**). The **cumulative injury cycle** causes decreased performance, myofascial adhesions (which further alter length-tension relationships and joint arthrokinematics), and eventually injury.

These predictable patterns of dysfunction are referred to as **movement impairments**. Movement impairment refers to the state in which the structural integrity of the HMS is compromised because the components are out of alignment, causing the body to make compensations that put it at a higher risk of injury. This places abnormal distorting forces on the structures in the HMS that are above and below the dysfunctional segment. If one segment in the HMS is out of alignment, then other movement segments have to compensate in an attempt to balance the force distribution of the dysfunctional segment. To avoid movement impairments and the chain reactions that one misaligned segment creates, the Corrective Exercise Specialist must

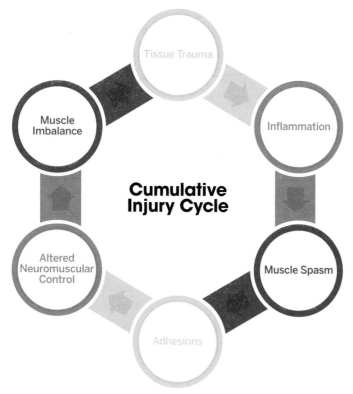

Figure 2-17   Cumulative injury cycle

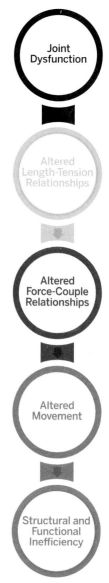

Figure 2-18   Joint dysfunction

emphasize optimal static, transitional, and dynamic postural control to maintain the structural integrity of the HMS during functional activities. Optimal movement system balance and alignment helps prevent movement impairment patterns and provides optimal shock absorption, weight acceptance, and transfer of force during functional movements (Page et al., 2010; Panjabi, 1992; Petersen et al., 2014).

Static Malalignments

Static malalignments are deviations from ideal posture that can be observed when standing still; essentially, they represent situations where an individual is said to have poor posture. Common static malalignments include joint dysfunction (excessive joint positioning) as well as myofascial adhesions that lead to or can be caused by chronic poor static posture. Joint dysfunction is one of the most common causes of pain in an individual (Fingleton et al., 2015; Scheper et al., 2015). Once a joint has lost normal function, the muscles around that joint may spasm and tighten to minimize the stress at the involved segment. Certain muscles become overactive/shortened to prevent movement and further injury. This process initiates the cumulative injury cycle. Therefore, a joint dysfunction causes altered length-tension relationships. This alters normal force-couple relationships, which alters normal movement patterns and leads to structural and functional inefficiency (**Figure 2-18**). Assessing a client's static posture will bring to light common patterns of static malalignments that could be influencing movement quality.

Static malalignments are frequently the result of **pattern overload** from either chronic sedentary positioning or repetitive stress injury. The most common example of this is seen in people with computer-based jobs where long days seated at desks can lead to chronically overactive/shortened hip flexors, putting the pelvis in a chronic anteriorly rotated position. Some other common examples include reduced dorsiflexion from the chronic wearing of high-heeled shoes,

Static malalignments

Deviations from ideal posture that can be seen when standing still.

Pattern overload

Occurs when a segment of the body is repeatedly moved or chronically held in the same way, leading to a state of muscle overactivity.

forward head posture from too many hours looking down at phone screens (text neck), an asymmetrical weight shift in students who carry their backpacks on the same side all day, or shoulder impingement in construction workers who repeatedly hammer overhead with the same arm.

Altered Muscle Recruitment

Static malalignments (altered length-tension relationships resulting from poor static posture, joint dysfunction, and myofascial adhesions) may lead to altered muscle recruitment patterns (altered force-couple relationships). This is caused by **altered reciprocal inhibition**. Altered reciprocal inhibition is the process by which a tight muscle (short, overactive, and myofascial adhesions) causes decreased neural drive, and therefore less-than-optimal recruitment of its functional antagonist. This process alters the normal force-couple relationships that should be present at all segments throughout the HMS. Furthermore, altered reciprocal inhibition can lead to **synergistic dominance**, which is the process in which a synergist compensates for a prime mover to maintain force production.

For example, a tight psoas major muscle decreases the neural drive (and therefore optimal recruitment) of the gluteus maximus. This altered recruitment and force production of the gluteus maximus (prime mover for hip extension) leads to compensation and substitution by the synergists (hamstrings) and stabilizers (erector spinae) (**Figure 2-19**). This can potentially lead to hamstring strains and LBP. In another example, if a client has a weak gluteus medius, then synergists (tensor fascia latae, adductor complex, and quadratus lumborum; i.e., LS) become synergistically dominant to compensate for the weakness. This altered muscle recruitment pattern further alters static alignment (alters normal joint alignment and normal length-tension relationships around the joint to which the muscles attach) and leads to injury (McGowan et al., 2009; Page et al., 2010; Steele, 2012).

Dynamic Malalignments

Static malalignments, altered muscle recruitment, or a combination of both can then lead to **dynamic malalignments** or deviations from optimal posture during functional movements. These are what are being referred to when discussing movement impairments as dynamic malalignments can only be observed when the body is in motion. Common lower extremity movement impairments include excessive foot pronation, knee valgus (knock-knees), and increased movement at the LPHC (extension or flexion) during functional movements. Common upper extremity movement impairments include rounded shoulders, a forward head posture, and improper scapulothoracic or glenohumeral kinematics during functional movements. These movement impairments are what the Corrective Exercise Specialist will be looking for during movement assessments with clients. Those observations will then be refined with targeted mobility assessments of joints involved with the observed compensation.

By viewing things through the lens of RI, it becomes clear how dysfunction at one point of the body can lead to movement impairments at another. The compensations in movement that the body makes in response to static and dynamic malalignments are known as relative flexibility. **Relative flexibility** represents the body's ability to find the path of least resistance to accomplish a task, even if that path requires altered muscle recruitment and creates dynamic malalignments. By keeping RI in mind, experienced Corrective Exercise Specialists can quickly link an observed movement impairment back to the altered muscle recruitment patterns that are causing it and pinpoint the muscle imbalances that can be improved through the application of the Corrective Exercise Continuum.

Altered reciprocal inhibition

Process whereby an overactive/shortened muscle causes decreased neural drive, and therefore less-than-optimal recruitment of its functional antagonist.

Synergistic dominance

The process by which a synergist compensates for an inhibited prime mover to maintain force production.

Dynamic malalignments

Deviations from optimal posture during functional movements.

Relative flexibility

The body's ability to find the path of least resistance to accomplish a task, even if that path creates dynamic malalignments.

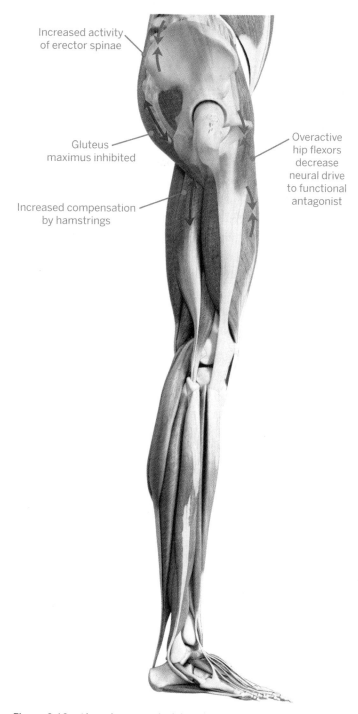

Increased activity of erector spinae

Gluteus maximus inhibited

Increased compensation by hamstrings

Overactive hip flexors decrease neural drive to functional antagonist

Figure 2-19 Altered reciprocal inhibition and synergistic dominance

The clearest example of relative flexibility in action is how an excessive forward lean at the hip can be caused by a lack of dorsiflexion down at the ankle when squatting to pick up a box from the ground. The down position of the squat requires optimal triple flexion of the legs (ankle, knee, and hip), but, in this case, the ankle cannot dorsiflex as much as it needs to. However, the task (picking up the box) still needs to be completed, so hip flexion naturally increases (bending over at the waist) to make up for the reduced range of motion at the ankle.

The Five Kinetic Chain Checkpoints

Identifying common impairments during the static postural and movement assessments requires the Corrective Exercise Specialist to look at the body in a systematic fashion so that consistency can be maintained from one assessment session to the next. Because movement happens at the joints, NASM recommends using the major joint locations of the body as the observation points when looking for static postural and movement impairments, starting at the ground and moving up. These key locations, known as the **kinetic chain checkpoints**, have been identified as the foot and ankle complex, the knees, the LPHC, the shoulders, and the head and neck. These checkpoints represent the links in the kinetic chain—links that, when not operating properly, can cause disruption to the entire interconnected system.

In order to better recognize impairments at each of the five kinetic chain checkpoints, it is important to understand what ideal posture looks like at each observational point while a client is standing still (**Figure 2-20**). This information can then be used as a frame of reference during both static and dynamic postural assessments.

Kinetic chain checkpoints

Key points on the body to observe and assess an individual's static and dynamic posture; feet/ankles, knees, LPHC, shoulders, and head/neck.

- **Foot and ankle**: Neutral arch of the foot (not flattened and toes not scrunched), feet parallel and pointing straight ahead, hip-to-shoulder width apart
- **Knee**: In line with the second and third toes of each foot and not flexed or hyperextended
- **Lumbo-pelvic-hip complex (LPHC)**: Neutral sagittal hip position (no excessive posterior or anterior tilt) and hips level in the frontal plane
- **Shoulders and thoracic spine**: Not rounded forward and in line with the hips and ears from a lateral viewpoint
- **Head and cervical spine**: Neutral cervical spine (no excessive forward positioning of the neck), ears in line with the shoulders, and a level chin

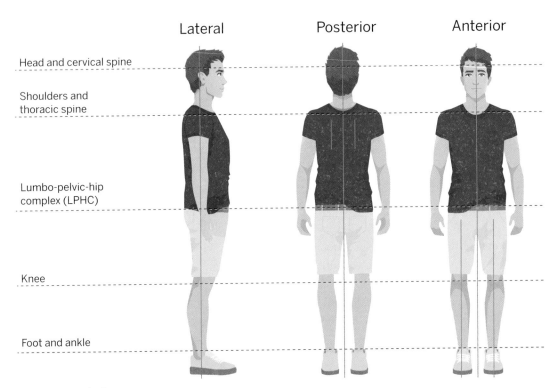

Head and cervical spine

Shoulders and thoracic spine

Lumbo-pelvic-hip complex (LPHC)

Knee

Foot and ankle

Lateral   Posterior   Anterior

Figure 2-20 Ideal posture

Human movement science is the study of how the HMS functions in an interdependent and interrelated scheme. The RI model, as it pertains to human movement, recognizes that for a person to fully function and successfully perform tasks in life, as well as in fitness training, coordinated and integrated action of all systems of the body is required. Thus, in order to fully address the HMS, the Corrective Exercise Specialist needs to first establish an assessment process that systematically observes a client's posture both statically and while in motion.

A corrective exercise program needs to always consider the foundations of motor behavior, because the goal is to improve movement quality by essentially reteaching optimal movement patterns. The HMS is an interconnected network of force-couples that need to function efficiently to produce the best possible movement. By integrating the foundational principles that govern muscular function, Corrective Exercise Specialists can better understand how disruptions to the kinetic chain can create movement impairments. The Corrective Exercise Continuum can then be applied to restore optimal length-tension relationships, leading to more efficiently functioning force-couples and the optimization of movement patterns.

REFERENCES

Biedert, R. M. (2000). Contribution of the three levels of nervous system motor control: Spinal cord, lower brain, cerebral cortex. In S. M. Lephart & F. H. Fu (Eds.), *Proprioception and neuromuscular control in joint stability* (pp. 23–30). Human Kinetics.

Buckland A. J., Miyamoto, R., Patel, R. D., Slover, J., & Razi, A. E. (2017). Differentiating hip pathology from lumbar spine pathology: Key points of evaluation and management. *Journal of the American Academy of Orthopaedic Surgeons, 25*(2), e23–e34. https://doi.org/10.5435/JAAOS-D-15-00740

Byström, M. G., Rasmussen-Barr, E., & Grooten, W. J. (2013). Motor control exercises reduces pain and disability in chronic and recurrent low back pain: A meta-analysis. *Spine, 38*(6), E350–E358. https://doi.org/10.1097/BRS.0b013e31828435fb

Coker, C. A. (2018). *Motor learning and control for practitioners* (4th ed.). Routledge.

Crossley, K., Bennell, K., Green, S., & McConnell, J. (2001). A systematic review of physical interventions for patellofemoral pain syndrome. *Clinical Journal of Sport Medicine, 11*(2), 103–110. https://doi.org/10.1097/00042752-200104000-00007

Dos Remedios, C., & Gilmour, D. (2017). An historical perspective of the discovery of titin filaments. *Biophysical Reviews, 9*(3), 179–188. https://doi.org/10.1007/s12551-017-0269-3

Feher, J. (2017). Skeletal muscle mechanics. In *Quantitative human physiology: An introduction* (2nd ed.; pp. 292–304). Academic Press/Elsevier. https://doi.org/10.1016/B978-0-12-800883-6.00027-6

Fingleton, C., Smart, K., Moloney, N., Fullen, B. M., & Doody, C. (2015). Pain sensitization in people with knee osteoarthritis: A systematic review and meta-analysis. *Osteoarthritis and Cartilage, 23*(7), 1043–1056. https://doi.org/10.1016/j.joca.2015.02.163

Friedberg, R. P., Fields, K. B., & Grayzel, J. (2017). Anterior cruciate ligament injury. *UpToDate.* https://www.uptodate.com/contents/anterior-cruciate-ligament-injury#H1

Fulkerson, J. P. (2002). Diagnosis and treatment of patients with patellofemoral pain. *The American Journal of Sports Medicine, 30*(3), 447–456. https://doi.org/10.1177/03635465020300032501

Hamill, J., Knutzen, K. M., & Derrick, T. R. (2014). *Biomechanical basis of human movement* (4th ed.). Wolters Kluwer Health.

Herzog, M. M., Kerr, Z. Y., Marshall, S. W., & Wikstrom, E. A. (2019). Epidemiology of ankle sprains and chronic ankle instability. *Journal of Athletic Training, 54*(6), 603–610. https://doi.org/10.4085/1062-6050-447-17

Ireland, M. L., Willson, J. D., Ballantyne, B. T., & Davis, I. M. (2003). Hip strength in females with and without patellofemoral pain. *Journal of Orthopaedic and Sports Physical Therapy, 33*(11), 671–676.

Irving, D. B., Cook, J. L., Young, M. A., & Menz, H. B. (2007). Obesity and pronated foot type may increase the risk of chronic plantar heel pain: A matched case-control study. *BMC Musculoskeletal Disorders, 8*(41). https://doi.org/10.1186/1471-2474-8-41

Kaya, D., Yosmaoglu, B., & Doral, M. N. (Eds.). (2018). *Proprioception in orthopaedics, sports medicine and rehabilitation.* Springer International.

Kopeinig, C., Gödl-Purrer, B., & Salchinger, B. (2015). Fascia as a proprioceptive organ and its role in chronic pain: A review of current literature. *Safety in Health, 1*(Suppl. 1). https://doi.org/10.1186/2056-5917-1-S1-A2

Kosashvili, Y., Fridman, T., Backstein, D., Safir, O., & Bar, Z. Y. (2008). The correlation between pes planus and anterior knee or intermittent low back pain. *Foot & Ankle International, 29*(9), 910–913. https://doi.org/10.3113/FAI.2008.0910

Leetun, D. T., Ireland, M. L., Wilson, J. D., Ballantyne, B. T., & Davis, I. M. (2004). Core stability measures as risk factors for lower extremity injury in athletes. *Medicine and Science in Sports and Exercise, 36*(6), 926–934.

Leversen, J. S. R., Haga, M., & Sigmundsson, H. (2012). From children to adults: Motor performance across the life-span. *PLoS One, 7*(6), e38830–e38830. https://doi.org/10.1371/journal.pone.0038830

Magill, R. A., & Anderson, D. I. (2016). *Motor learning and control: Concepts and applications.* (11th ed.). McGraw-Hill Education.

McGowan, C. P., Neptune, R. R., Clark, D. J., & Kautz, S. A. (2009). Modular control of human walking: Adaptations to altered mechanical demands. *Journal of Biomechanics, 43*(3), 412–419. https://doi.org/10.1016/j.jbiomech.2009.10.009

Michaud, T. C. (2011). *Human locomotion: The conservative management of gait-related disorders.* Newton Biomechanics.

National Institute of Neurological Disorders and Stroke. (2014). Low back pain fact sheet. NIH Publication No. 15-5161.

Neumann, D. (2016). *Kinesiology of the musculoskeletal system: Foundations for physical rehabilitation* (3rd ed.). Elsevier.

Nishikawa, K. C., Lindstedt, S. L., & LaStayo, P. C. (2018). Basic science and clinical use of eccentric contractions: History and uncertainties. *Journal of Sport and Health Science, 7*(3), 265–274. https://doi.org/10.1016/j.jshs.2018.06.002

Page, P., Frank, C. C., & Lardner, R. (2010). *Assessment and treatment of muscle imbalance: The Janda approach.* Human Kinetics.

Panjabi, M. M. (1992). The stabilizing system of the spine. Part I. Function, dysfunction, adaptation, and enhancement. *Journal of Spinal Disorders, 5*(4), 383–389. https://doi.org/10.1097/00002517-199212000-00001

Payne, K. A., Berg, K., & Latin, R. W. (1997). Ankle injuries and ankle strength, flexibility, and proprioception in college basketball players. *Journal of Athletic Training, 32*(3), 221–225. https://www.ncbi.nlm.nih.gov/pubmed/16558453

Petersen, W., Ellermann, A., Gösele-Koppenburg, A., Best, R., Rembitzki, I. V., Brüggemann, G. P., & Liebau, C. (2014). Patellofemoral pain syndrome. *Knee Surgery, Sports Traumatology, Arthroscopy, 22*(10), 2264–2274. https://doi.org/10.1007/s00167-013-2759-6

Regev, G. J., Kim, C. W., Tomiya, A., Lee, Y., Ghofrani, H., Garfin, S. R., Lieber, R. L., & Ward, S. (2011, Dec.). Psoas muscle architectural design, in vivo sarcomere length range, and passive tensile properties support its role as a lumbar spine stabilizer. *Spine, 36*(26), E1666–E1674. https://doi.org/10.1097/BRS.0b013e31821847b3

Richardson, C., Hodges, P. W., & Hides, J. (2004). *Therapeutic exercise for lumbopelvic stabilization: A motor control approach for the treatment and prevention of low back pain* (2nd ed.). Churchill Livingstone.

Sahrmann, S., Azevedo, D. C., & Van Dillen, L. (2017). Diagnosis and treatment of movement system impairment syndromes. *Brazilian Journal of Physical Therapy, 21*(6), 391–399. https://doi.org/10.1016/j.bjpt.2017.08.001

Scheper, M. C., de Vries, J. E., Verbunt, J., & Engelbert, R. H. (2015). Chronic pain in hypermobility syndrome and Ehlers–Danlos syndrome (hypermobility type): It is a challenge. *Journal of Pain Research, 8*, 591–601. https://doi.org/10.2147/JPR.S64251

Schmidt, R. A., & Lee, T. D. (2014). *Motor learning and performance: From principles to application* (5th ed.). Human Kinetics.

Schmidt, R. A., Lee, T., Winstein, C., Wulf, G., & Zelaznik, H. N. (2019). *Motor control and learning: A behavioral emphasis* (6th ed.). Human Kinetics.

Seeley, R. R., Stephens, T. D., & Tate, P. (2004). *Anatomy and physiology* (7th ed.). McGraw-Hill.

Steele, C. (Ed.). (2012). *Applications of EMG in clinical and sports medicine.* IntechOpen. https://doi.org/10.5772/2349

Sueki, D. G., Cleland, J. A., & Wainner, R. S. (2013). A regional interdependence model of musculoskeletal dysfunction: Research, mechanisms, and clinical implications. *Journal of Manual & Manipulative Therapy, 21*(2), 90–102. https://doi.org/10.1179/2042618612Y.0000000027

Thomeé, R., Renström, P., Karlsson, J., & Grimby, G. (1995). Patellofemoral pain syndrome in young women: A clinical analysis of alignment, pain parameters, common symptoms, functional activity level. *Scandinavian Journal of Medicine & Science in Sports, 5*(4), 237–244. https://doi.org/10.1111/j.1600-0838.1995.tb00040.x

Vleeming, A., Mooney, V., & Stoeckart, R. (2007). *Movement, stability & lumbopelvic pain: Integration of research and therapy* (2nd ed.). Churchill Livingstone.

Wainner, R. S., Whitman, J. M., Cleland, J. A., & Flynn, T. W. (2007). Regional interdependence: A musculoskeletal examination model whose time has come. *Journal of Orthopaedic & Sports Physical Therapy, 37*(11), 658–660. https://doi.org/10.2519/jospt.2007.0110

Waterman, B. R., Owens, B. D., Davey, S., Zacchilli, M. A., & Belmont, P. J., Jr. (2010). The epidemiology of ankle sprains in the United States. *Journal of Bone and Joint Surgery, American Volume, 92*(13), 2279–2284. https://doi.org/10.2106/JBJS.I.01537

Watkins, J. (2010). *Structure and function of the musculoskeletal system* (2nd ed.). Human Kinetics.

Wilke, J., Krause, F., Vogt, L., & Banzer, W. (2016). What is evidence-based about myofascial chains: A systematic review. *Archives of Physical Medicine and Rehabilitation, 97*(3), 454–461. https://doi.org/10.1016/j.apmr.2015.07.023

Wilson, J. M., Loenneke, J. P., Jo, E., Wilson, G. J., Zourdos, M. C., & Kim, J. (2012). The effects of endurance, strength, and power training on muscle fiber type shifting. *The Journal of Strength & Conditioning Research, 26*(6), 1724–1729. https://doi.org/10.1519/JSC.0b013e318234eb6f

SECTION 2

Corrective Exercise Techniques

CHAPTER 3

Inhibitory Techniques

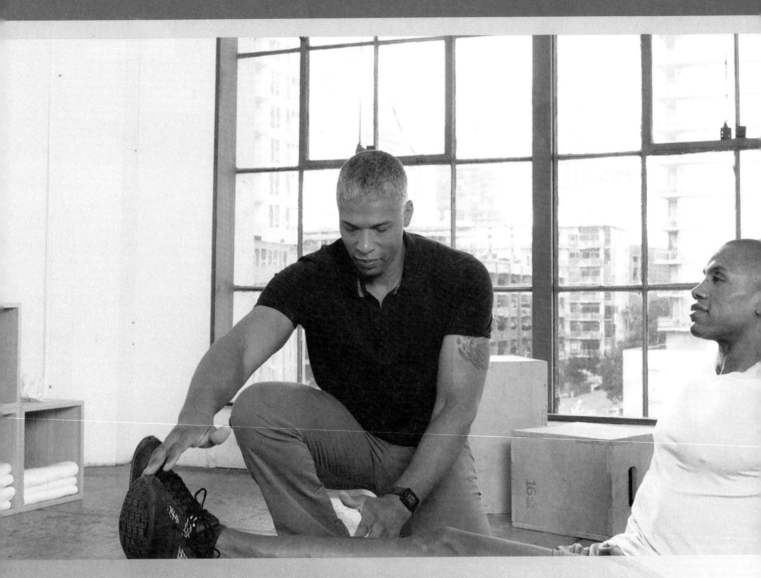

Learning Objectives

After reading this content, students should be able to demonstrate the following objectives:

- **Identify** current evidence supporting myofascial techniques.
- **Explain** the function of myofascial techniques in a corrective exercise program.
- **Identify** myofascial modalities and their uses.
- **Determine** appropriate strategies for implementing self-myofascial rolling.

Introduction

The first phase in the Corrective Exercise Continuum (**Figure 3-1**) is to inhibit or modulate activity of the nervous system that innervates the myofascia. One of the most common **self-myofascial techniques** (SMT) used to inhibit or modulate activity is myofascial rolling (aka self-myofascial rolling), previously referred to as self-myofascial release. This technique uses various tools such as a foam roller, roller ball, or handheld device. Allied health professionals may use other myofascial techniques, such as massage, instrument-assisted soft-tissue manipulation (IASTM), joint mobilization, and so forth to affect myofascial tissues.

> **Self-myofascial techniques**
>
> The category of flexibility techniques used to reduce tension in muscle fibers. Primarily used for overactive tissue.

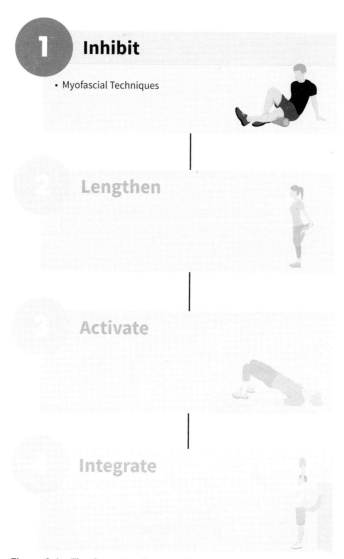

1 Inhibit
- Myofascial Techniques

Lengthen

Activate

Integrate

Figure 3-1 The Corrective Exercise Continuum: Inhibit

Myofascial Rolling

During the past decade the use of myofascial rolling techniques (i.e., foam-rolling muscles, as in **Figure 3-2**) has emerged to become a relatively common and practical intervention used within the health and fitness environment. The body of research has grown over the past 5 years, focusing on the therapeutic and physiological effects of the technique. The following sections will review the current research and discuss NASM's position on myofascial rolling.

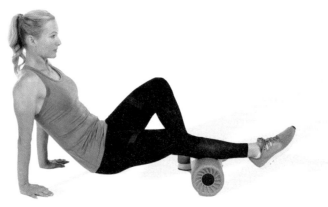

Figure 3-2 Foam rolling

Myofascial Rolling and the Cumulative Injury Cycle

It is essential for the health and fitness professional to understand that poor posture and repetitive overuse movements can create dysfunction within the connective tissues of the human movement system (HMS) (Iqbal & Alghadir, 2017). These dysfunctions eventually lead to an injury-and-repair response by the body termed the cumulative injury cycle (**Figure 3-3**) (Clark et al., 2010; Iqbal & Alghadir, 2017).

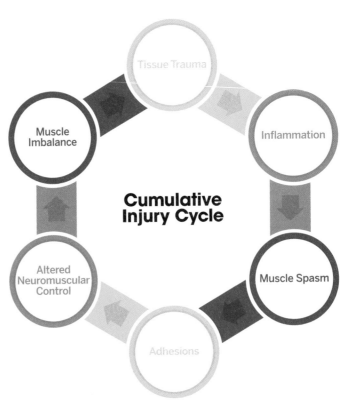

Figure 3-3 Cumulative injury cycle

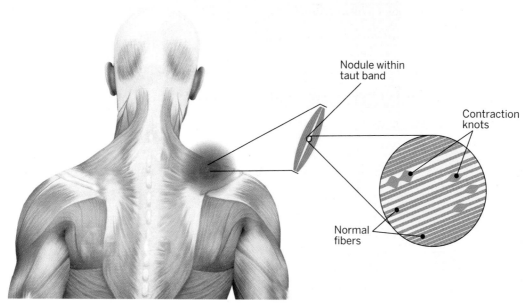

Figure 3-4 Myofascial adhesions

Current theory supports the idea that repetitive movements and long periods of poor posture lead to tissue trauma and inflammation. Inflammation, in turn, activates the body's pain response, which initiates a protective mechanism, increasing muscle tension and causing muscle spasm. These muscle spasms are not like a calf cramp. Heightened activity of the central nervous system (CNS) and tissue mechanoreceptors and nociceptors (e.g., pain receptors) in the injured area create a type of microspasm or tension (Jafri, 2014). As a result of the spasm, **adhesions** may begin to form within the myofascial tissues. These adhesions form a weak **inelastic** matrix that decreases normal mobility of the soft tissue (**Figure 3-4**) (Clark et al., 2010; Money, 2017). The result is alterations in neuromuscular control, length-tension relationships (leading to altered reciprocal inhibition), and force-couple relationships (leading to synergistic dominance), as well as arthrokinetic dysfunction (leading to altered joint motion) (Jafri, 2014; Zhuang et al., 2014). Left unchecked, these adhesions may begin to form structural changes in the soft tissue that are evident by Davis's law.

Davis's law states that soft tissue will model along the lines of stress (Cyron & Humphrey, 2017; Mueller & Maluf, 2002). Soft tissue remodels or rebuilds itself with a collagen matrix that forms in a random fashion and not in the same direction as the muscle fibers. If the myofascial tissues are not stimulated by movement, lengthening, and broadening, these connective tissue fibers may act as a roadblock, preventing soft tissue mobility. This creates alterations in normal tissue mobility and causes relative flexibility (Clark et al., 2010; Iqbal & Alghadir, 2017). Relative flexibility is the phenomenon of the human movement system seeking the path of least resistance during functional movement patterns (or movement compensation) (Clark et al., 2010). The body will move from point A to point B as ordered by the nervous system, and the ideal dynamic posture is abandoned to accommodate reduced tissue mobility. Continued movement compensation can lead to further muscle imbalances and potential injury.

Myofascial rolling techniques may help in modulating the local receptor activity, tension (microspasm), and CNS activity that develop from the traumatized tissue. Researchers and experts have postulated that myofascial rolling may help "break up" the myofascial adhesions, or "trigger points," that are created through the cumulative injury cycle (Behm & Wilke, 2019).

Myofascial adhesions

Knots in muscle tissue that can result in altered neuromuscular control.

Inelastic

Possessing the inability to stretch.

Davis's law

Law that states that soft tissue will model along the lines of stress.

However, current research does not fully support this theory and suggests that the post application improvements in tone may be due to local mechanical and neurophysiological mechanisms (Behm & Wilke, 2019). These theories will be discussed in subsequent sections.

Scientific Rationale for Myofascial Rolling

Myofascial rolling can be used for two primary reasons:

1. To affect local myofascial tissue dysfunction
2. To influence the autonomic nervous system

Myofascial Rolling and Myofascial Tissue Dysfunction

Myofascial rolling is classified as a compression technique where an external object (e.g., foam roller) compresses myofascial tissues. This type of intervention has traditionally been called self-myofascial release, which is considered outdated given the current research (Behm & Wilke, 2019). Specifically, the term *release* may be inaccurate as it refers to releasing a "knot," or myofascial trigger point. Current evidence suggests that direct compression by the object may produce a local mechanical and global neurophysiological response through afferent CNS pathways (Aboodarda et al., 2015; Behm & Wilke, 2019; Grabow et al., 2018; Young et al., 2018). External compression may stimulate afferent (sensory) receptors located throughout the muscle, fascia, and connective tissues of the HMS to override the dysfunctional yet protective mechanisms involved in the cumulative injury cycle. Thus, the term *myofascial rolling* is preferred and is used throughout the remainder of this textbook. Further, the term *self-myofascial rolling* is used to denote that, unless they are an appropriately licensed healthcare practitioner, fitness professionals teach their clients how to apply the techniques to themselves.

Myofascial Rolling: Local Mechanical and Neurophysiological Effects

With regard to the *local mechanical effects*, the direct roller pressure may change the viscoelastic properties of the local myofascia by mechanisms such as causing thixotropy (reduced viscosity), reducing myofascial restriction, promoting fluid changes (fascial hydration), and stimulating cellular responses (Behm & Wilke, 2019; Jay et al., 2014; Kelly & Beardsley, 2016). Researchers have also found that myofascial rolling reduces local arterial stiffness (Okamoto et al., 2014), increases arterial tissue perfusion (Hotfiel et al., 2017), and improves vascular endothelial function (Okamoto et al., 2014), which are all related to local physiological changes.

With regard to the *neurophysiological effects*, the direct roller pressure may influence tissue relaxation and pain in the local and surrounding tissues. For tissue relaxation, the roller pressure may induce a greater myofascial relaxation, or "stretch tolerance," through CNS afferent input from the Golgi tendon reflex, **gamma loop** modulation, and mechanoreceptors (**Figure 3-5**) (Aboodarda et al., 2015; Behm & Wilke, 2019; Cavanaugh et al., 2017; Cheatham & Kolber, 2017; Jay et al., 2014; Kelly & Beardsley, 2016; Monteiro et al., 2017; Nagi et al., 2011).

Researchers have postulated that roller pressure may modulate pain through stimulation of muscle and cutaneous receptors (e.g., interstitial type III and IV, free nerve endings, C-tactile fibers) (Aboodarda et al., 2015; Behm & Wilke, 2019; Nagi & Mahns, 2013; Nagi et al., 2011),

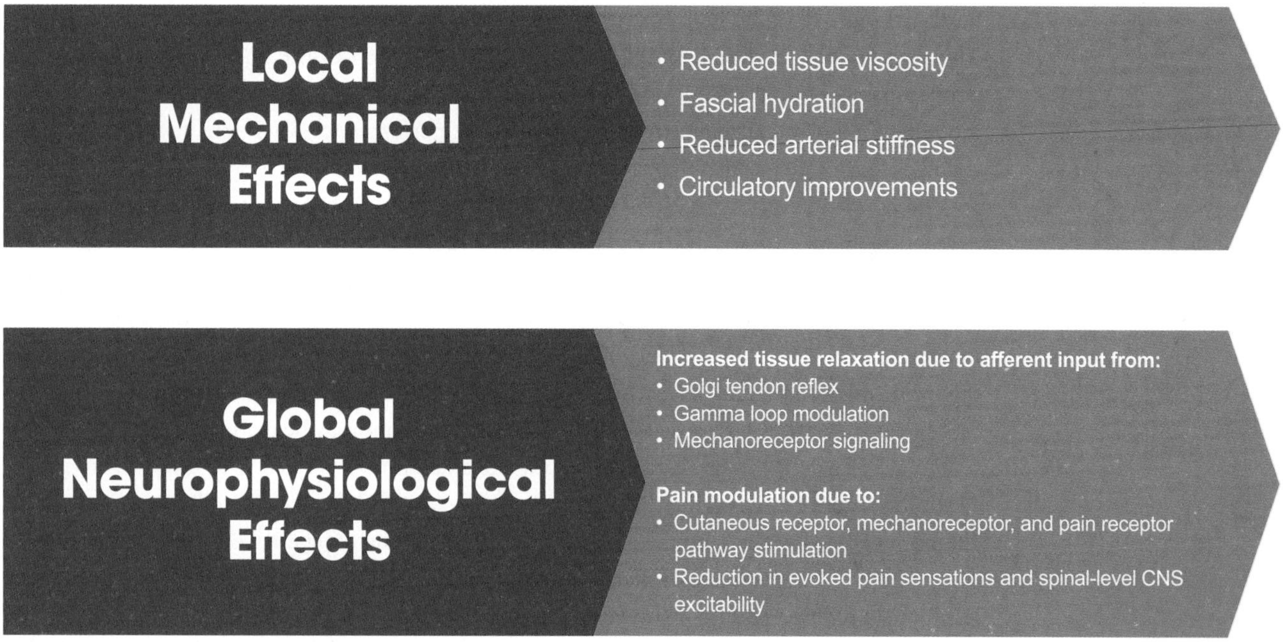

Local Mechanical Effects
- Reduced tissue viscosity
- Fascial hydration
- Reduced arterial stiffness
- Circulatory improvements

Global Neurophysiological Effects

Increased tissue relaxation due to afferent input from:
- Golgi tendon reflex
- Gamma loop modulation
- Mechanoreceptor signaling

Pain modulation due to:
- Cutaneous receptor, mechanoreceptor, and pain receptor pathway stimulation
- Reduction in evoked pain sensations and spinal-level CNS excitability

Figure 3-5 Local and global effects of myofascial rolling

mechanoreceptors (Young et al., 2018), afferent central nociceptive pathways (gate theory of pain) (Aboodarda et al., 2015; Cavanaugh et al., 2017), and descending antinociceptive pathways (diffuse noxious inhibitory control) (Aboodarda et al., 2015; Sullivan et al., 2013). Researchers have found that myofascial rolling decreases evoked pain (Cavanaugh et al., 2017) and reduces spinal-level excitability (Hoffman reflex) (Young et al., 2018), which provides evidence for these theories. These responses may be triggered by low, moderate, or high roller pressure, lending evidence to the sensitivity of myofascial tissues to external forces (Grabow et al., 2018).

The first phase in the NASM Corrective Exercise Continuum is to inhibit. By creating local mechanical changes to myofascial tissues and modulating the nervous system, the myofascia may have less "tone" and a greater mobility, which may provide a better pathway to the second phase in the continuum, which is to lengthen. The following sections will provide application guidelines for self-myofascial rolling programs.

Application Guidelines for Self-Myofascial Techniques

Myofascial rollers vary in shape, size, and density, which will have some influence on the overall effect. When choosing a myofascial tool, it is important to consider the pressure exerted by the object, which is the result of the object's diameter and density, and the force applied.

Pressure

The amount of pressure exerted by a myofascial roller is a product of its diameter and density; that is, a harder, smaller roller exerts more pressure than a larger, softer roller. No studies have been published to date that have explored the specific amount of pressure needed for optimal results. Curran et al. (2008) found that a rigid roller with a smaller contact size (i.e., smaller diameter) produced significantly more pressure than a traditional myofascial roller made of compressed foam. However, the subjects using the small, hard myofascial roller did not improve flexibility more than the subjects using the larger, softer myofascial roller (Curran et al., 2008). Although Grabow et al. (2018) did not specifically measure pressure, they had participants use a roller massager at 50%, 70%, and 90% of maximal perceived pain and found no differences in mobility nor any impairments in strength and jump performance. Therefore, more pressure (or rolling intensity) does not always lead to better results.

The ideal amount of pressure is dependent on the user's experience, pain threshold, and perception. In one study, Cheatham et al. (2018) had subjects rate their perception of pain while using a myofascial roller in two conditions: (1) while able to see the roller and (2) while blindfolded. They found that 40% of the participants rated the rollers differently on the pain scale. It is important to note that three rollers of different colors and densities were used. Thus, it appeared that color might have had at least some influence on the overall perceptions of pain. This concept needs to be investigated further before any assumptions may be made, but it is evident that preference and perception must be taken into consideration.

In the absence of changing the density or diameter of the myofascial roller, pressure can be altered by changing the amount of force applied to the myofascial roller. If using a handheld roller, such as a massage stick roller, the user can push with more force to increase pressure or less force to reduce pressure. However, increases in pressure are limited to the user's upper body strength and positioning, because it may be difficult to reach certain muscle groups. Overcoming these limitations is difficult with handheld myofascial rollers. To control pressure across different research subjects, Sullivan et al. (2013) constructed a constant pressure roller apparatus (CPRA). The use of the CPRA allowed researchers to attach 28.6 lb (13 kg) of weight plates, consistent across all subjects, for the myofascial rolling intervention. Such a device is not practical for the general population. Further, most handheld rollers that require both hands are limited to the lower extremities.

Another common method is to use myofascial rollers or balls and apply bodyweight pressure. Myofascial rollers and balls are not limited to the lower extremities, providing more options while not requiring the use of the hands. Bodyweight pressure is usually applied by either lying an extremity or targeted muscle across the myofascial roller or pinning a tool between the body and a wall. Thus, the most practical methods for applying pressure are the use of body weight (rollers, balls) and upper body strength (handheld rollers).

Density

Density plays a key role in the overall amount of pressure applied to the tissues. Individuals who have never used a myofascial roller should begin with a soft roller. Although denser rollers have frequently been promoted as better because they work deeper layers of tissue, research by Cheatham and Stull (2019) suggests that soft to moderate rollers may achieve better overall results. They found that high-density myofascial rollers may in fact increase the perception of pain with only minimal increases in joint mobility. Medium-density myofascial rollers appeared to show the best improvements in joint mobility and decreased the perception of pain, followed by mild-density myofascial rollers. The findings from this research further suggested that personal preference should be taken into consideration. The most effective myofascial roller is the one the individual will use regularly.

Over time, an individual can progress to using a denser myofascial roller, as needed. However, the goal should never be to cause or induce a significant amount of pain or discomfort. Myofascial techniques work to influence the nervous system. Thus, it is imperative that the user be able to breathe and relax while using myofascial techniques. Self-myofascial rollers that are too hard may interfere with overall relaxation and reduce the effectiveness of the techniques.

Diameter

The diameter of the myofascial roller also plays a role in the effect. Because pressure is a function of surface area, a smaller diameter elicits more acute pressure and may influence deeper layers of tissue. Conversely, a larger diameter myofascial roller has more surface area, which distributes the pressure more equally across the superficial tissues. Similar to the density of roller, the diameter of the roller can be progressed over time, as needed. Individuals just beginning to use myofascial rolling should begin with a larger diameter roller to become more accustomed to the practice before moving to smaller myofascial rollers.

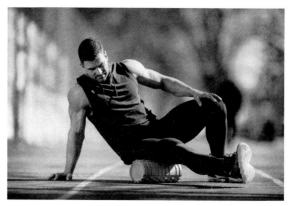

Foam roller
© Just Life/Shutterstock.

Texture

Like density and diameter, the texture of the myofascial roller also appears to have some influence on the overall effect. In a comparison of three myofascial rollers—one grid pattern, one random multilevel surface pattern, and one smooth—the two textured (patterned) rollers produced greater immediate effects (Cheatham & Stull, 2019). The textures used in this study were not large peaks or points but were simple changes in levels and crevices in the roller. Thus, the pressure applied to the tissue only changed slightly during rolling. It is not clear why a textured roller produced greater results, but Cheatham and Stull (2019) suggest that the textures may distort or "move" the tissues more than a smooth roller, which may stimulate the local receptors and CNS differently. It is important to note that a

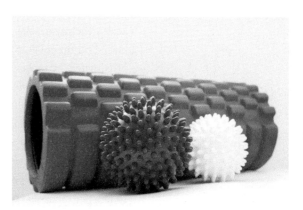

Rollers with different textures
© Mvjustina/Shutterstock

smooth roller also works very well. Therefore, a textured roller may be recommended, if available. If a textured roller is not available, then a smooth roller will still produce favorable results. For example, much of the early research showing improvements in mobility used self-made rollers made from materials such as polyvinyl chloride (PVC) pipe with a thin layer of smooth foam (MacDonald et al., 2014).

Application Guidelines

It is important to recognize that although the exact pressures applied to tissues by self-myofascial rollers have not been calculated, the fitness professional should still use caution. High-density and small-diameter myofascial rollers can apply a significant amount of pressure to the tissues, possibly resulting in tissue damage. Further, given that myofascial rolling requires a degree of relaxation, too much pressure may cause the user to tense up. Therefore, the fitness professional is encouraged to err on the side of caution by using less pressure via a larger, softer myofascial roller versus more pressure via a smaller, denser roller. Further, the fitness professional should monitor the user for normal relaxed breathing patterns and communicate with the user by asking whether the amount of pressure is comfortable or not. If the answer is no, then the fitness professional should immediately regress by reducing the pressure. Fitness professionals should begin clients on a large, soft, textured myofascial roller until they become more accustomed to self-myofascial rolling. Then, the fitness professional may choose to progress the client within their comfort level.

Myofascial Technique Tools

One of the most common and most recommended methods of self-myofascial rolling is the use of a cylindrical myofascial roller. Myofascial rollers are frequently termed "foam rollers," and they vary in material, size, shape, and length. As noted earlier, the size, material, and shape matter. The material a myofascial roller is constructed from will affect its density, and thus the total pressure applied. For this reason, "foam rolling" may be more appropriately termed *self-myofascial rolling*.

Myofascial Rollers

Myofascial rollers are usually cylindrical rollers of different shapes, sizes, and densities. Myofascial rollers appear to be the most practical for most clients and require the use of bodyweight pressure. A user will often sit or lie on the floor or stretching mat and place the targeted muscle across the myofascial roller. The pressure is then applied by adjusting the amount of weight placed on the roller. Myofascial rollers come in a variety of lengths, most commonly from approximately 12 inches to up to 36 inches (30 to 90 cm). The length of the roller has little influence on the overall effect, but longer rollers may feel more comfortable or stable to those who are new to myofascial rolling. Shorter rollers are often ideal for those who like to carry their roller with them, as it will fit nicely into a gym bag. A traveling fitness professional may like to have a shorter roller to carry, while a professional in a health club may choose to have the longer rollers. When referring to myofascial rollers, the foam (cylindrical) roller will be the most commonly discussed tool. The practice of myofascial rolling can also be performed with balls, handheld rollers (e.g., massage sticks), or other tools.

Myofascial Balls

Myofascial balls Spherical tools used for myofascial rolling that come in different sizes and densities; often called *massage balls*.

Myofascial balls, often called *massage balls*, are spherical rollers that come in different sizes and densities. Myofascial balls will generally elicit more pressure because of the reduced surface contact area compared to a myofascial roller of the same diameter and density. Therefore, a myofascial ball may be seen as a progression from a cylindrical myofascial roller. Myofascial balls are excellent tools for many areas of the body that a cylindrical roller may be too large to reach effectively. It is common to see lacrosse balls, tennis balls, baseballs, softballs, and golf balls used as myofascial tools due to their low cost. However, it is important to recognize that such balls are made for sport and not massage. Balls such as lacrosse balls and baseballs are very hard and are much more challenging for someone new to self-myofascial rolling to regulate the amount of pressure placed on the ball. For example, a new client attempting to roll the gluteals or piriformis on a lacrosse ball is going to experience a significant amount of pressure. Remember that the overall force applied is a function of density and diameter, so a small, hard ball will elicit a substantial amount of pressure directly into the tissues. Therefore, for clients with less experience, the fitness professional may want to use a larger, softer ball or a ball that is designed specifically for self-myofascial rolling.

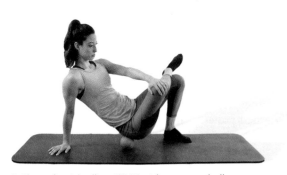

Self-myofascial rolling (SMR) with massage ball

Handheld Myofascial Rollers

Handheld myofascial rollers are a great alternative to regular myofascial rollers and balls. Handheld rollers that are designed for one hand are suitable for the entire body. Handheld rollers are constructed of a variety of materials, and although they come in varying sizes, handheld rollers are generally smaller than cylindrical foam rollers. Because handheld rollers are guided by the user, size and density are less of a concern because the pressure may be easily changed by increasing or decreasing the amount of force. Handheld rollers are a suitable option for users who are unable to get on the ground to use a traditional roller. Further, handheld rollers appear to be as effective as a traditional roller on hamstrings flexibility (DeBruyne et al., 2017).

Note, however, that handheld rollers do have a few limitations. First, those that are designed to be used in both hands may be limited to the lower extremities. Second, their use is limited by body positioning. Many users may have challenges reaching certain muscle groups while maintaining a safe posture. Third, the amount of pressure applied is limited by upper body strength. Clients may need to apply more pressure than they are capable of, whether due to an upper extremity injury or just a simple lack of strength, to achieve the desired effect. Therefore, if the user can get on the ground, it is recommended to use a cylindrical myofascial roller over a handheld one. If the user is unable to get on the ground, then the handheld is a suitable alternative. Furthermore, handheld rollers are available that can be compressed into a shorter length, and thus be more convenient for travel than a typical foam roller. Also, it is recommended that fitness professionals not use a handheld roller to apply pressure to their clients. The client should always be the one in control of the pressure; this enhances the safety of the technique and teaches the client to be self-reliant.

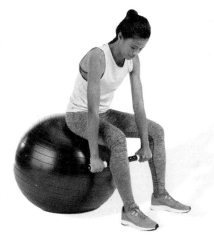

SMR with handheld roller—two hands

Vibration

The therapeutic effects of vibration are well known (Dong et al., 2019; Games et al., 2015; Park et al., 2018). However, much of this research used vibration plates or whole body vibration. The use of vibration in a more targeted device, such as a myofascial roller, also appears to be effective, but the specific ramifications are less well known. In a study comparing a myofascial roller with vibration to the same roller without vibration, those in the vibration group experienced greater improvements in flexibility and mobility (Cheatham, Stull, & Kolber, 2017; Han et al., 2017; Lim & Park, 2019; Romero-Moraleda et al., 2019) and reduction in the perception of pain (Cheatham, Kolber, & Cain, 2017; Han et al., 2017; Romero-Moraleda et al., 2019). Further, such improvements appeared to occur without negative effects on performance (Lim & Park, 2019; Romero-Moraleda et al., 2019; Sağiroğlui, 2017). It is important to note that these studies have been performed on different vibrating myofascial rollers that vibrate at different frequencies and with different amplitudes. Thus, the research is currently unable to prescribe a specific roller or frequency for a specific outcome. For example, setting a multispeed vibration roller to a lower setting does not appear to produce a different result than a higher frequency. More research is needed on vibration rollers before program standards can be recommended.

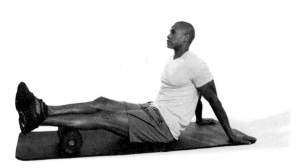

SMR with vibrating roller

A key takeaway from the current vibration roller research is the influence on the perception of pain. The vibration likely mitigates pain through an effect called *vibratory analgesia* (Hollins et al., 2014). Put simply, vibratory analgesia occurs when the vibration stimulates certain mechanoreceptors that temporarily interfere with the sensation of pain. It can be thought of as simply "turning the volume down" on the pain signal. It is important to note that the effect is temporary. However, this temporary reduction in the perception of pain provides a window of improved stretch tolerance for the Corrective Exercise Specialist to carry out the intended corrective strategies and exercises. The introduction of better movement patterns may, over time, produce favorable effects on pain.

Another perspective to consider is that the vibration will reduce the discomfort associated with myofascial rolling. When addressing more tender areas, such as the lateral thigh, a vibrating roller may be more comfortable, and thus the user may be more likely to stay on the tender area longer, leading to more positive overall results.

Cupping

Cupping

A form of myofascial therapy commonly practiced in Asian and Middle Eastern cultures that has recently become more popular in the United States.

Cupping is a form of myofascial therapy commonly practiced in Asian and Middle Eastern cultures that has recently become more popular in the United States (Al-Yousef et al., 2018). Cupping uses suction to help promote movement of blood and other fluids through the tissues. Asian and Middle Eastern cultures use cupping as a form of medical treatment for various conditions, and thus it is performed by appropriate healthcare providers and is heavily regulated (Al-Yousef et al., 2018). However, in the United States cupping has been positioned as an over-the-counter myofascial intervention technique. Research has supported the use of cupping for improving flexibility and mobility (Kim et al., 2017; Yim et al., 2017) and possibly helping to reduce pain (Kim et al., 2017; Yim et al., 2017; Yun-Ting et al., 2017). Further, companies have begun manufacturing cups and creating educational materials that may be more accessible to the general population. It is important to note that there are different methods of cupping that may produce different results.

At the time of this writing, there does not appear to be one specific cupping protocol that is best for myofascial intervention techniques; some use cupping passively (i.e., the client lies relaxed on a table), whereas others integrate an active approach (i.e., the client performs active flexion and extension movements). The active approach to cupping has been termed *myofascial decompression*. Decompression occurs by using the suction to "lift" the superficial tissue. Active movements are then used to mobilize and free up the underlying myofascial (RockTape, 2018). Due to the variability in techniques and

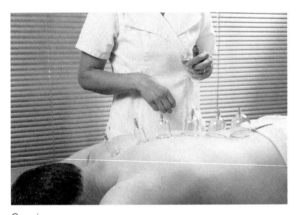

Cupping
© Sylv1rob1/Shutterstock

methods, it is recommended that the fitness professional seek out education and check local and state regulations regarding the use of cupping with clients.

Myofascial Flossing

Myofascial flossing

Method intended to increase flexibility by wrapping an elastic band around a region of the body and performing movements.

Myofascial flossing, otherwise termed *voodoo flossing* or simply *flossing*, is another method intended to increase flexibility and mobility. Myofascial flossing is performed by teaching the client to wrap a latex band around a body part using a 50% overlap pattern and using a stretch force of 50–90% (Cheatham & Baker, 2019; Kiefer et al., 2017). Once the band is applied, the client then performs up to 2 minutes of active or passive movements to induce tissue "flossing" (Borda & Selhorst, 2017; Cheatham & Baker, 2019). Myofascial flossing creates a tangential shearing or wringing-towel effect by creating compression around the muscle group. The movements are intended to help mobilize myofascial tissues. Although the research on myofascial flossing is still emerging, recent studies have indicated that the technique does improve flexibility, mobility, and performance (Driller et al., 2017; Driller & Overmayer, 2017; Mills et al., 2019; Ross & Kandassamy, 2017). Myofascial flossing has also shown promise as a technique to help speed up recovery by reducing the negative effects of delayed onset muscle soreness (DOMS) (Prill et al., 2019); it may also assist in speeding up recovery from specific injuries, such as Achilles tendinopathy (Borda & Selhorst, 2017). Note that the research methods and outcomes for myofascial flossing have not been consistent. Several studies have indicated no measurable improvement in mobility and flexibility (Keifer et al., 2017) or reduction in DOMS (Gorny & Stöggl, 2018). Due to this inconsistency, it is recommended that the fitness professional seek out education and check the legal requirements regarding the use of myofascial flossing with clients.

Note that myofascial flossing should not be confused with nerve flossing. Nerve flossing is an exercise that is intended to stretch irritated nerves and should only be prescribed by an appropriately licensed healthcare practitioner, such as a licensed physical therapist.

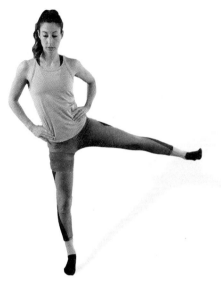

Voodoo flossing

Instrument-Assisted Soft Tissue Mobilization

Instrument-assisted soft tissue mobilization (IASTM) is a myofascial technique that uses specifically designed instruments to provide a mobilizing effect to scar tissue and myofascial adhesions (Cheatham et al., 2016). The use of instruments is thought to provide healthcare professionals with a mechanical advantage, allowing them to work myofascial tissue both deeper and differently than with their hands (Baker et al., 2013). IASTM has been promoted as an effective tool for removing scar tissue and promoting a return to normal function by inducing localized inflammation that restarts the healing process (Kim et al., 2017) and stimulates connective tissue remolding (Cheatham et al., 2016). The data on IASTM is mixed. However, some evidence suggests that the technique may improve short-term flexibility and mobility (Cheatham et al., 2016; Kim et al., 2017).

The recommended application of IASTM has also varied with many of the traditional methods, including a "scraping," which induces localized inflammation via microvascular and capillary hemorrhage (Kim et al., 2017). However, a recent study (Cheatham et al., 2019) found that a light "feather stroke" pressure performed for 90 seconds produced favorable results in subjects with DOMS 24 and 48 hours after strenuous exercise. The researchers suggested that the light pressure stimulates low threshold mechanoreceptors that innervate the skin, thus reducing the perception of pain (Cheatham et al., 2019). Further research is needed to help determine a recommended IASTM program.

It is important to note that IASTM is a myofascial technique that should be performed only by a licensed healthcare provider who has been trained on the tools.

Summary on Interventions

Many effective myofascial technique tools are available in the market today. Fitness professionals are encouraged to perform their research to decide which tool is the most practical for their specific clientele in their specific environment. In most cases, having a variety of myofascial tools

> **Instrument-assisted soft tissue mobilization (IASTM)**
>
> Specifically designed instruments to provide a mobilizing effect to scar tissue and myofascial adhesions.

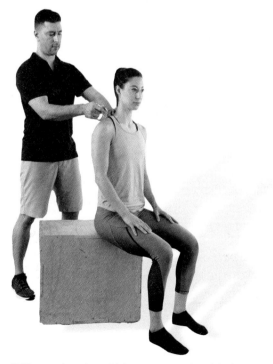

SMR to neck region with instrument-assisted device

on hand will provide fitness professionals the best opportunity to design effective self-myofascial intervention programs for the majority of their clients. The best myofascial technique tools are the ones that the client will consistently use. Also, the fitness professional should research local and state regulations regarding the use of certain myofascial tools.

Precautions and Contraindications for Self-Myofascial Rolling

Although the effects of self-myofascial rolling have been well documented, the potential precautions and contraindications have not been thoroughly investigated. Therefore, the precautions and contraindications of self-myofascial rolling have been taken from related myofascial therapies (Cheatham & Stull, 2018c). It is important to note that allied health professionals have been trained to specifically identify conditions that may warrant avoiding soft tissue work, and unless fitness professionals have received additional training, it is recommended that they use caution with all clients. If a client has an underlying condition, the fitness professional should have the client cleared through an appropriately licensed medical professional before proceeding with any myofascial techniques. Before beginning with self-myofascial rolling, the fitness professional must consider all precautions and contraindications, along with how the technique is being performed (Cheatham & Stull, 2019).

Self-myofascial rolling requires the client to apply bodyweight pressure on a myofascial roller, which may require the client to lie in different positions, such as side-lying, supine, prone, etc. Such positions may exacerbate the effects of certain precautions and contraindications. Further, self-myofascial rolling may produce some discomfort that results in clients holding their breath. In clients with hypertension, for example, a horizontal position combined with breath holding may result in a significant spike in blood pressure. Thus, a hypertensive client may need to perform self-myofascial rolling in a different position, such as seated using a handheld myofascial roller, and be encouraged to concentrate on slow, consistent breathing.

A *precaution*, as the name implies, means the fitness professional should proceed with extreme caution (**Table 3-1**). Clients with precautions can still perform self-myofascial rolling, but they may need to modify the position (e.g., seated instead of lying on the floor or mat), change the method of self-myofascial rolling (e.g., using a handheld instead of the traditional myofascial roller), or avoid rolling certain areas altogether. If for any reason a client with a precaution

TABLE 3-1 Self-Myofascial Rolling Precautions		
Hypertension (controlled)	Osteopenia	Pregnancy
Diabetes	Varicose veins	Bony prominences or regions
Abnormal sensations (e.g., numbness)	Sensitivity to pressure	Recent injury or surgery
Inability to position the body or perform myofascial rolling correctly	Young children	Elderly
Scoliosis or spinal deformity	Medications that may alter client sensations	Fibromyalgia (i.e., higher rolling pressures)

Reproduced from Cheatham, S. W., & Stull, K. R. (2018c). Roller massage: A commentary on clinical standards and survey of physical therapy professionals: Part 1. *International Journal of Sports Physical Therapy, 13*(4), 763–772. https://doi.org/10.26603/ijspt20180763

is not comfortable performing self-myofascial rolling, the fitness professional should not force the client to use the technique.

A *contraindication* differs from a precaution in that the risks likely outweigh the benefits. Self-myofascial rolling should not be conducted in the presence of a contraindication in order to ensure client safety (**Table 3-2**). It is important to note that some conditions, such as pregnancy, diabetes, varicose veins, recent injury or surgery, and hypertension, may be considered either precautionary or contraindicative depending on the client (Cheatham & Stull, 2018c). Therefore, a medical professional should be consulted before proceeding with self-myofascial rolling.

TABLE 3-2 Self-Myofascial Rolling Contraindications

Skin rash, open wounds, blisters, local tissue inflammation, bruises, or tumors	Deep vein thrombosis	Osteoporosis
Bone fracture of myositis ossificans	Cancer or malignancy	Hypertension (uncontrolled)
Acute or severe cardiac, liver, or kidney disease	Acute infection (viral or bacterial), fever, or contagious condition	Neurologic conditions resulting in loss or altered sensation
Bleeding disorders	Systemic conditions (e.g., diabetes)	Recent surgery or injury
Connective tissue disorders	Peripheral vascular insufficiency or disease	Medications that thin the blood or alter sensations
Direct pressure over surgical site or hardware	Chronic pain conditions (e.g., rheumatoid arthritis)	Direct pressure over face, eyes, arteries, veins (e.g., varicose veins), or nerves
Pregnancy (consult MD)	Direct pressure over bony prominences or regions (e.g., lumbar vertebrae)	Extreme discomfort or pain felt by client
Severe scoliosis or spinal deformity	Osteomyelitis	

Reproduced from Cheatham, S. W., & Stull, K. R. (2018c). Roller massage: A commentary on clinical standards and survey of physical therapy professionals: Part 1. *International Journal of Sports Physical Therapy, 13*(4), 763–772. https://doi.org/10.26603/ijspt20180763

Research is needed to validate these suggestions specific to self-myofascial rolling. The precautions and contraindications listed here are not all-inclusive and should be considered a starting point for the fitness professional (Cheatham & Stull, 2018c).

Key Points for Practical Application

Currently, consensus is lacking on optimal self-myofascial rolling programs, which has posed limitations on future research (Cheatham et al., 2015). Until recently, the research used a wide variety of myofascial rolling programs. Thus, no single program has emerged as "recommended." However, recall the earlier discussion about research that suggests that self-myofascial rolling appears to induce both nervous system and mechanical changes, which should be reflected in the program. Thus, a self-myofascial rolling program should include a two-step approach.

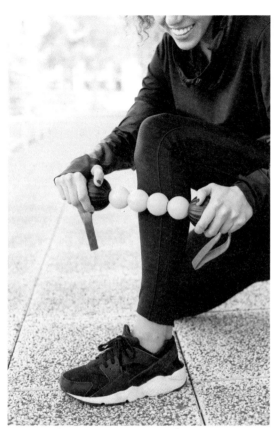

© Luna Vandoorne/Shutterstock

Step 1: Reduce Overall Tension

The first "intent" of self-myofascial rolling is to reduce the overactivity or tension in the targeted muscle (i.e., appeal to global neurophysiological effects). To do this, the user should roll the targeted muscle slowly to identify an uncomfortable spot and hold pressure. During this time, the user should be coached to breathe and relax for 30 to 60 seconds or until a reduction in discomfort is felt. While holding pressure, the user can apply pressure into the roller, but pain is not the goal. Thus, it is more important to relax and breathe than to apply heavy pressure to the point relaxation is no longer possible.

Step 2: Introduce Tissue Movement

Once a reduction in tension has been achieved, the next step is to appeal to the local mechanical aspect by introducing active movements. Active movements involve moving the targeted limb on the myofascial roller. Cheatham and Stull (2018a) demonstrated that performing knee flexion (contraction of the hamstrings) while pressure from a myofascial roller was applied to the quadriceps produced greater knee flexion mobility compared to no knee flexion. While the results of this study should not be generalized to all muscle groups, it is recommended that the fitness professional include active movements to investigate how each client responds. Other active movements may include dorsiflexion while rolling the calves, knee extensions while rolling the hamstrings, hip flexion and abduction/adduction while rolling the piriformis, scapular retraction while rolling the pectorals, and shoulder flexion while rolling the latissimus dorsi. Further research is needed to confirm any theories surrounding this method, but the improvements in mobility may be due to increased fluid movement through the myofascia, enhanced thixotropic effects (reduced viscosity) due to the tensile stresses and heat associated with muscle contractions, reduced fibrous band tension that has developed between the myofascia, and reciprocal inhibition from the contraction of the antagonist. Although no specific recommendations currently exist, performing four to six active movements, at a medium pace, may be easy for the individual to remember and execute effectively.

While this two-step approach is recommended by NASM to maximize both mechanical and neurophysiological mechanisms, individuals who have increased sensitivity or who find the steps too complex may choose to simply roll the target muscle continuously for 90 to 120 seconds. If this rolling method is used, the user should roll the entire muscle slowly (approximately 1 inch per second) for the desired time. For individuals just beginning a rolling program, it may be more important to ensure that they are comfortable rolling before prescribing a complex self-myofascial rolling program.

Length of Time for Self-Myofascial Rolling

In a survey of allied health professionals, respondents stated that they most commonly recommended that clients roll for a total of 5 to 10 minutes (rolling each muscle group for between

30 seconds and 2 minutes) at a pace of 2 to 5 seconds per roll (Cheatham, 2018). A series of studies have supported that self-myofascial rolling for approximately 2 minutes does produce favorable results (Cheatham, Stull, & Kolber, 2017; Cheatham & Baker, 2017; Cheatham, Kolber, & Cain et al., 2017; Cheatham & Stull, 2018a; Cheatham & Stull, 2018b; Cheatham & Stull, 2019). Monteiro et al. (2017) found that at least 90 seconds was needed to improve functional movements, such as a deep squat. Therefore, spending at least 90 seconds and no more than 2 minutes (total time) on a target muscle may produce the best results. However, again note the lack of research specifically comparing various myofascial rolling durations for optimal results.

Frequency of Self-Myofascial Rolling

Research suggests that self-myofascial rolling may be used as part of a warm-up and cooldown (Cheatham, 2018; Cheatham et al., 2015; Schroeder & Best, 2015; Wiewelhove et al., 2019). Self-myofascial rolling has also been shown to prolong warm-up effects (Hodgson et al., 2019). In the study by Hodgson et al. (2019), self-myofascial rolling was performed at 10-minute intervals for 30 minutes after a warm-up, maintaining knee flexion and hip flexion mobility improvements versus no additional self-myofascial rolling. This finding would be important for athletes who are not starters, for example, and who must sit on the bench for prolonged periods after the warm-up before entering the game or match. Persistent self-myofascial rolling at 10-minute intervals would ensure their warm-up–induced enhanced flexibility was sustained. Another study demonstrated that self-myofascial rolling during a halftime period within a simulated soccer match maintained sprint speed, whereas no self-myofascial rolling at halftime resulted in impaired sprint velocity (Kaya et al., 2019).

Although the acute effects of self-myofascial rolling are relatively short, consistent use may result in chronic effects. Self-myofascial rolling just two times per week over 4 weeks has been shown to improve functional movement patterns (Boguszewski et al., 2017). Further, performing self-myofascial rolling five times in 7 days improved hip extension in a functional lunge pattern (Bushell et al., 2015). Thus, performing myofascial rolling between two and five times per week may be enough to experience some positive results. It is important to note that Boguszewski et al. (2017) and Bushell et al. (2015) did not use self-myofascial rolling as part of an overall corrective exercise program. Given the available evidence of the benefits of myofascial rolling both as part of a warm-up and cooldown, and the integrated approach of corrective exercise, there is no reason to believe that self-myofascial rolling cannot be used on most days of the week, along with the corrective exercise program.

Body Position

It is imperative that users do their best to maintain safe body alignment while self-myofascial rolling to avoid increasing the chances of injury or causing musculoskeletal pain. Two common mistakes made while self-myofascial rolling are (1) allowing the lumbar spine to hyperextend (arched lower back) and the cervical spine to extend excessively (head falling forward) while rolling in a prone position and (2) elevating the shoulders (shoulder shrug) while in a seated position. During self-myofascial rolling, clients should be coached to keep their spine neutral (from the pelvis to the skull) and the shoulders in a safe and relaxed position. Modifications should be made, as needed, to ensure that the client can stay relaxed and in a neutral position. Proper kinetic chain alignment still applies during self-myofascial techniques.

- Follow the two-step approach:
  1. Hold pressure for 30 to 60 seconds.
  2. Perform active movements to "free up" or mobilize myofascial tissues.
- Spend between 90 seconds and 2 minutes (total) on each muscle group.
- Perform myofascial rolling on most days of the week as part of a corrective exercise program.
- Maintain a neutral spine and relaxed shoulders.
- Modify, as necessary, to maintain a relaxed and safe position.
- Roll slowly.

Acute Training Variables

To be effective, self-myofascial rolling must follow sound acute training variables, as shown in **Table 3-3**. At present, there are no known reasons that myofascial rolling cannot be performed daily or most days of the week. This is the current practice of NASM with apparently healthy individuals. However, this will ultimately be determined by the client, any possible precautions that exist, and the advice of a licensed medical professional. One set per noted body region or muscle group is sufficient. The myofascial roller (or other myofascial tool) should be held on the tender area for 30 to 60 seconds and then four to six active movements performed. The intensity should be such that there is some discomfort felt, but the user should be able to relax and breathe. Lastly, total myofascial rolling duration should be between 5 and 10 minutes, with 90 to 120 seconds per muscle group.

TABLE 3-3 Acute Training Variables for Self-Myofascial Rolling

Frequency	Sets	Repetitions	Intensity	Duration
Most days of the week (unless otherwise specified)	1	Hold areas of discomfort for 30 to 60 seconds Perform four to six repetitions of active movement	Should be some discomfort, but able to relax and breathe	5 to 10 minutes total time; 90 to 120 seconds per muscle group

Several different methods are available to teach clients how to effectively use the myofascial roller. In a 2017 study, Cheatham, Kolber, and Cain demonstrated that following the guidance of a live fitness professional produced the greatest increase in knee flexion mobility, followed closely by following video instruction, which was followed closely by self-guided instruction. However, all methods of instruction proved effective. While following live instruction may be best, the authors concluded that in the case of limited resources fitness professionals should trust that videos, as well as existing self-guided programs, may serve as suitable alternatives.

Self-Myofascial Roller Exercises

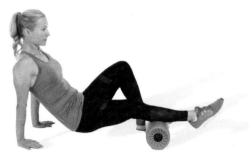

Gastrocnemius/soleus

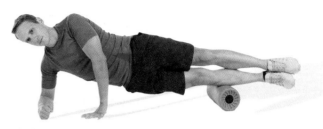

Fibularis (peroneal) complex

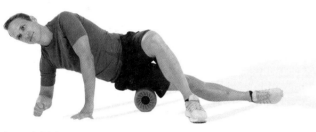

Lateral thigh

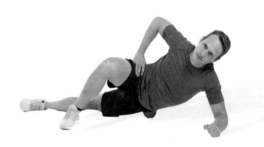

Tensor fascia latae

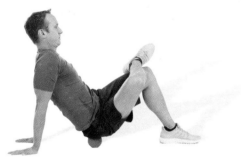

Piriformis

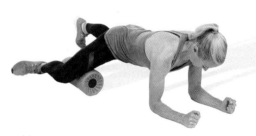

Adductors

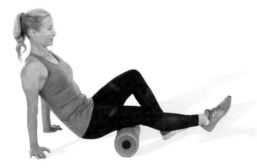

Hamstrings

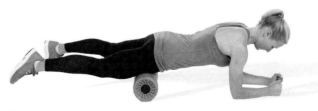

Quadriceps

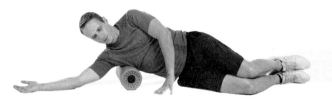
Latissimus dorsi

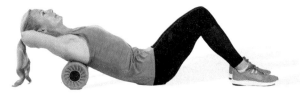
Thoracic spine

SUMMARY

Self-myofascial rolling is the primary inhibitory technique used in the first phase of the Corrective Exercise Continuum. Self-myofascial rolling is used to release tension or decrease activity of overactive myofascial tissues in the body and to introduce mobility between the myofascial tissues. A variety of myofascial rollers are available to choose from depending on the intended myofascial structures to be mobilized. Myofascial rollers will have varying effects depending on their size, shape, and construction. Additional considerations when choosing myofascial tools are ease of use and the ability to control depth of penetration into myofascial tissues. Self-myofascial rolling may be successfully performed by holding the tender area plus active movement (preferred), solely holding, or continuous rolling. Clients will achieve the desired effect of soft tissue mobilization, reestablish neuromuscular efficiency in the body, and avoid injury after they have been properly instructed in and follow the correct application of myofascial rolling.

REFERENCES

Aboodarda, S. J., Spence, A. J., & Button, D. C. (2015). Pain pressure threshold of a muscle tender spot increases following local and non-local rolling massage. *BMC Musculoskeletal Disorders, 16,* 265. https://doi.org/10.1186/s12891-015-0729-5

Al-Yousef, H. M., Wajid, S., & Sales, I. (2018). Knowledge, attitudes, and perceptions of cupping therapy (CT) in Saudi Arabia: A cross-sectional survey among the Saudi population. *Biomedical Research (0970-938X), 29*(17), 3351–3355. https://doi.org/10.4066/biomedicalresearch.29-18-1015

Baker, R. T., Nasypany, A., Seegmiller, J. G., & Baker, J. G. (2013). Instrument-assisted soft tissue mobilization treatment for tissue extensibility dysfunction. *International Journal of Athletic Therapy and Training, 18*(5), 16–21. https://doi.org/10.1123/ijatt.18.5.16

Behm, D. G., & Wilke, J. (2019). Do self-myofascial release devices release myofascia? Rolling mechanisms: A narrative review. *Sports Medicine, 49*(8), 1173–1181. https://doi.org/10.1007/s40279-019-01149-y

Boguszewski, D., Falkowska, M., Adamczyk, J. G., & Białoszewski, D. (2017). Influence of foam rolling on the functional limitations of the musculoskeletal system in healthy women. *Biomedical Human Kinetics, 9*(1), 75–81. https://doi.org/10.1515/bhk-2017-0012

Borda, J., & Selhorst, M. (2017). The use of compression tack and flossing along with lacrosse ball massage to treat chronic Achilles tendinopathy in an adolescent athlete: A case report. *Journal of Manual and Manipulative Therapy, 25*(1), 57–61. https://doi.org/10.1080/10669817.2016.1159403

Bushell, J. E., Dawson, S. M., & Webster, M. M. (2015). Clinical relevance of foam rolling on hip extension angle in a functional lunge position. *Journal of Strength and Conditioning Research, 29*(9), 2397–2403. https://doi.org/10.1519/JSC.0000000000000888

Cavanaugh, M. T., Doweling, A., Young, J. D., Quigley, P. J., Hodgson, D. D., Whitten, J. H., Reid, J. C., Aboodarda, S. J., & Behm, D. G. (2017). An acute session of roller massage prolongs voluntary torque development and diminishes evoked pain. *European Journal of Applied Physiology, 117*(1), 109–117. https://doi.org/10.1007/s00421-016-3503-y

Cheatham, S. W. (2018). Roller massage: A descriptive survey of allied health professionals. *Journal of Sport Rehabilitation, 28*(6), 1–10. https://doi.org/10.1123/jsr.2017-0366

Cheatham, S. W., & Baker, R. (2017). Differences in pressure pain threshold among men and women after foam rolling. *Journal of Bodywork and Movement Therapies, 21*(4), 978–982. https://doi.org/10.1016/j.jbmt.2017.06.006

Cheatham, S. W., & Baker, R. (2019). Technical report: Quantification of the Rockfloss˚ floss band stretch force at different elongation lengths. *Journal of Sport Rehabilitation, 29*(3), 377–380. https://doi.org/10.1123/jsr.2019-0034

Cheatham, S. W., & Kolber, M. J. (2017). Does self-myofascial release with a foam roll change pressure pain threshold of the ipsilateral lower extremity antagonist and contralateral muscle groups? An exploratory study. *Journal of Sport Rehabilitation, 27*(2), 1–18. https://doi.org/10.1123/jsr.2016-0196

Cheatham, S. W., Kolber, M. J., & Cain, M. (2017). Comparison of video-guided, live instructed, and self-guided foam roll interventions on knee joint range of motion and pressure pain threshold: A randomized controlled trial. *International Journal of Sports Physical Therapy, 12*(2), 242–249. https://www.ncbi.nlm.nih.gov/pmc/articles/PMC5380867/

Cheatham, S. W., Kolber, M. J., Cain, M., & Lee, M. (2015). The effects of self-myofascial release using a foam roll or roller massager on joint range of motion, muscle recovery, and performance: A systematic review. *International Journal of Sports Physical Therapy, 10*(6), 827–838. https://www.ncbi.nlm.nih.gov/pmc/articles/PMC4637917/

Cheatham, S. W., Kreiswirth, E., & Baker, R. (2019). Does a light pressure instrument assisted soft tissue mobilization technique modulate tactile discrimination and perceived pain in healthy individuals with DOMS? *Journal of the Canadian Chiropractic Association, 63*(1), 18–25. https://www.ncbi.nlm.nih.gov/pmc/articles/PMC6493209/

Cheatham, S. W., Lee, M., Cain, M., & Baker, R. (2016). The efficacy of instrument assisted soft tissue mobilization: a systematic review. *Journal of the Canadian Chiropractic Association, 60*(3), 200–211. https://www.ncbi.nlm.nih.gov/pmc/articles/PMC5039777/

Cheatham, S. W., & Stull, K. R. (2018a). Comparison of a foam rolling session with active joint motion and without joint motion: A randomized controlled trial. *Journal of Bodywork and Movement Therapies, 22*(3), 707–712. https://doi.org/10.1016/j.jbmt.2018.01.011

Cheatham, S. W., & Stull, K. R. (2018b). Comparison of three different density type foam rollers on knee range of motion and pressure pain threshold: A randomized controlled trial. *International Journal of Sports Physical Therapy, 13*(3), 474–482. https://doi.org/10.26603/ijspt20180474

Cheatham, S. W., & Stull, K. R. (2018c). Roller massage: A commentary on clinical standards and survey of physical therapy professionals: Part 1. *International Journal of Sports Physical Therapy, 13*(4), 763–772. https://doi.org/10.26603/ijspt20180763

Cheatham, S. W., & Stull, K. R. (2019). Roller massage: Comparison of three different surface type pattern foam rollers on passive knee range of motion and pain perception. *Journal of Bodywork and Movement Therapies, 23*(3), 555–560. https://doi.org/10.1016/j.jbmt.2019.05.002

Cheatham, S. W., Stull, K. R., & Kolber, M. J. (2017). Comparison of a vibrating foam roller and a non-vibrating foam roller intervention on knee range of motion and pressure pain threshold: A randomized controlled trial. *Journal of Sport Rehabilitation, 28*(1), 1–23. https://doi.org/10.1123/jsr.2017-0164

Cheatham, S. W., Stull, K. R., & Kolber, M. J. (2018). Roller massage: Is the numeric pain rating scale a reliable measurement and can it direct individuals with no experience to a specific roller density? *The Journal of the Canadian Chiropractic Association, 62*(3), 161–169. https://www.ncbi.nlm.nih.gov/pmc/articles/PMC6319431/

Clark, M., Lucett, S., & National Academy of Sports Medicine. (2010). *NASM essentials of corrective exercise training.* Lippincott Williams & Wilkins.

Curran, P. F., Fiore, R. D., & Crisco, J. J. (2008). A comparison of the pressure exerted on soft tissue by 2 myofascial rollers. *Journal of Sport Rehabilitation, 17*(4), 432–442. https://doi.org/10.1123/jsr.17.4.432

Cyron, C. J., & Humphrey, J. D. (2017). Growth and remodeling of load-bearing biological soft tissues. *Meccanica, 52*(3), 645–664. https://doi.org/10.1007/s11012-016-0472-5

DeBruyne, D. M., Dewhurst, M. M., Fischer, K. M., Wojtanowski, M. S., & Durall, C. (2017). Self-mobilization using a foam roller versus a roller massager: Which is more effective for increasing hamstrings flexibility? *Journal of Sport Rehabilitation, 26*(1), 94–100. https://doi.org/10.1123/jsr.2015-0035

Dong, Y., Wang, W., Zheng, J., Chen, S., Qiao, J., & Wang, X. (2019). Whole body vibration exercise for chronic musculoskeletal pain: A systematic review and meta-analysis of randomized controlled trials. *Archives of Physical Medicine and Rehabilitation, 100*(11), 2167–2178. https://doi.org/10.1016/j.apmr.2019.03.011

Driller, M., Mackay, K., Mills, B., & Tavares, F. (2017). Tissue flossing on ankle range of motion, jump and sprint performance: A follow-up study. *Physical Therapy in Sport: Official Journal of the Association of Chartered Physiotherapists in Sports Medicine, 28*, 29–33. https://doi.org/10.1016/j.ptsp.2017.08.081

Driller, M. W., & Overmayer, R. G. (2017). The effects of tissue flossing on ankle range of motion and jump performance. *Physical Therapy in Sport: Official Journal of the Association of Chartered Physiotherapists in Sports Medicine, 25*, 20–24. https://doi.org/10.1016/j.ptsp.2016.12.004

Games, K. E., Sefton, J. M., & Wilson, A. E. (2015). Whole-body vibration and blood flow and muscle oxygenation: A meta-analysis. *Journal of Athletic Training, 50*(5), 542–549. https://doi.org/10.4085/1062-6050-50.2.09

Gorny, V., & Stöggl, T. (2018). Tissue flossing as a recovery tool for the lower extremity after strength endurance intervals. *Sportverletzung Sportschaden: Organ Der Gesellschaft Fur Orthopadisch-Traumatologische Sportmedizin, 32*(1), 55–60. https://doi.org/10.1055/s-0043-122782

Grabow, L., Young, J. D., Alcock, L. R., Quigley, P. J., Byrne, J. M., Granacher, U., Skarabot, J., & Behm, D. G. (2018). Higher quadriceps roller massage forces do not amplify range of-motion increases or impair strength and jump performance. *Journal of Strength and Conditioning Research, 32*(11), 3059–3069. https://doi.org/10.1519/jsc.0000000000001906

Han, S.-W., Lee, Y.-S., & Lee, D.-J. (2017). The influence of the vibration form roller exercise on the pains in the muscles around the hip joint and the joint performance. *Journal of Physical Therapy Science, 29*(10), 1844–1847. https://doi.org/10.1589/jpts.29.1844

Hodgson, D. D., Quigley, P. J., Whitten, J. H. D., Reid, J. C., & Behm, D. G. (2019). Impact of ten-minute interval roller massage on performance and active range of motion. *Journal of Strength and Conditioning Research, 33*(6), 1512–1523. https://doi.org/10.1519/JSC.0000000000002271

Hollins, M., McDermott, K., & Harper, D. (2014). How does vibration reduce pain? *Perception, 43*(1), 70–84. https://doi.org/10.1068/p7637

Hotfiel, T., Swoboda, B., Krinner, S., Grim, C., Engelhardt, M., Uder, M., & Heiss, R. U. (2017). Acute effects of lateral thigh foam rolling on arterial tissue perfusion determined by spectral Doppler and power Doppler ultrasound. *Journal of Strength and Conditioning Research, 31*(4), 893–900. https://doi.org/10.1519/jsc.0000000000001641

Iqbal, Z. A., & Alghadir, A. H. (2017). Cumulative trauma disorders: A review. *Journal of Back and Musculoskeletal Rehabilitation, 30*(4), 663–666. https://doi.org/10.3233/bmr-150266

Jafri, M. S. (2014). Mechanisms of myofascial pain. *International Scholarly Research Notices, 2014.* https://doi.org/10.1155/2014/523924

Jay, K., Sundstrup, E., Sondergaard, S. D., Behm, D., Brandt, M., Saervoll, C. A., Jakobsen, M. D., & Andersen, L. L. (2014). Specific and cross over effects of massage for muscle soreness: Randomized controlled trial. *International Journal of Sports Physical Therapy, 9*(1), 82–91. https://www.ncbi.nlm.nih.gov/pmc/articles/PMC3924612/

Kaya, S., Cug, M., & Behm, D. G. (2019). The effect of foam rolling during the half-time period on second half simulated soccer-specific performance. *International Journal of Sports Physical Therapy.* [Under Review]

Kelly, S., & Beardsley, C. (2016). Specific and cross-over effects of foam rolling on ankle dorsiflexion range of motion. *International Journal of Sports Physical Therapy, 11*(4), 544–551. https://www.ncbi.nlm.nih.gov/pubmed/24567859

Kiefer, B. N., Lemarr, K. E., Enriquez, C. C., Tivener, K. A., & Daniel, T. (2017). A pilot study: Perceptual effects of the voodoo floss band on glenohumeral flexibility. *International Journal of Athletic Therapy and Training, 22*(4), 29–33. https://doi.org/10.1123/ijatt.2016-0093

Kim, J., Sung, D. J., & Lee, J. (2017). Therapeutic effectiveness of instrument-assisted soft tissue mobilization for soft tissue injury: Mechanisms and practical application. *Journal of Exercise Rehabilitation, 13*(1), 12–22.

Kim, J.-E., Cho, J.-E., Do, K.-S., Lim, S.-Y., Kim, H.-J., & Yim, J.-E. (2017). Effect of cupping therapy on range of motion, pain threshold, and muscle activity of the hamstring muscle compared to passive stretching. *Journal of the Korean Society of Physical Medicine, 12*(3), 23–32. https://doi.org/10.13066/kspm.2017.12.3.23

Lim, J.-H., & Park, C.-B. (2019). The immediate effects of foam roller with vibration on hamstring flexibility and jump performance in healthy adults. *Journal of Exercise Rehabilitation, 15*(1), 50–54. https://doi.org/10.12965/jer.1836560.280

Macdonald, G. Z., Button, D. C., Drinkwater, E. J., & Behm, D. G. (2014). Foam rolling as a recovery tool after an intense bout of physical activity. *Medicine and Science in Sports and Exercise, 46*(1), 131–142. https://doi.org/10.1249/MSS.0b013e3182a123db

Mills, B., Mayo, B., Tavares, F., & Driller, M. (2019). The effect of tissue flossing on ankle range of motion, jump, and sprint performance in elite rugby union athletes. *Journal of Sport Rehabilitation,* 1–18. https://doi.org/10.1123/jsr.2018-0302

Money, S. (2017). Pathophysiology of trigger points in myofascial pain syndrome. *Journal of Pain and Palliative Care Pharmacotherapy, 31*(2), 158–159. https://doi.org/10.1080/15360288.2017.1298688

Monteiro, E. R., Škarabot, J., Vigotsky, A. D., Brown, A. F., Gomes, T. M., & Novaes, J. D. (2017). Acute effects of different self-massage volumes on the FMS™ overhead deep squat performance. *International Journal of Sports Physical Therapy, 12*(1), 94–104. https://www.ncbi.nlm.nih.gov/pmc/articles/PMC5294950/

Mueller, M. J., & Maluf, K. S. (2002). Tissue adaptation to physical stress: A proposed "physical stress theory" to guide physical therapist practice, education, and research. *Physical Therapy, 82*(4), 383–403. https://doi.org/10.1093/ptj/82.4.383

Nagi, S. S., & Mahns, D. A. (2013). C-tactile fibers contribute to cutaneous allodynia after eccentric exercise. *Journal of Pain, 14*(5), 538–548. https://doi.org/10.1016/j.jpain.2013.01.009

Nagi, S. S., Rubin, T. K., Chelvanayagam, D. K., Macefield, V. G., & Mahns, D. A. (2011). Allodynia mediated by C-tactile afferents in human hairy skin. *Journal of Physiology, 589*(Pt 16), 4065–4075. https://doi.org/10.1113/jphysiol.2011.211326

Okamoto, T., Masuhara, M., & Ikuta, K. (2014). Acute effects of self-myofascial release using a foam roller on arterial function. *Journal of Strength and Conditioning Research, 28*(1), 69–73. https://doi.org/10.1519/JSC.0b013e31829480f5

Park, Y. J., Park, S. W., & Lee, H. S. (2018). Comparison of the effectiveness of whole body vibration in stroke patients: A meta-analysis. *BioMed Research International, 2018,* 5083634. https://doi.org/10.1155/2018/5083634

Prill, R., Schulz, R., & Michel, S. (2019). Tissue flossing: A new short-term compression therapy for reducing exercise-induced delayed-onset muscle soreness. A randomized, controlled and double-blind pilot crossover trial. *Journal of Sports Medicine and Physical Fitness, 59*(5), 861–867. https://doi.org/10.23736/S0022-4707.18.08701-7

RockTape. (2018). RockPods course notes [Lecture notes]. https://www.rocktape.com/medical/education/fmt-rockfloss-rockpods/

Romero-Moraleda, B., González-García, J., Cuéllar-Rayo, Á., Balsalobre-Fernández, C., Muñoz-García, D., & Morencos, E. (2019). Effects of vibration and non-vibration foam rolling on recovery after exercise with induced muscle damage. *Journal of Sports Science and Medicine, 18*(1), 172–180. https://www.ncbi.nlm.nih.gov/pmc/articles/PMC6370959/

Ross, S., & Kandassamy, G. (2017). The effects of 'tack and floss' active joint mobilisation on ankle dorsiflexion range of motion using Voodoo Floss bands. *Journal of Physical Therapy, 25,* 20–24. https://research.edgehill.ac.uk/en/publications/the-effects-of-tack-and-floss-active-joint-mobilisation-on-ankle--2

Sağiroğlui, İ. (2017). Acute effects of applied local vibration during foam roller exercises on lower extremity explosive strength and flexibility performance. *European Journal of Physical Education and Sport Science, 3*(1), 20–31. https://oapub.org/edu/index.php/ejep/article/view/1041

Schroeder, A. N., & Best, T. M. (2015). Is self myofascial release an effective preexercise and recovery strategy? A literature review. *Current Sports Medicine Reports, 14*(3), 200–208. https://doi.org/10.1249/JSR.0000000000000148

Sullivan, K. M., Silvey, D. B. J., Button, D. C., & Behm, D. G. (2013). Roller-massager application to the hamstrings increases sit-and-reach range of motion within five to ten seconds without performance impairments. *International Journal of Sports Physical Therapy, 8*(3), 228–236. https://www.ncbi.nlm.nih.gov/pmc/articles/PMC3679629/

Wang, Y. T., Qi, Y., Tang, F. Y., Li, F. M., Li, Q. H., Xu, C. P., Xie, G. P., & Sun, H. T. (2017). The effect of cupping therapy for low back pain: A meta-analysis based on existing randomized controlled trials. *Journal of Back and Musculoskeletal Rehabilitation, 30*(6), 1187–1195. https://doi.org/10.3233/BMR-169736

Wiewelhove, T., Döweling, A., Schneider, C., Hottenrott, L., Meyer, T., Kellmann, M., Pfeiffer, M., & Ferrauti, A. (2019). A meta-analysis of the effects of foam rolling on performance and recovery. *Frontiers in Physiology, 10*, 376. https://doi.org/10.3389/fphys.2019.00376

Yim, J., Park, J., Kim, H., Woo, J., Joo, S., Lee, S., & Song, J. (2017). Comparison of the effects of muscle stretching exercises and cupping therapy on pain thresholds, cervical range of motion and angle: A cross-over study. *Physical Therapy Rehabilitation Science, 6*(2), 83–89. https://doi.org/10.14474/ptrs.2017.6.2.83

Young, J. D., Spence, A. J., & Behm, D. G. (2018). Roller massage decreases spinal excitability to the soleus. *Journal of Applied Physiology, 124*(4), 950–959. https://doi.org/10.1152/japplphysiol.00732.2017

Zhuang, X., Tan, S., & Huang, Q. (2014). Understanding of myofascial trigger points. *Chinese Medical Journal (Engl), 127*(24), 4271–4277. http://doi.org/10.3760/cma.j.issn.0366-6999.20141999

Lengthening Techniques

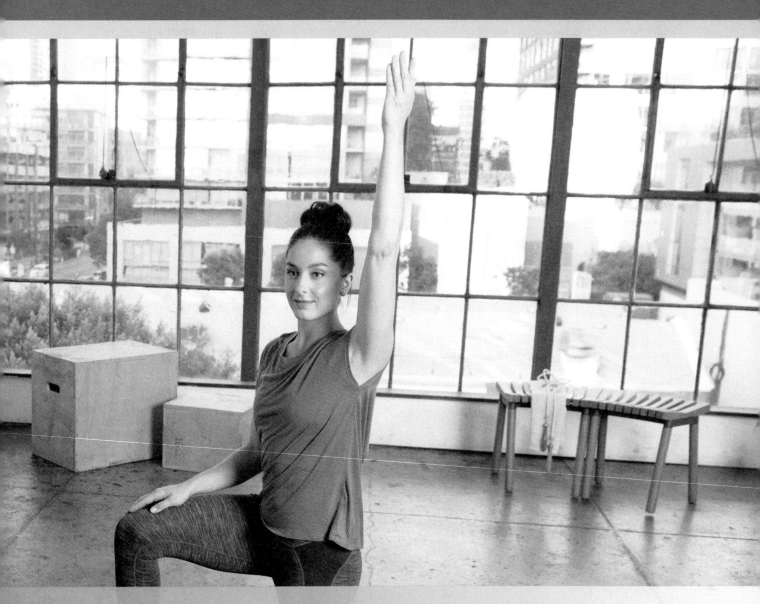

Learning Objectives

After reading this content, students should be able to demonstrate the following objectives:

- **Define** *flexibility*, *extensibility*, and *muscle length*.
- **Explain** the function of lengthening techniques in a corrective exercise program.
- **Describe** the application guidelines for various stretching techniques.

Introduction

Inhibitory techniques are used in the first phase of the Corrective Exercise Continuum to decrease overactivity of myofascial tissue and thus prepare the tissue for other corrective exercise techniques. The second phase in the Corrective Exercise Continuum is to lengthen overactive muscles and myofascial tissues (**Figure 4-1**). Lengthening refers to the elongation of mechanically shortened muscle and connective tissue to reduce their resistance to stretch and increase range of motion (ROM) at the tissue and joint. Several stretching methods are available to accomplish this; however, the focus of this chapter and the Corrective Exercise Specialist will be on the most common methods of stretching: **static stretching**, **dynamic stretching**, and **neuromuscular stretching (NMS)** (**Table 4-1**). Although the goal of each form of stretching is the same (improving available ROM at a joint, increasing tissue extensibility, decreasing muscle and tendon injury risk, and enhancing neuromuscular efficiency), each method can be used separately or integrated with other techniques to achieve individualized program goals.

Static stretching

The process of passively taking a muscle to the point of tension and holding the stretch for a minimum of 30 seconds.

Dynamic stretching

The active extension of a muscle, using a muscle's force production and the body's momentum, to take a joint through the full available range of motion.

Neuromuscular stretching (NMS)

A flexibility technique that incorporates varied combinations of isometric contraction and static stretching of the target muscle to create increases in range of motion. Also called proprioceptive neuromuscular facilitation (PNF).

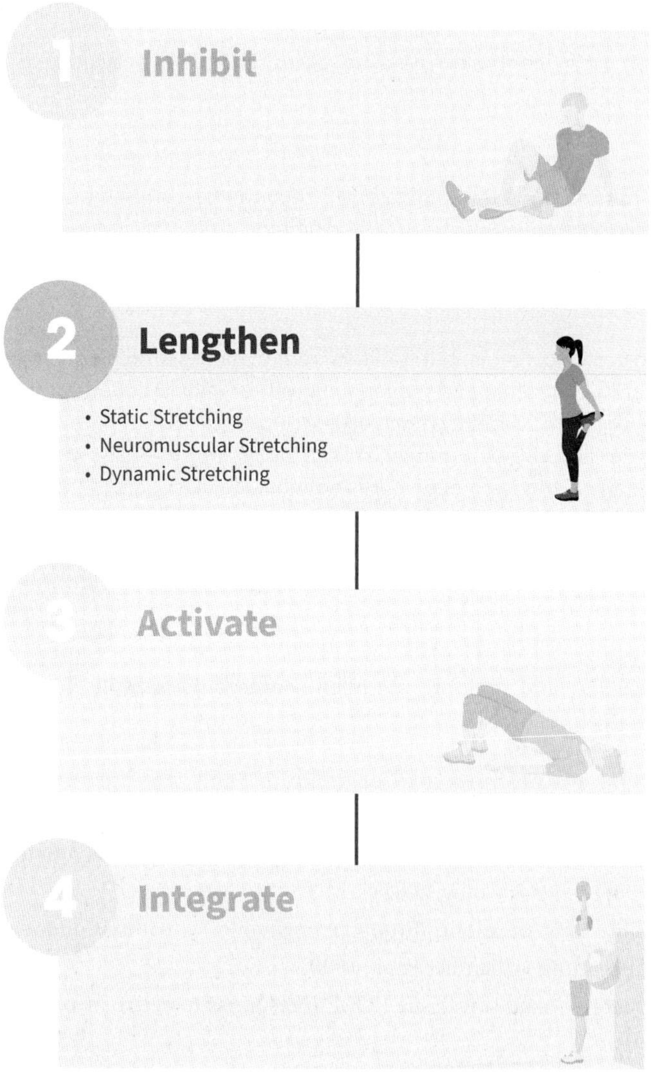

1 Inhibit

2 Lengthen
- Static Stretching
- Neuromuscular Stretching
- Dynamic Stretching

3 Activate

4 Integrate

Figure 4-1 Corrective Exercise Continuum—lengthen

TABLE 4-1 Description of Stretching Techniques

Technique	Description
Lengthening Techniques Used in Corrective Exercise Strategies	
Static stretching	Static stretching combines low-to-moderate forces with long duration using a variety of neural, mechanical, and psycho-physiological mechanisms. This form of stretching, performed alone or with a partner, allows for relaxation and concomitant elongation of muscle. To properly perform static stretching, the stretch is held at the first point of tension or resistance barrier for a specific time period (e.g., 30 seconds). It is theorized that this form of flexibility decreases muscle spindle activity and motor neuron excitability (neural), muscle compliance and changes in fascicle angles and orientation (mechanical), and increased stretch tolerance (psycho-physiological).
Neuromuscular stretching	Neuromuscular stretching (NMS; commonly called proprioceptive neuromuscular facilitation, or PNF) involves taking the muscle to its end-ROM (point of joint compensation), holding that position for 10 to 30 seconds, and then actively contracting the stretched muscle for 5 to 10 seconds. NMS often needs a partner but can be performed with stretch bands.
Dynamic stretching	Dynamic stretching uses a controlled movement through the full or nearly full joint ROM.
Other Techniques	
Active stretching	Active stretching uses multiple repetitions of a 2-second static stretch but emphasizes a contraction of the antagonist to induce reciprocal inhibition. This intervention is used to move muscles that tend to be overactive through available ranges of motion and to prepare them for work.
Ballistic stretching	Ballistic stretching is also dynamic, but it differs from dynamic stretching in that ballistic stretching incorporates higher-speed movements with bouncing actions at the end of the ROM. Due to the higher movement velocities and less control of the movement with ballistic stretching, it is riskier and carries a greater chance for injury, especially when a proper active warm-up is not incorporated beforehand. It is not considered a part of the corrective exercise strategy. It is used by competitive athletes in a warm-up in an attempt to activate the central nervous system and muscle.

Flexibility

The present state or ability of a joint to move through a range of motion.

Stretching

An active process to elongate muscles and connective tissues in order to increase the present state of flexibility.

The terms *flexibility* and *stretching* are often confused. **Flexibility** has been defined in the following ways in the literature:

- As the ROM available to a joint or group of joints (DeVries, 1986; Hebbelink, 1988; Hubley-Kozey, 1991; Liemohn, 1988; Stone & Kroll, 1991)
- As the ability to move a joint smoothly and easily through its complete pain-free ROM (Kent, 1998; Kisner & Colby, 2002)
- As the ability to move a joint through a normal ROM without undue stress to the musculotendinous unit (Chandler et al., 1990)
- As a normal joint and soft tissue ROM in response to active or passive stretch (Halvorson, 1989)

Thus, the term *flexibility* generally refers to the present state or ability of a joint to move through a ROM. **Stretching**, however, is an active or passive process to elongate muscles and connective tissues in order to increase that present state of flexibility.

Types of Stretching Techniques

Stretching as a technique to lengthen muscle and tendon has been the subject of debate for several decades, leading researchers to continue to study the effects, duration, and methodologies behind stretching. To date, this subject might be one of the most widely diverse and profusely studied topics related to human performance. The traditional thought is that regular stretching improves flexibility, which results in improved injury resistance and performance with some activities (Hartig & Henderson, 1999; Witvrouw et al., 2007). Consequently, regular stretching is a recommended component of exercise programs, such as during a warm-up or cool-down. The following techniques represent methods by which tissue extensibility and range of motion may be improved. The technique(s) to be used will be determined by the Corrective Exercise Specialist based on the area being stretched, effectiveness, client goals, and the level of client adherence to the program.

Static Stretching

Arguably, during the last half-century, static stretching has been the most common flexibility training technique used by health and fitness professionals (Alter, 2004; Behm, 2018; Behm et al., 2016; Behm & Chaouachi, 2011; Kay & Blazevich, 2012). Static stretching represents a group of flexibility techniques used to increase the extensibility of muscle and connective tissue (lengthening), and thus ROM at a joint (Alter, 2004; Behm, 2018; Behm et al., 2016; Behm & Chaouachi, 2011; Kay & Blazevich, 2012). In practice, static stretching is characterized by the following (Alter, 2004; Nelson & Bandy, 2005):

- Elongation of muscle and myofascial tissue to an end-range and statically holding that position for a period of time
- Maximal control of structural alignment
- Minimal acceleration into and out of the elongated (stretch) position

This form of flexibility training is associated with the lowest risk for injury during the stretching routine and deemed the safest to use because individuals can perform static stretching on their own with the slow, minimal-to-no motion required (Smith, 1994). Evidence has documented that static stretching can reduce the incidence of lower body muscle and tendon injuries, especially with high-velocity contractions and rapid change of direction activities (Behm, 2018; McHugh & Cosgrave, 2010). Additionally, although static stretching can be done with another person, it is commonly performed alone, so it can be easily incorporated into any integrated exercise program (**Figure 4-2**).

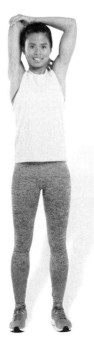

Figure 4-2 Static stretching

MECHANICAL ADAPTATIONS

Although the exact mechanisms responsible for the efficacy of static stretching are not fully understood, it is believed that static stretching may produce mechanical, neural, and psycho-physiological adaptations that result in increased joint ROM (Alter, 2004; Behm, 2018; Behm et al., 2016; Behm & Chaouachi, 2011; Kay & Blazevich, 2012). Mechanically, static stretching appears to affect the **viscoelastic** component of myofascial tissue (Guissard et al., 2001; Magnusson, Simonsen, Aagaard, Sorensen, & Kjaer, 1996). More specifically, there may be a decrease in the passive resistance a muscle has to stretching. It is this reduction in stretch resistance that allows greater tissue extensibility (Cornwell et al., 2002; Kubo et al., 2001, 2002). In general, it is thought that static stretching causes an acute viscoelastic stress relaxation response, allowing for an immediate increase in ROM (Behm, 2018; Behm et al., 2016; Behm & Chaouachi, 2011).

NEUROLOGICAL ADAPTATIONS

Neurologically, static stretching of muscle and myofascial tissues to the end-ROM appears to decrease motor neuron excitability. With passive static stretching, the muscle is typically extended at a slow-to-moderate rate into an elongated position and held for an extended period of time (Alter, 2004; Behm, 2018; Behm et al., 2016). Recall that specialized organs, called muscle spindles, are located within the muscle that detect changes in the extent and rate of change in muscle length. Within the muscle spindle, **nuclear chain fibers** preferentially respond to changes in muscle elongation, whereas the **nuclear bag fibers** respond to both the extent and rate of elongation (Matthews, 1981). Muscle reflexes occur in response to the amount and rate of muscle lengthening (**Figure 4-3**). However, when the static stretch is held for a prolonged period (e.g., 30 to 60 seconds), these reflexes are less active (**disfacilitation**), and thus the muscle can relax more, providing less resistance to lengthening or stretching. Even with less than a 10-second stretch, the nuclear bag fibers should decrease their discharge rate because there would be no change in the rate of the stretch.

Cutaneous (i.e., skin) nerve fibers, when activated by mechanical stress (e.g., tension, pressure, or vibration), can also contribute to an increase in ROM (Jenner & Stephens, 1982). These cutaneous receptors can also help reduce muscle reflex activity (pre- and postsynaptic inhibition), but they only continue for a few seconds after stretching (Morelli et al., 1999). Joint and cutaneous receptors do not play a significant role in reflex inhibition with small stretch lengthening but can provide a minor contribution during large-amplitude stretches. In the research, large-amplitude stretches have been defined as movements progressing beyond specific markers (e.g., > 10 degrees dorsiflexion) (Guissard & Duchateau, 2006; Guissard et al., 1988).

Other possible neurological stretch mechanisms are **Golgi tendon organs (GTOs)** and Renshaw cells. GTOs are activated by tension exerted on the muscle tendon (Chalmers, 2004; Houk et al., 1980), contributing to reflex inhibition (autogenic inhibition). However, it has been shown that GTOs are not highly sensitive to the tension associated with static stretching. Contributions to muscle relaxation with GTOs are more likely to occur with dynamic stretches that use large ranges of motion (Guissard & Duchateau, 2006) such as leg swings. Furthermore, GTO inhibition stops around 60 to 100 milliseconds after stretching, so its effect would not persist after ending the stretch (Houk et al., 1980). Thus, because GTOs are more active during active muscle contractions, their inhibition effect would contribute more during dynamic stretching than with a passive holding of a stretch.

Renshaw cells can also contribute to muscle relaxation or inhibition with large-amplitude stretches (recurrent inhibition). Recurrent inhibition plays a greater role with weak dynamic contractions (Katz & Pierrot-Deseilligny, 1999). Renshaw cells should provide some inhibition

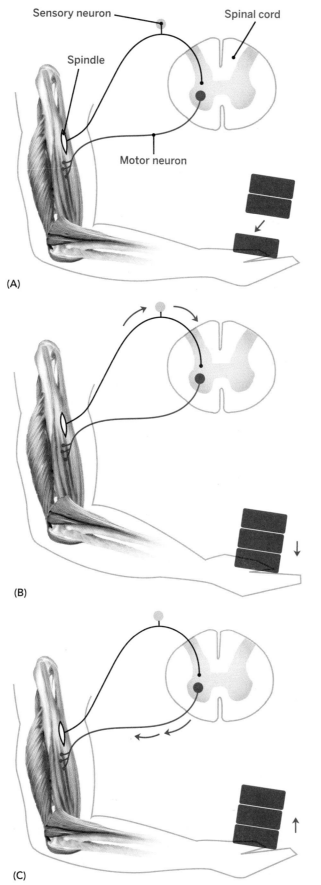

Sensory neuron

Spinal cord

Spindle

Motor neuron

(A)

(B)

(C)

Figure 4-3 **(A)** Add load to muscle; **(B)** Spindle senses stretch and reflexively signals contraction; **(C)** Muscle contracts to restore arm position

with full ROM dynamic stretching and lesser effects with static stretching. Thus, static stretching can inhibit or relax the muscle by muscle spindle disfacilitation (reduced discharge frequency of the nuclear bag and chain fibers), whereas Renshaw cell inhibition is a more important contributor to the increases in ROM with dynamic stretching.

TRY THIS

Sit down with knees extended and reach as far as possible to your toes (or past). Hold that position for 30 seconds. Now see if you can reach farther. It is likely that you can because of the disfacilitation (decreased discharge) of the nuclear chain and bag fibers that caused your muscle to relax more.

PSYCHO-PHYSIOLOGICAL ADAPTATIONS

In addition to mechanical and neural responses to stretching, psycho-physiological mechanisms, specifically, can lead to increases in stretch tolerance. Some researchers believe that stretch tolerance is the greatest contributor to increased ROM (Magnusson, Simonsen, Aagaard, & Kjaer, 1996; Magnusson, Simonsen, Aagaard, Sorensen, & Kjaer, 1996; Magnusson, Simonsen, Dyhre-Poulsen, Aagaard, Mohr, & Kjaer, 1996). The term *stretch tolerance* means the client or athlete can tolerate greater discomfort and then push themselves through a greater ROM.

This effect can be psychological as the person becomes more accustomed to the discomfort as they hold a static stretch for a longer period of time (e.g., 30 to 60 seconds). It can also be physiological as prolonged activation of the pain receptors can decrease their firing frequency or discharge as well as signal the release of endorphins and enkephalins (opioids made by the body) that will reduce pain and discomfort throughout the body (Melzack & Wall, 1965). Thus, increased stretch tolerance is considered *psycho-physiological* because both psychological and physiological factors may contribute.

CHRONIC ADAPTATIONS TO STATIC STRETCHING

All previously mentioned adaptations to static stretching (mechanical, neurological, and psycho-physiological) can occur acutely with a single stretching session, whereas long-term flexibility training would cause chronic changes across many of the factors. The discussed changes

GETTING TECHNICAL

Sometimes, research literature may use the term *neuromyofascial* tissue. Of course, myofascia has nervous system connections, but, in terms of stretching, nerves are not very extensible and can only elongate to a certain point. The perineurium, which is the connective sheath surrounding a bundle of nerves, can elongate 6–20% of its resting length (Alter, 2004; Sunderland, 1978, 1991).

When the maximum nerve length is reached, the nerve can be injured. A nerve that is stretched by only 6% can inhibit nerve conduction (Grewal et al., 1996; Wall et al., 1992). Additionally, a nerve elongated by just 8% can reduce blood flow, while complete blood occlusion occurs at 15% nerve elongation (Lundborg, 1975; Lundborg & Rydevik, 1973; Ogata & Naito, 1986).

However, nerves usually follow an undulating (curvy) path within myofascial tissue (Smith, 1966). When stretching, nerves do not actually elongate to a great extent, they just straighten out. Therefore, muscles can be stretched to a great degree without damaging the nerves.

in viscoelasticity would only be short-term and not influence long-term training improvements in flexibility. However, research has shown that muscle spindle discharge can be chronically reduced, leading to a more relaxed muscle (Blazevich et al., 2012). This neural adaptation might be attributed to a more compliant (i.e., less stiff) muscle that would cause less activation of the spindles.

Researchers have also reported that the neural adaptations (i.e., less reflex activity) can occur independently of changes in muscle and tendon stiffness (Guissard & Duchateau, 2004). Chronic, training-induced decreases in muscle stiffness (increased compliance) are attributed to plastic (semi-permanent) changes in the muscle fiber angles, changes in the structure of tissue components (e.g., fewer collagen cross-linkages), and other factors.

Additionally, when muscles or connective tissue are subjected to a constant stretch, the tissues can experience a creep phenomenon. **Tissue creep** means that the muscles and tendons do not return to their original length after prolonged stretching because of physical changes in the proteins, such as collagen (Wallmann et al., 2012). Furthermore, increases in stretch tolerance can also be a chronic training adaptation leading to the ability to withstand the discomfort of greater ROM.

Tissue creep

An initial rapid increase in strain followed by a slower increase in strain at a constant stress.

 CRITICAL

Improvements in joint ROM are always due to several factors:

- Mechanical (muscle and tendon factors affecting compliance or stiffness)
- Neural (inhibition of the central nervous system to help the muscle relax)
- Psycho-physiological (stretch tolerance)

Neuromuscular Stretching

Neuromuscular stretching (NMS), also known as proprioceptive neuromuscular facilitation (PNF), has received greater attention during the past 20 years as an optimal method for lengthening myofascial tissues. NMS is a technique that involves a process of isometrically contracting a desired muscle in a lengthened position to induce a relaxation response on the tissue, allowing it to further elongate (Behm, 2018; Burke et al., 2000).

Many clinicians and researchers believe that this form of stretching combines the mechanisms and benefits of both static and active stretching while keeping the risk of tissue injury low (Bonnar et al., 2004; Burke et al., 2000). Most of the current research has demonstrated that NMS stretching is equally effective at increasing ROM when compared with static stretching (Bonnar et al., 2004; Burke et al., 2000; Higgs & Winter, 2009). Furthermore, some studies have shown NMS to be more effective and to have a reduced negative effect on muscular power than static stretching (Marek et al., 2005; Young & Elliott, 2001).

NMS is usually characterized by four stages:

1. Taking the target muscle to its end-range ROM (point of joint compensation) and holding for 10 seconds
2. Actively contracting the target muscle to be stretched (5- to 10-second submaximal intensity contraction)
3. Passively (or actively) elongating the target muscle to a new end-range
4. Statically holding the new position for 20 to 30 seconds and repeating the contract-relax cycle up to a total of three times

There can be slight variations on the four stages of NMS. The two most common variations are the contract–relax technique and contract–relax–agonist–contract (CRAC) technique (Sady et al., 1982; Sharman et al., 2006). The contract–relax method includes static stretching of the target muscle followed immediately by an isometric contraction of the stretched (target) muscle, followed with another stretch of the target muscle. In CRAC, the target muscle being lengthened is considered the antagonist. This technique involves an additional contraction of the agonist muscle (i.e., the muscle opposing the target muscle) immediately following the isometric contraction and prior to the additional stretching of the target muscle.

One advantage that NMS has over static stretching is that the contraction of the stretched muscle places more mechanical stress on the tendon than with passive static stretching. Because the muscle is already in an elongated position, the subsequent contraction will emphasize the elongation of the tendon (tissue creep), providing an additional mechanical factor (reduced tendon stiffness) not emphasized with static stretching and further helping to increase joint ROM (Behm, 2018). A traditional weakness of NMS compared to static stretching is that it usually requires the assistance of another person (help from a partner or supervision of a professional). However, it can also be performed as a self-applied technique where the target muscle is contracted against a stretch band (Behm et al., 2019) (**Figure 4-4**).

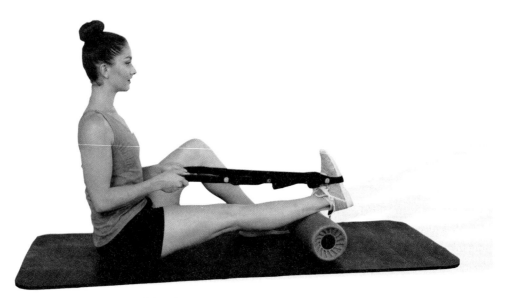

Figure 4-4 NMS with stretch band

MECHANISMS OF NEUROMUSCULAR STRETCHING

Autogenic inhibition

The process by which neural impulses that sense tension are greater than the impulses that cause muscles to contract, providing an inhibitory effect to the muscle spindles.

In the past, it was proposed that a variety of reflex inhibition techniques might be involved with NMS. It was believed that the contraction of the opposing muscle would activate reciprocal inhibition and relax the muscle being stretched (e.g., activating the quadriceps causes the hamstrings to relax and elongate, allowing the knees to straighten and hips to flex). It was also believed that the subsequent contraction of the target muscle to be stretched would activate the GTOs (**autogenic inhibition**) (Chalmers, 2004; Hindle et al., 2012; Houk et al., 1980). However, evidence is lacking as to whether this reflex activity plays an important role in NMS (Chalmers, 2004; Chalmers & Knutzen, 2004; Hindle et al., 2012; Sharman et al., 2006).

However, while holding the muscle in a stretched position (Stage 4 of NMS), there is a substantial decrease in motor neuron excitability that is said to last up to 15 seconds, and thus acts in the same manner as static stretching. Similarly, increased stretch tolerance (Mitchell et al., 2007), decreased tissue viscosity, and increased muscle compliance (reduced stiffness)

(Kay et al., 2015; Magnusson, Simonsen, Aagaard, Dyhre-Poulsen et al., 1996) contribute to an observable increase in joint ROM.

Early research indicated that NMS joint ROM increases were primarily due to neurological mechanisms, such as reciprocal inhibition, autogenic inhibition, and other factors. More recent evidence points to additional contributions from mechanical and psycho-physiological (increased stretch tolerance) factors (Whalen et al., 2019). In general, NMS provides similar-to-greater improvements in joint ROM as static stretching. While NMS experiences similar changes as static stretching, such as changes in viscoelasticity and increased muscle compliance, the additional contraction of an already stretched muscle places more stress on the tendon, providing greater lengthening stresses (i.e., reduced tendon stiffness and increased tissue creep) that are not experienced to a similar extent with static stretching.

TRY THIS

For NMS, lay on your back and static stretch your hamstrings (flex your hip) as far as you can for 30 seconds. Now see how much farther you flex the hip. Next contract your hamstrings against a partner for 5 to 10 seconds (not a maximal contraction). Now again see how much farther your ROM has achieved. This greater ROM is because the contraction put stress on and elongated the tendon, which normally does not get stretched to the same extent with passive static stretching.

Dynamic Stretching

Dynamic stretching has become more popular in the last 20 years, proving to be an important addition to many a client's warm-up routine. Dynamic stretching uses a controlled movement through the entire ROM of the active joints (Fletcher, 2010): for example, single-leg squatting (**Figure 4-5**), multiplanar sequences (**Figure 4-6**), or moving the arms in circles (shoulder circumduction) (**Figure 4-7**).

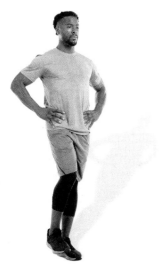

Figure 4-5A Dynamic stretch example: single-leg squat touchdown—start

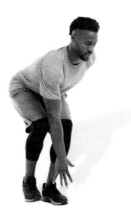

Figure 4-5B Dynamic stretch example: single-leg squat touchdown—finish

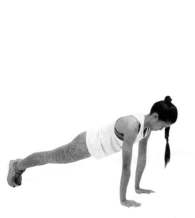

Figure 4-6A Dynamic stretch example: world's greatest stretch—start

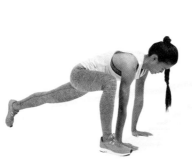

Figure 4-6B Dynamic stretch example: world's greatest stretch—movement

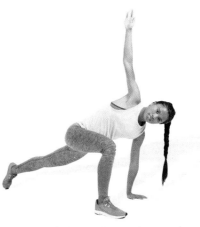

Figure 4-6C Dynamic stretch example: world's greatest stretch—finish

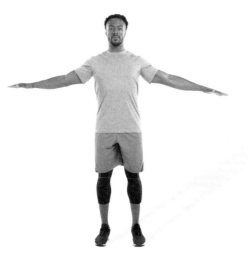

Figure 4-7A Dynamic stretch example: arm circles—start

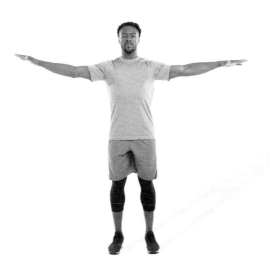

Figure 4-7B Dynamic stretch example: arm circles—finish

Dynamic stretching differs from ballistic stretching, because ballistic stretching uses higher-velocity movements with bouncing actions at the end of the joint ROM (Bacurau et al., 2009; Nelson & Kokkonen, 2001). Whereas static stretching tends to inhibit the nervous system to relax the muscle, dynamic stretching activates or excites the nervous system (Guissard & Duchateau, 2004, 2006; Guissard et al., 1988). Dynamic stretching has advantages over static stretching and NMS when used before sports performance or more demanding exercise because it can be training or movement specific (training movement matches the movement of the activity) (Behm & Sale, 1993; Sale & MacDougall, 1981). In addition, the muscle contractions increase metabolic activity, thus elevating muscle temperature (Bishop, 2003; Fletcher & Jones, 2004; Young, 2007; Young & Behm, 2002), contributing to improved muscle viscoelasticity. Thus, the shear and compressive stresses placed on the stretched muscles with dynamic stretching (similar to static and NMS) induce improvements in viscoelasticity, which contribute to increased muscle lengthening and joint ROM. Furthermore, dynamic stretching tends to improve, or at least has no detrimental effects on, subsequent performance in comparison to the reports regarding prolonged static stretching or NMS performed in isolation without a full warm-up.

CRITICAL

Whereas static stretching and NMS inhibit muscle activation by decreasing the nuclear bag and nuclear chain muscle spindle receptor activity (Ia afferents), dynamic stretching excites the central nervous system. The higher rate and amount of muscle lengthening with dynamic stretching increases myotatic reflex activity, and thus counterbalances the inhibitory effects of static stretching on subsequent performance.

Inhibiting muscle activation of overactive tissues is a key component of the Corrective Exercise Continuum. **Thus, static stretching and/or NMS should be used prior to activity when muscle imbalances are present.**

The Scientific Rationale for Stretching

The proposed mechanism for the use of stretching as it relates to muscle injury risk is illustrated in **Figure 4-8**. The compliance (or flexibility) of the musculotendinous unit affects the relative amount of energy absorbed by the muscle and tendon (Safran et al., 1988). Although tissue compliance will not change the total or absolute force applied to muscles and tendons, it will influence how those forces are distributed over time. With a more compliant (i.e., more flexible) musculotendinous unit, muscles and tendons will absorb forces over a longer duration, reducing the peak forces applied to them. Less compliant tissues will absorb forces over a shorter duration, which increases the peak forces they experience. It is like the difference between dropping a weight onto a stiff board versus a trampoline. While the absolute force (i.e., the weight) applied is the same in both instances, the surfaces absorb that force differently because of how compliant (or noncompliant) they are. More peak forces absorbed by muscles and tendons may increase the trauma experienced by the tissue over time, increasing the risk for injury. Thus, increasing musculotendinous flexibility through stretching will lead to a decrease in peak muscle

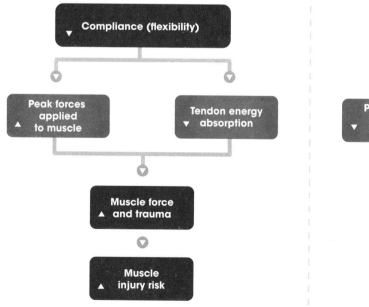
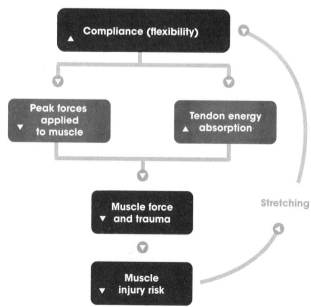

Figure 4-8 Proposed mechanism for the use of stretching as it relates to reducing injury risk

energy absorption and trauma to muscle fibers, with a decrease in muscle and tendon injury risk being the potential result. The relationship between musculotendinous compliance and force absorption is summarized below:

- **High compliance (↑ flexibility)** = Forces absorbed by muscles and tendons over a longer duration (reduction in peak forces applied to musculotendinous unit)
- **Low compliance (↓ flexibility)** = Forces absorbed by muscles and tendons over a shorter duration (increase in peak forces applied to the musculotendinous unit)
- **↑ Muscle and tendon peak force absorption over shorter durations** = ↑ Force and trauma to muscle and tendon fibers

The proposed mechanism for the use of stretching as it relates to performance centers around the relationship between the stiffness of the musculotendinous unit and its influence on the work required to move the limb. If the muscle and tendon are not optimally extensible because of increased stiffness, then the force of contraction required to create motion is greater; that is, the stiffer the muscle and tendon, the more resistant they are to motion. This inefficiency may have a negative effect on performance (**Figure 4-9**). The relationship between musculotendinous stiffness and performance is summarized as follows:

- High stiffness (↓ flexibility) → ↑ Resistance to motion = ↑ Work required
- Low stiffness (↑ flexibility) → ↓ Resistance to motion = ↓ Work required
- ↓ Flexibility limits joint range of motion, which creates altered movement patterns

Therefore, decreasing muscle stiffness through stretching will decrease the work required to perform an activity and potentially increase overall performance.

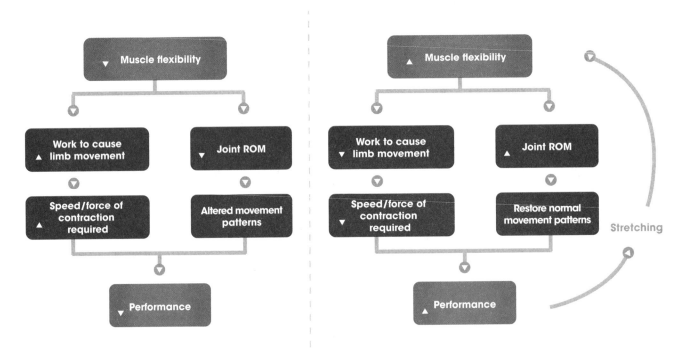

Figure 4-9 Proposed mechanism for the use of stretching as it relates to performance

Conversely, research spanning the late 1990s through the second decade of the 2000s indicates that prolonged, pre-activity, static stretching could negatively affect force and power production, as well as sprint and balance performance, among other measures. The proposed mechanism for how stretching is thought to negatively affect force production is illustrated in **Figure 4-10**.

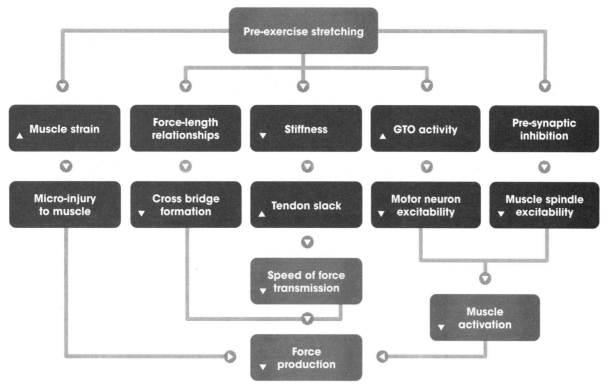

Figure 4-10   Proposed mechanism of pre-exercise stretching and force production

The general theory is that prolonged static stretching in isolation (without a full dynamic warm-up) can affect the structural and neurological components of muscle, which can lead to decrements in the ability of the muscle to effectively generate force. However, recent research has highlighted the limitations of these previous studies and the importance of performing static stretching in combination with dynamic stretching and activities (Behm et al., 2016; Blazevich et al., 2018; Murphy et al., 2010; Reid et al., 2018). This preservation of muscular force generation is an additional reason why exercises like those performed in phases three and four of the Corrective Exercise Continuum occur after lengthening techniques.

Conflict between traditional theory and recent research on pre-exercise stretching has created confusion among professionals and the industry, with the common question being: "Should static stretching be performed to improve performance and decrease the risk of injury?" The following section will discuss what the evidence has shown on the effects of stretching for improving ROM, performance enhancement, and injury prevention.

Improving ROM

Stretching exercises are primarily used to increase the available joint ROM, specifically if the range at that joint is limited by overactive and shortened myofascial tissues. The scientific literature strongly supports the use of all stretching exercises both acutely and chronically (with training) to achieve this goal (Alter, 2004; Behm, 2018; Behm et al., 2016; Behm & Chaouachi, 2011; Kay & Blazevich, 2012). Although static stretching and NMS have been reported to produce greater joint ROM than dynamic stretching, other studies have shown that dynamic stretching provides similar increases in joint ROM as with static and NMS (Beedle & Mann, 2007). Thus, based on the scientific evidence, it cannot be conclusively stated that one stretching technique is definitively better than the others for improving joint ROM.

Additionally, the degree of improvement may be relative to the total available ROM at the joint. For example, hip flexion is typically 100 to 130 degrees of motion, and ankle dorsiflexion is commonly limited to 15 to 20 degrees of motion. In comparison, thoracolumbar extension has a range of 20 to 30 degrees and flexion of 60 to 80 degrees, respectively (Behm, 2018). Therefore, although stretching is still important for areas such as the lumbar spine, the gains in flexibility cannot be expected to be as great as for the hip or shoulders, which are both ball-and-socket joints.

Several researchers suggest that each joint and muscle group may respond differently to stretching protocols; thus, each tissue to be stretched should be carefully evaluated, and the stretching protocol may need to be different for each ROM limitation found. For instance, a 6-week stretching program for the hamstring complex effectively increased ROM, but the same program applied to the gastrocnemius muscle did not result in a change of ROM (Bandy & Irion, 1994; Bandy et al., 1997; Youdas, Krause, Egan et al., 2005). Fitness professionals should carefully evaluate movement through the appropriate assessments and frequently reevaluate, to determine whether a selected protocol is effective for the desired outcome. Fitness professionals should strive to find the right combination of lengthening techniques that maximize the effectiveness and adherence for each client.

DURATION AND FREQUENCY

Much of the debate surrounding the use of stretching protocols has involved the necessary duration and frequency of stretching to produce a change in ROM. For example, excellent studies by Bandy and colleagues found that static hamstring stretches need to be held for 30 seconds and performed five times per week for 6 weeks to produce significant changes in knee extension ROM (Bandy & Irion, 1994; Bandy et al., 1997; Behm, 2018). Many other studies have found that durations of 15 to 30 seconds can produce significant changes in ROM, both acutely and chronically (Behm, 2018).

To ensure significant improvements in ROM without adversely affecting performance, Behm and colleagues (Behm, 2018; Behm et al., 2016) recommend less than 60 seconds of stretching per muscle group within a single stretching session, whereas Thomas and colleagues (2018), in their meta-analysis review, recommend a minimum duration of 5 minutes per week for each muscle group. It is still unclear whether stretching should be performed daily or whether it can be performed as few as three times a week to produce significant changes (Bandy & Irion, 1994; Bandy et al., 1997; Ford et al., 2005; Godges et al., 1993).

More recently, a study by Caldwell et al. (2019) compared stretching once versus twice per day for 2 weeks. They did not find an increase in passive, static ROM, but did find improvements with dynamic and ballistic ROM, as well as strength and power (jump) improvements. They suggest that it is possible for overtraining to occur with excessive stretching frequencies, which may be reflected in the lack of increases in static ROM, at least with recreationally active participants.

INTENSITY

The appropriate stretching intensity also remains a question. Many individuals and studies (Behm et al., 2001, 2004, 2006, 2011; Behm & Kibele, 2007) recommend stretching to the point of discomfort. This is also referred to as stretching to the elastic limit. The elastic limit is the minimum amount of stress placed on tissue to elicit permanent strain. Going farther than the elastic limit could cause the tissue to not return to its original length (Alter, 2004), and thus contribute to strains (muscle) and sprains (ligaments).

CRITICAL

Stretching an injured or fatigued muscle or tendon to the point of discomfort can lead to additional injury!

Conversely, a number of static stretching studies have demonstrated that stretching to less than the point of discomfort provides similar flexibility improvements as stretching to the point of discomfort (Behm & Kibele, 2007; Knudson et al., 2001, 2004; Manoel et al., 2008; Young et al., 2006). Research has suggested that high-force (i.e., stretching to the point of discomfort), shorter-duration stretches may emphasize elastic (short-term or temporary) tissue deformation, whereas low-force (i.e., less than or near the point of discomfort), prolonged stretching emphasizes plastic (long-term or semi-permanent) changes in tissue length (Apostolopoulos, 2001; Laban, 1962; Sun et al., 1995; Warren et al., 1971, 1976).

Individuals have different levels of pain tolerance; therefore, an individual with a high pain threshold could put more strain on the muscles and tendons than someone with a lower pain tolerance. Considering the general population, it may be safer, and reportedly equally effective, to recommend stretching just below the point of discomfort. In general, it is recommended that individuals should approach their point of discomfort momentarily and then reduce that elongation by about 10% (i.e., go near the point of discomfort but not to the point of discomfort) for the static or NMS stretch duration.

TRAINING TIP

Although ROM will increase with short-duration stretching (5 to 15 seconds), the recommended duration for each muscle is 30 to 60 seconds. Stretch to the onset of or near the point of discomfort, but there is no need to elicit great discomfort or pain. Just place moderate stretch tension on the muscle. ROM can be improved within 2 to 6 weeks if performed 3 to 5 days per week.

STRETCHING PROGRAM DURATION

The chronic duration of ROM gains (how long the increased ROM persists) has yet to be fully investigated. Although some studies suggest that ROM improvements are negated after 4 weeks of no stretching (Willy et al., 2001), others have found that stretching does improve long-lasting ROM (Harvey et al., 2002). The majority of this research has been performed using static stretching, so the durations, frequencies, and long-term changes that are attributable to dynamic or NMS stretching need further study. Some initial evidence suggests that NMS or dynamic stretching protocols can produce greater gains in ROM compared with static stretching, and these gains may occur more quickly (Etnyre & Lee, 1988; Fasen et al., 2009; Sady et al., 1982; Schuback et al., 2004). However, other studies have found no differences in ROM gains between active, NMS, or static stretching (Bandy et al., 1998; Davis et al., 2005; Lucas & Koslow, 1984; Winters et al., 2004).

TABLE 4-2 Suggested Warm-Up Components

Myofascial Rolling	Static Stretching	Dynamic Stretching	Task-Specific Activities
90 seconds to 2 minutes of myofascial rolling per muscle group to increase muscle temperatures, decrease tissue viscoelasticity, increase inhibition, and other factors.	< 60 seconds per muscle group if participating in high-intensity exercise or athletic activity. No need to go to the point of discomfort or pain. Stretch major muscle groups and specific muscle groups to the activity. Focus on muscles identified as overactive/shortened during assessment stages.	≤ 90 seconds per muscle group. Use full range of motion with a controlled movement at moderate speeds.	5 to 15 minutes. Practice movements that are associated with the sport or task at velocities close to the actual movement. This may include exercises performed during the Activate and Integrate phases of the Corrective Exercise Continuum.

NOTE: Most research studies have used a general cardio warm-up as a method to both prepare the tissue for stretching and for standardization of protocols. However, NASM suggests beginning with self-myofascial techniques (myofascial roller or another myofascial tool) in an effort to improve blood flow and tissue mobility prior to stretching protocols. In the presence of muscle imbalance and dysfunctional movement, myofascial rolling may prevent exacerbating tissue overload and reinforcing dysfunctional patterns.

The few studies that involve a full warm-up do not report performance decrements and show that stretching may even provide some performance improvements (Little & Williams, 2006; Murphy et al., 2010; Samson et al., 2012; Taylor et al., 2013; Wallmann et al., 2008). The lack of static stretching deficits when a full warm-up is included could be due to postactivation potentiation (enhanced force and power after prior muscle contractions) effects of the dynamic activities (Kummel et al., 2016; Turki et al., 2011). In addition, Blazevich et al. (2018) found that including static or dynamic stretching into a warm-up led to greater participant confidence for their following sports performance. Because psychological effects are so important for performance, this is another reason to include short-to-moderate durations of static stretching (< 60 seconds) into a complete warm-up prior to competition.

 GETTING TECHNICAL

Psychological Benefits of Stretching

Although most clinicians and patients focus on the physical changes produced by stretching, the psychological benefits may be just as great. Several researchers have studied the effects of stretching programs on muscle tension (measured by electromyographic [EMG] activity), self-reported emotions, feelings of muscle tension, and levels of stress-related hormones within the saliva (Carlson et al., 1990; Carlson & Curran, 1994; Hamaguchi et al., 2008; Sugano & Nomura, 2000). These studies have found that stretching reduces both physiological (EMG) and self-reported muscle tension, results in decreased feelings of sadness, and can decrease levels of stress-related hormones (Carlson et al., 1990; Carlson & Curran, 1994; Hamaguchi et al., 2008; Sugano & Nomura, 2000). Blazevich et al. (2018) incorporated 30 seconds of static stretching into a full warm-up and reported increased ROM but no impairments in jumping, sprinting, or agility tests. However, the authors also included a psychological measure and found that including static or dynamic stretching into a warm-up instilled greater participant confidence regarding their performance in the ensuing sports-related tests. Anecdotally, many individuals report similar feelings of reduced tension after routine stretching and feel that this mentally prepares them for physical activity. Thus, although stretching itself may not significantly affect athletic performance, the psychological benefit may be an important consideration when working with clients.

In a 2012 study, Sandberg et al. demonstrated that stretching the antagonist muscles of a jump (i.e., dorsiflexors, knee flexors, and hip flexors) resulted in enhanced jump height and power. The research notes that the effect size was small, indicating that there was not a huge difference between the groups. However, when it comes to athletic performance, even small ROM improvements can make a big difference in competition.

Chronic, long-term stretching protocols have produced varied effects on athletic performance. Various physiological factors affecting performance are positively influenced by stretch training. Stretching can enhance muscle and tendon compliance (less stiffness), which augments the **stretch–shortening cycle** (i.e., used in jumping, sprinting) by enhancing the ability to store elastic energy (Medeiros & Lima, 2017; Wilson et al., 1992). This enhancement is more apparent with longer-duration eccentric (muscle lengthening) to concentric (muscle shortening) contractions, such as a rebound chest press (Wilson et al., 1992), but it might not have such a benefit on brief duration stretch–shortening cycle activities like sprinting.

Another advantage of stretch training is greater force production at longer muscle lengths (Behm et al., 2016; Medeiros & Lima, 2017). A number of stretching studies have found enhanced eccentric peak **torque**, which, during stretch–shortening cycle activities, potentiates the subsequent concentric contraction (Cappa & Behm, 2011, 2013). And although one study found a decrease in vertical jump performance, sprint speed, or reaction time (Chaouachi et al., 2008), others have demonstrated increases in vertical jump, muscular strength, power, and balance ability after a regular stretching program (Gajdosik et al., 2005; Hunter & Marshall, 2002; Kokkonen et al., 2007; LaRoche et al., 2008; Shrier, 2004; Wilson et al., 1992).

Stretch-shortening cycle

An active stretch (eccentric contraction) of a muscle followed by an immediate shortening (concentric contraction) of that same muscle.

Torque

A force that produces rotation; most commonly measured in Newton-meters (Nm).

TRY THIS

Stretch–Shortening Cycle
Perform a vertical jump from a squat position and measure the height jumped. Now, jump again either from a 2-foot platform or with a countermovement jump. Notice how much higher the jump was with the drop jump or countermovement jump. The landing phase of the jump (eccentric contraction) stored elastic energy in the muscle that was used in the concentric phase to allow for a higher jump. A more compliant (flexible) muscle allows for more energy storage over a longer period of time.

Effect of Stretching on Improving Injury Resistance

Many fitness professionals and athletes perform stretching as part of a routine warm-up before activity, prompted by the belief that stretching can reduce certain injuries. The evidence suggests that pre-exercise static stretching does not have a significant influence on all-cause injury risk or rates (Pope et al., 1998, 2000; Small et al., 2008), although the effects of chronic, long-term static stretching protocols tend to lead to decreased muscle and tendon injury rates (Amako et al., 2003; Andrish et al., 1974; Hartig & Henderson, 1999; Hilyer et al., 1990; Pope et al., 2000; Thacker et al., 2004).

Confusion in the literature exists regarding the lack of static stretching effects upon all-cause injury risk versus muscle and tendon injury risk. All-cause injury risk can include problems such as bone fractures, knee cartilage lesions, bursitis, overtraining injuries, and many other problems. Stretching cannot normally prevent a bone fracture, but, as mentioned earlier, it can increase muscle and tendon energy absorption capabilities, which can help decrease the high and rapid forces associated with sprinting and agility movements, thereby improving client or athlete durability at these forces.

Several authors and researchers have shown that regular, long-term static stretching can lead to a decreased incidence of muscle and tendon injury (18–43% decreased rate) and decreased cost of time lost from injury, and fewer severe muscle/tendon injuries occurred in the stretched subjects compared with control subjects (Fradkin et al., 2006; Hartig & Henderson, 1999; Woods et al., 2007). Behm et al. (2016) reported a 54% injury risk reduction of muscle and tendon injuries with static stretching. In their review, Behm et al. (2016) recommend that pre-activity static and dynamic stretching of 5 minutes or more should be beneficial for sprint running injury rate reduction, but others note that it is less effective for endurance running activities (overuse injuries) (Baxter et al., 2017). In all of the studies cited, there do not appear to be any negative consequences relative to injury risk when implementing a regular or pre-exercise stretching program.

CRITICAL

Remember to distinguish between all-cause injuries and musculotendinous injuries. Stretching cannot decrease the incidence of all-cause injuries (e.g., concussions, fractured bones, etc.). However, static stretching can reduce the incidence of muscle and tendon injuries, especially with high-velocity and change-of-direction activities, as is common in athletics or higher-intensity exercise.

Summary of the Evidence

As indicated by the aforementioned review of research and literature surrounding flexibility, the following guidelines have been determined:

- There is strong evidence to indicate that regular stretching of all types (static, NMS, or dynamic) improves ROM.
- There is a moderate level of evidence that dynamic stretch training can positively affect strength and performance, whereas static stretching can decrease muscle and tendon injury risk in healthy individuals without identified limitations in flexibility.
- There is moderate evidence to indicate that acute, prolonged (> 60 seconds per muscle group), pre-exercise static stretching and NMS performed in isolation (i.e., without a complete warm-up sequence) can decrease strength and performance by 3–7%. However, when placed within the context of a comprehensive warm-up and/or the phases of the Corrective Exercise Continuum, static stretching and NMS will have a trivial chance of impairing subsequent performance and do not increase injury risk in healthy individuals without identified limitations in flexibility.

In review of the literature surrounding stretching, some limitations come to light:

1. Research was not performed on individuals with limited flexibility.
   - Pre-exercise stretching may have positive effects on performance and injury risk in those who are inflexible at the outset.
2. Research focused primarily on stretching as the sole exercise.
   - Flexibility is only one piece to maximizing performance and decreasing injury risk.
   - Much of the research investigated impractical (lack of ecological validity) durations of stretching.
   - An integrated continuum may have different results:
     Inhibit → Stretch (Lengthen) → Activate → Integrate into Functional Movement
3. Research has not addressed an individual's specific needs based on an assessment.
   - Research has taken a one-size-fits-all approach.
   - Research needs to investigate the effects of pre-exercise stretching on inflexible muscle groups.
4. A customized corrective exercise strategy may be most effective in improving performance and decreasing the risk of injury.

Application Guidelines for Lengthening Techniques

The use of stretching, like any other form of exercise, should be pursued with an understanding of any potential risks involved. The precautions and contraindications listed in **Table 4-3** may prevent stretching from being used only in a particular muscle or muscle group and not necessarily for all possible muscles for a client.

TABLE 4-3 Precautions and Contraindications for Stretching

Precautions	Contraindications
- Special populations (e.g., pregnant women, osteoarthritis, and rheumatoid arthritis) - Seniors - Hypertensive patients - Neuromuscular disorders - Joint replacements - Fibromyalgia - Marfan syndrome	- Acute injury or muscle strain or tear of the muscle being stretched - Recent musculoskeletal surgery or treatment (i.e., shoulder dislocations, ligament repairs, or fractures) - Acute rheumatoid arthritis of the affected joint - Osteoporosis

The Corrective Exercise Specialist should explain to the client that pain should not be experienced during the stretching protocol, but that mild discomfort may be experienced. The evidence shows that it is unnecessary to static stretch to the point of extreme discomfort regardless of the health status of the client (Apostolopoulos, 2001; Laban, 1962; Sun et al., 1995; Warren et al., 1971,

1976). Whether the client is healthy, recovering from injury, or involved in rehabilitation, mild discomfort is expected. Dynamic stretching should be included later in a rehabilitation process, as the momentum from dynamic movement can place excessive stress on recovering tissue. Dynamic stretching should always be performed so the movement is under control (slow and deliberate movement).

Static Stretching Acute Training Variables

Most studies on static stretching have shown a frequency of 5 days per week using one to four repetitions of durations of 15 to 30 seconds to be most beneficial for the apparently healthy population between 15 and 45 years of age (Alter, 2004; Behm, 2018; Behm et al., 2016). Although there is a range in the evidence, most research confirms that 20 to 30 seconds of stretch duration may, in fact, produce more reliable, and possibly quicker, results (Bandy et al., 1997, 1998; Shrier & Gossal, 2000). In clients age 65 years and older, it was shown that longer durations of 60 seconds may produce better and longer-lasting results (Feland et al., 2001).

For practical application purposes, the Corrective Exercise Specialist should recommend a stretch duration that maximizes results and adherence to the flexibility routine (**Table 4-4**). Moreover, static stretching should only be applied to muscles that have been determined to be overactive/shortened during the assessment process.

TABLE 4-4   Acute Training Variables for Static Stretching

Frequency	Sets	Repetitions	Duration
Daily (unless specified otherwise)	n/a	1 to 4*	20- to 30-second hold 60-second hold for older clients (≥ 65 years)

*Perform no more than 60 seconds of static stretching per muscle group if completed before an athletic competition or high-intensity activity.

STATIC STRETCHES

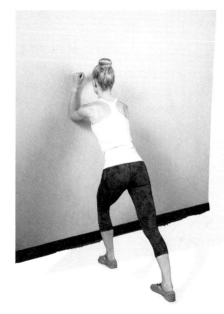

Static gastrocnemius stretch

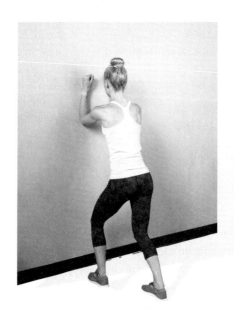

Static soleus stretch

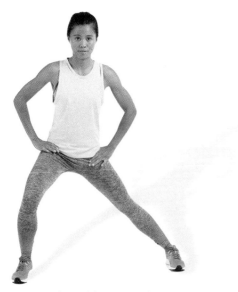

Static standing adductor stretch

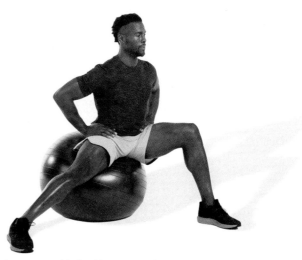

Static seated ball adductor stretch

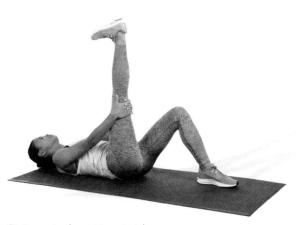

Static supine hamstring stretch

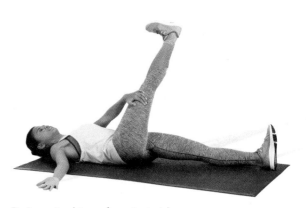

Static supine biceps femoris stretch

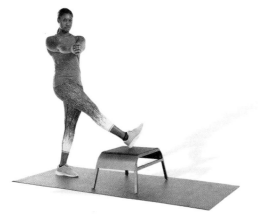

Static standing biceps femoris stretch

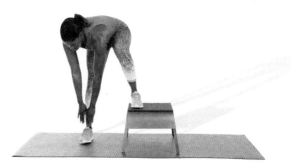

Static adductor magnus stretch

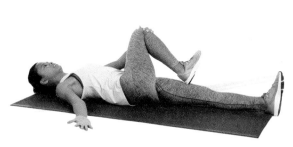

Static piriformis stretch

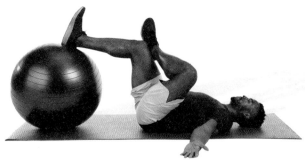

Static supine ball piriformis stretch

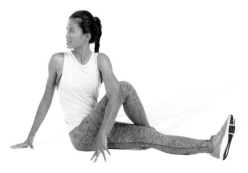

Static erector spinae stretch

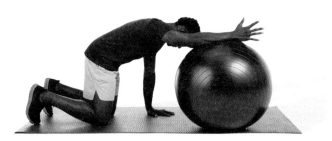

Static ball latissimus dorsi stretch

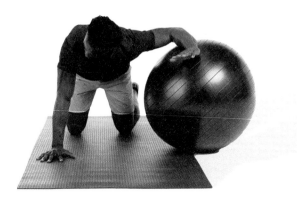

Static ball pectoral stretch

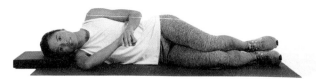

Static posterior shoulder stretch

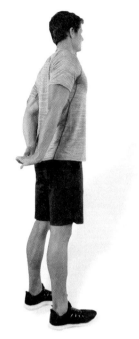

Static long head of biceps stretch

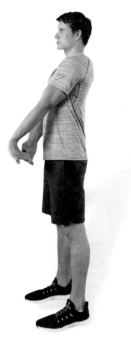

Static wrist flexor stretch

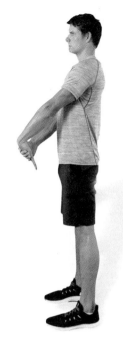

Static wrist extensor stretch

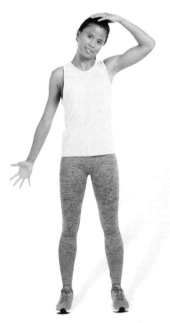

Static upper trapezius stretch

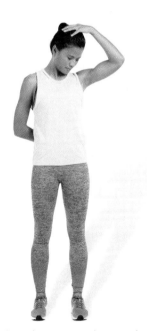

Static levator scapulae stretch

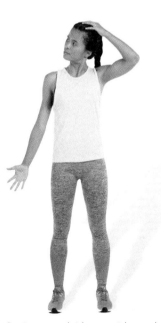

Static sternocleidomastoid stretch

CHAPTER 4: LENGTHENING TECHNIQUES | 113

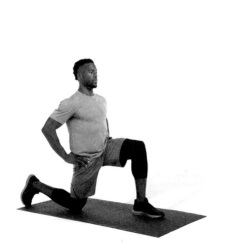

Static kneeling hip flexor stretch—start

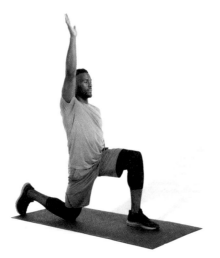

Static kneeling hip flexor stretch—movement

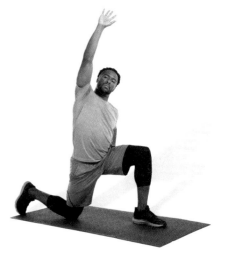

Static kneeling hip flexor stretch—finish

STATIC STRETCHES: STATIC STANDING HIP FLEXOR STRETCH

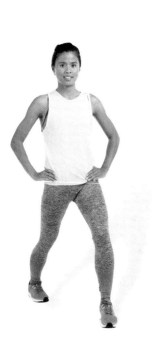

Static standing hip flexor stretch—start

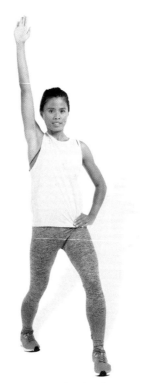

Static standing hip flexor stretch—movement

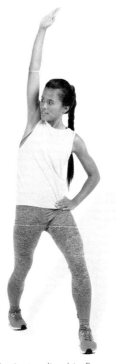

Static standing hip flexor stretch—finish

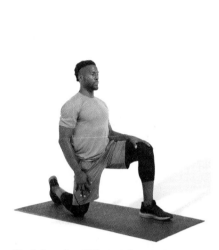

Static kneeling TFL stretch—start

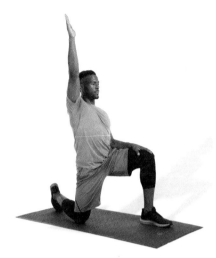

Static kneeling TFL stretch—movement

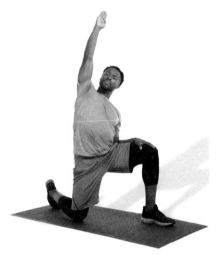

Static kneeling TFL stretch—finish

Neuromuscular Stretching Acute Training Variables

NMS can be performed daily unless otherwise stated. Typically, one to three repetitions or cycles of contract–relax (CR) are used per stretch with an isometric contraction time ranging from 7 to 15 seconds, with at least 10 seconds being ideal (Bonnar et al., 2004; Davis et al., 2005; Guissard et al., 2001; Rowlands et al., 2003). Acutely, it appears that there is no significant difference between 3-, 6-, and 10-second isometric holds (Bonnar et al., 2004). However, for chronic gains, it appears that longer durations produce better results (Rowlands et al., 2003). Research has also shown that a submaximal isometric contraction intensity of 20% is effective to produce significantly increased ROM (Feland & Marin, 2004). Based on the variance in the current body of research, and for the purposes of the Corrective Exercise Specialist, we recommend an isometric contraction of 7–10 seconds. Based on some of the static stretching research, holding the passive stretch for 20 to 30 seconds may produce the greatest results.

Like static stretching, NMS should only be applied to muscles that have been determined to be overactive during the assessment. The examples provided illustrate self-applied NMS with the assistance of an inelastic stretch band or firm object (e.g., foam roller). The exerciser will isometrically contract the target muscle against the band or object and also use the band (if applicable) to pull the target muscle into relaxation during those stages of NMS.

NEUROMUSCULAR STRETCHES

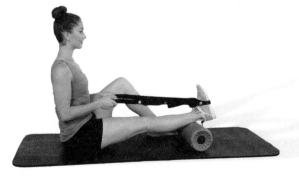

NMS gastrocnemius/soleus complex

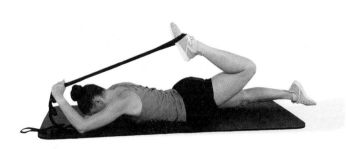

NMS hip flexor complex

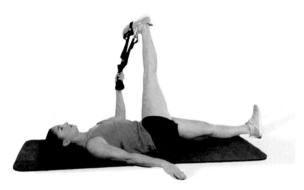

NMS biceps femoris

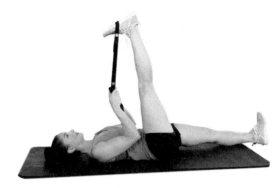

NMS hamstrings complex

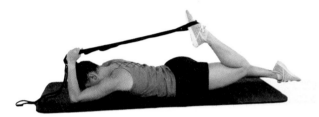

NMS quadriceps

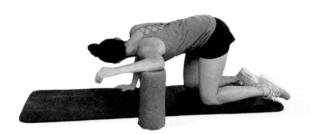

NMS pectorals

Dynamic Stretching Acute Training Variables

A systematic review by Behm and Chaouachi (2011) recommends that no more than 90 seconds of dynamic stretching should be performed for each muscle group, if the goal is to preserve performance. The same review indicates dynamic stretching for more than 90 seconds may elicit increases in performance; however, this is inconclusive. The velocity of the dynamic movement should be under active control (unlike ballistic stretching), and thus is typically performed at one cycle per second (e.g., hip flexion and extension should take approximately 1 second). Dynamic stretching can be performed 3 to 6 days per week. Dynamic stretching should be specific to the task at hand and reflect the more complex movement to be performed during the bulk of the workout.

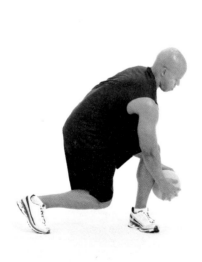

Medicine ball lift and chop—start

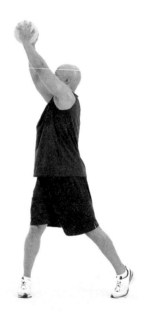

Medicine ball lift and chop—finish

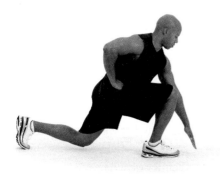

Multiplanar lunge with reach—sagittal

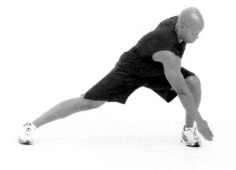

Multiplanar lunge with reach—frontal

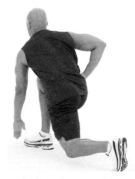

Multiplanar lunge with reach—transverse

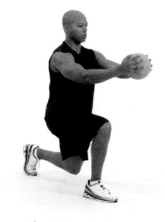

Lunge with rotation—start

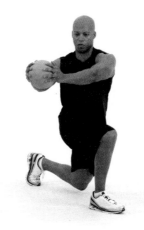

Lunge with rotation—finish

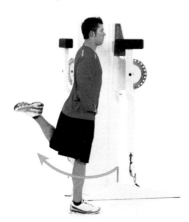

Leg swings—front to back

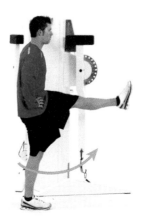

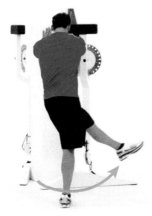

Leg swings—side to side

SUMMARY

Stretching is one of the most commonly used modalities by health and fitness professionals, yet it is still widely misused and misunderstood. As with all components of the Corrective Exercise Continuum, proper application of stretching depends on the needs of the client and the goals of the fitness program. Stretching should be used to correct faulty movement patterns (found during the integrated assessment process), specifically to lengthen shortened myofascial tissues and improve stretch tolerance. Stretching should not be used without conducting a movement assessment first. The different types of stretching techniques (static, NMS, or dynamic) can each produce improvements in ROM. When integrated with inhibition, activation, and integration exercises, stretching can be used to effectively enhance the fitness and well-being of clients.

REFERENCES

Allander, E., Bjornsson, O. J., Olafsson, O., Sigfusson, N., & Thorsteinsson, J. (1974). Normal range of joint movements in shoulder, hip, wrist and thumb with special reference to side: A comparison between two populations. *International Journal of Epidemiology, 3*(3), 253–261. https://doi.org/10.1093/ije/3.3.253

Alter, M. J. (2004). *Science of flexibility*. Human Kinetics.

Amako, M., Oda, T., Masuoka, K., Yoko, H., & Campisi, P. (2003). Effect of static stretching on prevention of injuries for military recruits. *Military Medicine, 168*(6), 442–446.

Andrish, J. T., Bergeld, J. A., & Walheim, J. (1974). A prospective study on the management of shin splints. *Journal of Bone and Joint Surgery, 56*(8), 1697–1700.

Apostolopoulos, N. (2001). Performance flexibility. In B. Foran (Ed.), *High-performance sports conditioning* (pp. 49–61). Human Kinetics.

Bacurau, R. F., Monteiro, G. A., Ugrinowitsch, C., Tricoli, V., Cabral, L. F., & Aoki, M. S. (2009). Acute effect of a ballistic and a static stretching exercise bout on flexibility and maximal strength. *Journal of Strength and Conditioning Research, 23*(1), 304–308.

Bandy, W. D., & Irion, J. M. (1994). The effect of time on the static stretch of the hamstrings muscles. *Physical Therapy, 74*(9), 845–850.

Bandy, W. D., Irion, J. M., & Briggler, M. (1997). The effect of time and frequency of static stretching on flexibility of the hamstring muscles. *Physical Therapy, 77*(10), 1090–1096.

Bandy, W. D., Irion, J. M., & Briggler, M. (1998). The effect of static stretch and dynamic range of motion training on the flexibility of the hamstring muscles. *Journal of Orthopaedic and Sports Physical Therapy, 27*(4), 295–300.

Baxter, C., Mc Naughton, L. R., Sparks, A., Norton, L., & Bentley, D. (2017). Impact of stretching on the performance and injury risk of long-distance runners. *Research in Sports Medicine, 25*(1), 78–90. https://doi.org/10.1080/15438627.2016.1258640

Beedle, B. B., & Mann, C. L. (2007). A comparison of two warm-ups on joint range of motion. *Journal of Strength and Conditioning Research, 21*(3), 776–779.

Behm, D. G. (2018). *The science and physiology of flexibility and stretching: Implications and applications in sport performance and health*. Routledge.

Behm, D. G., Bambury, A., Cahill, F., & Power, K. (2004). Effect of acute static stretching on force, balance, reaction time, and movement time. *Medicine & Science in Sports & Exercise, 36*(8), 1397–1402. https://doi.org/10.1249/01.mss.0000135788.23012.5f

Behm, D. G., Blazevich, A. J., Kay, A. D., & McHugh, M. (2016). Acute effects of muscle stretching on physical performance, range of motion, and injury incidence in healthy active individuals: A systematic review. *Applied Physiology, Nutrition, and Metabolism, 41*(1), 1–11. https://doi.org/10.1139/apnm-2015-0235

Behm, D. G., Bradbury, E. E., Haynes, A. T., Hodder, J. N., Leonard, A. M., & Paddock, N. R. (2006). Flexibility is not related to stretch-induced deficits in force or power. *Journal of Sports Science and Medicine, 5*(1), 33–42.

Behm, D. G., Button, D. C., & Butt, J. C. (2001). Factors affecting force loss with prolonged stretching. *Canadian Journal of Applied Physiology, 26*(3), 261–272.

Behm, D. G., & Chaouachi, A. (2011). A review of the acute effects of static and dynamic stretching on performance. *European Journal of Applied Physiology, 111*(11), 2633–2651. https://doi.org/10.1007/s00421-011-1879-2

Behm, D. G., & Kibele, A. (2007). Effects of differing intensities of static stretching on jump performance. *European Journal of Applied Physiology, 101*(5), 587–594. https://doi.org/10.1007/s00421-007-0533-5

Behm, D. G., Lau, R. J., O'Leary, J. J., Rayner, M. C. P., Burton, E. A., & Lavers, L. (2019). The acute effects of unilateral self-administered static stretching on contralateral limb performance. *Journal of Performance Health Research, 3*(1), 1–7. https://doi.org/10.25036/jphr.2019.3.1.behm

Behm, D. G., Plewe, S., Grage, P., Rabbani, A., Beigi, H. T., Byrne, J. M., & Button, D. C. (2011). Relative static stretch-induced impairments and dynamic stretch-induced enhancements are similar in young and middle-aged men. *Applied Physiology, Nutrition, and Metabolism, 36*(6), 790–797. https://doi.org/10.1139/h11-107

Behm, D. G., & Sale, D. G. (1993). Velocity specificity of resistance training. *Sports Medicine, 15*(6), 374–388.

Bishop, D. (2003). Warm up II: Performance changes following active warm up and how to structure the warm up. *Sports Medicine, 33*(7), 483–498.

Blazevich, A. J., Cannavan, D., Waugh, C. M., Fath, F., Miller, S. C., & Kay, A. D. (2012). Neuromuscular factors influencing the maximum stretch limit of the human plantar flexors. *Journal of Applied Physiology, 113*(9), 1446–1455. https://doi.org/10.1152/japplphysiol.00882.2012

Blazevich, A. J., Gill, N. D., Kvorning, T., Kay, A. D., Goh, A., Hilton, B., Drinkwater, E. J., & Behm, D. G. (2018). No effect of muscle stretching within a full, dynamic warm-up on athletic performance. *Medicine & Science in Sports & Exercise, 50*(6), 1258–1266. https://doi.org/10.1249/MSS.0000000000001539

Bonnar, B. P., Deivert, R. G., & Gould, T. E. (2004). The relationship between isometric contraction durations during hold-relax stretching and improvement of hamstring flexibility. *Journal of Sports Medicine and Physical Fitness, 44*(3), 258–261.

Burke, D. G., Culligan, C. J., & Holt, L. E. (2000). The theoretical basis of proprioceptive neuromuscular facilitation. *Journal of Strength and Conditioning Research, 14*(4), 496–500.

Caldwell, S. L., Bilodeau, R. L. S., Cox, M. J., & Behm, D. G. (2019). Cross education training effects are evident with twice daily, self-administered band stretch training. *Journal of Sports Science and Medicine, 18*(3), 544–551.

Cappa, D. F., & Behm, D. G. (2011). Training specificity of hurdle vs. countermovement jump training. *Journal of Strength and Conditioning Research, 25*(10), 2715–2720. https://doi.org/10.1519/JSC.0b013e318208d43c

Cappa, D. F., & Behm, D. G. (2013). Neuromuscular characteristics of drop and hurdle jumps with different types of landings. *Journal of Strength and Conditioning Research, 27*(11), 3011–3020. https://doi.org/10.1519/JSC.0b013e31828c28b3

Carlson, C. R., Collins, F. L., Nitz, A. J., Sturgis, E. T., & Rogers, J. L. (1990). Muscle stretching as an alternative relaxation training procedure. *Journal of Behavior Therapy and Experimental Psychiatry, 21*(1), 29–38.

Carlson, C. R., & Curran, S. L. (1994). Stretch-based relaxation training. *Patient Education and Counseling, 23*(1), 5–12.

Chalmers, G. (2004). Re-examination of the possible role of Golgi tendon organ and muscle spindle reflexes in proprioceptive neuromuscular facilitation muscle stretching. *Sports Biomechanics, 3*(1), 159–183.

Chalmers, G. R., & Knutzen, K. M. (2004). Recurrent inhibition in the soleus motor pool of elderly and young adults. *Electromyography Clinical Neurophysiology, 44*(7), 413–421.

Chandler, T. J., Kibler, W. B., Uhl, T. L., Wooten, B., Kiser, A., & Stone, E. (1990). Flexibility comparisons of junior elite tennis players to other athletes. *American Journal of Sports Medicine, 18*(2), 134–136. https://doi.org/10.1177/036354659001800204

Chaouachi, A., Chamari, K., Wong, P., Castagna, C., Chaouachi, M., Moussa-Chamari, I., & Behm, D. G. (2008). Stretch and sprint training reduces stretch-induced sprint performance deficits in 13- to 15-year-old youth. *European Journal of Applied Physiology, 104*(3), 515–522. https://doi.org/10.1007/s00421-008-0799-2

Clark, S., Christiansen, A., Hellman, D. F., Hugunin, J. W., & Hurst, K. M. (1999). Effects of ipsilateral anterior thigh soft tissue stretching on passive unilateral straight-leg raise. *Journal of Orthopaedic and Sports Physical Therapy, 29*(1), 4–9; discussion 10–12. https://doi.org/10.2519/jospt.1999.29.1.4

Cornwell, A., Nelson, A. G., & Sidaway, B. (2002). Acute effects of stretching on the neuromechanical properties of the triceps surae muscle complex. *European Journal of Applied Physiology, 86*(5), 428–434.

Davis, D. S., Ashby, P. E., McHale, K. L., McQuain, J. A., & Wine, J. M. (2005). The effectiveness of 3 stretching techniques on hamstring flexibility using consistent stretching parameters. *Journal of Strength and Conditioning Research, 19*(1), 27–32.

DeVries, H. A. (1986). *Physiology of exercise for physical education and athletics* (4th ed.). William C. Brown.

Ebben, W. P., & Blackard, D. O. (2001). Strength and conditioning practices of National Football League strength and conditioning coaches. *Journal of Strength and Conditioning Research, 15*(1), 48–58.

Ebben, W. P., Carroll, R. M., & Simenz, C. J. (2004). Strength and conditioning practices of National Hockey League strength and conditioning coaches. *Journal of Strength and Conditioning Research, 18*(4), 889–897.

Ebben, W. P., Hintz, M. J., & Simenz, C. J. (2005). Strength and conditioning practices of Major League Baseball strength and conditioning coaches. *Journal of Strength and Conditioning Research, 19*(3), 538–546.

Etnyre, B. R., & Lee, E. J. (1988). Chronic and acute flexibility of men and women using three different stretching techniques. *Research Quarterly for Exercise and Sport, 59*(3), 222–228.

Fasen, J. M., O'Connor, A. M., Schwartz, S. L., Watson, J. O., Plastaras, C. T., Garvan, C. W., Bulcao, C., Johnson, S. C., & Akuthota, V. (2009). A randomized controlled trial of hamstring stretching: comparison of four techniques. *Journal of Strength and Conditioning Research, 23*(2), 660–667. https://doi.org/10.1519/JSC.0b013e318198fbd1

Feland, J. B., & Marin, H. N. (2004). Effect of submaximal contraction intensity in contract-relax proprioceptive neuromuscular facilitation stretching. *British Journal of Sports Medicine, 38*(4), E18.

Feland, J. B., Myrer, J. W., Schulthies, S. S., Fellingham, G. W., & Measom, G. W. (2001). The effect of duration of stretching of the hamstring muscle group for increasing range of motion in people aged 65 years or older. *Physical Therapy, 81*(5), 1110–1117.

Fletcher, I. M. (2010). The effect of different dynamic stretch velocities on jump performance. *European Journal of Applied Physiology, 109*(3), 491–498. https://doi.org/10.1007/s00421-010-1386-x

Fletcher, I. M., & Jones, B. (2004). The effect of different warm-up stretch protocols on 20 meter sprint performance in trained rugby union players. *Journal of Strength and Conditioning Research, 18*(4), 885–888.

Ford, G. S., Mazzone, M. A., & Taylor, K. (2005). The effect of 4 different durations of static hamstring stretching on passive knee-extension range of motion. *Journal of Sport Rehabilitation, 14*(2), 95–107. https://doi.org/10.1123/jsr.14.2.95

Fowles, J. R., Sale, D. G., & MacDougall, J. D. (2000). Reduced strength after passive stretch of the human plantar flexors. *Journal of Applied Physiology, 89*(3), 1179–1188.

Fradkin, A. J., Gabbe, B. J., & Cameron, P. A. (2006). Does warming up prevent injury in sport? The evidence from randomised controlled trials? *Journal of Science and Medicine in Sport, 9*(3), 214–220. https://doi.org/10.1016/j.jsams.2006.03.026

Gabbard, C., & Tandy, R. (1988). Body composition and flexibility among prepubescent males and females. *Journal of Human Movement Studies, 4*(14), 153–159.

Gajdosik, R. L., Vander Linden, D. W., McNair, P. J., Williams, A. K., & Riggin, T. J. (2005). Effects of an eight-week stretching program on the passive-elastic properties and function of the calf muscles of older women. *Clinical Biomechanics, 20*(9), 973–983.

Godges, J. J., MacRae, P. G., & Engelke, K. A. (1993). Effects of exercise on hip range of motion, trunk muscle performance, and gait economy. *Physical Therapy, 73*(7), 468–477. https://doi.org/10.1093/ptj/73.7.468

Grewal, R., Xu, J., Sotereanos, D. G., & Woo, S. L. (1996). Biomechanical properties of peripheral nerves. *Hand Clinics, 12*(2), 195–204.

Guissard, N., & Duchateau, J. (2004). Effect of static stretch training on neural and mechanical properties of the human plantar-flexor muscles. *Muscle and Nerve, 29*(2), 248–255.

Guissard, N., & Duchateau, J. (2006). Neural aspects of muscle stretching. *Exercise and Sport Science Reviews, 34*(4), 154–158.

Guissard, N., Duchateau, J., & Hainaut, K. (1988). Muscle stretching and motoneuron excitability. *European Journal of Applied Physiology, Occupational Physiology, 58*(1–2), 47–52.

Guissard, N., Duchateau, J., & Hainaut, K. (2001). Mechanisms of decreased motoneurone excitation during passive muscle stretching. *Experimental Brain Research, 137*(2), 163–169.

Haley, S. M., Tada, W. L., & Carmichael, E. M. (1986). Spinal mobility in young children. A normative study. *Physical Therapy, 66*(11), 1697–1703.

Halvorson, G. A. (1989). Principles of rehabilitating sports injuries. In C. C. Teitz (Ed.), *Scientific foundations of sports medicine* (pp. 345–371). Mosby.

Hamaguchi, T., Fukudo, S., Kanazawa, M., Tomiie, T., Shimizu, K., Oyama, M., & Sakurai, K. (2008). Changes in salivary physiological stress markers induced by muscle stretching in patients with irritable bowel syndrome. *BioPsychoSocial Medicine, 2*, 20.

Hartig, D., & Henderson, J. M. (1999). Increasing hamstring flexibility decreases lower extremity overuse injuries in military basic trainees. *American Journal of Sports Medicine, 27*(2), 173–176.

Harvey, L., Herbert, R., & Crosbie, J. (2002). Does stretching induce lasting increases in joint ROM? A systematic review. *Physiotherapy Research International, 7*(1), 1–13.

Hebbelink, M. (1988). *Flexibility*. Blackwell Scientific.

Higgs, F., & Winter, S. L. (2009). The effect of a four-week proprioceptive neuromuscular facilitation stretching program on isokinetic torque production. *Journal of Strength and Conditioning Research, 23*(5), 1442–1447.

Hilyer, J. C., Brown, K. C., Sirles, A. T., & Peoples, L. (1990). A flexibility intervention to reduce the incidence and severity of joint injuries among municipal firefighters. *Journal of Occupational Medicine, 32*(7), 631–637.

Hindle, K. B., Whitcomb, T. J., Briggs, W. O., & Hong, J. (2012). Proprioceptive neuromuscular facilitation (PNF): Its mechanisms and effects on range of motion and muscular function. *Journal of Human Kinetics, 31*, 105–113.

Houk, J. C., Crago, P. E., & Rymer, W. Z. (1980). Functional properties of the Golgi tendon organs. In J. E. Desmedt (Ed.), *Spinal and supraspinal mechanisms of voluntary motor control and locomotion* (Vol. 8, pp. 33–43). Karger.

Hubley-Kozey, C. L. (1991). Testing flexibility. In J. D. MacDougall, H. A. Weger, & H. J. Green (Eds.), *Physiological testing of the high-performance athlete* (2nd ed., pp. 309–359). Human Kinetics.

Hunter, J. P., & Marshall, R. N. (2002). Effects of power and flexibility training on vertical jump technique. *Medicine & Science in Sports & Exercise, 34*(3), 478–486.

Jenner, J. R., & Stephens, J. A. (1982). Cutaneous reflex responses and their central nervous pathways studied in man. *Journal of Physiology, 333*, 405–419.

Jones, M. A., Buis, J. M., & Harris, I. D. (1986). Relationships of race and sex to physical and motor measures. *Perceptual and Motor Skills, 63*(1), 169–170. https://doi.org/10.2466/pms.1986.63.1.169

Katz, R., & Pierrot-Deseilligny, E. (1999). Recurrent inhibition in humans. *Progress in Neurobiology, 57*(3), 325–355.

Kay, A. D., & Blazevich, A. J. (2012). Effect of acute static stretch on maximal muscle performance: A systematic review. *Medicine & Science in Sports & Exercise, 44*(1), 154–164. https://doi.org/10.1249/MSS.0b013e318225cb27

Kay, A. D., Husbands-Beasley, J., & Blazevich, A. J. (2015). Effects of contract-relax, static stretching, and isometric contractions on muscle-tendon mechanics. *Medicine & Science in Sports & Exercise, 47*(10), 2181–2190. https://doi.org/10.1249/MSS.0000000000000632

Kent, M. (1998). *The Oxford dictionary of sports science and medicine* (2nd ed.). Oxford University Press.

Kisner, C., & Colby, L. A. (2002). *Therapeutic exercise: Foundations and techniques* (4th ed.). F. A. Davis.

Knudson, D., Bennett, K., Corn, R., Leick, D., & Smith, C. (2001). Acute effects of stretching are not evident in the kinematics of the vertical jump. *Journal of Strength and Conditioning Research, 15*(1), 98–101.

Knudson, D. V., Noffal, G. J., Bahamonde, R. E., Bauer, J. A., & Blackwell, J. R. (2004). Stretching has no effect on tennis serve performance. *Journal of Strength and Conditioning Research, 18*(3), 654–656.

Kokkonen, J., Nelson, A. G., Eldredge, C., & Winchester, J. B. (2007). Chronic static stretching improves exercise performance. *Medicine & Science in Sports & Exercise, 39*(10), 1825–1831.

Kubo, K., Kanehisa, H., & Fukunaga, T. (2001). Is passive stiffness in human muscles related to the elasticity of tendon structures? *European Journal of Applied Physiology, 85*(3–4), 226–232.

Kubo, K., Kanehisa, H., & Fukunaga, T. (2002). Effect of stretching training on the viscoelastic properties of human tendon structures in vivo. *Journal of Applied Physiology, 92*(2), 595–601.

Kummel, J., Kramer, A., Cronin, N. J., & Gruber, M. (2016). Postactivation potentiation can counteract declines in force and power that occur after stretching. *Scandinavian Journal of Medicine & Science in Sports, 27*(12), 1750–1760. https://doi.org/10.1111/sms.12817

Laban, M. M. (1962). Collagen tissue: Implications of its response to stress in vitro. *Archives of Physical Medicine and Rehabilitation, 43*, 461–466.

LaRoche, D. P., Lussier, M. V., & Roy, S. J. (2008). Chronic stretching and voluntary muscle force. *Journal of Strength and Conditioning Research, 22*(2), 589–596. https://doi.org/10.1519/JSC.0b013e3181636aef

Liemohn, W. P. (1988). Flexibility and muscular strength. *Journal of Physical Education, Recreation & Dance, 59*(7), 37–40.

Little, T., & Williams, A. G. (2006). Effects of differential stretching protocols during warm-ups on high-speed motor capacities in professional soccer players. *Journal of Strength and Conditioning Research, 20*(1), 203–207.

Lucas, R. C., & Koslow, R. (1984). Comparative study of static, dynamic, and proprioceptive neuromuscular facilitation stretching techniques on flexibility. *Perceptual and Motor Skills, 58*(2), 615–618. https://doi.org/10.2466/pms.1984.58.2.615

Lundborg, G. (1975). Structure and function of the intraneural microvessels as related to trauma, edema formation, and nerve function. *Journal of Bone and Joint Surgery. American Volume, 57*(7), 938–948.

Lundborg, G., & Rydevik, B. (1973). Effects of stretching the tibial nerve of the rabbit. A preliminary study of the intraneural circulation and the barrier function of the perineurium. *Journal of Bone and Joint Surgery. British Volume, 55*(2), 390–401.

Magnusson, S. P., Simonsen, E. B., Aagaard, P., Dyhre-Poulsen, P., McHugh, M. P., & Kjaer, M. (1996). Mechanical and physiological responses to stretching with and without preisometric contraction in human skeletal muscle. *Archives of Physical Medicine and Rehabilitation, 77*(4), 373–378. https://doi.org/10.1016/s0003-9993(96)90087-8

Magnusson, S. P., Simonsen, E. B., Aagaard, P., & Kjaer, M. (1996). Biomechanical responses to repeated stretches in human hamstring muscle in vivo. *American Journal of Sports Medicine, 24*(5), 622–627.

Magnusson, S. P., Simonsen, E. B., Aagaard, P., Sorensen, H., & Kjaer, M. (1996). A mechanism for altered flexibility in human skeletal muscle. *Journal of Physiology, 497*(Pt 1), 291–298.

Magnusson, S. P., Simonsen, E. B., Dyhre-Poulsen, P., Aagaard, P., Mohr, T., & Kjaer, M. (1996). Viscoelastic stress relaxation during static stretch in human skeletal muscle in the absence of EMG activity. *Scandinavian Journal of Medicine & Science in Sports, 6*(6), 323–328.

Manoel, M. E., Harris-Love, M. O., Danoff, J. V., & Miller, T. A. (2008). Acute effects of static, dynamic, and proprioceptive neuromuscular facilitation stretching on muscle power in women. *Journal of Strength and Conditioning Research, 22*(5), 1528–1534.

Marek, S. M., Cramer, J. T., Fincher, A. L., Massey, L. L., Dangelmaier, S. M., Purkayastha, S., Fitz, K. A., & Culbertson, J. Y. (2005). Acute effects of static and proprioceptive neuromuscular facilitation stretching on muscle strength and power output. *Journal of Athletic Training, 40*(2), 94–103.

Matthews, P. B. (1981). Muscle spindles: Their messages and their fusimotor supply. In V. B. Brooks (Ed.), *Handbook of physiology. Section 1: The nervous system* (Vol. II, pp. 189–288). American Physiological Society.

McGill, S. M. (2002). *Low back disorders: Evidence based prevention and rehabilitation.* Human Kinetics.

McHugh, M. P., & Cosgrave, C. H. (2010). To stretch or not to stretch: The role of stretching in injury prevention and performance. *Scandinavian Journal of Medicine & Science in Sports, 20*(2), 169–181. https://doi.org/10.1111/j.1600-0838.2009.01058.x

Medeiros, D. M., & Lima, C. S. (2017). Influence of chronic stretching on muscle performance: Systematic review. *Human Movement Science, 54*, 220–229. https://doi.org/10.1016/j.humov.2017.05.006

Melzack, R., & Wall, P. D. (1965). Pain mechanisms: A new theory. *Science, 150*(3699), 971–979.

Mitchell, U. H., Myrer, J. W., Hopkins, J. T., Hunter, I., Feland, J. B., & Hilton, S. C. (2007). Acute stretch perception alteration contributes to the success of the PNF "contract-relax" stretch. *Journal of Sport Rehabilitation, 16*(2), 85–92.

Morelli, M., Chapman, C. E., & Sullivan, S. J. (1999). Do cutaneous receptors contribute to changes in the amplitude of the H-reflex during massage? *Electromyography Clinical Neurophysiology, 39*(7), 441–447.

Murphy, J. R., Di Santo, M. C., Alkanani, T., & Behm, D. G. (2010). Aerobic activity before and following short-duration static stretching improves range of motion and performance vs. a traditional warm-up. *Applied Physiology, Nutrition, and Metabolism, 35*(5), 679–690. https://doi.org/10.1139/H10-062

Nelson, R. T., & Bandy, W. D. (2005). An update on flexibility. *Strength Conditioning Journal, 27*(1), 10–16.

Nelson, A. G., & Kokkonen, J. (2001). Acute ballistic muscle stretching inhibits maximal strength performance. *Research Quarterly for Exercise and Sport, 72*(4), 415–419. https://doi.org/10.1080/02701367.2001.10608978

Ogata, K., & Naito, M. (1986). Blood flow of peripheral nerve effects of dissection, stretching and compression. *Journal of Hand Surgery. British & European Volume, 11*(1), 10–14.

Pope, R. P., Herbert, R. D., & Kirwan, J. D. (1998). Effects of ankle dorsiflexion range and pre-exercise calf muscle stretching on injury risk in army recruits. *Australian Journal of Physiotherapy, 44*(3), 165–177.

Pope, R. P., Herbert, R. D., Kirwan, J. D., & Graham, B. J. (2000). A randomized trial of preexercise stretching for prevention of lower-limb injury. *Medicine & Science in Sports & Exercise, 32*(2), 271–277.

Power, K., Behm, D., Cahill, F., Carroll, M., & Young, W. (2004). An acute bout of static stretching: Effects on force and jumping performance. *Medicine & Science in Sports & Exercise, 36*(8), 1389–1396.

Reid, J. C., Greene, R., Young, J. D., Hodgson, D. D., Blazevich, A. J., & Behm, D. G. (2018). The effects of different durations of static stretching within a comprehensive warm-up on voluntary and evoked contractile properties. *European Journal of Applied Physiology, 118*(7), 1427–1445. https://doi.org/10.1007/s00421-018-3874-3

Rowlands, A. V., Marginson, V. F., & Lee, J. (2003). Chronic flexibility gains: Effect of isometric contraction duration during proprioceptive neuromuscular facilitation stretching techniques. *Research Quarterly for Exercise and Sport, 74*(1), 47–51.

Sady, S. P., Wortman, M., & Blanke, D. (1982). Flexibility training: Ballistic, static or proprioceptive neuromuscular facilitation? *Archives of Physical Medicine and Rehabilitation, 63*(6), 261–263.

Safran, M. R., Garrett, W. E., Jr., Seaber, A. V., Glisson, R. R., & Ribbeck, B. M. (1988). The role of warmup in muscular injury prevention. *American Journal of Sports Medicine, 16*(2), 123–129.

Sale, D., & MacDougall, D. (1981). Specificity in strength training: A review for the coach and athlete. *Canadian Journal of Applied Sport Sciences, 6*(2), 87–92.

Samson, M., Button, D. C., Chaouachi, A., & Behm, D. G. (2012). Effects of dynamic and static stretching within general and activity specific warm-up protocols. *Journal of Sports Science and Medicine, 11*(2), 279–285.

Sandberg, J. B., Wagner, D. R., Willardson, J. M., & Smith, G. A. (2012). Acute effects of antagonist stretching on jump height, torque, and electromyography of agonist musculature. *Journal of Strength and Conditioning Research, 26*(5), 1249–1256. https://doi.org/10.1519/JSC.0b013e31824f2399

Schuback, B. H., Hooper, J., & Salisbury, L. G. (2004). A comparison of a self-stretch incorporating proprioceptive neuromuscular facilitation components and a therapist-applied PNF-technique on hamstring flexibility. *Physiotherapy, 90*(3), 151–157. https://doi.org/10.1016/j.physio.2004.02.009

Sharman, M. J., Cresswell, A. G., & Riek, S. (2006). Proprioceptive neuromuscular facilitation stretching: Mechanisms and clinical implications. *Sports Medicine, 36*(11), 929–939.

Shrier, I. (2004). Does stretching improve performance? A systematic and critical review of the literature. *Clinical Journal of Sport Medicine, 14*(5), 267–273.

Shrier, I., & Gossal, K. (2000). Myths and truths of stretching. *The Physician and Sports Medicine, 28*(8), 57–63.

Simenz, C. J., Dugan, C. A., & Ebben, W. P. (2005). Strength and conditioning practices of National Basketball Association strength and conditioning coaches. *Journal of Strength and Conditioning Research, 19*(3), 495–504.

Small, K., Mc Naughton, L., & Matthews, M. (2008). A systematic review into the efficacy of static stretching as part of a warm-up for the prevention of exercise-related injury. *Research in Sports Medicine, 16*(3), 213–231. https://doi.org/10.1080/15438620802310784

Smith, C. A. (1994). The warm-up procedure: To stretch or not to stretch. A brief review. *Journal of Orthopedic & Sports Physical Therapy, 19*(1), 12–17.

Smith, J. W. (1966). Factors influencing nerve repair. I. Blood supply of peripheral nerves. *Archives of Surgery, 93*(2), 335–341.

Smith, N. P., Barclay, C. J., & Loiselle, D. S. (2005). The efficiency of muscle contraction. *Progress in Biophysics & Molecular Biology, 88*(1), 1–58. https://doi.org/10.1016/j.pbiomolbio.2003.11.014

Soucie, J. M., Wang, C., Forsyth, A., Funk, S., Denny, M., Roach, K. E., Boone, D., & Hemophilia Treatment Center Network. (2010). Range of motion measurements: Reference values and a database for comparison studies. *Haemophilia, 17*(3), 500–507. https://doi.org/10.1111/j.1365-2516.2010.02399.x

Stone, W. J., & Kroll, W. A. (1991). *Sports conditioning and weight training: Programs for athletic competition* (3rd ed.). William C. Brown.

Sugano, A., & Nomura, T. (2000). Influence of water exercise and land stretching on salivary cortisol concentrations and anxiety in chronic low back pain patients. *Journal of Physiological Anthropology and Applied Human Science, 19*(4), 175–180. https://doi.org/10.2114/jpa.19.175

Sullivan, M. K., Dejulia, J. J., & Worrell, T. W. (1992.). Effect of pelvic position and stretching method on hamstring muscle flexibility. *Medicine & Science in Sports & Exercise, 24*(12), 1383–1389.

Sun, J.-S., Tsuang, Y.-H., Liu, T.-K., Hang, Y.-S., Cheng, C.-K., & Lee, W. W.-L. (1995). Viscoplasticity of rabbit skeletal muscle under dynamic cyclic loading. *Clinical Biomechanics, 10*(5), 258–262.

Sunderland, S. (1978). Traumatized nerves, roots and ganglia: Musculoskeletal factors and neuropathological consequences. In I. M. Korr (Ed.), *The neurobiologic mechanisms in manipulative therapy* (pp. 137–138). Plenum Press.

Sunderland, S. (1991). *Nerve injuries and their repair. A critical appraisal* (3rd ed.). Churchill Livingstone.

Taylor, J. M., Weston, M., & Portas, M. D. (2013). The effect of a short practical warm-up protocol on repeated sprint performance. *Journal of Strength and Conditioning Research, 27*(7), 2034–2038. https://doi.org/10.1519/JSC.0b013e3182736056

Thacker, S. B., Gilchrist, J., Stroup, D. F., & Kimsey, C. D., Jr. (2004). The impact of stretching on sports injury risk: A systematic review of the literature. *Medicine & Science in Sports & Exercise, 35*(3), 371–378.

Thomas, E., Bianco, A., Paoli, A., & Palma, A. (2018). The relation between stretching typology and stretching duration: The effects on range of motion. *International Journal of Sports Medicine, 39*(4), 243–254. https://doi.org/10.1055/s-0044-101146

Turki, O., Chaouachi, A., Drinkwater, E. J., Chtara, M., Chamari, K., Amri, M., & Behm, D. G. (2011). Ten minutes of dynamic stretching is sufficient to potentiate vertical jump performance characteristics. *Journal of Strength and Conditioning Research, 25*(9), 2453–2463. https://doi.org/10.1519/JSC.0b013e31822a5a79

Wall, E. J., Massie, J. B., Kwan, M. K., Rydevik, B. L., Myers, R. R., & Garfin, S. R. (1992). Experimental stretch neuropathy. Changes in nerve conduction under tension. *Journal of Bone and Joint Surgery. British Volume, 74*(1), 126–129.

Wallmann, H. W., Christensen, S. D., Perry, C., & Hoover, D. L. (2012). The acute effects of various types of stretching static, dynamic, ballistic, and no stretch of the iliopsoas on 40-yard sprint times in recreational runners. *International Journal of Sports Physical Therapy, 7*(5), 540–547.

Wallmann, H. W., Mercer, J. A., & Landers, M. R. (2008). Surface electromyographic assessment of the effect of dynamic activity and dynamic activity with static stretching of the gastrocnemius on vertical jump performance. *Journal of Strength and Conditioning Research, 22*(3), 787–793. https://doi.org/10.1519/JSC.0b013e3181660e27

Warren, C. G., Lehmann, J. F., & Koblanski, J. N. (1971). Elongation of rat tail tendon: Effect of load and temperature. *Archives of Physical Medicine and Rehabilitation, 52*(10), 465–474.

Warren, C. G., Lehmann, J. F., & Koblanski, J. N. (1976). Heat and stretch procedures: An evaluation using rat tail tendon. *Archives of Physical Medicine and Rehabilitation, 57*(3), 122–126.

Whalen, A., Farrell, K., Roberts, S., Smith, H., & Behm, D. G. (2019). Topical analgesic improved or maintained ballistic hip flexion range of motion with treated and untreated legs. *Journal of Sports Science and Medicine, 18*(3), 552–558.

Willy, R. W., Kyle, B. A., Moore, S. A., & Chleboun, G. S. (2001). Effect of cessation and resumption of static hamstring muscle stretching on joint range of motion. *Journal of Orthopaedic & Sports Physical Therapy, 31*(3), 138–144. https://doi.org/10.2519/jospt.2001.31.3.138

Wilson, G. J., Elliot, B. C., & Wood, G. A. (1992). Stretch shorten cycle performance enhancement through flexibility training. *Medicine & Science in Sports & Exercise, 24*(1), 116–123.

Winters, M. V., Blake, C. G., Trost, J. S., Marcello-Brinker, T. B., Lowe, L. M., Garber, M. B., & Wainner, R. S. (2004). Passive versus active stretching of hip flexor muscles in subjects with limited hip extension: A randomized clinical trial. *Physical Therapy, 84*(9), 800–807.

Witvrouw, E., Mahieu, N., Roosen, P., & McNair, P. (2007). The role of stretching in tendon injuries. *British Journal of Sports Medicine, 41*(4), 224–226.

Woods, K., Bishop, P., & Jones, E. (2007). Warm-up and stretching in the prevention of muscular injury. *Sports Medicine, 37*(12), 1089–1099.

Youdas, J. W., Krause, D. A., Egan, K. S., Therneau, T. M., & Laskowski, E. R. (2005). The effect of static stretching of the calf muscle-tendon unit on active ankle dorsiflexion range of motion. *Journal of Orthopedic Sports Physiology Therapy, 33*(7), 408–417.

Youdas, J. W., Krause, D. A., Hollman, J. H., Harmsen, W. S., & Laskowski, E. (2005). The influence of gender and age on hamstring muscle length in healthy adults. *Journal of Orthopaedic & Sports Physical Therapy, 35*(4), 246–252. https://doi.org/10.2519/jospt.2005.35.4.246

Young, W. B., & Behm, D. (2002). Should static stretching be used during a warm-up for strength and power activities? *Strength and Conditioning Journal, 24*(6), 33–37. https://doi.org/10.1519/00126548-200212000-00006

Young, W., Elias, G., & Power, J. (2006). Effects of static stretching volume and intensity on plantar flexor explosive force production and range of motion. *Journal of Sports Medicine and Physical Fitness, 46*(3), 403–411.

Young, W., & Elliott, S. (2001). Acute effects on static stretching, proprioceptive neuromuscular facilitation stretching, and maximum voluntary contractions on explosive force production and jumping performance. *Research Quarterly for Exercise and Sport, 72*(3), 273–279.

Young, W. B. (2007). The use of static stretching in warm-up for training and competition. *International Journal of Sports Physiology and Performance, 2*(2), 212–216.

CHAPTER 5

Activation Techniques

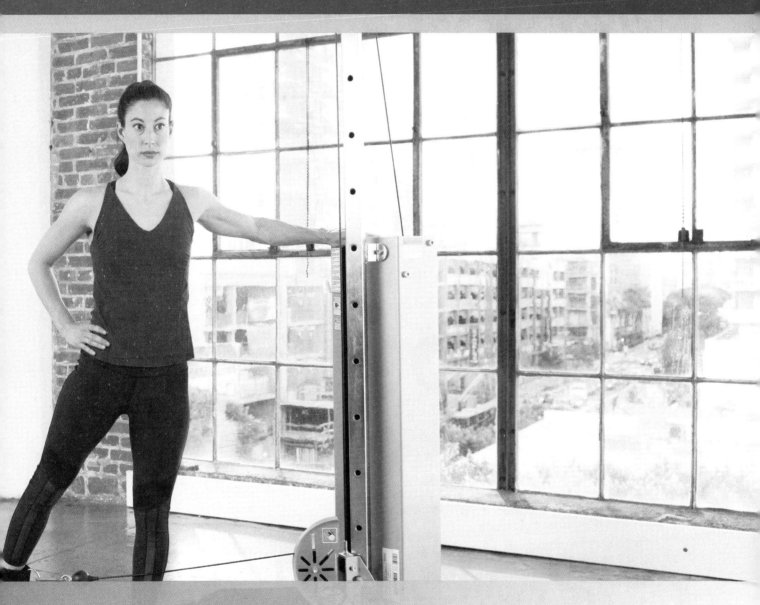

Learning Objectives

After reading this content, students should be able to demonstrate the following objectives:

- **Explain** the function of activation techniques in a corrective exercise program.
- **Identify** activation techniques for use in corrective exercise programming.
- **Describe** the application guidelines for activation techniques.

Introduction

The first two phases of the Corrective Exercise Continuum address the overactive/shortened myofascial tissue that can restrict optimal joint range of motion (ROM) and ultimately decrease movement ability. The third phase of the Corrective Exercise Continuum is activate (**Figure 5-1**). Activation refers to the stimulation (or reeducation) of underactive/lengthened myofascial tissue. Because human movement system impairments (muscle imbalances) include both overactive and underactive muscles, a comprehensive corrective strategy must also address the underactive muscles.

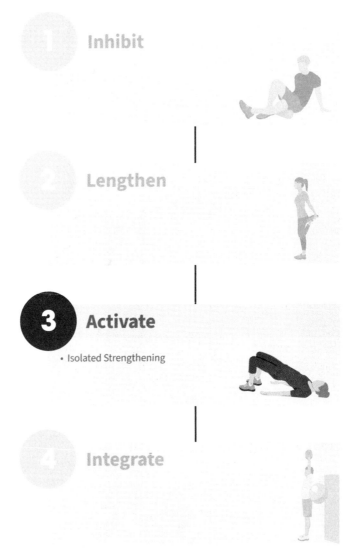

Figure 5-1 Corrective Exercise Continuum—activate

Isolated Strengthening

Isolated strengthening exercises are used to isolate particular muscles to increase the force production capabilities through concentric, isometric, and eccentric muscle actions. These exercises are applied to potentially underactive muscles as indicated through the assessment process.

Scientific Rationale for Isolated Strengthening

Isolated strengthening is a technique used to increase **intramuscular coordination** of specific muscles. This is achieved through a combination of enhanced **motor unit activation**, **synchronization**, and **firing rate**. Each of these parameters is known to increase the strength of a muscle contraction (Enoka, 2015). Intramuscular coordination is known to be developed through resistance exercises focusing on a particular muscle (Bruhn et al., 2004). More important, however, is the increased activation of the muscle throughout the full available ROM of a joint or joints associated with the particular muscle. This is important to achieve before performing integrated exercises to avoid compensation of synergistic muscles (synergistic dominance) during the final phase of the Corrective Exercise Continuum.

Isolated strengthening exercises can be performed immediately after inhibitory and lengthening techniques. Favorable results are produced in professional practice, and Bell et al. (2013) demonstrated the effectiveness of activation techniques following inhibitory and lengthening techniques on knee valgus. For example, the combination of overactivity of the tensor fascia latae and underactivity of the gluteus medius may contribute to knee valgus observed during a squat pattern. If activation of the gluteus medius were to be performed first, before the inhibition and lengthening of the TFL, the TFL may synergistically try to dominate hip abduction. However, when the TFL is inhibited and lengthened, it is less apt to interfere with the gluteus medius during hip abduction activation exercises. Additionally, if the adductors limit hip abduction, providing inhibition and stretches to the adductors can allow for a greater end-range of motion for the gluteus medius to work through. Although the benefits of isolated muscle activation do not require inhibition and lengthening to achieve results, NASM suggests following the Corrective Exercise Continuum to optimize muscle synergies and client and athlete outcomes.

CHECK IT OUT

Mennell's Four Basic Truisms
Mennell's (1964) truisms provide a theoretical basis for the following hypothesis: Attempting to strengthen muscles when joint motion restriction is present will provide less-than-optimal results, and limited joint ROM needs to be considered during any exercise application.

1. When a joint is not free to move, the muscles that move it cannot be free to move it.
2. Muscles cannot be restored to normal if the joints that they move are not free to move.
3. Normal muscle function is dependent on normal joint movement.
4. Impaired muscle function perpetuates and may cause deterioration in abnormal joints.

These four truisms are some of the reasons to perform inhibitory and lengthening techniques (first two phases of the Corrective Exercise Continuum) before isolated strengthening exercises.

An example of an isolated strengthening exercise is a standing cable hip abductor exercise, as shown in **Figure 5-2**. The idea is to position the client and the resistance in the best line of action for an optimal recruitment of each desired muscle. In the case of the standing cable hip

Intramuscular coordination

The ability of the neuromuscular system to allow optimal levels of motor unit recruitment and synchronization within a muscle.

Motor unit activation

The progressive activation of a muscle by successive recruitment of contractile units (motor units) to accomplish increasing gradations of contractile strength.

Synchronization

The synergistic activation of multiple motor units.

Firing rate

The frequency at which a motor unit is activated.

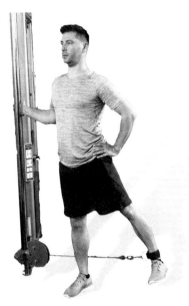

Figure 5-2 Hip abduction isolated strengthening exercise

abductor exercise, the desired movement is hip abduction; thus, the resistance must be set up to directly oppose this motion. These exercises can be performed with manual resistance (neuromuscular facilitation and positional isometrics), cables, body weight, elastic tubing, dumbbells, and machines.

The eccentric phase of the muscle contraction is slower during isolated strengthening. Many reasons for slow-tempo eccentrics will be discussed. Eccentric-focused exercise has been increasingly utilized for corrective strategies because of physiological and mechanical properties (Hody et al., 2019). The eccentric component involved with isolated strengthening has been proven to play a role in the recovery of muscle injury (Lepley & Butterfield, 2017; Shadle & Cacolice, 2017; Tyler et al., 2017) and tendinopathies (de Souza & Araújo, 2016; Lorenz & Reiman, 2011), decreases the risk of muscle strains (Shadle & Cacolice, 2017), and is even involved in immunochemistry (Reidy et al., 2018). Eccentric muscle actions provide greater strength gains compared to concentric muscle actions in isolation (Gois et al., 2014; Maeo et al., 2018; Roig et al., 2009). Interestingly, evidence suggests that eccentric exercise on a muscle on one side of the body increases strength of the contralateral muscle on the unexercised limb (Lepley & Palmieri-Smith, 2014). The same cross-education strength outcomes were not found for concentric-only exercise. Additional benefits of eccentric training are substantial gains in cross-sectional area, promotion of optimal fiber length, increased pennation angle, and targeting of type II muscle fibers while improving variables related to strength, power, and speed performance (Douglas et al., 2017; Lepley et al., 2017).

Eccentric exercise is also associated with muscle damage and increased delayed onset muscle soreness (DOMS; Deli et al., 2017; Hody et al., 2019). However, the first bout of eccentric exercise and subsequent DOMS has a protective effect on the muscle tissue that minimizes soreness and aids in faster recovery during future workouts (Prasartwuth et al., 2019). The goal is to practice slow and controlled submaximal eccentric muscle recruitment and to progressively increase intensity over time (Hody et al., 2019). When performed at the tempo under the Corrective Exercise Continuum, the eccentric phase is approximately 4 seconds. Because eccentric training can lead to muscular soreness, even corrective exercise should be progressive in nature in order to minimize the client's DOMS response.

 GETTING TECHNICAL

Muscle Weakness and Knee Injuries

Knee overuse injuries are common injuries in exercisers, and they are common topics of study. One meta-analysis found that overuse injuries in enrolled military persons showed lower absolute strength of the hip external rotators, knee extensors, and knee flexors and lower normalized hip extensors, external rotators, and abductors (Kollock et al., 2016). A meta-analysis of patellofemoral pain showed associated common findings, including increased hip adduction, internal rotation, and gluteal weakness, as well as neuromuscular impairment (Mirzaie et al., 2016).

A systematic review with meta-analysis of individuals with symptomatic knee osteoarthritis suggested significant hip muscular strength deficits (Deasy et al., 2016). An additional review of hip strength that also reviewed core stability and strength showed that strength limitations in both regions were associated with patellofemoral pain (Earl-Boehm et al., 2018). Strengthening of the hip and core musculature is a corrective strategy for the knee and should be considered a valuable and necessary intervention.

Application Guidelines for Isolated Strengthening Techniques

Once the first two phases of the Corrective Exercise Continuum have been implemented to focus on increased mobility, isolation exercises are used to strengthen targeted musculature selected based on the assessment process. All areas of movement impairment should follow the Corrective Exercise Continuum to help optimize movement efficiency throughout the entire system.

Precautions and Contraindications

Precautions for isolated strengthening exercises follow those for most forms of training (**Table 5-1**). Precautions are used to make the fitness professional aware of possible associations of contraindications, although they are not contraindications alone. However, contraindications serve as a reason to withhold an otherwise indicated exercise recommendation until clearance is obtained from the client's physician. Pain is an immediate indicator to cease the offending activity.

TABLE 5-1 Precautions and Contraindications for Isolated Strengthening

Precautions	Contraindications
- Special populations - Neuromuscular disorders - Clients with poor core stabilization strength	- Acute injury or muscle strain or tear of the muscle being strengthened - Acute rheumatoid arthritis of the affected joint - Impaired joint motion - Pain produced during the movement

Acute Training Variables

Isolated strengthening can be performed 3 to 5 days per week depending on the intensity and volume used with one to two sets of 10 to 15 repetitions being suitable before an integrated exercise program. Each repetition will consist of a 4-second eccentric component, 2-second isometric hold at the end-ROM, and a 1-second concentric component (**Table 5-2**) (ACSM, 2009). With

TABLE 5-2 Acute Training Variables for Isolated Strengthening

Frequency	Sets	Repetitions	Duration of Repetition
3 to 5 days per week	1 to 2	10 to 15	4/2/1 4 seconds eccentric 2 seconds isometric hold at end-range 1 second concentric

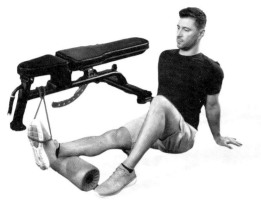

Posterior tibialis—start

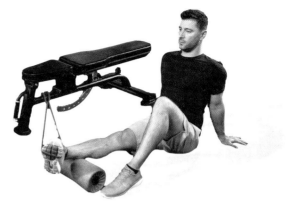

Posterior tibialis—finish

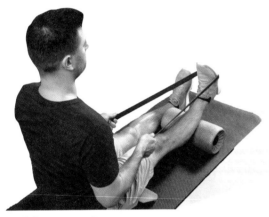

Medial gastrocnemius—start

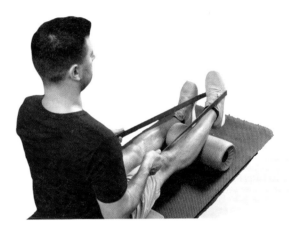

Medial gastrocnemius—finish

Hip and Knee

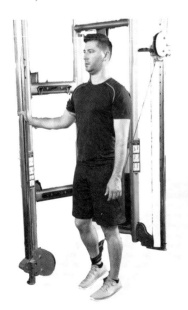

Standing quadriceps—start

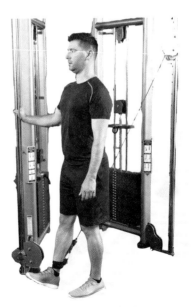

Standing quadriceps—finish

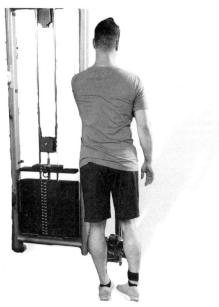

Medial hamstrings complex (knee flexion)—start

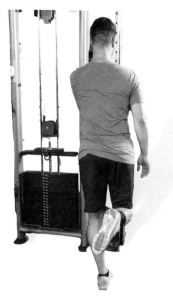

Medial hamstrings complex (knee flexion)—finish

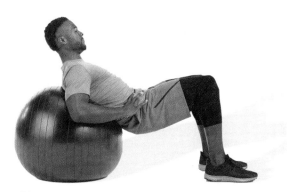

Ball bridge—start

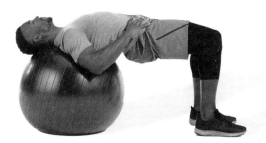

Ball bridge—finish

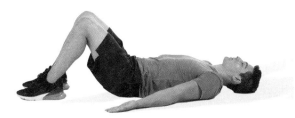

Floor bridge—start

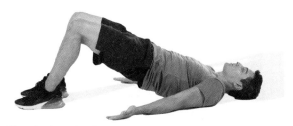

Floor bridge—finish

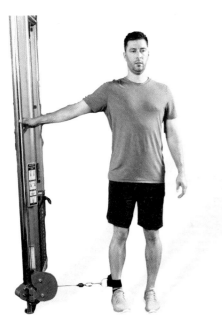

Adductor—start

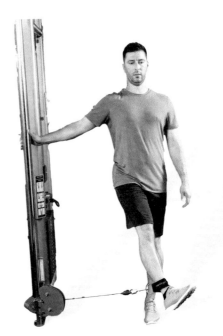

Adductor—finish

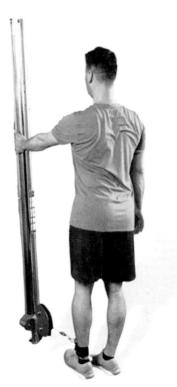

Standing gluteus maximus—start

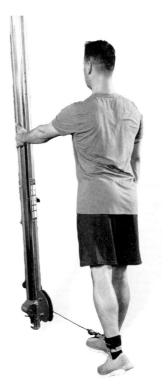

Standing gluteus maximus—finish

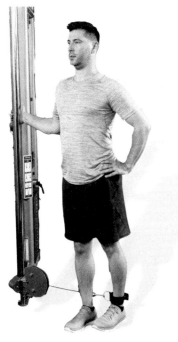

Standing gluteus medius—start

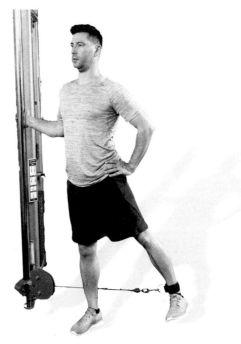

Standing gluteus medius—finish

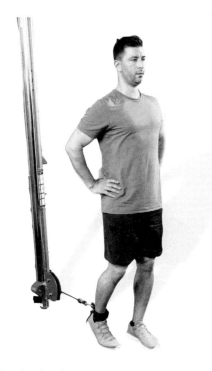

Standing hip flexor—start

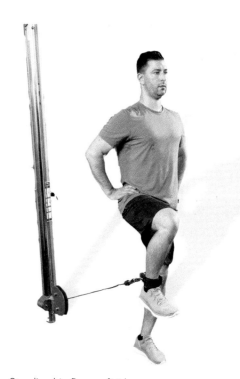

Standing hip flexor—finish

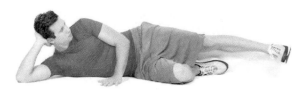

Wall slides—start

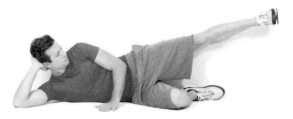

Wall slides—finish

Abdominals/Intrinsic Core Stabilizers

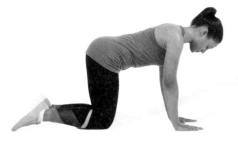

Quadruped marching—start

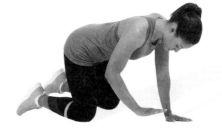

Quadruped marching—finish

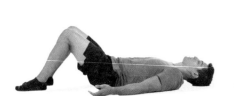

Supine marching—start

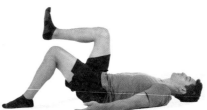

Supine marching—movement 1

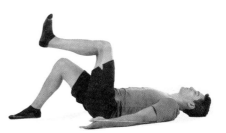

Supine marching—movement 2

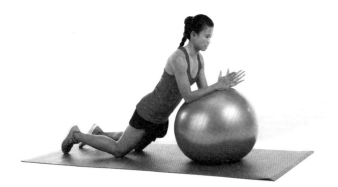

Ball roll outs—start

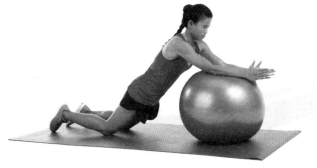

Ball roll outs—finish

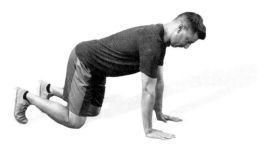

Quadruped arm/opposite leg raise—start

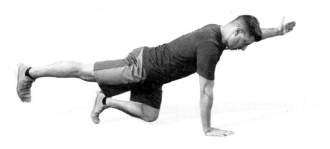

Quadruped arm/opposite leg raise—finish

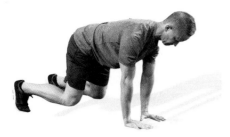

Four-point quadruped arm/opposite leg raise—start

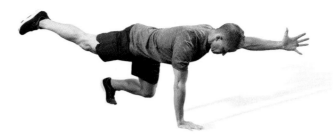

Four-point quadruped arm/opposite leg raise—finish

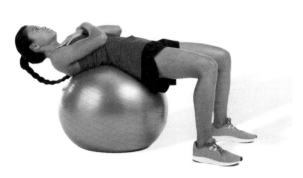

Ball crunch—start

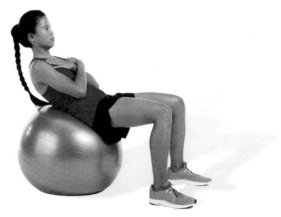

Ball crunch—finish

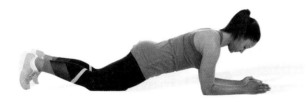

Short lever plank

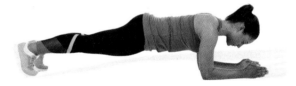

Long lever plank

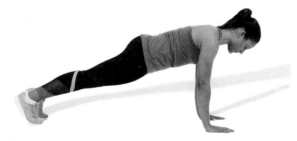

Straight arm plank

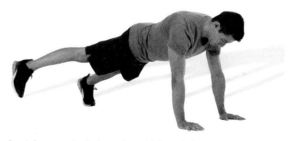

Straight arm plank, leg raise with hip abduction

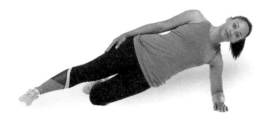

Short lever side plank

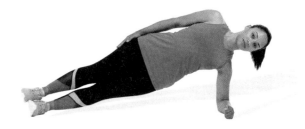

Long lever side plank

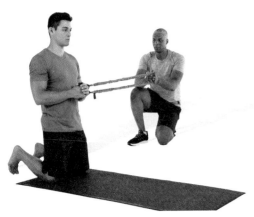

Pallof press—start

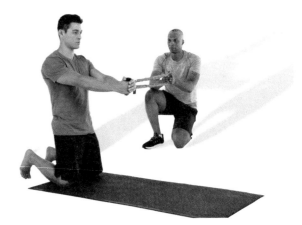

Pallof press—finish

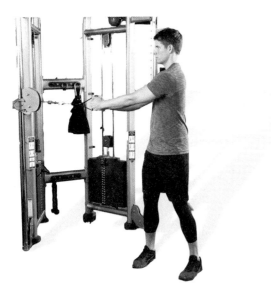

Standing cable rotation—start

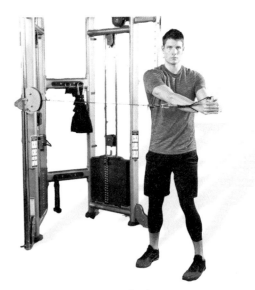

Standing cable rotation—finish

Optimizing the Plank

A study by Choi et al. (2019) showed differences in abdominal muscles of those with low-back pain by changing ankle positioning during a plank. Abdominal activity was significantly increased for those performing isometric dorsiflexion compared to those performing a traditional plank, isometric plantarflexion plank, or no ankle involvement (block under distal shins). Perhaps cueing active dorsiflexion during a prone plank hold can help fitness clients with decreased core stability and overall core strength.

In another study the length of the lever increased a challenge to the global musculature during a plank (Schoenfeld et al., 2014). The study also showed increase in core musculature activation when performing a posterior tilt. Thus, cueing a posterior tilt while also performing isometric dorsiflexion may increase local and global muscle activation while minimizing stress on the lumbar spine that can be felt by some people and populations.

Shoulder

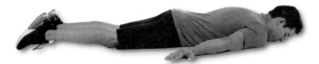

Floor cobra—start

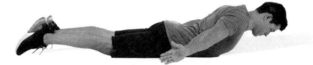

Floor cobra—finish

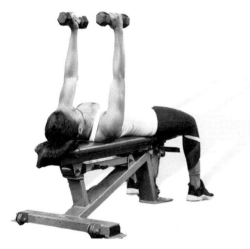

Serratus anterior—start

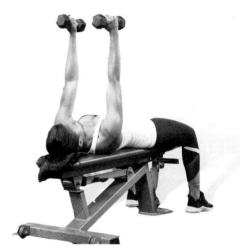

Serratus anterior—finish

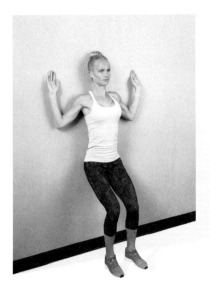

Wall angels—start

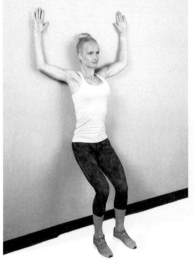

Wall angels—finish

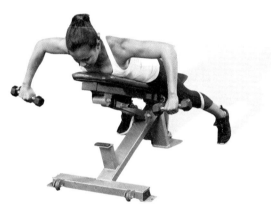

Prone shoulder external rotation—start

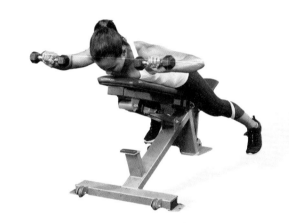

Prone shoulder external rotation—finish

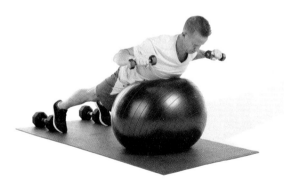

Prone military press—start

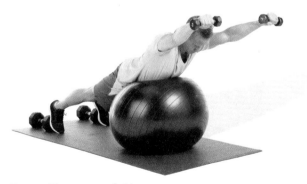

Prone military press—finish

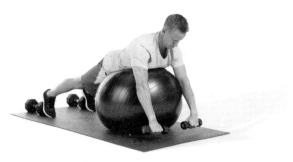

Ball combo 1—start

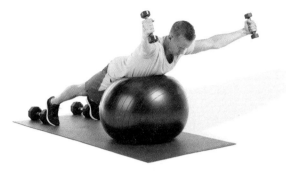

Ball combo 1—scaption

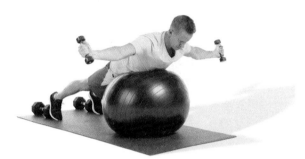

Ball combo 1—retraction

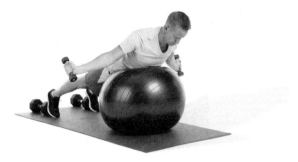

Ball combo 1—cobra (finish)

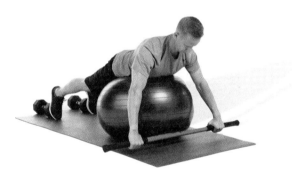

Ball combo 2 with dowel rod—start

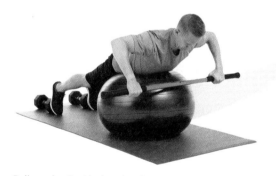

Ball combo 2 with dowel rod—row

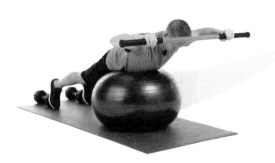

Ball combo 2 with dowel rod—rotate

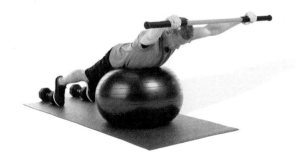

Ball combo 2 with dowel rod—press

Elbow and Wrist

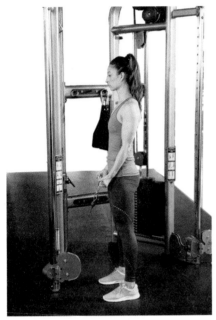

Standing elbow flexion—start

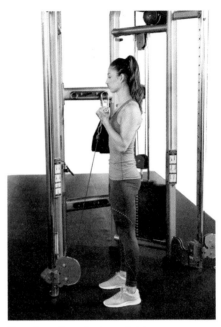

Standing elbow flexion—finish

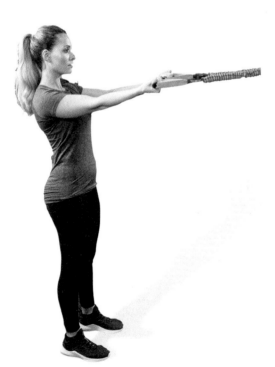

Standing elbow flexion with shoulder
flexed—start

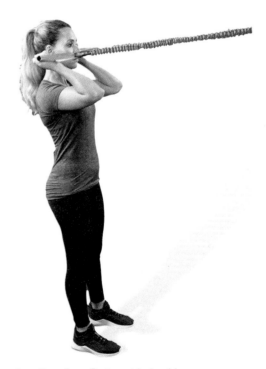

Standing elbow flexion with shoulder
flexed—finish

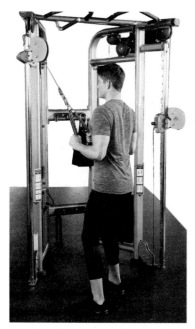
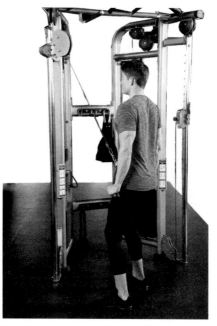

Standing elbow extension—start

Standing elbow extension—finish

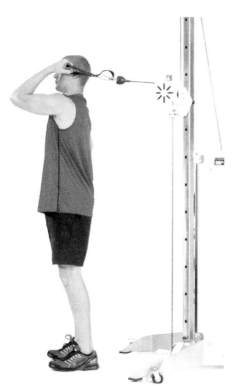
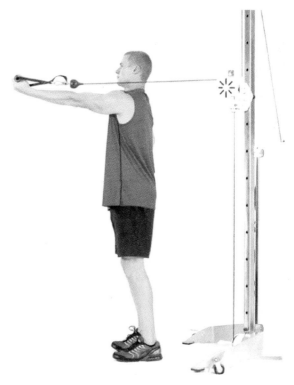

Standing elbow extension with shoulder flexed—start

Standing elbow extension with shoulder flexed—finish

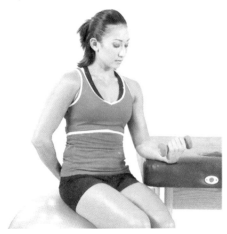

Wrist flexion

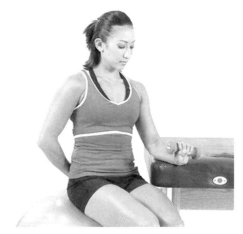

Wrist extension

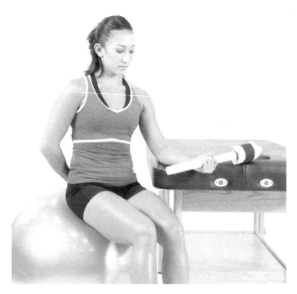

Wrist supination

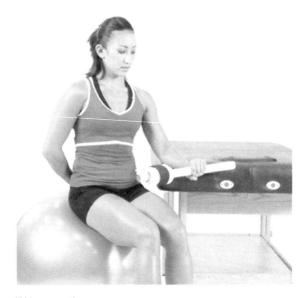

Wrist pronation

Cervical Spine

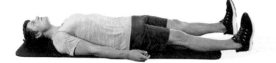

Supine chin tuck—start

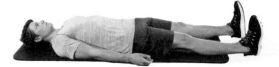

Supine chin tuck—finish

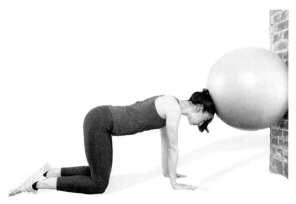

Quadruped chin tucks with stability ball—start

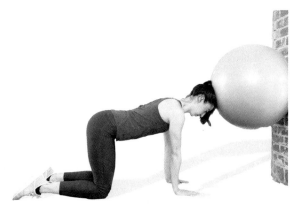

Quadruped chin tucks with stability ball—finish

SUMMARY

The assessment process provides insights into muscular over- and underactivity. Once the muscles that limit optimal range of motion are inhibited and lengthened via the first two phases in the Corrective Exercise Continuum, muscles that are identified as too underactive to stabilize or eccentrically decelerate unwanted movement should be strengthened. This strengthening takes place with isolated, preferential muscle activation. These repetitions are slow with a focus on eccentric control. If the primary muscle to be activated is not isolated, synergists can take control as a substitute prime mover and perpetuate imbalance. Isolated activation of a targeted muscle increases intramuscular coordination, motor unit activation, synchronization, and firing rate. Once strength has been provided to an underactive muscle through potentially a new range of motion, the Corrective Exercise Specialist can move to integrated training to train intermuscular coordination and refinement of global movement patterns.

REFERENCES

American College of Sports Medicine (ACSM). (2009). Progression models in resistance training for healthy adults. *Medicine & Science in Sports & Exercise, 41*(3), 687–708. https://doi.org/10.1249/mss.0b013e3181915670

Bell, D. R., Oates, D. C., Clark, M. A., & Padua, D. A. (2013). Two- and 3-dimensional knee valgus are reduced after an exercise intervention in young adults with demonstrable valgus during squatting. *Journal of Athletic Training, 48*(4), 442–449. https://doi.org/10.4085/1062-6050-48.3.16

Bruhn, S., Kullmann, N., & Gollhofer, A. (2004). The effects of a sensorimotor training and a strength training on postural stabilisation, maximum isometric contraction and jump performance. *International Journal of Sports Medicine, 25*(1), 56–60.

Choi, J. H., Kim, D. E., & Cynn, H. S. (2019). Comparison of trunk muscle activity between traditional plank exercise and plank exercise with isometric contraction of ankle muscles in subjects with chronic low back pain. *Journal of Strength and Conditioning Research.* https:doi.org/10.1519/JSC.0000000000003188

de Souza, R. V., & Araújo, V. L. (2016). The effect of eccentric training on tissue repair in individuals with Achilles tendinopathy: A literature review. *Manual Therapy, Posturology & Rehabilitation Journal, 14*, 1–8. https://doi.org/10.17784/mtprehabJournal.2016.14.378

Deasy, M., Leahy, E., & Semciw, A. I. (2016). Hip strength deficits in people with symptomatic knee osteoarthritis: A systematic review with meta-analysis. *Journal of Orthopaedic & Sports Physical Therapy, 46*(8), 629–639.

Deli, C. K., Fatouros, I. G., Paschalis, V., Georgakouli, K., Zalavras, A., Avloniti, A., Koutedakis, Y., & Jamurtas, A. Z. (2017). A comparison of exercise-induced muscle damage following maximal eccentric contractions in men and boys. *Pediatric*

Exercise Science, 29(3), 316–325. https://doi.org/10.1123/pes.2016-0185

Douglas, J., Pearson, S., Ross, A., & McGuigan, M. (2017). Chronic adaptations to eccentric training: A systematic review. *Sports Medicine, 47*(5), 917. https://doi.org/10.1007/s40279-016-0628-4

Earl-Boehm, J. E., Bolgla, L. A., Emory, C., Hamstra-Wright, K. L., Tarima, S., & Ferber, R. (2018). Treatment success of hip and core or knee strengthening for patellofemoral pain: Development of clinical prediction rules. *Journal of Athletic Training, 53*(6), 545–552. https://doi.org/10.4085/1062-6050-510-16

Enoka, R. M. (2015). *Neuromechanics of human movement* (5th ed.). Human Kinetics.

Gois, M. O., Campoy, F. A., Alves, T., Ávila, R. P., Vanderlei, L. C., & Pastre, C. M. (2014). The influence of resistance exercise with emphasis on specific contractions (concentric vs. eccentric) on muscle strength and post-exercise autonomic modulation: a randomized clinical trial. *Brazilian Journal of Physical Therapy, 18*(1), 30–37.

Hody, S., Croisier, J.-L., Bury, T., Rogister, B., & Leprince, P. (2019). Eccentric muscle contractions: Risks and benefits. *Frontiers in Physiology, 10*, 536. https://doi.org/10.3389/fphys.2019.00536

Kollock, R. O., Andrews, C., Johnston, A., Elliott, T., Wilson, A. E., Games, K. E., & Sefton, J. M. (2016). A meta-analysis to determine if lower extremity muscle strengthening should be included in military knee overuse injury-prevention programs. *Journal of Athletic Training, 51*(11), 919–926. https://doi.org/10.4085/1062-6050-51.4.09

Lepley, L. K., & Butterfield, T. A. (2017). Shifting the current clinical perspective: isolated eccentric exercise as an effective intervention to promote the recovery of muscle after injury. *Journal of Sport Rehabilitation, 26*(2), 122–130. https://doi.org/10.1123/jsr.2017-0008

Lepley, L. K., Lepley, A. S., Onate, J. A., & Grooms, D. R. (2017). Eccentric exercise to enhance neuromuscular control. *Sports Health, 9*(4), 333–340. https://doi.org/10.1177/1941738117710913

Lepley, L. K., & Palmieri-Smith, R. M., (2014). Cross-education strength and activation after eccentric exercise. *Journal of Athletic Training, 49*(5), 582–589. https://doi.org/10.4085/1062-6050-49.3.24

Lorenz, D., & Reiman, M. (2011). The role and implementation of eccentric training in athletic rehabilitation: Tendinopathy, hamstring strains, and ACL reconstruction. *International Journal of Sports Physical Therapy, 6*(1), 27–44.

Maeo, S., Shan, X., Otsuka, S., Kanehisa, H., & Kawakami, Y. (2018). Neuromuscular adaptations to work-matched maximal eccentric versus concentric training. *Medicine & Science in Sports & Exercise, 50*(8), 1629–1640. https://doi.org/10.1249/MSS.0000000000001611

Mennell, J. M. (1964). *Joint pain: Diagnosis and treatment using manipulative techniques.* Little Brown & Co.

Mirzaie, G., Kajbafvala, M., Rahimi, A., Manshadi, F. D., & Kalantari, K. K. (2016). Altered hip mechanics and patellofemoral pain. A review of literature. *Ortopedia, Traumatologia, Rehabilitacja, 18*(3), 215–221.

Prasartwuth, O., Suteebut, R., Chawawisuttikool, J., Yavuz, U. S., & Turker, K. S. (2019). Using first bout effect to study the mechanisms underlying eccentric exercise induced force loss. *Journal of Bodywork and Movement Therapies, 23*(1), 48–53. https://doi.org/10.1016/j.jbmt.2017.11.008

Reidy, P. T., Lindsay, C. C., McKenzie, A. I., Fry, C. S., Supiano, M. A., Marcus, R. L., LaStayo, P. C., & Drummond, M. J. (2018, July). Aging-related effects of bed rest followed by eccentric exercise rehabilitation on skeletal muscle macrophages and insulin sensitivity. *Experimental Gerontology, 107*, 37–49. https://doi.org/10.1016/j.exger.2017.07.001

Roig, M., O'Brien, K., Kirk, G., Murray, R., McKinnon, P., Shadgan, B., & Reid, W. D. (2009). The effects of eccentric versus concentric resistance training on muscle strength and mass in healthy adults: A systematic review with meta-analysis. *British Journal of Sports Medicine, 43*(8), 556–568. https://doi.org/10.1136/bjsm.2008.051417

Schoenfeld, B. J., Contreras, B., Tiryaki-Sonmez, G., Willardson, J. M., & Fontana, F. (2014). An electromyographic comparison of a modified version of the plank with a long lever and posterior tilt versus the traditional plank exercise. *Sports Biomechanics, 13*(3), 296–306. https:doi.org/10.1080/14763141.2014.942355

Shadle, I. B., & Cacolice, P. A. (2017). Eccentric exercises reduce hamstring strains in elite adult male soccer players: A critically appraised topic. *Journal of Sport Rehabilitation, 26*(6), 573–577. https://doi.org/10.1123/jsr.2015-0196

Tyler, T. F., Schmitt, B. M., Nicholas, S. J., & McHugh, M. P. (2017). Rehabilitation after hamstring-strain injury emphasizing eccentric strengthening at long muscle lengths: Results of long-term follow-up. *Journal of Sport Rehabilitation, 26*(2), 131–140. https://doi.org/10.1123/jsr.2015-0099

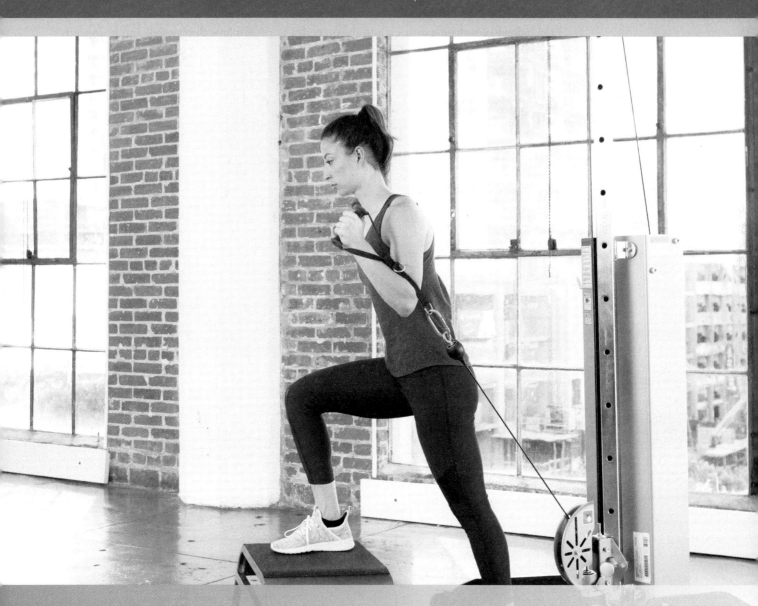

CHAPTER 6

Integration Techniques

Learning Objectives

After reading this content, students should be able to demonstrate the following objectives:

- **Explain** the function of integration techniques in a corrective exercise program.
- **Identify** integration techniques for use in corrective exercise programming.
- **Describe** the application guidelines for integration techniques.

Introduction

The fourth and final phase of the Corrective Exercise Continuum culminates with integration techniques (**Figure 6-1**). Integration techniques are used to reeducate the human movement system (HMS) back into a functional synergistic movement pattern. The use of multiple joint actions and multiple muscle synergies helps to reestablish neuromuscular control, promoting coordinated movement among the involved muscles. The first three phases of the Corrective Exercise Continuum are similar to pulling out individual instruments of an orchestra to work on the reeducation and refinement of individual performances. The fourth phase of the model adds the individual instruments back into the orchestra to relearn how to play well and in concert with others as a single integrated unit.

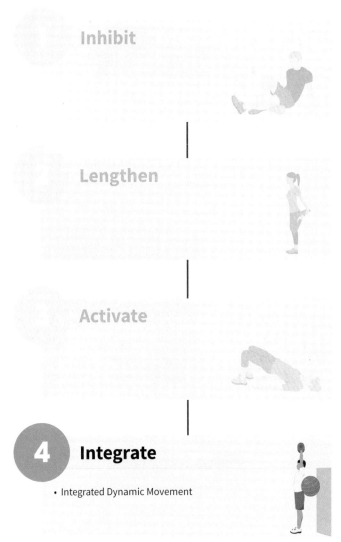

Figure 6-1   Corrective Exercise Continuum—integrate

During the client intake and assessment process, the Corrective Exercise Specialist receives valuable information about the client's goals and needs. Perhaps the client's goal is to increase sprint speed but, during the assessment, poor lower extremity mechanics are identified. Although the ultimate goal is still to help increase sprinting speed, initially sprint training may be limited, with the focus on establishing structural integrity and neuromuscular efficiency.

The initial three phases of the Corrective Exercise Continuum provide attention to individual muscles; the integrated portion of the model focuses on refinement of coordinated movement patterns where degrees of freedom are controlled. Movement efficiency is initially practiced with limited resistance, slower tempos, and high repetitions so that the client can modify and rehearse quality movement before progressing complexity or velocity.

Integrated Dynamic Movement

Once the appropriate muscles have been inhibited and lengthened and others have been activated via preferential isolated strengthening, integration techniques can be performed through the use of integrated dynamic movement. Integrated dynamic movement involves the use of dynamic total-body exercises where the lower body, lumbo-pelvic-hip complex (LPHC), and upper body each have coordinated responsibilities. Collectively, integrated dynamic movement enhances the functional capacity of the HMS by increasing multiplanar neuromuscular control. This is achieved by using exercises that focus on the synergistic function of agonists, antagonists, synergists, stabilizers, and neutralizer muscles during movement. The remainder of this chapter will review the scientific rationale for integrated dynamic movement and provide application guidelines for integrated dynamic movement exercises.

Scientific Rationale for Integrated Dynamic Movement

Focused movements in a controlled setting provide practice and rehearsal for the ability to eccentrically decelerate, stabilize, and concentrically accelerate movement. As performance and neuromuscular control improve over time, integrated movements change with more progressive dynamics such as added speed, resistance, impact forces, and multivariant and directional patterns. It is suggested that some lower extremity injuries occur in relation to poor eccentric control (deceleration) of the hip, knee, and trunk in the frontal and transverse planes resulting from hip musculature weakness (Boling & Padua, 2013). Integrated exercise focuses on initially practicing eccentric deceleration slowly so that adjustments can be made. During the eccentric phase, more strength gains are made compared to concentric muscle actions in isolation (Gois et al., 2014; Maeo et al., 2018; Roig et al., 2008), but also where most muscle damage, inflammation, impaired muscle function, and muscular soreness occurs; hence, the limited number of sets, especially for the newer exerciser (Ives et al., 2017).

As a reminder, during movement, the agonists are the prime movers of a specific joint action regardless of concentric or eccentric muscle action. For instance, the pectoralis major is the primary concentric mover in shoulder horizontal adduction during a chest pressing movement. The same muscle is also the primary decelerator of the eccentric portion of a chest press. Synergists support the agonist. Antagonists are the opposing muscles of a specific joint action. Stabilizers are the muscles that limit or cease undesirable action of the fixed attachment of the muscle. Neutralizers limit or cease the undesirable action of the mobile attachment site of the muscle. All of these primary functions of muscles throughout the muscle action spectrum of the HMS during total-body integrated exercise are called on to provide and control degrees of freedom to obtain neuromuscular efficiency and optimization of human movement.

Challenges to the HMS come in a variety of ways. Multijoint motions are often used because they promote and require greater **intermuscular coordination** to achieve the desired outcome (Enoka, 2015). Intermuscular coordination is the ability of different muscles in the body to work together to allow coordination of global and refined movements. Both unilateral and bilateral exercises are effective at increasing performance measures, and unilateral exercise has a

Intermuscular coordination

The ability of different muscles in the body to work together to allow coordination of global and refined movements.

greater influence on unilateral performance (McCurdy et al., 2005). Interestingly, the strengthening of one side unilaterally can also increase the strength of the contralateral limb (Manca et al., 2017). Though there are many applications of this, it may make sense to exercise the dominant limb first as a primer to better prepare the nondominant limb for recruitment, if applicable for the client or athlete. Overhead (often used in integrated dynamic movements), standing, and unilateral and bilateral exercises place increased stress on the core musculature (Saeterbakken & Fimland, 2012). For example, unilateral chest press exercises have a greater influence on core muscular recruitment (Bray et al., 2010). When dynamic exercises implement upper and lower body, unilateral and bilateral exercises, the core musculature integrates upper/lower and right/left, allowing for extensive overall intermuscular coordination.

Multijoint exercises in all planes of motion from both bilateral and unilateral stances help increase intermuscular coordination and reeducate the neuromuscular system to maintain proper postural alignment during functional activity. Thus, the objective of integrated dynamic movements is to promote high levels of intermuscular coordination (neuromuscular efficiency) in a progressive manner to align with a client's functional needs. By doing this, postural control is reestablished and resistance to injury is increased.

Integrated dynamic movement involves low load and controlled movement in ideal posture. This ensures that joints start and remain in proper alignment, muscles function in their proper length-tension relationships, and synergistic muscle recruitment is optimal. Integration techniques may also be a primer exercise for more-advanced exercise programming later in the workout. An example of integrated dynamic movement may include a ball squat with an overhead press (**Figure 6-2**).

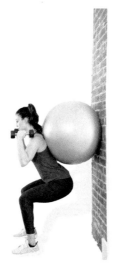 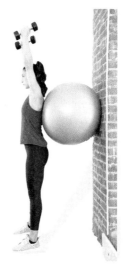

Figure 6-2A Ball squat with overhead press—start

Figure 6-2B Ball squat with overhead press—finish

The importance of integrated dynamic movement lies not just in the movement patterns themselves, but in the progression of the movement patterns as well. For example, a base exercise would consist of a two-legged exercise with minimal challenge to stability (i.e., dumbbell squat). Progression from here would be to an alternating or staggered stance exercise (i.e., step-up), and then progress to a lunge and then to a single-leg base of support exercise (i.e., single-leg squat) to more dynamic movements (such as hopping) (**Figures 6-3** through **6-5**). This progression can be performed first in the sagittal plane and then progress to the frontal (side to side) and transverse (rotation) planes. The incorporation of upper body movement, plane of motion, and challenge to stability can also be added.

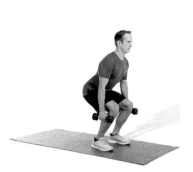

Figure 6-3 Sample integrated dynamic movement progression—two leg

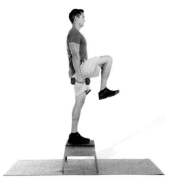

Figure 6-4 Sample integrated dynamic movement progression—alternating leg

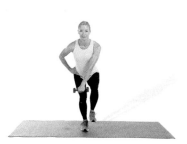

Figure 6-5 Sample integrated dynamic movement progression—single leg

 GETTING TECHNICAL

The Use of Resistance Training Exercises in Unstable Environments
Many tools are available that provide unstable surfaces on which to perform exercises, such as half foam rollers, wobble boards, soft mats, and air-filled bladders. Research shows that these are not ideal for producing strength or power, but they may be indicated for increasing motor control via coactivations and anticipatory postural adjustments. The increase in antagonistic cocontractions may help to increase joint stiffness and has a place in low-back discomfort and other rehabilitative applications (Behm & Colado, 2012). A meta-analysis by Behm et al. (2015) showed varied training outcomes based on age as a result of exercising in unstable environments. Adolescents and young adults experienced different improvements in strength, strength endurance, and power. In contrast, older adults experienced the greatest improvements in static and dynamic balance. While unstable environments should not be the primary means to produce high levels of strength or power, they may be beneficial in supporting various training outcomes for multiple populations; assuming the client qualifies to perform them.

Application Guidelines for Integration Techniques

Once the first three components of the Corrective Exercise Continuum have been implemented to focus on increased ROM and to strengthen isolated musculature to provide strength to the newly achieved ROM, an integrated movement pattern is implemented. This implementation allows the upper body, the LPHC, and lower body to work together to practice movement efficiency and support motor learning and control. If the compensation only shows lower extremity dysfunction, it is still important to practice a total-body integrated movement so that this area practices moving well with other parts of the body. The same is true for the upper extremity or the LPHC. All areas of movement compensation should follow the Corrective Exercise Continuum to help optimize movement efficiency throughout the entire system.

Precautions and Contraindications

Precautions and contraindications for integrated dynamic movement exercises follow the same general guidelines for all exercise and can be seen in **Table 6-1**. Again, it is important to perform an assessment for each client before integrated dynamic movement exercises to ensure that the exercises selected are appropriate and safe.

TABLE 6-1 Precautions and Contraindications for Integrated Dynamic Movement	
Precautions	**Contraindications**
■ Special populations ■ Neuromuscular disorders	■ Acute injury or muscle strain or tear of the muscle being worked ■ Acute rheumatoid arthritis of the affected joint ■ Position of exercise (prone, supine, or decline position) relative to the client's condition (pregnancy, coronary heart disease, etc.) ■ Acute injury to joint involved during movement ■ Pain

Integration Considerations for the Lower Extremities

Jumping tasks may be used as lower body integration phase progressions. It is important that clients are prepared to exhibit neuromuscular control at varying speeds in multiple planes. However, not all individuals will have the physical capabilities to perform many of the jump task progressions during this phase of their corrective program. The Corrective Exercise Specialist may need to modify the integrative movements to accommodate the client and ensure safety. This section provides suggestions for functional movement progressions for clients who do not initially qualify for jumping activities and/or want to work toward them, along with coaching suggestions to improve performance.

Functional Movement Progressions

For clients who cannot participate in jumping exercises, a basic functional movement progression that incorporates total-body exercises in multiple planes can be used as integrated dynamic movements. This progression could begin with ball squats, then to step-ups, then to lunges, then to single-leg squats (from more stable/less dynamic to more unstable/more dynamic). For each exercise, it will be important to cue the individual to keep the knee(s) in line with the toes and to not allow the knee to move medially or laterally relative to the foot to ensure proper arthrokinematics and neuromuscular control.

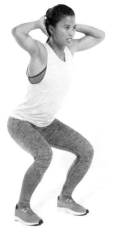

Squatting

Step-up

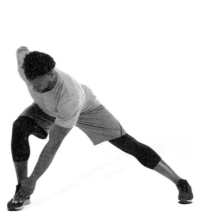

Lunging

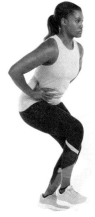

Single-leg squatting

Lower Extremity Progressions and Neuromusculoskeletal Control

Neuromusculoskeletal control imbalances are often evident in clients during athletic movements that include **ligament dominance**, **quadriceps dominance**, and **leg dominance** (Hewett & Bates, 2017; Padua et al., 2018). These terms encompass lower extremity movement observations resulting from instability, poor control, and/or recruitment asymmetries. Many movement types can be used to reinforce proper integration of the foot and ankle, knee, and LPHC, starting from training the athletic position and progressing through multiple jumping tasks to cutting maneuvers.

To target ligament dominance deficits, the fitness professional should instruct the individual to visualize and guide the knee as a single-plane (sagittal) hinge joint allowing flexion and extension, not valgus (medial displacement) and varus (lateral displacement) motion (Hewett & Bates, 2017; Padua et al., 2018). They should also use training movements that will facilitate both identification and correction of unwanted knee motions in the frontal plane.

Teaching dynamic control of knee motion in the sagittal plane may be achieved through progressive exercises that challenge the neuromusculoskeletal system (Hewett & Bates, 2017; Padua et al., 2018). To target the deficits described as ligament dominance, the fitness professional must first make the individual aware of proper form and technique as well as undesirable and potentially dangerous positions as identified in **Table 6-2**. To achieve this awareness, individuals can be video recorded using a tablet, smartphone camera, or another recording device, or placed in front of a mirror to improve their awareness of undesirable medial/lateral knee alignments during movement (Hewett & Bates, 2017; Padua et al., 2018; Taylor et al., 2017). Second, the health and fitness professional must be diligent in providing adequate feedback of correct technical performance to facilitate the desirable neuromusculoskeletal alterations. If inadequate or inappropriate feedback is provided, then the client or athlete may be reinforcing improper techniques while training (Hewett & Bates, 2017; Padua et al., 2018; Taylor et al., 2017).

Ligament dominance

Decreased lower extremity frontal plane stability, usually evidenced by valgus and varus positioning, causing connective tissues to be the limiting factor of end range of motion control.

Quadriceps dominance

Decreased strength or recruitment of the posterior chain musculature relative to anterior chain musculature.

Leg dominance

Limb-to-limb asymmetries in neuromusculoskeletal control or muscle recruitment.

TABLE 6-2 Neuromusculoskeletal Control Imbalances and Verbal Feedback

Imbalance	Verbal Cueing Suggestions
Ligament dominance: valgus, varus	▪ "Keep your knees in line with your second and third toes of your feet."
Knee (quadriceps) dominance	▪ "Bend your knees and hips as you land." ▪ "Keep your knees in line with your second and third toes." ▪ "Soft landing/feet." ▪ "Absorb your landing with your hips."
Leg dominance	▪ "Maintain equal weight on both legs as you land." ▪ "Have your feet touch down softly at the same time when landing."

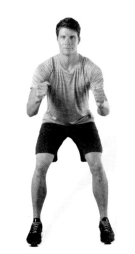

Figure 6-6 Athletic position

ATHLETIC POSITION

Before teaching dynamic movement exercises, individuals should be shown the proper athletic position. The athletic position is a functionally stable position with the knees comfortably flexed, shoulders back, eyes up, feet approximately shoulder-width apart, and the body mass balanced over the balls of the feet. The knees should be over the balls of the feet and the chest should be over the knees (Hewett et al., 1996; Myer et al., 2004). This is the individual's ready position and should be considered the functional starting and finishing position for most jumping tasks required during athletic performance (**Figure 6-6**).

WALL JUMPS

Wall jumps are an example of an integrated dynamic movement exercise that could be used to target ligament dominance deficits. This low-to-moderate intensity jump movement allows the fitness professional to begin analysis of the athlete's degree of valgus or varus motion in the knee (Myer et al., 2005). During wall jumps, the individual does not go through deep knee flexion angles, with most of the vertical movement provided by active ankle plantar flexion (Myer et al., 2005). The relatively straight knee makes even slight amounts of medial knee motion easy to identify. When medial knee motion is observed, the fitness professional should begin to give verbal feedback cues to the individual during this low-to-moderate intensity exercise. This feedback allows the athlete to cognitively process the proper knee motion required to perform the exercise. Neuromusculoskeletal control of medial knee motion is critical when landing with knee angles close to full extension as this is a commonly reported mechanism of injury (Lopes et al., 2018).

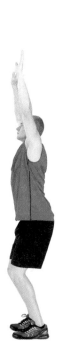

Wall jumps—start
© Courtesy of National Academy of Sports Medicine

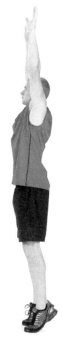

Wall jumps—finish
© Courtesy of National Academy of Sports Medicine

TUCK JUMP

Another useful exercise to target the ligament-dominant athlete is the tuck jump. Although sometimes used as an assessment, the tuck jump can also be used as an exercise that is on the opposite end of the intensity spectrum from the wall jump and requires a high effort level from the individual. During the tuck jump exercise, the fitness professional can quickly identify an individual who may demonstrate abnormal levels of frontal plane knee displacement during jumping and landing because the individual usually devotes minimal attention to technique on the first few repetitions (Myer et al., 2005; Stroube et al., 2013).

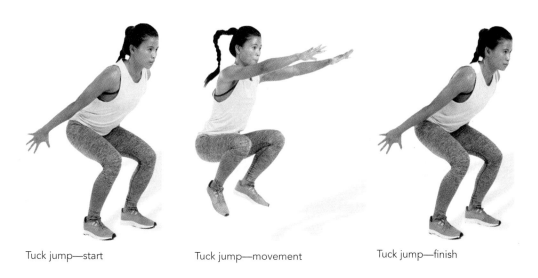

Tuck jump—start   Tuck jump—movement   Tuck jump—finish

HORIZONTAL JUMP TEST

The horizontal jump test exercise (also called a long jump with a double-leg stance) allows the fitness professional to assess the individual's knee motion while they progress through movements in the sagittal plane. The achievement of dynamic knee control during tasks performed in all planes of movement is critical to address deficits that may transfer into competitive sports participation or everyday activities. During competition, athletes may display "dynamic valgus," a position of hip adduction, tibial external rotation, and ankle eversion that is the result of muscular actions rather than ground reaction forces (Hewett et al., 2005; Myer et al., 2005). The horizontal jump is a moderate-intensity integrated, dynamic movement exercise that can provide another opportunity for the fitness professional to assess active valgus and provide feedback on more desirable techniques that can assist the individual's cognitive recognition during each jump to perfect technique. When performing the horizontal jump, individuals may

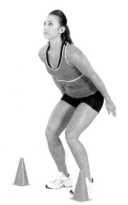

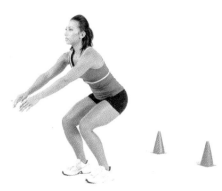

Horizontal jump test—start
© Courtesy of National Academy of Sports Medicine

Horizontal jump test—finish
© Courtesy of National Academy of Sports Medicine

demonstrate dynamic valgus when taking off from a jump rather than landing. This movement deficit should be identified and corrected during training. In addition, individuals should be instructed to hold the landing (stabilize) for 5 seconds, which forces the individual to gain and maintain dynamic knee control for a more prolonged period (Myer et al., 2005). The prolonged deep hold may facilitate feedback-driven lower extremity alignment adjustments and ultimately improve frontal plane alignment of the knee.

180-DEGREE JUMP

The 180-degree jump is an integrated dynamic movement exercise that is incorporated into dynamic movement training to teach dynamic body and lower-extremity control while the body is rotating in the transverse plane. The rotational forces created by the 180-degree jump must be quickly absorbed and redirected in the opposite direction (Myer et al., 2005). This movement is important to teach the individual to recognize and control dangerous rotational forces that can improve body awareness and control, which will reduce injury risk and also improve measures of performance (Lopes et al., 2018; Padua et al., 2018).

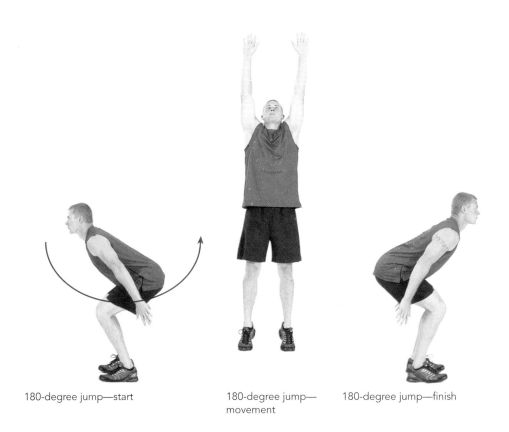

180-degree jump—start

180-degree jump—movement

180-degree jump—finish

SINGLE-LEG HORIZONTAL JUMP TEST

Once the individual has been trained to maintain appropriate knee alignment during the jump, land, and hold of the long-jump exercise with double-leg stance, the single-leg hop and hold exercise can be incorporated into the training. Most noncontact ACL injuries occur when landing or decelerating on a single limb (Ford et al., 2006; Lopes et al., 2018; Myer et al., 2013; Paterno et al., 2010; Stroube et al., 2013; Taylor et al., 2017). The single-leg hop and hold exercise roughly mimics a mechanism of an ACL injury during competitive play (Myer et al., 2005). When initiating the single-leg hop and hold exercise, the individual should be instructed to jump only a few inches and land with deep knee flexion. As they master the low-intensity jumps, the distance can be progressively increased, as long as they can continue to maintain deep knee flexion when landing and control unwanted frontal plane motion at the knee. Proper progression into the single-leg hop and hold is critical to ensure athlete safety during training. This point is salient for the health and fitness professional, because ACL injury risk reduction techniques should not introduce inappropriate risk of injury during training.

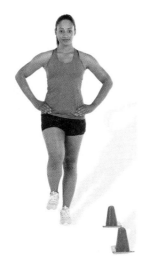 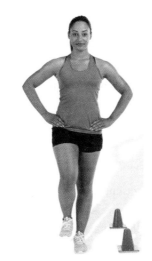

Single-leg horizontal jump test—start   Single-leg horizontal jump test—finish

CUTTING MANEUVERS

The end stages of training targeted toward ligament-dominance deficits are achieved through the use of unanticipated cutting movements. Before teaching unanticipated cutting, individuals should first be able to attain proper athletic position proficiently. This ready position is the goal position to achieve before initiating a directional cut. Adding the directional cues to the unanticipated part of training can be as simple as pointing or as sports specific as using partner mimic or ball retrieval drills (Hewett et al., 2005; Myer et al., 2005).

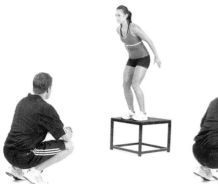 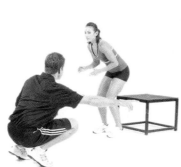 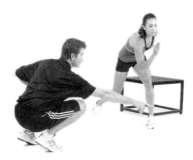

Cutting maneuvers—start   Cutting maneuvers—movement   Cutting maneuvers—finish

Single-faceted sagittal plane training and conditioning protocols that do not incorporate cutting maneuvers will not provide similar levels of external varus or valgus or rotational loads that are seen during sport-specific cutting maneuvers. Training programs that incorporate safe levels of lateral control may induce more muscle-dominant neuromusculoskeletal adaptations. Such adaptations may prepare the individual for the multidirectional movement demands that occur during sport competition, which can improve performance and reduce risk of lower-extremity injury (Ford et al., 2006; Hewett et al., 2006; Lopes et al., 2018; Myer et al., 2005, 2008; Paterno et al., 2010; Stroube et al., 2013; Taylor et al., 2017).

Recent evidence demonstrates that training that incorporates unanticipated movements can reduce lower-extremity injury risk. Additionally, training individuals to preactivate their musculature before landing may facilitate **kinematic adjustments** (Hewett & Bates, 2017; Kajiwara et al., 2019; Padua et al., 2018). Training the individual to use safe cutting techniques in unanticipated sport situations or everyday activities may also help impart technique adaptations that will integrate into the client's competitive movements during sport competition or during daily living activities. If naturally ligament-dominant individuals achieve muscular-dominant movement strategies, their future risk of ACL and other knee injuries will likely be reduced (Hewett & Bates, 2017; Kajiwara et al., 2019; Padua et al., 2018).

Kinematic adjustments

Small alterations in movement pattern execution made in response to repetitive or novel performance conditions.

Acute Training Variables

Training variables for integrated dynamic movement can be seen in **Table 6-3** (Voight & Cook, 2007). These exercises can be safely performed anywhere from 3 to 5 days per week depending on the intensity and volume used. Generally, only one integrated dynamic movement is necessary, although others can be incorporated, if desired. For example, if using corrective exercise as part of movement prep, one integrated exercise should suffice. However, if developing a corrective exercise session as a full workout, three to four integrated exercises, performed for up to three sets, may be warranted.

TABLE 6-3 Acute Training Variables for Integrated Dynamic Movement

Frequency	Sets	Repetitions	Duration of Rep
3 to 5 days per week	1 to 3	10 to 15	Controlled

Integrated Dynamic Movement Exercises

Almost any exercise requiring multijoint control and activity may be considered an integrated dynamic movement. The Corrective Exercise Specialist will take multiple factors into account when selecting exercises, such as client goals, preferences, current movement compensations, and workout objectives. The individual's physical capabilities should also be taken into consideration when selecting an integrated dynamic movement. While by no means an exhaustive list, the exercises shown provide examples of integrated dynamic movements.

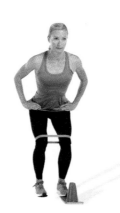

Lateral tube walking—start

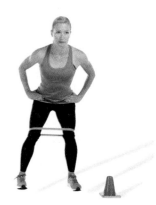

Lateral tube walking—movement

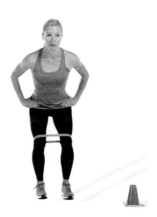

Lateral tube walking—finish

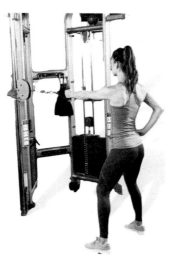

Single-arm row to arrow position—start

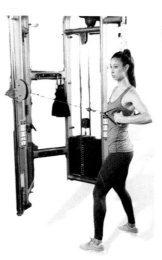

Single-arm row to arrow position—finish

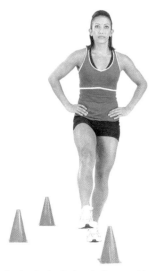

Sagittal: single-leg balance with multiplanar reach

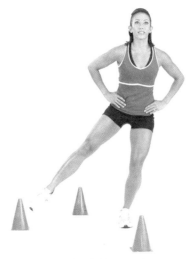

Frontal: single-leg balance with multiplanar reach

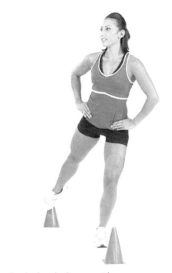

Transverse: single-leg balance with multiplanar reach

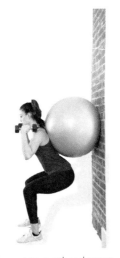

Ball squat to overhead press—start

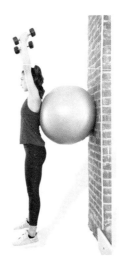

Ball squat to overhead press—finish

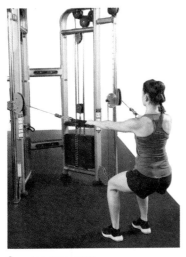

Squat to row—start

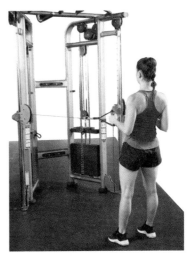

Squat to row—finish

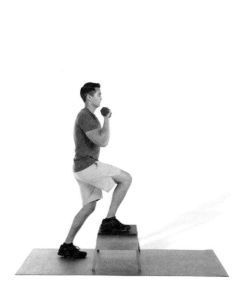
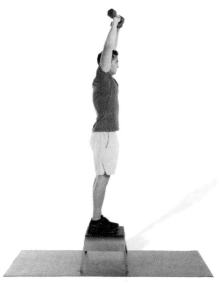

Step up to overhead press—start

Step up to overhead press—finish

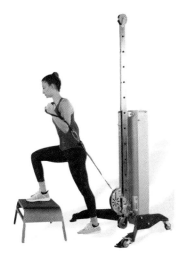
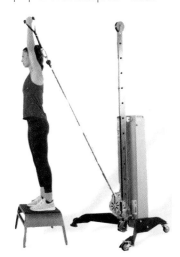

Step up with cable press—start

Step up with cable press—finish

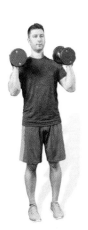
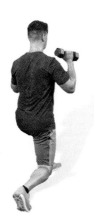
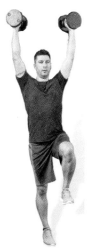

Transverse lunge to overhead press—start

Transverse lunge to overhead press—movement

Transverse lunge to overhead press—finish

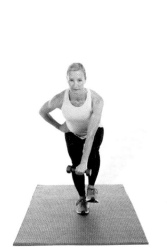
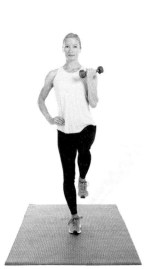
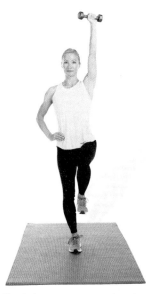

Single-leg squat to overhead press—start

Single-leg squat to overhead press—movement

Single-leg squat to overhead press—finish

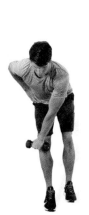
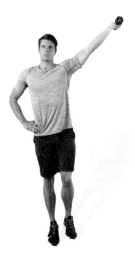

Single-leg Romanian deadlift to PNF pattern—start

Single-leg Romanian deadlift to PNF pattern—finish

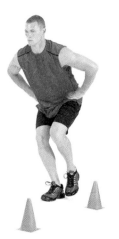
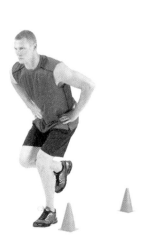

Hop with stabilization—start

Hop with stabilization—finish

SUMMARY

The integration phase completes the Corrective Exercise Continuum. This chapter offers the rationale, peer-reviewed support, and descriptions of various techniques to address the reintegration of muscles once reeducation has been performed. This optimizes synergistic and functional movement patterns and completes a comprehensive program for both corrective exercise and preparation of more advanced training models such as the NASM OPT® Model. The Corrective Exercise Continuum can be used by Corrective Exercise Specialists to provide greater value to their current training clients as well as increase marketability to a larger prospect base in general. The repeatability of this continuum allows for one system to be utilized with great success with many different body types, goals, and skill and activity levels. The model is simple, but its application will require a deeper understanding of assessment and functional anatomy. It will require patience and practice for new users to optimize its utility, but the outcomes are worth any possible challenges to implementation.

REFERENCES

Behm, D., & Colado, J. C. (2012). The effectiveness of resistance training using unstable surfaces and devices for rehabilitation. *International Journal of Sports Physical Therapy, 7*(2), 226–241.

Behm, D. G., Muehlbauer, T., Kibele, A., & Granacher, U. (2015). Effects of strength training using unstable surfaces on strength, power and balance performance across the lifespan: A systematic review and meta-analysis. *Sports Medicine, 45*(12), 1645–1669. https://doi.org/10.1007/s40279-015-0384-x

Boling, M., & Padua, D. (January 01, 2013). Relationship between hip strength and trunk, hip, and knee kinematics during a jump-landing task in individuals with patellofemoral pain. *International Journal of Sports Physical Therapy, 8*(5), 661–669.

Bray, W. P., Lake, J. P., & Shorter, K. (2010). Can muscle activation be increased when modifying the dumbbell chest press? An electromyographic comparison. *International Symposium on Biomechanics in Sports: Conference Proceedings Archive, 28*, 1–2. https://ojs.ub.uni-konstanz.de/cpa/article/view/4595

Enoka, R. M. (2015). *Neuromechanics of human movement* (5th ed.). Human Kinetics.

Ford, K. R., Myer G. D., Smith, R. L., Vianello, R. M., Seiwert, S. L., & Hewett, T. E. (2006). A comparison of dynamic coronal plane excursion between matched male and female athletes when performing single leg landings. *Clinical Biomechanics, 21*(1), 33–40.

Gois, M. O., Campoy, F. A., Alves, T., Ávila, R. P., Vanderlei, L. C., & Pastre, C. M. (2014). The influence of resistance exercise with emphasis on specific contractions (concentric vs. eccentric) on muscle strength and post-exercise autonomic modulation: A randomized clinical trial. *Brazilian Journal of Physical Therapy, 18*(1), 30–37. https://doi.org/10.1590/s1413-35552012005000141

Hewett, T. E., & Bates, N. A. (2017). Preventive biomechanics: A paradigm shift with a translational approach to biomechanics.

American Journal of Sports Medicine, 45(11), 2654–2664. https://doi.org/10.1177/0363546516686080

Hewett, T. E., Ford, K. R., & Myer, G. D. (2006). Anterior cruciate ligament injuries in female athletes: Part 2, A meta-analysis of neuromuscular interventions aimed at injury prevention. *American Journal of Sports Medicine, 34*(3), 490–498.

Hewett, T. E., Myer, G. D., Ford, K. R., Heidt, R. S., Colosimo, A. J., McLean, S. G., van den Bogert, A. J., Paterno, M. V., & Succop, P. (2005). Biomechanical measures of neuromuscular control and valgus loading of the knee predict anterior cruciate ligament injury risk in female athletes: A prospective study. *American Journal of Sports Medicine, 33*(4), 492–501. 10.1177/0363546504269591

Hewett, T. E., Stroupe, A. L., Nance., T. A., & Noyes, F. R. (1996). Plyometric training in female athletes: Decreased impact forces and increased hamstring torques. *American Journal of Sports Medicine, 24*(6), 765–773.

Ives, S. J., Bloom, S., Matias, A., Morrow, N., Martins, N., Roh, Y., Ebenstein, D., O'Brien, G., Escudero, D., Brito, K., Glickman, L., Connelly, S., & Arciero, P. J. (2017). Effects of a combined protein and antioxidant supplement on recovery of muscle function and soreness following eccentric exercise. *Journal of the International Society of Sports Nutrition, 14*, 21. https://doi.org/10.1186/s12970-017-0179-6

Kajiwara, M., Kanamori, A., Kadone, H., Endo, Y., Kobayashi, Y., Hyodo, K., Takahashi, T., Arai, N., Taniguchi, Y., Yoshioka, T., & Yamazaki, M. (2019). Knee biomechanics changes under dual task during single-leg drop landing. *Journal of Experimental Orthopaedics, 6*(1).

Lopes, T. J. A., Ferrari, D., Ioannidis, J., Simic, M., Mícolis de Azevedo, F., & Pappas, E. (2018). Reliability and validity of frontal plane kinematics of the trunk and lower extremity measured with 2-dimensional cameras during athletic tasks: A systematic review with meta-analysis. *The Journal of Orthopaedic and Sports Physical Ther apy, 48*(10), 812–822. https://doi.org/10.2519/jospt.2018.8006

Maeo, S., Shan, X., Otsuka, S., Kanehisa, H., & Kawakami, Y. (2018). Neuromuscular adaptations to work-matched maximal eccentric versus concentric training. *Medicine & Science in Sports & Exercise, 50*(8), 1629–1640. https://doi.org/10.1249/mss.0000000000001611

Manca, A., Dragone, D., Dvir, Z., & Deriu, F. (2017). Cross-education of muscular strength following unilateral resistance training: A meta-analysis. *European Journal of Applied Physiology, 117*(11), 2335–2354. https://doi.org/10.1007/s00421-017-3720-z

McCurdy, K. W., Langford, G. A., Doscher, M. W., Wiley, L. P., & Mallard, K. G. (2005). The effects of short-term unilateral and bi-lateral lower-body resistance training on measures of strength and power. *Journal of Strength and Conditioning Research, 19*(1), 9–15. https://doi.org/10.1519/14173.1

Myer, G. D., Ford, K. R., & Hewett, T. E. (2004). Rationale and clinical techniques for anterior cruciate ligament injury prevention among female athletes. *Journal of Athletic Training, 39*(4), 352–364.

Myer, G. D., Ford, K. R., Palumbo, J. P., & Hewett, T. E. (2005). Neuromuscular training improves performance and lower-extremity biomechanics in female athletes. *Journal of Strength and Conditioning Research, 19*(1), 51–60.

Myer, G. D., Paterno M. V., Ford, K. R., Hewett, T.E. (2008). Neuromuscular training techniques to target deficits before return to sport after anterior cruciate ligament reconstruction. *Journal of Strength and Conditioning Research, 22*(3), 987–1014.

Myer, G. D., Stroube, B. W., DiCesare, C. A., Brent, J. L., Ford, K. R., Heidt, R. S. J., & Hewett, T. E. (2013). Augmented feedback supports skill transfer and reduces high-risk injury landing mechanics: A double-blind, randomized controlled laboratory study. *American Journal of Sports Medicine, 41*(3), 669–677.

Padua, D. A., DiStefano, L. J., Hewett, T. E., Garrett, W. E., Marshall, S. W., Golden, G. M., Shultz, S. J., & Sigward, S. M. (2018). National Athletic Trainers' Association position statement: Prevention of anterior cruciate ligament injury. *Journal of Athletic Training, 53*(1), 5–19. https://doi.org/10.4085/1062-6050-99-16

Roig, M., Obrien, K., Kirk, G., Murray, R., Mckinnon, P., Shadgan, B., & Reid, W. D. (2008). The effects of eccentric versus concentric resistance training on muscle strength and mass in healthy adults: A systematic review with meta-analysis. *British Journal of Sports Medicine, 43*(8), 556–568. https://doi.org/10.1136/bjsm.2008.051417

Saeterbakken, A. H., & Fimland, M. S. (2012). Muscle activity of the core during bilateral, unilateral, seated and standing resistance exercise. *European Journal of Applied Physiology, 112*(5), 1671–1678. https://doi.org/10.1007/s00421-011-2141-7

Stroube, B. W., Myer, G. D., Brent, J. L., Ford, K. R., Heidt, R. S., & Hewett, T. E. (January 01, 2013). Effects of task-specific augmented feedback on deficit modification during performance of the tuck-jump exercise. *Journal of Sport Rehabilitation, 22*(1), 7–18.

Taylor, J. B., Nguyen, A. D., Paterno, M. V., Huang, B., & Ford, K. R. (2017). Real-time optimized biofeedback utilizing sport techniques (ROBUST): A study protocol for a randomized controlled trial. *BMC Musculoskeletal Disorders, 18*(1), 71. https://doi.org/10.1186/s12891-017-1436-1

Voight, M. L., & Cook, G. (2007). Impaired neuromuscular control: Reactive neuromuscular training. In M. L. Voight, B. J. Hoogenboom, & W. E. Prentice (Eds.), *Muscular skeletal interventions: Techniques for therapeutic exercise* (pp. 181–214). McGraw-Hill.

SECTION 3

Client Assessment

CHAPTER 7

Client Intake and Assessment

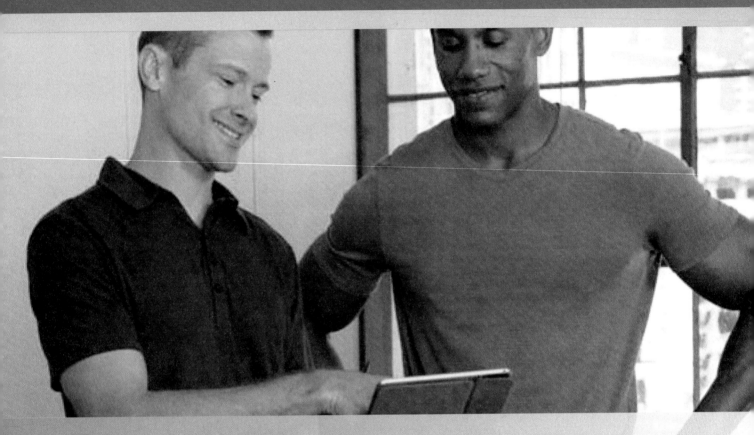

Learning Objectives

After reading this content, students should be able to demonstrate the following objectives:

- **Identify** the various assessments used for corrective exercise programming.
- **Determine** the appropriate assessment strategies based on client type.
- **Describe** client intake procedures.
- **Identify** instances warranting referral to health professionals.
- **Identify** legal and ethical considerations in working with clients.
- **Describe** effective and appropriate coaching and communication strategies during client intake and beyond.

Introduction

The initial session with a client is probably the most critical. During this first encounter, the Corrective Exercise Specialist will conduct several assessments related to physical readiness, general lifestyle information, medical history, goals, and other physical and psychological behaviors. They will also ensure that all legal and ethical forms and procedures are signed and completed.

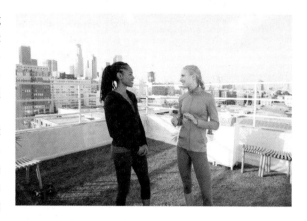

More important, the initial session is the time to build a rapport with the client. This rapport will serve as the backbone for the entire corrective exercise experience. To foster a positive rapport, the client needs to feel as though they are a part of the process, and this should begin prior to starting any assessments. Encouraging the client to become an active participant will build motivation and create new behaviors open to change. Once a mutual bond is developed, the assessment process can begin.

Assessments are crucial in the design of a safe, individualized corrective exercise program and include the client intake screening, static postural assessment, movement assessments, and targeted mobility assessments. Positive communication of this process will help foster client buy-in, creating long-lasting, profitable relationships.

Client Communication

Even after its initial development with the goal of improving muscle balance, the implementation of corrective exercise techniques by industry professionals has varied. Because of this, clients may have a different understanding of what corrective exercise is and who needs it. One of the most critical parts of using corrective exercise with clients is how to effectively communicate the process and its benefits.

The Corrective Exercise Specialist has the responsibility to communicate with empathy from the first meeting with the client to create trust and understanding, which reinforces adherence over time. They need to be clear about the benefits of corrective exercise programming to the individual client (i.e., what's in it for them) and how taking the time to work on optimal movement will impact their results for the better.

In fact, the Corrective Exercise Specialist may even refrain from using the term *corrective exercise* during client conversations, as this may suggest that something is wrong with the client that requires fixing. Many clients make the decision to undertake fitness programs with a set of issues in mind that they already want to improve, thus adding an additional layer of correction can negatively impact their excitement and outlook on the process. Although terminology like *compensation*, *impairment*, and *dysfunction* are well-known to fitness professionals, technical industry terms are not the best words to use with clients.

A discussion on the Corrective Exercise Continuum begins with an explanation of assessments and how they will inform corrective program design. The Corrective Exercise Specialist needs to use common language to explain what each assessment is and to create an environment that is free from judgment. The client needs to understand that before any comprehensive workout plan can be developed, a baseline understanding of how their body prefers to move is needed. Time should also be taken to explain that while seeking ideal movement is important for improvements in function, mobility, and comfort, nobody is perfect. Everyone is looking to improve something, and refining quality of movement should be no more daunting than losing a few pounds or gaining strength.

Static posture

The starting point from which an individual moves.

Dynamic posture

How an individual is able to maintain an erect posture while performing functional tasks or in motion.

Compensatory movement

A nonideal movement strategy employed by the kinetic chain to fulfill the desired movement pattern.

As clients begin their workout plan with integration of the Corrective Exercise Continuum, they should be provided with reminders of why and how the posture-improving program will help them achieve their goals in the safest and most effective manner possible. Corrective Exercise Specialists should communicate to the client that this is done by addressing movement efficiency and recruiting the proper muscles at the proper time. They should also explain that using this format of conditioning (at least in the beginning of the program and for warm-up protocols) decreases the chances the client will overtrain and lays the groundwork for optimal progression through the NASM Optimum Performance Training® (OPT®) model. This can be explained to the client by saying something like the following:

By understanding your body's movement habits and preferences, we can design an individualized movement prep segment for your workouts that ensures the right muscle groups are working at the right time. This maximizes your body's response to exercise, has a positive impact on your results, and helps to keep you safe as you undertake more intense exercises.

Types of Assessments

A number of subjective and objective assessments must be administered before designing a corrective exercise protocol for clients. Each assessment should be conducted in a manner that is efficient and thorough. **Table 7-1** provides a brief overview of each of the key assessment types used by Corrective Exercise Specialists.

TABLE 7-1 Assessment Types

Assessment Type	Description
Client intake screen	The client intake screen is the first step in the overall assessment process. This screen collects valuable subjective information and notes any "red flags" related to physical readiness, general lifestyle, and medical history. This subjective information will provide a first glimpse at potential movement impairments that may come to light later in the assessment process.
Static postural assessment	Static postural assessment is a visual observation of the client's posture when standing still. Proper **static posture** allows for optimal mobility and joint kinematics, whereas poor posture is indicative of either a structural problem or poor musculoskeletal recruitment patterns.
Movement assessments	Movement assessments are designed to evaluate a person's **dynamic posture**, which refers to the structural alignment of the musculoskeletal system when the body is in motion. **Compensatory movement** can be observed through a series of movement assessments such as the overhead squat assessment and other transitional, dynamic, and loaded movement assessments.
Mobility assessments	Mobility assessments are used to identify deficits in joint range of motion and help refine observations discovered in the static and movement assessments used with the client. Human movement requires a combination of soft-tissue flexibility, joint range of motion, and neuromuscular control. Any lack of neuromuscular control or restriction in a body segment's mobility will alter movement patterns and lead to impairments throughout the kinetic chain.

Effective assessments are critical to the corrective exercise programming process. The information gathered from these assessments creates a roadmap for the Corrective Exercise Specialist. In an ideal world, each client would pass each assessment with no red flags noted. In the real world, this is not always the case. Therefore, what is needed to further aid in the programming process is a systematic approach to implementing the assessment process.

The Corrective Exercise Specialist Assessment Flow

The Corrective Exercise Specialist (CES) Assessment Flow is the roadmap for a comprehensive, individualized postural and movement evaluation for each client (**Figure 7-1**). As with all new fitness training clients, the process begins with the client intake screen. Once the client has been cleared to begin formal increased activity, the next step is static assessment to identify structural malalignments. Next, a series of movement assessments is conducted to evaluate the body's alignment during common movement patterns. Then, based on the findings from the static and movement assessments, specific mobility assessments are used to refine the observations and pinpoint which muscles need **inhibition (phase 1), lengthening (phase 2),** and **activation (phase 3)** when working within the Corrective Exercise Continuum.

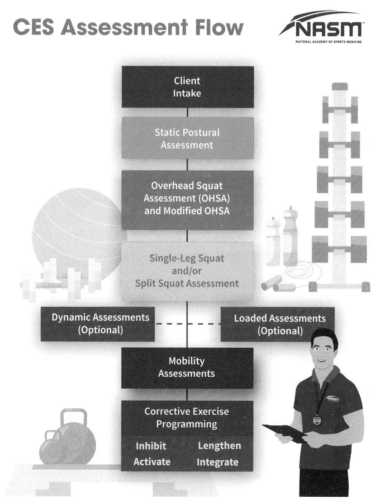

Figure 7-1 CES Assessment Flow

Does the entire assessment flow need to be used with every client? The answer is *maybe*. The assessment process should be individualized and guided by client goals, functional abilities, impairments, and the degree of observed compensations. For some clients, static posture observations and the overhead squat assessment will provide everything needed to effectively design a corrective program. When movement compensations are obvious in these early stage assessments, performing more-advanced tests may bring increased risk. However, other more-advanced clients who present with relatively efficient posture may need to drill down with more difficult tests (e.g., the single-leg squat, depth jump assessment).

This makes it critical to use the CES Assessment Flow to map out the assessment path (static > movement > mobility) for clients based on both what they need *and* what they want to accomplish. The observations from each will provide a guide for what to do next.

Client Intake Screen

The client intake screen is the first step in the client assessment process. It is also the most critical step for earning client buy-in and developing a long-term, profitable relationship. Throughout the initial session, the Corrective Exercise Specialist has many opportunities to build strong rapport while learning about the client.

The client intake screen should be as thorough and detailed as possible. Corrective Exercise Specialists should gather as much information as possible during the initial evaluation of a client to help formulate a clear direction. Key components of a thorough client intake screen include the Physical Activity Readiness Questionnaire (PAR-Q), questions about the client's general lifestyle (e.g., occupation, hobbies, etc.), a review of the client's relevant medical history, and a discussion of the client's health and fitness goals.

The client intake screen (**Figure 7-2**) can be turned into a comprehensive questionnaire and can be completed prior to the client's first visit or in person during the first meeting. Whichever method the professional chooses to implement, it is important to conduct a one-on-one interview with the client during the first appointment to discuss the information gathered, build rapport and personal connection, and outline key components of the assessment process. By doing so, the Corrective Exercise Specialist creates a client-centric environment in which the client is viewed as a key member of the Corrective Exercise Continuum team. This aids in building motivation and a commitment to change for the client.

Readiness for Activity

Physical Activity Readiness Questionnaire for Everyone (PAR-Q+)

Series of questions designed to determine if a person is ready to undertake more strenuous physical activity.

Before any exercise program can start, new clients need to be cleared for physical activity. One of the easiest methods of doing so is to use the **Physical Activity Readiness Questionnaire for Everyone (PAR-Q+)** (**Figure 7-3**; complete form is shown in Appendix B), which was designed to help determine if a person is ready to undertake low-to-moderate-to-high activity levels (Warburton et al., 2014). Furthermore, it aids in identifying people for whom certain activities may not be appropriate or who may need further medical attention.

The PAR-Q+ is directed toward detecting any possible cardiorespiratory dysfunction, such as coronary heart disease, and is a good beginning point for gathering personal background information regarding a client's health status. If the client answers yes to any of the questions on the PAR-Q+, they need to be referred to a qualified medical professional for clearance prior to beginning their exercise regimen. However, the PAR-Q+ is only one component of a thorough

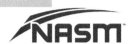

Client Intake Screen

Name _____ Date_____

Occupation

Does your occupation require extended periods of sitting?

YES   NO

Does your occupation require repetitive movements? (If YES, please explain.)
_____

YES   NO

Does your occupation require you to wear shoes with a heel (e.g., dress shoes)?

YES   NO

Does your occupation require heavy lifting?

YES   NO

Does your occupation cause you mental stress?

YES   NO

Lifestyle

Do you have any stressors in your personal life? (If yes, please explain.)
_____

YES   NO

Do you get 8 or more hours of sleep per night? (If no, please explain.)
_____

YES   NO

Do you feel energized throughout the day and prior to activities? (If no, please explain.)
_____

YES   NO

Do you believe you are drinking enough fluids?

YES   NO

Recreation

Do you partake in any recreational physical activities (golf, skiing, etc.)? (If YES, please explain.)
_____

YES   NO

Do you have any additional hobbies (reading, video games, etc.)? (If YES, please explain.)
_____

YES   NO

Medical

Have you ever had an injury to your ankles, knees, back, or shoulders? (If YES, please explain.)
_____

YES   NO

Have you ever had any surgeries? (If YES, please explain.)
_____

YES   NO

Figure 7-2 Client intake screen

client intake screen. While this information is extremely important to ensure safety on the exercise floor, other questions need to be asked to uncover information relating to variables in life that impact a client's posture and movement efficiency. This includes questions about an individual's general lifestyle and medical history.

2020 PAR-Q+

The Physical Activity Readiness Questionnaire for Everyone

The health benefits of regular physical activity are clear; more people should engage in physical activity every day of the week. Participating in physical activity is very safe for MOST people. This questionnaire will tell you whether it is necessary for you to seek further advice from your doctor OR a qualified exercise professional before becoming more physically active.

GENERAL HEALTH QUESTIONS

Please read the 7 questions below carefully and answer each one honestly: check YES or NO.	YES	NO
1) Has your doctor ever said that you have a heart condition ☐ OR high blood pressure ☐?	☐	☐
2) Do you feel pain in your chest at rest, during your daily activities of living, OR when you do physical activity?	☐	☐
3) Do you lose balance because of dizziness OR have you lost consciousness in the last 12 months? Please answer NO if your dizziness was associated with over-breathing (including during vigorous exercise).	☐	☐
4) Have you ever been diagnosed with another chronic medical condition (other than heart disease or high blood pressure)? PLEASE LIST CONDITION(S) HERE: _____	☐	☐
5) Are you currently taking prescribed medications for a chronic medical condition? PLEASE LIST CONDITION(S) AND MEDICATIONS HERE: _____	☐	☐
6) Do you currently have (or have had within the past 12 months) a bone, joint, or soft tissue (muscle, ligament, or tendon) problem that could be made worse by becoming more physically active? Please answer NO if you had a problem in the past, but it does not limit your current ability to be physically active. PLEASE LIST CONDITION(S) HERE: _____	☐	☐
7) Has your doctor ever said that you should only do medically supervised physical activity?	☐	☐

☑ **If you answered NO to all of the questions above, you are cleared for physical activity.**
Please sign the PARTICIPANT DECLARATION. You do not need to complete Pages 2 and 3.

- ▶ Start becoming much more physically active – start slowly and build up gradually.
- ▶ Follow Global Physical Activity Guidelines for your age (https://apps.who.int/iris/handle/10665/44399).
- ▶ You may take part in a health and fitness appraisal.
- ▶ If you are over the age of 45 yr and NOT accustomed to regular vigorous to maximal effort exercise, consult a qualified exercise professional before engaging in this intensity of exercise.
- ▶ If you have any further questions, contact a qualified exercise professional.

PARTICIPANT DECLARATION
If you are less than the legal age required for consent or require the assent of a care provider, your parent, guardian or care provider must also sign this form.

I, the undersigned, have read, understood to my full satisfaction and completed this questionnaire. I acknowledge that this physical activity clearance is valid for a maximum of 12 months from the date it is completed and becomes invalid if my condition changes. I also acknowledge that the community/fitness center may retain a copy of this form for its records. In these instances, it will maintain the confidentiality of the same, complying with applicable law.

NAME _____ DATE _____

SIGNATURE _____ WITNESS _____

SIGNATURE OF PARENT/GUARDIAN/CARE PROVIDER _____

◉ **If you answered YES to one or more of the questions above, COMPLETE PAGES 2 AND 3.**

⚠ **Delay becoming more active if:**

- You have a temporary illness such as a cold or fever; it is best to wait until you feel better.
- You are pregnant - talk to your health care practitioner, your physician, a qualified exercise professional, and/or complete the ePARmed-X+ at www.eparmedx.com before becoming more physically active.
- Your health changes - answer the questions on Pages 2 and 3 of this document and/or talk to your doctor or a qualified exercise professional before continuing with any physical activity program.

Figure 7-3 Opening page of the PAR-Q+
Reprinted with permission from the PAR-Q+ Collaboration (www.eparmedx.com) and the authors of the PAR-Q+ (Dr. Darren Warburton, Dr. Norman Gledhill, Dr. Veronica Jamnik, Dr. Roy Shephard, and Dr. Shannon Bredin)

General Lifestyle Information

Asking some very basic questions concerning an individual's occupation and lifestyle can provide a wealth of information. Aside from cases of acute injury, the majority of compensations seen in the static postural and movement assessments will stem from clients' day-to-day habits as many situations in modern life put the body in chronically compromised positions (e.g., sitting at a desk all day). When the body is chronically kept in a certain position or when the same task is performed repeatedly, it adapts and becomes accustomed to those patterns. By uncovering a client's daily movement patterns (or lack thereof), fitness professionals can pinpoint the habits that may have compromised the client's posture in the first place. Fitness professionals with keen behavior-change coaching skills can then work with clients to help break those habits and support all the hard work being done throughout their fitness program.

OCCUPATION

Knowing a client's occupation can provide the fitness professional with great insight into the client's movement capacity and the kinds of movement patterns that are repeatedly performed throughout the day. By obtaining this information, they can begin to recognize important clues about the overall function of a client. Each question provides relevant information about daily movement patterns and can identify potential compensations to look for during the next steps of the assessment process. Examples of typical questions are shown in **Figure 7-4**.

Occupation

Does your occupation require extended periods of sitting?

        YES   NO

Does your occupation require repetitive movements? (If YES, please explain.)

        YES   NO

_____

Does your occupation require you to wear shoes with a heel (e.g., dress shoes)?

        YES   NO

Does your occupation require heavy lifting?

        YES   NO

Does your occupation cause you mental stress?

        YES   NO

Figure 7-4 Client occupation questions

EXTENDED PERIODS OF SITTING

Sedentary behavior, or prolonged sitting, has been associated with an increased risk of adverse health outcomes (Baker et al., 2018; Biswas et al., 2015; Cuéllar & Lanman, 2017; Fares et al., 2017; Page et al., 2010). Cardiovascular disease, cancer, type 2 diabetes, obesity, hypertension, and mortality rates associated which each disease have been shown to increase with sedentary behavior (Baker et al., 2018; Biswas et al., 2015; Brown et al. 2003; Lee & Wong, 2015). Furthermore, clients who are required to sit most of the day as are those working at a computer, are potentially prone to musculoskeletal adaptations such as a decrease in spinal posture and increase in musculoskeletal discomfort (Baker et al., 2018; Mackenzie et al., 2018; Mörl & Bradl, 2013). Postural imbalances within the lumbo-pelvic-hip complex have a strong influence throughout the kinetic chain.

REPETITIVE MOVEMENTS

Repetitive movements can create a pattern overload to muscles and joints, which may lead to tissue trauma resulting in pain and eventually kinetic chain dysfunction (Falla et al., 2017; Fares

food groups from their diet as this can lead to inadequate micronutrients needed to support health (Thomas et al., 2016).

Hydration habits are just as important as nutritional habits to assess. The best way to assess fluid status is through urine color, which should be somewhere between the color of light lemonade and clear water when the body is adequately hydrated. It is recommended that clients consume adequate amounts of fluid before, during, and after activity to mitigate the effects of sweat loss, but the simple and most important practice is to simply drink **ad libidum**, always reaching for a glass of water when thirsty. Additionally, the consumption of fluids that aid in electrolyte replacement is recommended for exercise activities lasting longer than 1 hour (Thomas et al., 2016). Failure to maintain proper hydration levels will lead to a decrease in performance and overall health, creating fatigue and potentially further compensatory movement.

RECREATION

Recreation refers to an individual's physical activities outside of the work environment. By finding out what recreational activities an individual performs, Corrective Exercise Specialists can better design a program to fit client needs. For example, many people like to golf, ski, play tennis, or engage in a variety of other sporting activities in their spare time. Proper program strategies must be incorporated to ensure that individuals are trained in a manner that optimizes the efficiency of the human movement system while addressing potential muscle imbalances that may be a result of their activity.

For example, golfers are prone to LPHC and shoulder compensations due to poor swing mechanics (Zouzias et al., 2018). Alpine skiers are subjected to knee valgus forces and, as a result, may develop compensations in the ankle, knee, and LPHC (Owens et al., 2018). Tennis athletes are more susceptible to overuse injuries of the upper extremity, specifically the elbow and shoulder (e.g., tennis elbow). Changes to racquet grip or racquet properties as well as the repetitive swing motion could alter the biomechanics of the kinetic chain (Abrams et al., 2012).

HOBBIES

Hobbies refer to activities that an individual may partake in regularly but are not necessarily athletic in nature. Examples include gardening, working on cars, reading, watching television, and playing video games. As discussed previously, repetitive movement can lead to a disturbance in the kinetic chain. Gardening and working on cars require a significant amount of time spent in a hunched over position, potentially on the hands and knees or contorted to access hard to reach nuts and bolts. Reading, watching television, using mobile phones, and playing video games are all often associated with a forward head and rounded shoulders and upper back posture. These positions, if not corrected, can lead to injury over time. Therefore, it is important for the Corrective Exercise Specialist to assess all activity to mitigate the risk of compensatory movement secondary to tissue overload. If a client is performing the same movement at work, during recreational activities, and with the hobbies they enjoy, the cumulative effect can frequently lead to the development of muscle imbalances.

Medical History

Learning a client's medical history is crucial for the corrective exercise process. While the PAR-Q+ will provide information about potential cardiorespiratory issues that could make exercise dangerous, that tool is simply used for clearance for activity. The Corrective Exercise Specialist, additionally, needs information about the structure and function of the individual by uncovering important medical information like past injuries, surgeries, and chronic conditions. See **Figure 7-6** for sample questions about a client's medical history.

Ad libidum

Latin phrase that translates to "as desired"; refers to eating or drinking as you are normally driven to (i.e., not purposely overeating or undereating).

Introduction

Following client intake, posture analysis is the first part of the corrective exercise assessment process (**Figure 8-1**). Posture is an observable assessment of how a client places their body in different positions (Lee et al., 2017). Posture can be observed during static positions (e.g., standing or sitting) or dynamic movement (e.g., lifting a box). Static posture represents how an individual physically presents themselves without movement and is a reference for the alignment of the body. Static posture is considered the base for movement because it requires isometric contractions from many different muscles to maintain muscle tension to hold the specific position (Bokaee et al., 2016; Oliveira & Silva, 2016). Movement originates from an individual's static posture, which provides the first clues toward a comprehensive understanding of their overall mobility and neuromuscular control capabilities. It is likely that the client's kinetic chain tendencies while static will be observed during later assessment stages.

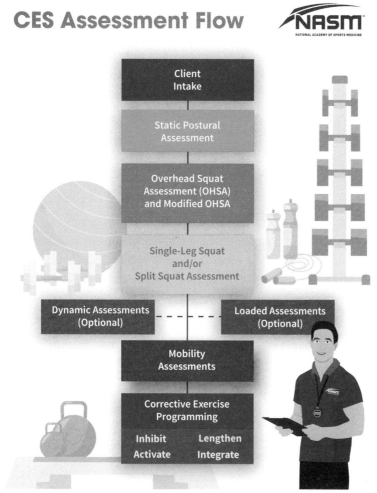

Figure 8-1 CES Assessment Flow

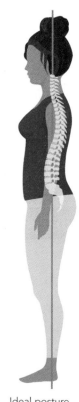

Ideal posture

Importance of Posture as It Relates to Injury

Static postural assessment is the first step toward identifying muscle imbalances (**altered length-tension relationships**) throughout the body. Although static assessment may not be able to specifically identify the root cause of a movement impairment, it provides insight into

Altered length-tension relationships

Occur when the resting length of a muscle is too short or too long to generate optimal force.

which muscles are being held in chronically shortened or lengthened positions and sheds light on related impairments in other areas of the body that may be contributing to a dysfunction (per the Regional Interdependence model).

A strong relationship exists between a rounded shoulder posture and the degree of forward head posture a person exhibits (Kim & Kim, 2016). This correlation led to the identification of Janda's upper crossed syndrome and can eventually lead to musculoskeletal injury if not corrected (Arshadi et al., 2019). Corrective Exercise Specialists are encouraged to look for causative factors during the comprehensive assessment in order to help link the client's subjective reports (e.g., an area of discomfort) with potential causes (e.g., sitting at a desk all day). This will help create a more effective corrective program that empowers the client to change everyday habits on top of the work performed in the fitness facility.

HELPFUL HINT

Remember to always keep the Regional Interdependence (RI) model in mind and consider the body as one interdependent system (i.e., the kinetic chain); an impairment in one area of the body can affect regions both above and below it (Sueki et al., 2013). Using this mindset during the static postural assessment will help determine what to look for in other areas of the body during the next steps of evaluating movement quality and available mobility.

For example, during a static postural assessment, a client demonstrates flat feet and also stands with the hip and knee in an internally rotated position. That chronic internal rotation of the leg could either be a contributing factor to flat feet or it could be caused by it. At this stage of the process, there is no way to tell, making it vital to assess postural alignment both when standing still and while in motion.

Muscle Imbalance

A number of different factors can cause changes in joint alignment, mobility of the myofascia, and muscle function. Whatever the reason, the body will continually adapt in an attempt to produce the functional outcome that is requested by the central nervous system (i.e., relative flexibility). This is often seen after soft tissue injuries that are a result of **pattern overload** (Verhagen et al., 2013). For example, a desk worker may suffer from neck pain due to a forward head posture during prolonged computer work. The computer monitor may not be at an optimal position, requiring the individual to assume a forward head. Unfortunately, this adaptability will lead to muscle imbalances that can move beyond a dysfunction and into tissue damage. As the muscle adapts to this chronic positioning, the myofascial system (e.g., muscles and connective tissue) will shorten or lengthen in response to the increasing stressor demands (Page et al.,

Pattern overload

Occurs when a segment of the body is repeatedly moved or chronically held in the same way, leading to a state of muscle overactivity.

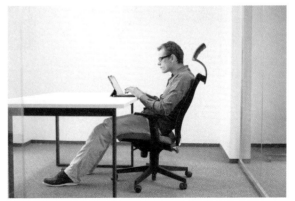

© Marcin Balcerzak/Shutterstock

2010). This can result in cervical stabilizer muscles being less efficient as they are pulled out of optimal alignment.

Muscle imbalance is a condition in which there is a lack of balance between muscles surrounding a joint (Mersmann et al., 2017) and may be caused by altered reciprocal inhibition, synergistic dominance, arthrokinematic dysfunction, and/or overall decreased neuromuscular control (**Figure 8-2**). However, regardless of the cause, muscle imbalance represents altered length-tension relationships within the muscles surrounding a joint that cause the joint to rest in a suboptimal position (i.e., muscles are overactive/shortened on one side of the joint and underactive/lengthened on the other). This incorrect joint positioning then causes normal force-couples to fall out of optimal function, causing a cascading effect throughout the entire kinetic chain.

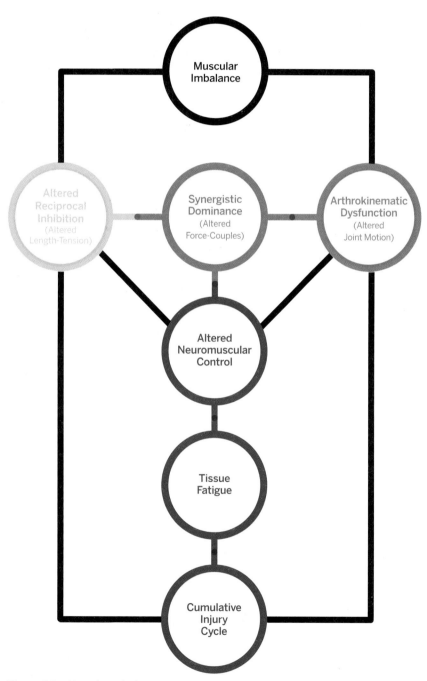

Figure 8-2 Muscular imbalance

It has been demonstrated that certain muscles have a tendency to be overactive/shortened while other muscles are commonly underactive/lengthened (**Table 8-1**) (Kendall et al., 2014; Page et al., 2010). These commonalities are typically caused by chronic suboptimal positioning and repetitive motions that most people encounter every day in modern society, such as sitting at a desk all day, looking down at phones, wearing high-heeled shoes, or carrying a bag on the same shoulder, just to name a few (Tegtmeier, 2018). Because of this, specific patterns of **postural distortion** have been identified, such as Dr. Vladimir Janda's upper, lower, and layered crossed syndromes, and the various common posture types as described by Florence Kendall (Kendall et al., 2014; Page et al., 2010).

TABLE 8-1 Muscles Prone to Imbalance

Overactive/Shortened	Underactive/Lengthened
Upper Body	
Cervical extensors	Deep cervical flexors (longus coli and capitis)
Latissimus dorsi	Middle and lower trapezius
Levator scapulae	Rhomboids
Pectorals (major and minor)	Serratus anterior
Scalenes	
Sternocleidomastoid	
Upper trapezius	
LPHC and Lower Body	
Gastrocnemius	Gluteus maximus and medius
Hamstrings	Fibularis (peroneal) muscles
Hip adductors	Rectus abdominis
Piriformis	Tibialis anterior and posterior
Psoas	Transverse abdominis
Quadratus lumborum	Vastus medialis and lateralis
Rectus femoris	
Soleus	
Tensor fascia latae	

Factors Related to Postural Imbalance

Numerous factors can lead to the development of muscle imbalances and postural impairments. The following are the main factors that influence a person's posture:

- Chronic suboptimal postures
- Habitual repetitive movements
- Acute injuries
- Recovery from surgery
- Incompletely rehabilitated past injuries

ALTERED MOVEMENT PATTERNS FROM CHRONIC SUBOPTIMAL POSTURES

Corrective Exercise Specialists must understand posture and the importance it has in people's lives. Individuals may have developed poor postural habits without even realizing it. Office workers are particularly susceptible due to long periods of desk work and looking at computer screens (Intolo et al., 2019; Shiri & Falah-Hassani, 2015). Workstations both at home and at the office frequently contribute to neck and arm dysfunction. Incorrect positioning of the computer monitor, the keyboard, and the chair all work to create an environment for the development of postural deviations (Bruno Garza & Young, 2015; Intolo et al., 2019)

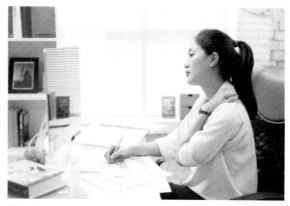
© Torwaistudio/Shutterstock

ALTERED MOVEMENT PATTERNS FROM HABITUAL REPETITIVE MOVEMENT

Repetitive movements can lead to chronic overuse and eventually injury, which can lead to changes in myofascial mobility (Clark et al., 2010). Poor posture and a lack of daily movement are also considered a contributing factor (Tegtmeier, 2018). Muscles that are repeatedly placed in a shortened position, such as the hip flexors during sitting, will eventually adapt and tend to remain short. Repetitive movements can cause imbalances by placing demands on certain muscle groups more predominantly. This is evident when looking at different athletes such as swimmers. Due to the repetitive horizontal adduction needed for most types of swimming, they often exhibit overemphasized pectoral muscles in relation to the scapular retractors, giving them a rounded shoulder posture (Lynch et al., 2010; Struyf et al., 2017).

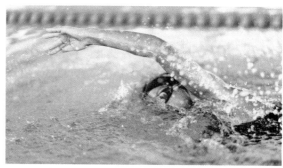
© Microgen/Shutterstock

Athletes are not the only ones at risk. Repetitive movement also affects people in everyday life, such as a construction worker who hammers with the same hand day in and day out. Food servers often carry large trays with the same arm, and students tend to favor one shoulder over the other when carrying a backpack. A parent usually carries their child on the same hip.

Postural imbalances are also seen in the gym with people who focus on certain muscle groups more than others. This is evident in individuals who overemphasize chest, shoulder, and biceps work. This often results in rounded shoulders, a forward head, and internal rotation at the shoulder joint (Kolber et al., 2014, 2017).

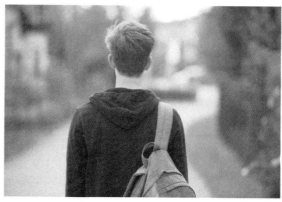
© Nejc Vesel/Shutterstock

ALTERED MOVEMENT PATTERNS FROM ACUTE INJURY

Acute injury may also result in chronic muscle imbalances. In the presence of a healing injury, an individual may assume adaptive postures to avoid pain or to *create function* using relative flexibility for daily tasks (Trulsson et al., 2016). Even after the pain has subsided and motion restrictions or strength has returned, the individual may not change their adaptive movement strategies unless reminded to return to a more efficient movement pattern. The continued use of compensatory patterns alters loads across the joints and recruitment strategies of muscles unrelated to the injury, all leading to compounding muscular imbalances that are reflected in postural changes.

Soft tissue injury may also result in tissue that becomes chronically restricted. Immobilization through splinting or self-immobilization due to pain (i.e., guarding behavior) may cause the local tissues to become shortened. Without restoring mobility, the shortened tissues may not function properly, forcing compensatory muscle activity and motions at the regions above or below the injured area. For example, a client with right foot pain may limp during gait and use greater hip muscle activity. This may abnormally load the lower extremity on the noninjured side and lead to new muscle imbalances and cumulative injury if not corrected.

ALTERED MOVEMENT PATTERNS AFTER SURGERY

After surgery, the body repairs itself with scar tissue. Surgical scars can become dysfunctional and result in compensatory altered movement patterns and postural changes if not addressed. Collagen fibers from healing scars often develop in a random fashion and can bind to the local myofascia and alter joint and muscle function (Alvira-Lechuz et al., 2017). Scar mobilization through proper movement, manual therapies (e.g., massage), and stretching should be done throughout the healing process to ensure proper mobility is maintained (Alvira-Lechuz et al., 2017).

ALTERED MOVEMENT PATTERNS FROM INCOMPLETELY REHABILITATED PAST INJURIES

At times, clients with injuries may not be able to complete their rehabilitation due to reasons such as insurance limits, work demands, and finances. These individuals may be at a higher risk of re-injury if not fully recovered or if all related issues (e.g., muscle imbalances) have not been successfully corrected. For example, clients may want to return to the gym and self-rehabilitate, which could put them in danger if not guided properly by a qualified health professional. Prior to working with such a client, the Corrective Exercise Specialist should contact the client's rehabilitation or medical professional to obtain proper guidelines and clearance. Client safety is the first priority in such a situation.

Systematic Approach to Assess Static Posture

Static postural assessment requires the practitioner to have strong visual observation skills. This can be developed with time and practice. Commonly, static postural assessments begin at the feet and travel upward to the head. Often, alterations or deviations observed in the lower part of the body are reflected further up the kinetic chain. Many of these impairments can be uncovered through a comprehensive static postural assessment (**Figure 8-3**).

Static Postural Assessment

1 Client Intake

2 Static Postural Assessment

3 Overhead Squat Assessment (OHSA) and Modified OHSA

4 Single-Leg Squat and/or Split Squat Assessment

4a Dynamic Assessments
OPTIONAL

4b Loaded Assessments
OPTIONAL

5 Mobility Assessments

6 Corrective Exercise Programming
INHIBIT · LENGTHEN
ACTIVATE · INTEGRATE

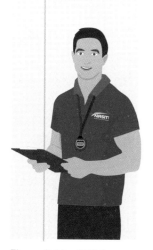

Observe static posture focusing on kinetic chain checkpoints below.

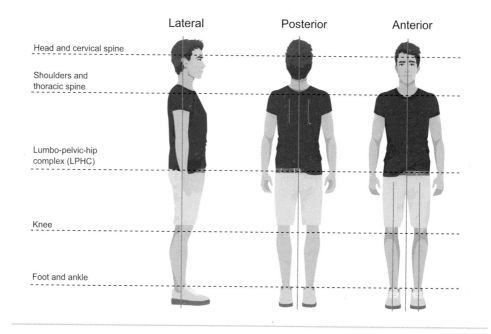

Compare client to postural distortion patterns below.

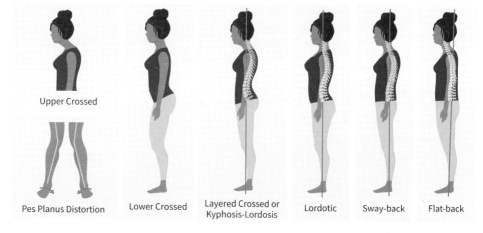

Identify potentially overactive and underactive muscles based on the postural patterns they most closely match.

Figure 8-3A CES Assessment Flow: static postural assessment

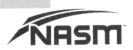

Static Postural Assessment

Name_____ Date_____

OBSERVATIONAL FINDINGS

CHECKPOINT	STATIC POSITION	POTENTIAL OVERACTIVE/ SHORTENED MUSCLES	POTENTIAL UNDERACTIVE/ LENGTHENED MUSCLES
Foot and Ankle	☐ Feet: straight/parallel ☐ Feet: externally rotated ☐ Arch: neutral ☐ Arch: flattened (pes planus) ☐ Arch: raised (pes cavus) ☐ Lower leg is vertical ☐ Lower leg posteriorly displaced (plantar flexed)		
Knee	☐ In line w/ 2nd & 3rd toes ☐ Valgus (knock-kneed) ☐ Varus (bowlegged) ☐ Neutral (straight) ☐ Flexed ☐ Hyperextended		
LPHC	☐ Pelvis: level ☐ Pelvis: anterior tilt ☐ L-spine: normal curve ☐ Pelvis: posterior tilt ☐ L-spine: exc. lordosis ☐ Hips: neutral ☐ L-spine: red. lordosis ☐ Hips: extended ☐ L-spine: lateral shift ☐ Hips: flexed		
Shoulders and Thoracic Spine	☐ Shoulders: level ☐ Shoulders: elevated ☐ Shoulders: in line w/ hips & ears ☐ Shoulders: rounded forward ☐ T-spine: normal curve ☐ T-spine: exc. kyphosis		
Head and Cervical Spine	☐ Head: neutral (not tilted or rotated) ☐ Head: forward in cervical extension ☐ C-spine: normal curve		
Pes Planus Distortion	☐ Yes ☐ No		

Additional Notes

_____

_____

_____

Figure 8-3B Static postural assessment observations form

To perform a static postural assessment, Corrective Exercise Specialists should have their clients remove their shoes and then simply stand in what the client feels to be their most neutral, relaxed position. That standing position is the client's static posture. It is recommended that the client wear relatively form-fitting clothing (so long as they are comfortable), because baggy clothes can hide critical details. The client will be observed from front (anterior), side (lateral), and rear (posterior) viewpoints. Their observed posture will then be compared to ideal standing posture. Any deviations from that ideal will represent a static postural impairment.

HELPFUL HINT

After completing all components of the CES Assessment Flow, muscles identified as overactive/shortened will be inhibited and lengthened in the first two phases of the Corrective Exercise Continuum. Muscles identified as underactive/lengthened will be activated in phase 3. The newly balanced length-tension relationships are then integrated into functional movement patterns in phase 4 to restore optimal force-couples throughout the body. Note that static postural assessment is just the first part of the comprehensive corrective exercise process.

CRITICAL

Removing shoes is essential to accurately view a client's posture in the most natural setting; specifically, in relation to impairments at the foot and ankle. However, it is understood that some facilities have specific dress codes in place that may prevent this from happening. In addition, some clients may simply not feel comfortable removing their shoes.

The most important thing is consistency from one assessment session to the next. If a client's initial assessment was performed with shoes on, then all reassessments later in the program should be performed with shoes on as well. This will ensure that progressions can be clearly tracked without any confounding variables.

Kinetic Chain Checkpoints

Postural assessments require observation of the kinetic chain. To structure this observation, NASM has devised the use of kinetic chain checkpoints to allow the professional to systematically view the body during motion. The kinetic chain checkpoints refer to major joint regions of the body, including the following:

- Foot and ankle
- Knee
- Lumbo-pelvic-hip complex (LPHC)
- Shoulders and thoracic spine
- Head and cervical spine

When viewing a client from the front, the following represents ideal posture at each of the kinetic chain checkpoints. It should be noted that the term *neutral* may have varying definitions and a level of subjectivity. The Corrective Exercise Specialist is advised to use the ideal postures described at each kinetic chain checkpoint as the reference point for neutral positioning. Any deviations from these ideals will represent static postural impairments:

- **Foot and ankle:** Straight and parallel, not flattened or externally rotated
- **Knees:** In line with the second and third toes, not valgus or varus
- **LPHC:** Pelvis level to the horizon
- **Shoulders:** Level, not elevated or rounded
- **Head:** Neutral position, neither tilted nor rotated

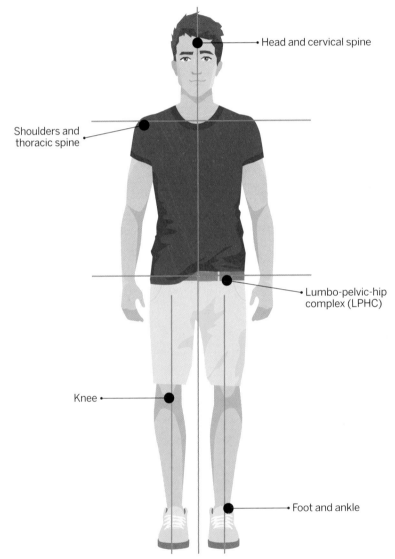

Kinetic chain checkpoints—anterior view

LATERAL VIEW

When viewing ideal posture from a lateral viewpoint, an imaginary line should run from the ankle, through the middle of the femur, hip, center of shoulder, and middle of the ear. Specific lateral posture at the five kinetic chain checkpoints is as follows:

- **Foot and ankle:** Neutral position, leg vertical at a right angle to the sole of foot
- **Knees:** Neutral position, not flexed nor hyperextended
- **LPHC:** Pelvis in neutral position, not anteriorly nor posteriorly rotated
- **Shoulders:** In line with the hips and ears
- **Head:** Neutral position, not in cervical extension (jutting forward)

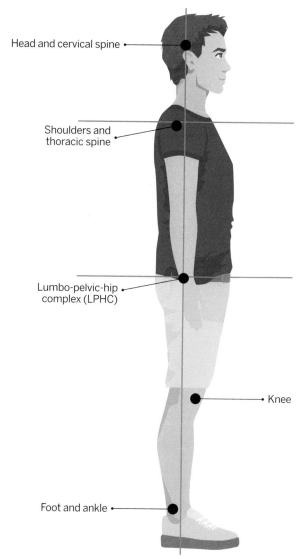

Kinetic chain checkpoints—lateral view

Static posture should also be assessed from a rear viewpoint. Ideal posture from a posterior viewpoint appears as follows:

- **Foot and ankle:** Heels are straight and parallel, not overly pronated (flattened)
- **Knees:** Neutral position, neither valgus nor varus
- **LPHC:** Pelvis level to the horizon
- **Shoulders/scapulae:** Level, not elevated nor rounded forward
- **Head:** Neutral position, neither tilted nor rotated

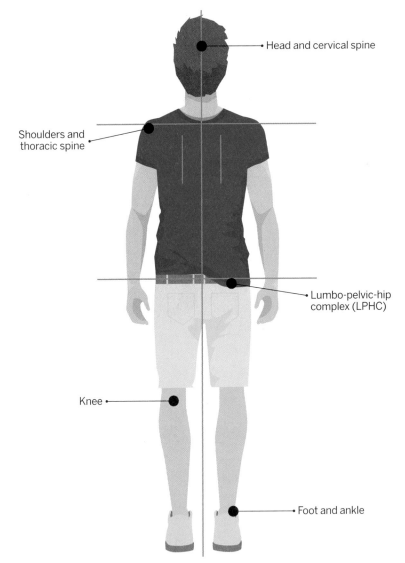

Kinetic chain checkpoints—posterior view

Common Patterns of Postural Distortion

Because everything in the body is connected, static postural impairments tend to not present one at a time. For this reason, static postural impairments are typically grouped into patterns based on how they relate. For example, a person with an anterior pelvic tilt will almost certainly have excessive lumbar lordosis (excessive low-back arch). Furthermore, due to commonalities of lifestyle and occupation within the population, a handful of common patterns of postural distortion provide the basis of what to look for during the static postural assessment. These observations will then provide insight into potential movement dysfunctions that may be observed during the later movement assessments (Kendall et al., 2014).

Although they are not the only ones in existence, two of the most commonly referenced postural classification paradigms are *Janda's postural distortion syndromes* and *Kendall's posture classifications* (Kendall et al., 2014; Page et al., 2010). Both have identified specific muscle or muscle group imbalances that are typically related to observed patterns of postural distortion (Kendall et al., 2014; Page et al., 2010) and will serve as the posture types to identify during the static assessment process for corrective exercise.

 TRAINING TIP

Each client has unique characteristics and may not simply fall within one common paradigm. Corrective Exercise Specialists must refine their static postural observations with movement and targeted mobility assessments in order to form the clearest picture possible and inform the most effective exercise selection.

The most popular postural classifications are Janda's syndromes, which describe three distortion patterns (Page et al., 2010). The second-most popular paradigm, Kendall's postures, describes four distortion patterns (Kendall et al., 2014). Additionally, pes planus distortion syndrome is another muscle imbalance pattern that it is often observed in both clinical practice and in fitness facilities with clients.

 HELPFUL HINT

Both Janda's and Kendall's common patterns of postural distortion are observed from the lateral viewpoint.

Janda's Syndromes

In 1979, Vladimir Janda, MD, DSc, defined the upper, lower, and layered crossed syndromes. His classifications were derived from many years of treating patients with polio and different chronic pain syndromes. Janda's approach focused on identifying and addressing neuromuscular imbalances through static postural assessment, movement-based testing, and evaluating gait mechanics (Page et al., 2010).

 CHECK IT OUT

Kyphosis and **lordosis** are the technical terms for the natural curvatures of the spine. The lumbar spine's normal curve toward the front of the body is termed *lordosis*, whereas the thoracic spine's normal curve to the rear is called *kyphosis*. Many postural impairments will be related to excessive or reduced positioning of the spine's lordotic and kyphotic curves. *Excessive lumbar lordosis* refers to an excessive curve of the lower back, whereas *excessive thoracic kyphosis* refers to a rounded upper back. *Reduced lordosis* or *reduced kyphosis* means there is a flattening of the spine's natural lumbar or thoracic curves, respectively.

Kyphosis

Natural curvature of the thoracic spine toward the back of the body.

Lordosis

Natural curvature of the lumbar or cervical spine toward the front of the body.

Individuals who spend long periods of time sitting often present with lower crossed syndrome (LCS) due to chronic anterior positioning of the hip (Key, 2010). An individual with Janda's LCS presents with a combination of excessive lumbar lordosis and an anterior pelvic tilt. Individuals with LCS may also demonstrate a lateral lumbar shift, knees slightly flexed or hyperextended, and feet plantar flexed. The LCS postural distortion pattern can inhibit deep stabilizing muscles, requiring compensatory activation of superficial muscles to help stabilize the spinal segments.

CHECK IT OUT

The "crossed" in Janda's upper and lower crossed syndromes comes from how the locations of the overactive/shortened and underactive/lengthened muscles "cross" at the affected joint when looking at the body from a lateral viewpoint. For example, in lower crossed syndrome, the hip flexors and lumbar extensors are overactive (drawing a diagonal line across the hip from anterior bottom to posterior top), while the abdominals and gluteus maximus/medius are underactive (drawing a diagonal line across the hip from anterior top to posterior bottom), forming an X when the locations are connected with lines. The same applies to upper crossed syndrome with the muscles of the upper back, chest, and neck.

LCS also influences the body's kinetic chain above and below the hip. The spine responds to increased lumbar lordosis with subsequent increases in thoracic kyphosis and cervical lordosis—leading to rounding of the upper back and possible forward head posture in some individuals—while the lower extremity can sometimes respond to the pelvic tilt with hyperextension of the knees and chronically plantar flexed feet (Page et al., 2010).

GETTING TECHNICAL

Although an anterior pelvic tilt is the cornerstone static malalignment of LCS, individual differences in lumbar spine mobility led Janda to further detail LCS into two subtypes based on how the kinetic chain responds to the pelvic tilt, labeled LCS-A and LCS-B. These subtypes account for the related static malalignments that can potentially be seen above and below the hip (e.g., hyperextended knees, plantar flexed feet, rounded shoulders, and forward head) in those with LCS.

In LCS-A, individuals compensate for the anterior pelvic tilt with a considerable increase in lumbar lordosis (i.e., excessive low-back arch) and an increase in thoracolumbar kyphosis (i.e., rounding of the mid-to-upper back) without visibly affecting the alignment of the knees and cervical spine (Page et al., 2010). Those presenting with LCS-B have a more mobile lower back and abdominal area; therefore, the lumbar spine responds to the anterior pelvic tilt with less prominent lumbar lordosis and more visible compensatory malalignment in the upper back, head and neck, and knees, presenting more prominent kyphosis in the thoracic spine, knee hyperextension (i.e., recurvatum), and forward head posture (Page et al., 2010).

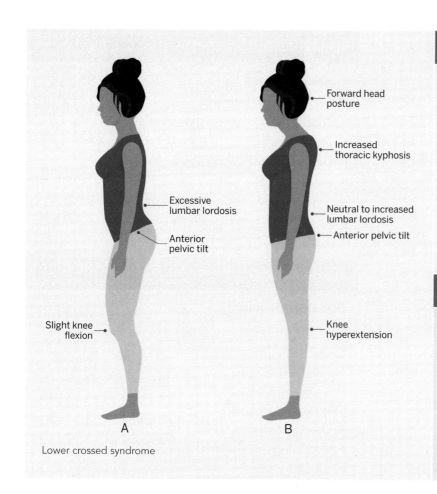

Static Positions

- **Head:** Neutral to forward
- **Cervical spine:** Normal to extended
- **Thoracic spine:** Normal to rounded
- **Shoulders:** Neutral to rounded
- **Lumbar spine:** Neutral to excessive lordosis, possible lateral shift
- **Pelvis:** Anterior tilt
- **Hip joints:** Flexed or neutral
- **Knee joints:** Flexed or hyperextended
- **Ankle joints:** Neutral or plantar flexed

Muscle Activity

Overactive/shortened
- Hip flexors
- Lumbar extensors
- Gastrocnemius/soleus

Underactive/lengthened
- Abdominals
- Gluteus maximus and medius
- Hamstrings

Forward head posture

Increased thoracic kyphosis

Excessive lumbar lordosis

Neutral to increased lumbar lordosis

Anterior pelvic tilt

Anterior pelvic tilt

Slight knee flexion

Knee hyperextension

A

B

Lower crossed syndrome

 CHECK IT OUT

One might think that plantar flexion when standing still means the individual is performing a heel raise. For people with proper knee joint alignment, you would be right! However, if a person's knees hyperextend, the posterior displacement of the tibia/fibula puts the ankles into a chronic, slightly plantar flexed position even when standing with feet flat on the ground. While standing upright, the lower leg will not be at a right angle to the sole of the foot when observed from the lateral view.

UPPER CROSSED SYNDROME

An individual with Janda's upper crossed syndrome (UCS) may present with a forward head, hyperextended cervical spine, and rounded shoulders. Individuals with UCS may also present with excessive thoracic kyphosis, elevated shoulders, rotated or abducted shoulders, and winging of the scapulae. UCS may lead to joint dysfunction at the atlanto-occipital joint (cervical vertebra C1), cervical vertebral segments C4 through C5, the cervicothoracic joint, the glenohumeral joint, and thoracic vertebra T4 through T5 segments (Page et al., 2010).

Static Positions

- **Head:** Forward
- **Cervical spine:** Extended
- **Thoracic spine:** Excessive kyphosis
- **Shoulders:** Rounded, elevated (scapular winging)
- **Lumbar spine:** Normal curve or extended
- **Pelvis:** Neutral
- **Hip joints:** Neutral or slightly flexed
- **Knee joints:** Neutral or slightly flexed
- **Ankle joints:** Neutral

Muscle Activity

Overactive/shortened
- Cervical extensors
- Pectorals (major and minor)
- Upper trapezius
- Levator scapulae

Underactive/lengthened
- Deep neck flexors
- Rhomboids, middle/lower trapezius
- Serratus anterior

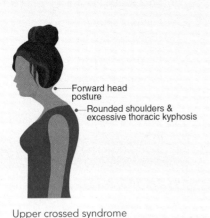

Forward head posture

Rounded shoulders & excessive thoracic kyphosis

Upper crossed syndrome

GETTING TECHNICAL

A UCS posture can decrease shoulder joint (glenohumeral) stability as the glenoid fossa (joint) becomes more vertical due to an underactive serratus anterior, which can lead to shoulder abduction, rotation, and scapular winging. This decreased stability increases activation of the levator scapulae and upper trapezius to maintain an optimal (centralized) shoulder joint position. This can often lead to neck discomfort and shoulder injuries (Page et al., 2010).

LAYERED CROSSED SYNDROME

Individuals with Janda's layered crossed syndrome may present with both components of UCS and LCS (subtype A or B). In the upper body, individuals may present with the primary findings: forward head, excessive thoracic kyphosis, rounded and elevated shoulders, shoulder rotation or abduction, and winging of the scapulae. In the lower body, individuals may present with the following primary findings: excessive lumbar lordosis, anterior pelvic tilt, lateral lumbar shift, lateral leg rotation, flexed hips, knee hyperextension, and ankle plantar flexion (Page et al., 2010). Individuals with layered crossed syndrome may present with mobility and motor dysfunction that has compounded over time.

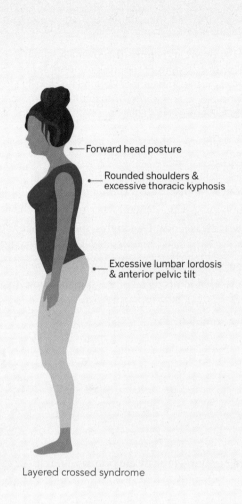

- Forward head posture

- Rounded shoulders & excessive thoracic kyphosis

- Excessive lumbar lordosis & anterior pelvic tilt

Layered crossed syndrome

Static Positions

- **Head:** Forward
- **Cervical spine:** Extended
- **Thoracic spine:** Excessive kyphosis
- **Shoulders:** Rounded, elevated, possible scapular winging
- **Lumbar spine:** Excessive lordosis, possible lateral shift
- **Pelvis:** Anterior tilt
- **Hip joints:** Flexed
- **Knee joints:** Flexed or hyperextended
- **Ankle joints:** Neutral or plantar flexed

Muscle Activity

Overactive/shortened

- Cervical extensors
- Pectorals (major and minor)
- Upper trapezius
- Levator scapulae
- Hip flexors
- Lumbar extensors
- Gastrocnemius/soleus

Underactive/lengthened

- Deep neck flexors
- Rhomboids, middle/lower trapezius
- Serratus anterior
- Anterior abdominals
- Hip extensors (hamstrings)
- Gluteus maximus and medius

 TRAINING TIP

Notice that there are many overlaps among the postural impairment syndromes identified by Janda. This is due to the concept of regional interdependence and how impairments at one point on the kinetic chain can have a cascading influence throughout the body.

When observing a client's static posture, look for the most prominent static malalignments first. For example, if an anterior pelvic tilt is excessive, with less noticeable (but still present) associated malalignments above or below the hip, the client would be best matched with LCS (with the additional malalignments then pointing them toward either LCS-A or LCS-B).

If malalignments at the shoulders, neck, and head are more prominent than malalignments below the thoracic region, the client would be best matched to UCS. Layered crossed syndrome then represents a situation where the client has equally prominent malalignments from both LCS and UCS at the same time.

Remember, it is not a fitness professional's job to "diagnose" their client with a postural syndrome. Rather, by matching a client's static posture to the syndrome to which they most closely align, probable overactive/underactive relationships can be identified, providing foundational (broad) information that will then be refined with movement (more specific) and joint mobility (most specific) assessments.

For adults, Janda suggests that muscle imbalance may begin distally at the pelvis and continue proximally to the shoulder and neck region. This may be evident in individuals who sit with poor posture at the desk for long periods of time. For adolescents and teens, this progression is reversed with proximal muscle imbalances continuing distally into the extremities (Page et al., 2010). This may be evident among individuals who play video games or use their smartphone with poor posture, which is often called *text neck* (Cuellar & Lanman, 2017; Fares et al., 2017).

Kendall's Posture Types

In 1949, Florence Kendall, a physical therapist, published a textbook identifying the link between muscle imbalances, postural distortions, and pain. Kendall was a pioneer in the field and an influence for other great minds to follow, such as Janda. Due to this, there are many similarities between Janda's syndromes and the four posture types identified by Kendall. The difference lies in that Kendall was only looking at posture in regard to the shape of the spine, whereas Janda's newer syndrome classifications considered joints distal of the spinal column (e.g., knee hyperextension in individuals with LCS-B). Nevertheless, Kendall's four posture types are still frequently referenced in the exercise science community and include:

- Lordotic posture
- Flat-back posture
- Sway-back posture
- Kyphosis-lordosis posture

LORDOTIC POSTURE

Individuals with Kendall's lordotic posture may present with the primary findings of excessive lumbar lordosis and an anterior pelvic tilt. Individuals may also assume other compensatory

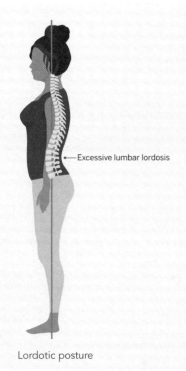

—Excessive lumbar lordosis

Lordotic posture

Static Positions

- **Head:** Neutral position
- **Cervical spine:** Normal curve
- **Thoracic spine:** Normal curve
- **Lumbar spine:** Excessive lordosis
- **Pelvis:** Anteriorly tilted
- **Hip joints:** Flexed
- **Knee joints:** Slightly flexed or hyperextended
- **Ankle joints:** Slightly plantar flexed

Muscle Activity

Overactive/shortened
- Hip flexors
- Internal obliques (upper)
- Lumbar extensors

Underactive/lengthened
- Abdominals (external obliques)
- Hip extensors (hamstrings)

positions such as a lateral lumbar shift, lateral leg rotation, and knees slightly flexed or hyperextended. Kendall's lordotic posture has components of Janda's LCS. The upper body typically has a neutral head position and normal cervical and thoracic curves (Kendall et al., 2014).

FLAT-BACK POSTURE

An individual with Kendall's flat-back posture may have both upper- and lower-body postural issues. For the upper body, the individual may present with a forward head, hyperextended cervical spine, excessive upper thoracic kyphosis (rounding), reduced lower thoracic kyphosis (flattening), and rounded shoulders. For the lower body, the individual may have reduced lumbar lordosis (flattening), a posteriorly tilted pelvis, extended hips, extended knees, and slightly plantar flexed ankles (Kendall et al., 2014; Key, 2010).

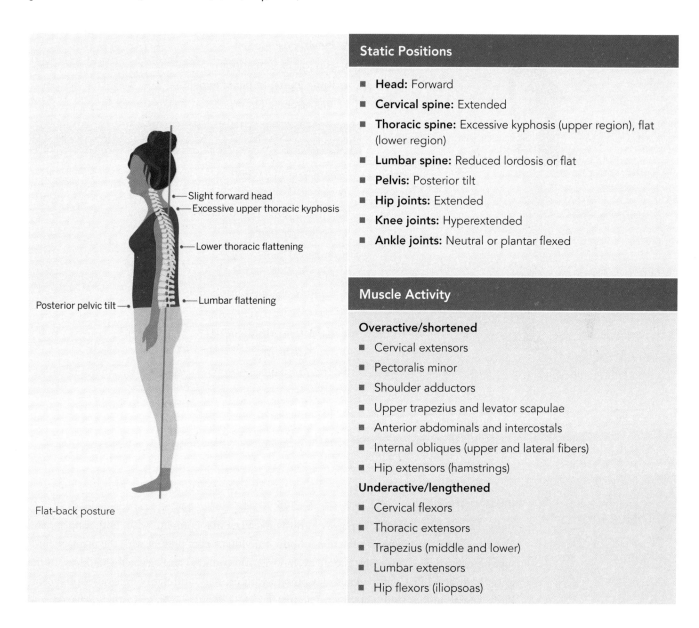

Slight forward head
Excessive upper thoracic kyphosis
Lower thoracic flattening
Posterior pelvic tilt
Lumbar flattening

Flat-back posture

Static Positions

- **Head:** Forward
- **Cervical spine:** Extended
- **Thoracic spine:** Excessive kyphosis (upper region), flat (lower region)
- **Lumbar spine:** Reduced lordosis or flat
- **Pelvis:** Posterior tilt
- **Hip joints:** Extended
- **Knee joints:** Hyperextended
- **Ankle joints:** Neutral or plantar flexed

Muscle Activity

Overactive/shortened
- Cervical extensors
- Pectoralis minor
- Shoulder adductors
- Upper trapezius and levator scapulae
- Anterior abdominals and intercostals
- Internal obliques (upper and lateral fibers)
- Hip extensors (hamstrings)

Underactive/lengthened
- Cervical flexors
- Thoracic extensors
- Trapezius (middle and lower)
- Lumbar extensors
- Hip flexors (iliopsoas)

SWAY-BACK POSTURE

Individuals with sway-back posture may present with both upper- and lower-body postural issues. For the upper body, the individual may present with a forward head, extended cervical spine, and excessive thoracic kyphosis (posterior displacement). For the lower body, the individual may have reduced lumbar lordosis (flattening), a posteriorly tilted pelvis, extended hips, hyperextended knees, and neutral ankles (Kendall et al., 2014). Other muscle imbalances may be present and should be considered by the professional.

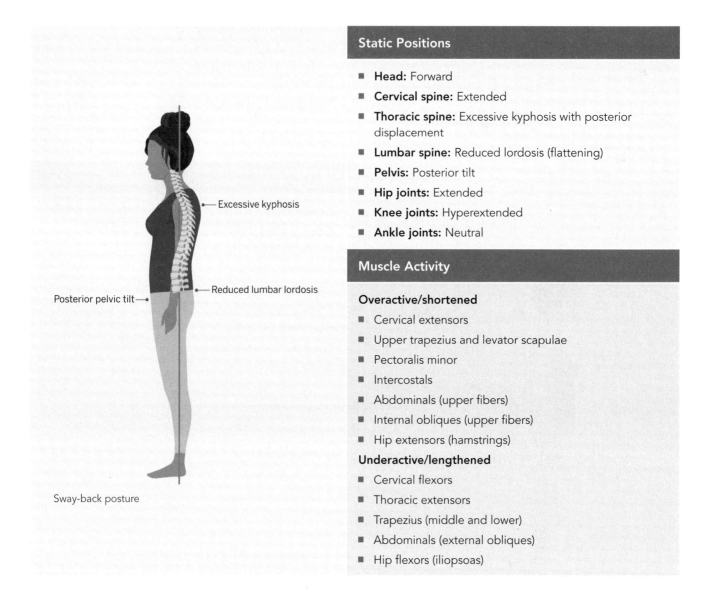

Excessive kyphosis

Reduced lumbar lordosis

Posterior pelvic tilt

Sway-back posture

Static Positions

- **Head:** Forward
- **Cervical spine:** Extended
- **Thoracic spine:** Excessive kyphosis with posterior displacement
- **Lumbar spine:** Reduced lordosis (flattening)
- **Pelvis:** Posterior tilt
- **Hip joints:** Extended
- **Knee joints:** Hyperextended
- **Ankle joints:** Neutral

Muscle Activity

Overactive/shortened
- Cervical extensors
- Upper trapezius and levator scapulae
- Pectoralis minor
- Intercostals
- Abdominals (upper fibers)
- Internal obliques (upper fibers)
- Hip extensors (hamstrings)

Underactive/lengthened
- Cervical flexors
- Thoracic extensors
- Trapezius (middle and lower)
- Abdominals (external obliques)
- Hip flexors (iliopsoas)

KYPHOSIS-LORDOSIS POSTURE

Individuals with Kendall's kyphosis-lordosis posture may present with both upper- and lower-body postural issues. In the upper body, individuals may present with the primary findings of forward head, excessive thoracic kyphosis, and rounded and elevated shoulders. In the lower body and LPHC, individuals may present with primary findings of excessive lumbar lordosis, lateral lumbar shift, anterior pelvic tilt, flexed hips, knees hyperextended or flexed, and ankle plantar flexion (Kendall et al., 2014).

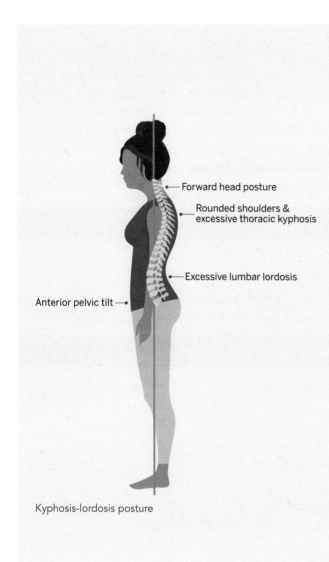

Forward head posture

Rounded shoulders & excessive thoracic kyphosis

Excessive lumbar lordosis

Anterior pelvic tilt

Kyphosis-lordosis posture

Static Positions

- **Head:** Forward
- **Cervical spine:** Extended
- **Thoracic spine:** Excessive kyphosis
- **Shoulders:** Rounded, elevated
- **Lumbar spine:** Excessive lordosis, possible lateral shift
- **Pelvis:** Anterior tilt
- **Hip joints:** Flexed
- **Knee joints:** Flexed or hyperextended
- **Ankle joints:** Neutral or plantar flexed

Muscle Activity

Overactive/shortened

- Cervical extensors
- Upper trapezius and levator scapulae
- Shoulder adductors
- Intercostals
- Pectoralis minor
- Internal obliques (upper and lateral)
- Hip flexors (iliopsoas)
- Lumbar extensors

Underactive/lengthened

- Cervical flexors
- Thoracic extensors
- Trapezius (middle and lower)
- Anterior abdominals (external obliques)
- Hip extensors (hamstrings)

 TRAINING TIP

Use Kendall's posture types in the same way as Janda's syndromes. Simply compare a client's static posture to the type that most closely matches in order to form a broad picture of the probable muscle imbalances the client might have. Subsequent movement and mobility assessments will then be used to focus that view to a much more detailed understanding of which muscles are in fact overactive/shortened or underactive/lengthened.

Pes Planus Distortion Syndrome

Pes planus distortion syndrome

A postural distortion pattern characterized by flat feet, knee valgus, and an anterior pelvic tilt.

Another common pattern of static postural impairment seen in the greater population is pes planus distortion. Similar to impairments seen in Janda's LCS, individuals with **pes planus distortion syndrome** may present with a combination of excessive pes planus (flat feet), knee flexion (reduced knee extension ROM), hip and knee internal rotation, knee valgus (knock-kneed), and an anterior pelvic tilt (Barwick et al., 2012; Fritz, 2013). Essentially, pes planus distortion syndrome represents the cascading influence that flat feet have on the kinetic chain. Pes planus distortion syndrome may lead to joint dysfunction at the big toe, ankle

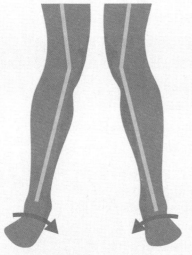

Pes planus distortion syndrome

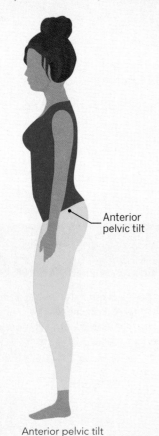

Anterior pelvic tilt

Anterior pelvic tilt

Static Positions

- **Pelvis:** Anterior tilt
- **Hip joints:** Internally rotated
- **Knee joints:** Valgus, flexed
- **Ankle joints:** Pronated (flattened, pes planus)

Muscle Activity

Overactive/shortened
- Gastrocnemius and soleus
- Peroneals
- Adductors
- Iliotibial band
- Iliopsoas
- Hamstrings

Underactive/lengthened
- Posterior and anterior tibialis
- Vastus medialis
- Gluteus maximus and medius
- Hip external rotators
- Hip flexors
- Thoracolumbar paraspinals

joints, sacroiliac joint, and lumbar spine. Individuals with this posture may develop injuries such as, but not limited to, plantar fasciitis, medial tibial stress syndrome (shin splints), patellar tendinitis, and low-back pain (Barwick et al., 2012; Chuter & Janse de Jonge, 2012; Neal et al., 2014; Okunuki et al., 2019).

Kinetic Check Points and Postural Distortion Syndromes

As the Corrective Exercise Specialist conducts the static postural assessment, they note any deviations from ideal static positions at each kinetic checkpoint. The totality of those observations should align to a postural distortion pattern. Professionals should consider that clients may or may not fall within one of the classifications. They may present with components of one or more classifications. The postural distortion classifications provide a starting point and framework for fitness professionals prior to other tests and measures such as with movement-based assessments. **Tables 8-2** and **8-3** provide a summary of the common muscle imbalances for each of the respective postural distortion patterns.

TABLE 8-2 Janda's Syndromes

	Lower Crossed Syndrome	Upper Crossed Syndrome	Layered Crossed Syndrome
Foot and Ankle	**Overactive:** Gastrocnemius/ soleus	**Overactive:** NC	**Overactive:** Gastrocnemius/ soleus
	Underactive: NC	**Underactive:** NC	**Underactive:** NC
Knee	**Overactive:** See foot and ankle	**Overactive:** NC	**Overactive:** See foot and ankle
	Underactive: NC	**Underactive:** NC	**Underactive:** NC
Lumbo-Pelvic-Hip Complex	**Overactive:** Hip flexors, lumbar extensors	**Overactive:** NC	**Overactive:** Hip flexors, lumbar extensors
	Underactive: Abdominals, hip extensors, gluteus maximus and medius	**Underactive:** NC	**Underactive:** Abdominals, hip extensors, gluteus maximus and medius

(continues)

posture. *Journal of Physical Therapy Science, 28*(10), 2929–2932. https://doi.org/10.1589/jpts.28.2929

Kolber, M. J., Cheatham, S. W., Salamh, P. A., & Hanney, W. J. (2014). Characteristics of shoulder impingement in the recreational weight-training population. *Journal of Strength & Conditioning Research, 28*(4), 1081–1089. https://doi.org/10.1519/jsc.0000000000000250

Kolber, M. J., Hanney, W. J., Cheatham, S. W., Salamh, P. A., Masaracchio, M., & Liu, X. (2017). Shoulder joint and muscle characteristics among weight-training participants with and without impingement syndrome. *Journal of Strength & Conditioning Research, 31*(4), 1024–1032. https://doi.org/10.1519/jsc.0000000000001554

Lee, C. H., Lee, S., & Shin, G. (2017). Reliability of forward head posture evaluation while sitting, standing, walking and running. *Human Movement Science, 55*, 81–86. https://doi.org/10.1016/j.humov.2017.07.008

Lynch, S. S., Thigpen, C. A., Mihalik, J. P., Prentice, W. E., & Padua, D. (2010). The effects of an exercise intervention on forward head and rounded shoulder postures in elite swimmers. *British Journal of Sports Medicine, 44*(5), 376–381. https://doi.org/10.1136/bjsm.2009.066837

McCann, R. S., Crossett, I. D., Terada, M., Kosik, K. B., Bolding, B. A., & Gribble, P. A. (2017). Hip strength and star excursion balance test deficits of patients with chronic ankle instability. *Journal of Science and Medicine in Sport, 20*(11), 992–996. https://doi.org/10.1016/j.jsams.2017.05.005

Mersmann, F., Bohm, S., & Arampatzis, A. (2017). Imbalances in the development of muscle and tendon as risk factor for tendinopathies in youth athletes: A review of current evidence and concepts of prevention. *Frontiers in Physiology, 8*, 987. https://doi.org/10.3389/fphys.2017.00987

Neal, B. S., Griffiths, I. B., Dowling, G. J., Murley, G. S., Munteanu, S. E., Franettovich Smith, M. M., Collins, N. J., & Barton, C. J. (2014). Foot posture as a risk factor for lower limb overuse injury: A systematic review and meta-analysis. *Journal of Foot and Ankle Research, 7*(1), 55. https://doi.org/10.1186/s13047-014-0055-4

Okunuki, T., Koshino, Y., Yamanaka, M., Tsutsumi, K., Igarashi, M., Samukawa, M., Saitoh, H., & Tohyama, H. (2019). Forefoot and hindfoot kinematics in subjects with medial tibial stress syndrome during walking and running. *Journal of Orthopaedic Research, 37*(4), 927–932. https://doi.org/10.1002/jor.24223

Oliveira, A. C., & Silva, A. G. (2016). Neck muscle endurance and head posture: A comparison between adolescents with and without neck pain. *Manual Therapy, 22*, 62–67. https://doi.org/10.1016/j.math.2015.10.002

Page, P., Frank, C. C., & Lardner, R. (2010). *Assessment and treatment of muscle imbalance: The Janda approach.* Human Kinetics.

Shiri, R., & Falah-Hassani, K. (2015). Computer use and carpal tunnel syndrome: A meta-analysis. *Journal of the Neurological Sciences, 349*(1–2), 15–19. https://doi.org/10.1016/j.jns.2014.12.037

Struyf, F., Tate, A., Kuppens, K., Feijen, S., & Michener, L. A. (2017). Musculoskeletal dysfunctions associated with swimmers' shoulder. *British Journal of Sports Medicine, 51*(10), 775–780. https://doi.org/10.1136/bjsports-2016-096847

Sueki, D. G., Cleland, J. A., & Wainner, R. S. (2013). A regional interdependence model of musculoskeletal dysfunction: Research, mechanisms, and clinical implications. *Journal of Manual & Manipulative Therapy, 21*(2), 90–102. https://doi.org/10.1179/2042618612y.0000000027

Tegtmeier, P. (2018). A scoping review on smart mobile devices and physical strain. *Work, 59*(2), 273–283. https://doi.org/10.3233/wor-172678

Trulsson, A., Miller, M., Gummesson, C., & Garwicz, M. (2016). Associations between altered movement patterns during single-leg squat and muscle activity at weight-transfer initiation in individuals with anterior cruciate ligament injury. *BMJ Open Sport & Exercise Medicine, 2*(1), e000131. https://doi.org/10.1136/bmjsem-2016-000131

Verhagen, A. P., Bierma-Zeinstra, S. M., Burdorf, A., Stynes, S. M., de Vet, H. C., & Koes, B. W. (2013). Conservative interventions for treating work-related complaints of the arm, neck or shoulder in adults. *The Cochrane Database of Systematic Reviews,* (12), Cd008742. https://doi.org/10.1002/14651858.CD008742.pub2

CHAPTER 9

Movement Assessments

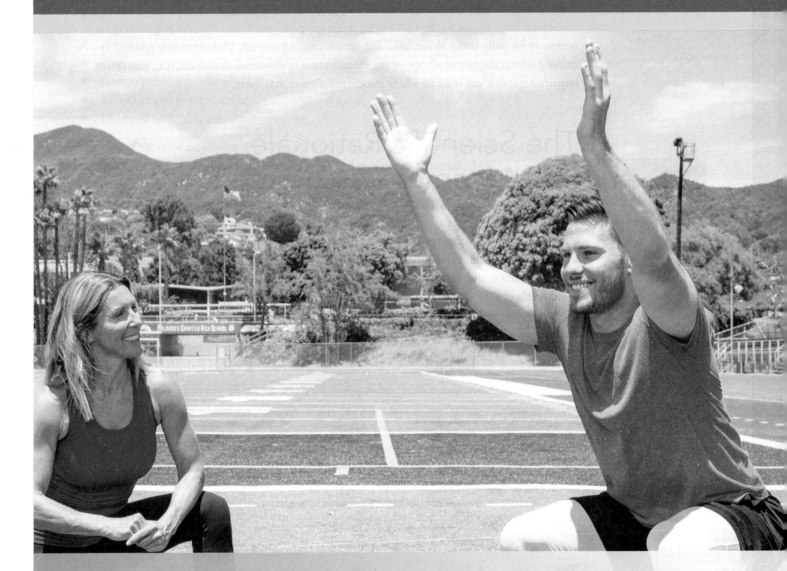

Learning Objectives

After reading this content, students should be able to demonstrate the following objectives:

- **Explain** the function of a movement assessment.
- **Differentiate** between transitional, loaded, and dynamic movement assessments.
- **Explain** the relationship between muscle imbalances and movement impairments.
- **Identify** the steps for performing movement assessments.

- Hinge
- Split stance
- Single leg and stepping

Correct performance of these movement patterns is an indication that the client can likely maintain correct form during common exercises and activities. The primary movement patterns should be observed throughout all workouts and assessed for kinetic chain alignment. The specific patterns of squat, push, pull, and overhead press can be performed as separate formal loaded assessments included as part of the CES Assessment Flow. Additionally, if a client refuses or is unable to perform the necessary transitional movement assessments, the Corrective Exercise Specialist can include these specific loaded movement assessments within the client's workouts. During the set, the Corrective Exercise Specialist can assess the client's movement quality and overall capabilities. Further, these loaded movements can serve as an initial "workout" to the client provided they can safely perform each movement. Loaded movement assessments include the following:

- Loaded squat
- Standing push
- Standing pull
- Standing overhead dumbbell press

DYNAMIC MOVEMENT ASSESSMENTS

Dynamic movement assessments

Assessments that involve movement with a change in the base of support.

Dynamic movement assessments involve movement with a change in one's base of support. This would include movements such as walking and jumping. Just like the loaded assessments, they can be seen as an optional advanced component of the corrective exercise assessment process, and include the following:

- Gait (walking) assessment
- Depth jump assessment
- The Davies test

Dynamic assessments can be used in two ways. The first is as a method of refinement and confirmation for what was observed in the transitional assessments. This is the primary purpose of the gait assessment. For example, if excessive pronation is observed in a client who enjoys walking and running for exercise, the gait assessment can be used to see how that compensation translates to everyday life and affects their performance.

Another use of the dynamic movement assessments is to add additional challenge to the movement assessment process for more advanced clients. As clients progress through their corrective exercise journey, transitional assessments may no longer provide any new and actionable information. Once movement impairments are relatively improved, clients will be able to perform tasks like the OHSA showing little-to-no compensation in their movement

⚠ CRITICAL

The depth jump assessment and Davies test should be considered advanced movements that pose a high demand on the musculoskeletal system. These dynamic assessments are often performed at a faster tempo, which can increase the risk of injury among clients who may not be prepared for such complex movements. Clients should always be instructed to perform dynamic assessments in the fastest manner that can be safely controlled and discouraged from rushing through the movement carelessly.

patterns. The depth jump assessment and Davies test both serve this optional need. Further, the higher-intensity movements, such as the depth jump and Davies test, place a greater demand on the musculoskeletal system and may be best reserved for those clients ready for plyometric or sport-specific activities.

Kinetic Chain Checkpoints

Just like during the static postural assessment, movement assessments require observation of the five kinetic chain checkpoints from multiple viewpoints. Although each region of the body will be assessed individually, the Corrective Exercise Specialist should always think of the body in relation to the Regional Interdependence (RI) model: as an interrelated system, where one joint or region has an influence on the others (Sueki et al., 2013).

Although a movement impairment may be noted for a given joint, the cause of that impairment may actually be coming from a lack of mobility or strength in a completely different region (Sueki et al., 2013). For example, knee valgus may be marked in a client assessment, but the cause of that movement impairment could be increased hip adduction and internal rotation and/or excessive foot and ankle pronation.

Each joint or body region has a specific biomechanical motion that it produces based on its structure and function, as well as the joints above and below it (Nakagawa et al., 2012a, 2012b; Powers, 2010; Sueki et al., 2013). When that specific motion deviates from its normal path, it is considered a movement impairment and can be used to presume possible muscle imbalance or joint dysfunction (Bolgla et al., 2008; Nakagawa et al., 2012b; Powers, 2010). In order to efficiently assess each movement, the following viewpoints should be used:

- **Anterior**: The anterior view is used to assess frontal and transverse plane movements (adduction, abduction, elevation, and rotation) (**Figure 9-1**).

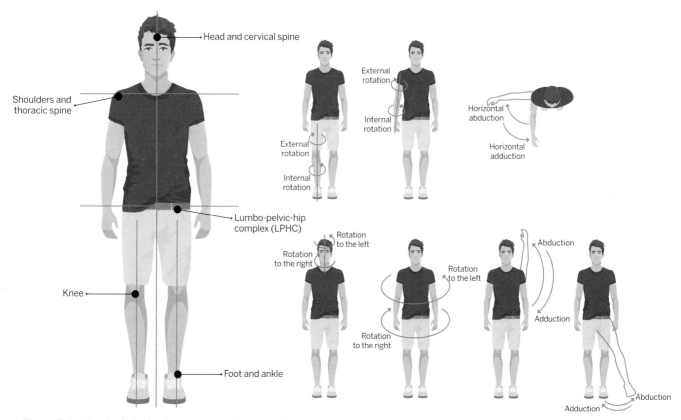

Figure 9-1 Kinetic chain checkpoints—anterior view with movement

- **Lateral**: The lateral view is used to assess sagittal plane movements (flexion and extension) (**Figure 9-2**).
- **Posterior**: The posterior view is used to assess foot and ankle pronation, asymmetrical weight shift, and scapular elevation (**Figure 9-3**).

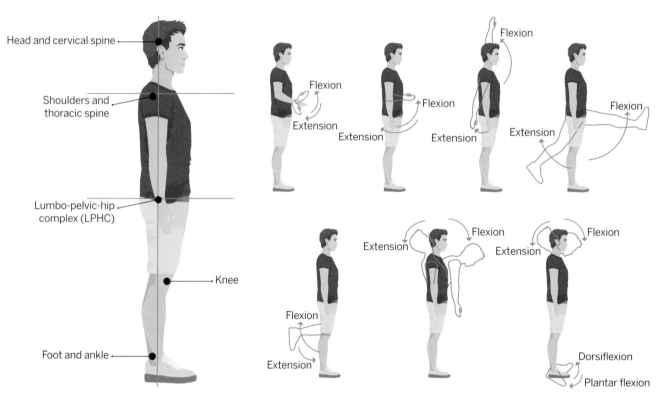

Figure 9-2 Kinetic chain checkpoints—lateral view with movement

Common Movement Impairments

No matter what movement assessment is being performed, there is a common collection of movement impairments that may be seen throughout the kinetic chain. Note that each of the following movement impairments may be caused by, or associated with, other movement impairments due to the concepts of regional interdependence.

Note that the term *movement impairment* is simply being used to describe a client's movement strategy as it deviates from optimal dynamic postural alignment. These observable impairments represent the body's compensatory strategies for accomplishing functional movement patterns in the presence of muscle imbalances. The relationship may be characterized as:

muscle imbalances → compensatory strategies → observable movement impairments

Table 9-1 includes the most common movement impairments that can be improved through corrective exercise.

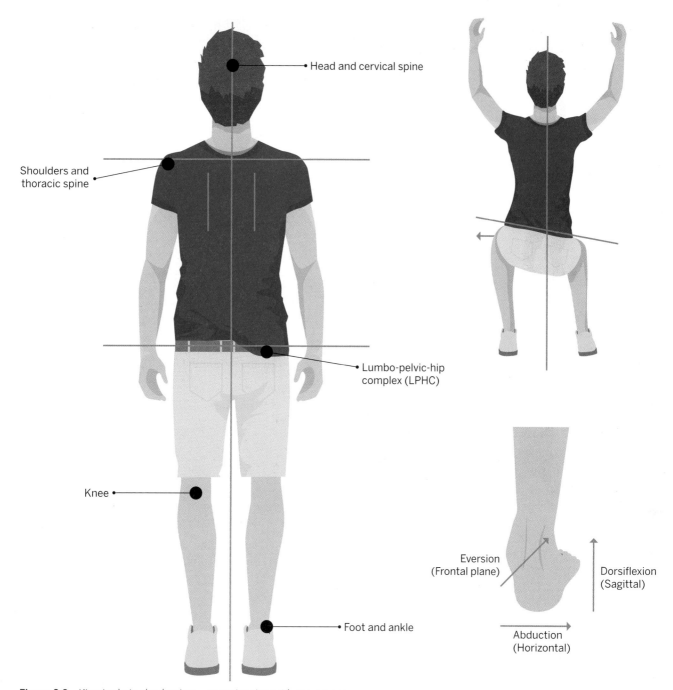

Figure 9-3 Kinetic chain checkpoints—posterior view with movement

 CRITICAL

The fitness professional should be careful when explaining movement impairments to their client. Jargon should be avoided, and the results should be communicated in a way that does not discourage the client. A friendly discussion of their movement quality, observed impairments, and corrective exercise plan is a great way to empower clients to be successful with their program. Use of terms such as *compensation*, *dysfunction*, and *impairment* may sound negative to the client. Referring to compensations as "movement strategies" or "habits that their body prefers" will not only make more sense to the client, but also avoid sounding too negative, clinical, or serious.

TABLE 9-1 Common Movement Impairments

	Excessive pronation	Look for the arch of the foot to collapse and flatten, eversion of the heel, or malalignment of the Achilles tendon.
	Feet turn out	Look for the toes to rotate laterally during the movement (aka foot abduction).
	Heel rise	Look for the heel to come off of the ground during the movement.
	Knee valgus	Look for the knees to collapse inward.

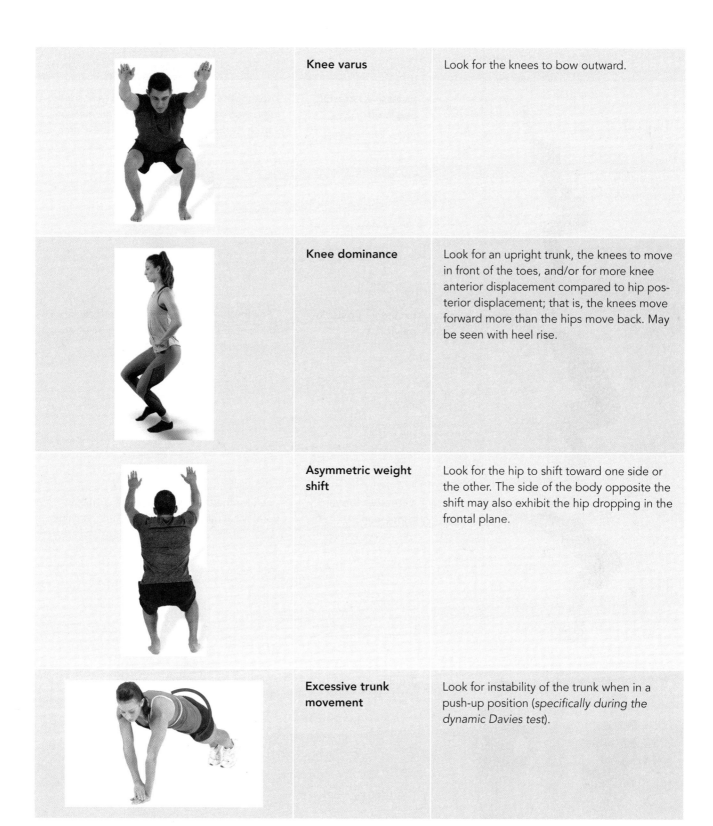

	Knee varus	Look for the knees to bow outward.
	Knee dominance	Look for an upright trunk, the knees to move in front of the toes, and/or for more knee anterior displacement compared to hip posterior displacement; that is, the knees move forward more than the hips move back. May be seen with heel rise.
	Asymmetric weight shift	Look for the hip to shift toward one side or the other. The side of the body opposite the shift may also exhibit the hip dropping in the frontal plane.
	Excessive trunk movement	Look for instability of the trunk when in a push-up position (*specifically during the dynamic Davies test*).

(continues)

TABLE 9-1 Common Movement Impairments (*continued*)

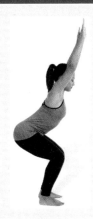

Excessive anterior pelvic tilt

Look for the pelvis to roll forward and for the lumbar spine to extend beyond normal curvature, creating a prominent low-back arch.

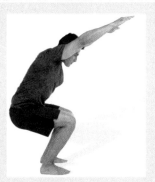

Excessive posterior pelvic tilt

Look for the pelvis to roll backward and for the lumbar spine to flex, creating a flattening or rounding of the lower back.

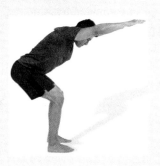

Excessive forward trunk lean

Look for the trunk to lean forward and beyond ideal parallel alignment with the shins.

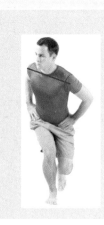 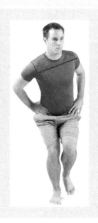

Trunk rotation

Look for the trunk of the body to rotate internally or externally during single-leg movements.

	Scapular elevation	Look for the shoulders to move up toward the ears.
	Scapular winging	Look for the scapulae to protrude excessively from the back, seen most prominently in a push-up position (*specifically during the dynamic Davies test or when pushing*).
	Arms fall forward	Look for the arms to fall forward to no longer be aligned with the torso and ears.
	Excessive cervical extension (forward head)	Look for the head to migrate forward, moving the ears out of alignment with the shoulders.

For each observable movement impairment, **Table 9-2** can be used to identify which muscles are potentially overactive/shortened and which are underactive/lengthened, causing the movement impairment to happen. Additionally, it will provide suggested mobility assessments related to each observed movement impairment. Table 9-2 is to be used as the solutions reference for all movement assessments in the corrective exercise process.

TABLE 9-2 Movement Assessment Solutions				
Checkpoint	View	Movement Impairment	Potential Contributors	Suggested Mobility Assessments*
Foot and ankle	Anterior	Feet turn out	**Overactive/shortened** ■ Biceps femoris (short head) ■ Gastrocnemius (lateral) ■ Soleus **Underactive/lengthened** ■ Anterior tibialis ■ Gastrocnemius (medial) ■ Gluteus maximus ■ Gluteus medius ■ Hamstrings complex (medial) ■ Posterior tibialis	■ Active knee extension ■ Ankle dorsiflexion ■ Hip abduction and external rotation ■ Modified Thomas test ■ Seated hip internal and external rotation
	Lateral	Heel rise	**Overactive/shortened** ■ Quadriceps complex ■ Soleus **Underactive/lengthened** ■ Anterior tibialis ■ Gluteus maximus	■ Active knee flexion ■ Ankle dorsiflexion
	Posterior	Excessive pronation	**Overactive/shortened** ■ Fibularis (peroneal) complex ■ Gastrocnemius (lateral) ■ Tensor fascia latae **Underactive/lengthened** ■ Anterior tibialis ■ Gastrocnemius (medial) ■ Gluteus maximus ■ Gluteus medius ■ Intrinsic foot muscles ■ Posterior tibialis	■ Ankle dorsiflexion ■ Modified Thomas test ■ Seated hip internal and external rotation
Knee	Anterior	Valgus (inward)	**Overactive/shortened** ■ Adductor complex ■ Biceps femoris (short head) ■ Gastrocnemius ■ Soleus ■ Tensor fascia latae ■ Vastus lateralis	■ Active knee extension ■ Ankle dorsiflexion ■ Hip abduction and external rotation

Checkpoint	View	Movement Impairment	Potential Contributors	Suggested Mobility Assessments*
Knee (*continued*)			**Underactive/lengthened** ■ Anterior tibialis ■ Gluteus maximus ■ Gluteus medius ■ Hamstrings complex (medial) ■ Posterior tibialis ■ Vastus medialis oblique (VMO)	■ Modified Thomas test ■ Seated hip internal and external rotation
	Anterior	Varus (outward)	**Overactive/shortened** ■ Adductor magnus (posterior fibers) ■ Anterior tibialis ■ Biceps femoris (long head) ■ Piriformis ■ Posterior tibialis ■ Tensor fascia latae **Underactive/lengthened** ■ Adductor complex ■ Gluteus maximus ■ Hamstrings complex (medial)	■ Active knee extension ■ Lumbar flexion ■ Modified Thomas test ■ Passive hip internal rotation ■ Seated hip internal and external rotation
	Lateral	Knee dominance	**Overactive/shortened^** ■ Adductor magnus ■ Piriformis ■ Quadriceps complex ■ Soleus **Underactive/lengthened^** ■ Core stabilizers ■ Gluteus maximus	■ Active knee flexion ■ Ankle dorsiflexion ■ Hip abduction and external rotation ■ Modified Thomas test ■ Passive hip internal rotation

LPHC	Anterior or posterior	Asymmetric weight shift	**Overactive/shortened**
			■ Same side as shift
			  • Adductor complex
			  • Tensor fascia latae
			■ Opposite side of shift
			  • Biceps femoris
			  • Gastrocnemius/soleus
			  • Piriformis
			Underactive/lengthened
			■ Core stabilizers
			■ Same side as shift
			  • Gluteus medius
			■ Opposite side of shift
			  • Adductor complex
				■ Active knee extension
				■ Ankle dorsiflexion
				■ Hip abduction and external rotation
				■ Modified Thomas test
				■ Seated hip internal and external rotation

(continues)

TABLE 9-2 Movement Assessment Solutions (*continued*)

Checkpoint	View	Movement Impairment	Potential Contributors	Suggested Mobility Assessments*
LPHC (*continued*)	Anterior or posterior	Excessive trunk movement during testing (Davies test)	**Overactive/shortened** ■ N/A **Underactive/lengthened** ■ Local core stabilizers	N/A
	Lateral	Excessive anterior pelvic tilt (increased lumbar extension)	**Overactive/shortened** ■ Adductor complex (anterior fibers) ■ Latissimus dorsi ■ Psoas ■ Rectus femoris ■ Spinal extensor complex (erector spinae, quadratus lumborum) ■ Tensor fascia latae **Underactive/lengthened** ■ External obliques ■ Gluteus maximus ■ Hamstrings complex ■ Local core stabilizers ■ Rectus abdominis	■ Active knee flexion ■ Hip abduction and external rotation ■ Lumbar flexion and extension ■ Modified Thomas test ■ Shoulder flexion
	Lateral	Excessive posterior pelvic tilt (increased lumbar flexion)	**Overactive/shortened** ■ Adductor magnus ■ External obliques ■ Hamstrings complex ■ Piriformis ■ Rectus abdominis **Underactive/lengthened** ■ Gluteus maximus ■ Latissimus dorsi ■ Local core stabilizers ■ Psoas ■ Rectus femoris ■ Spinal extensor complex (erector spinae, quadratus lumborum) ■ Tensor fascia latae	■ Active knee extension ■ Hip abduction and external rotation ■ Lumbar flexion and extension ■ Seated hip internal and external rotation

Checkpoint	View	Movement Impairment	Potential Contributors	Suggested Mobility Assessments*
LPHC (continued)	Lateral	Excessive forward trunk lean	**Overactive/shortened** ■ Adductor complex (anterior fibers) ■ External obliques (if observed with lumbar flexion) ■ Gastrocnemius ■ Psoas ■ Rectus abdominis (if observed with lumbar flexion) ■ Rectus femoris ■ Soleus ■ Tensor fascia latae **Underactive/lengthened** ■ Anterior tibialis ■ Gluteus maximus ■ Hamstrings complex ■ Local core stabilizers ■ Spinal extensor complex (erector spinae, quadratus lumborum)	■ Active knee flexion ■ Ankle dorsiflexion ■ Modified Thomas test
	Anterior	Inward trunk rotation (single-leg and split squat)	**Overactive/shortened** ■ Adductor complex ■ Tensor fascia latae **Underactive/lengthened** ■ Gluteus maximus ■ Gluteus medius ■ Local core stabilizers	■ Hip abduction and external rotation ■ Modified Thomas test ■ Seated hip internal and external rotation
	Anterior	Outward trunk rotation (single-leg and split squat)	**Overactive/shortened** ■ Adductor magnus (posterior fibers) ■ Hamstrings complex (lateral) ■ Piriformis **Underactive/lengthened** ■ Adductor complex (anterior fibers) ■ Gluteus maximus ■ Gluteus medius ■ Local core stabilizers	■ Hip abduction and external rotation ■ Modified Thomas test ■ Seated hip internal and external rotation

(continues)

TABLE 9-2 Movement Assessment Solutions (*continued*)

Checkpoint	View	Movement Impairment	Potential Contributors	Suggested Mobility Assessments*
Shoulders and thoracic spine	Anterior or posterior	Scapular elevation	**Overactive/shortened** ■ Levator scapulae ■ Pectoralis minor ■ Upper trapezius **Underactive/lengthened** ■ Lower trapezius ■ Serratus anterior	■ Cervical flexion and extension ■ Cervical lateral flexion ■ Cervical rotation ■ Seated thoracic rotation ■ Shoulder retraction ■ Thoracic extension
	Lateral	Scapular winging (Davies test and push assessment)	**Overactive/shortened** ■ Latissimus dorsi ■ Pectoralis minor ■ Upper trapezius **Underactive/lengthened** ■ Lower trapezius ■ Middle trapezius ■ Serratus anterior	■ Seated thoracic rotation ■ Shoulder flexion ■ Shoulder retraction ■ Thoracic extension
	Lateral	Arms fall forward	**Overactive/shortened** ■ Latissimus dorsi ■ Pectoralis major ■ Pectoralis minor ■ Teres major **Underactive/lengthened** ■ Infraspinatus ■ Lower trapezius ■ Middle trapezius ■ Posterior deltoids ■ Rhomboids ■ Teres minor	■ Cervical flexion and extension ■ Cervical rotation ■ Cervical lateral flexion ■ Shoulder extension ■ Shoulder flexion ■ Shoulder internal and external rotation ■ Shoulder retraction ■ Seated thoracic rotation ■ Thoracic extension
Head and cervical spine	Lateral	Excessive cervical extension (forward head)	**Overactive/shortened** ■ Cervical extensors (suboccipital) ■ Levator scapulae ■ Sternocleidomastoid ■ Upper trapezius **Underactive/lengthened** ■ Deep cervical flexors ■ Lower trapezius ■ Middle trapezius ■ Rhomboids	■ Cervical flexion and extension ■ Cervical lateral flexion ■ Cervical rotation

*It is not necessary to perform all of the listed mobility assessments associated with each movement impairment. The mobility assessments provided are a starting point that is narrowed down based on the results of the OHSA, modified OHSA, and other movement assessments. It is likely that only a few mobility assessments will be needed.

^Movement competency, pain avoidance, or balance strategies should be ruled out prior to assuming over- and underactive muscles as contributing factors to knee dominance.

Note that the list of movement assessment solutions presented in Table 9-2 is not exhaustive. Advanced or clinical professionals may include muscle groups not listed here. Muscles listed as overactive/shortened and underactive/lengthened are ones that best meet the following criteria:

- Biomechanical properties (i.e., the motion created or allowed by the muscle)
- Tendencies of muscle group activity (e.g., the gluteus maximus is usually underactive)
- Solution practicality in most settings (e.g., it is not realistic to program inhibition of the subscapularis in a nonclinical setting)
- Programming efficiency in most scenarios (e.g., performing activation of the medial hamstrings will also involve other tibial internal rotators)

Corrective exercise programming using the provided movement impairments and muscle groups, when further refined by later assessment stages, will optimize the movement quality and injury resistance of any client or athlete.

TRAINING TIP

Similar to pes planus distortion syndrome while static, pronation distortion syndrome (PDS) is an additional pattern of movement impairments commonly noted among fitness professionals with the OHSA and the SLS (Post et al., 2017; Räisänen et al., 2016). A client with PDS will demonstrate a combination of excessive foot/ankle pronation, knee valgus, and hip adduction and internal rotation during motion.

Transitional Movement Assessments

After completing a static postural assessment, the next step in the CES Assessment Flow is to use transitional movement assessments to evaluate dynamic posture. Transitional assessments use movements without a change in one's base of support. The Corrective Exercise Specialist will assess the client's posture and alignment during the ascent and descent of each movement, viewing from the front, side, and rear, and make note of any movement impairments that occur.

The Corrective Exercise Specialist should first explain how to correctly set up and perform the movement and then have the client perform the movement without providing any feedback. This will provide insight into the client's ability to perform the movement naturally. Transitional movements should be completed in a slow, controlled manner, and without significant effort by the client.

TRAINING TIP

During assessment, clients may choose to perform the movements differently based on their confidence, experience, motor control, and mobility. Due to the variations among individuals, NASM recommends using a standardized sequence for each assessment to allow for the highest levels of consistency and a direct comparison over time (McMillian et al., 2016; Warner et al., 2019). The recommended testing procedures are detailed for each movement assessment.

Overhead Squat Assessment

The overhead squat assessment (OHSA) is designed to assess dynamic posture, core stability, mobility, and neuromuscular control of the whole body during a squatting motion (Post et al., 2017; Rabin & Kozol, 2017). It is the first movement assessment that will be used for all clients and will serve as the qualifier to determine which additional movement assessments should be used (see **Figure 9-4**).

The OHSA has been shown to be a reliable, valid, and repeatable transitional movement assessment for movement impairments for one or more professionals who administer the test (Post et al., 2017; Rabin & Kozol, 2017). That is to say, even if a client is trained by different fitness professionals, the OHSA will remain a reliable measure to consistently assess progress. Assessment of this movement is essential to create a focused corrective exercise plan that considers the biomechanical and range of motion variations that will be assessed among different clients (Mauntel et al., 2015; Vidal et al., 2018).

NASM CES Assessment Flow

1 Client Intake

2 Static Postural Assessment

3 Overhead Squat Assessment (OHSA) and Modified OHSA

4 Single-Leg Squat and/or Split Squat Assessment

4a Dynamic Assessments
OPTIONAL

4b Loaded Assessments
OPTIONAL

5 Mobility Assessments

6 Corrective Exercise Programming
INHIBIT · LENGTHEN
ACTIVATE · INTEGRATE

Overhead Squat Assessment (OHSA)

NASM
NATIONAL ACADEMY OF SPORTS MEDICINE

Perform OHSA from anterior, lateral, and posterior views and note movement compensations.

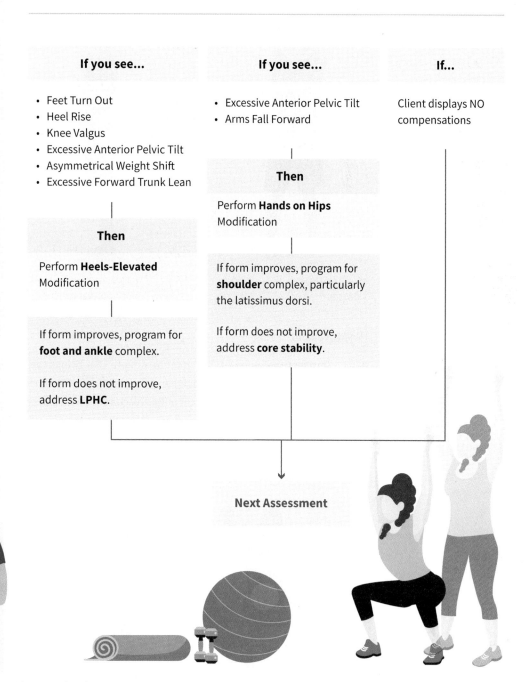

If you see...

- Feet Turn Out
- Heel Rise
- Knee Valgus
- Excessive Anterior Pelvic Tilt
- Asymmetrical Weight Shift
- Excessive Forward Trunk Lean

Then

Perform **Heels-Elevated** Modification

If form improves, program for **foot and ankle** complex.

If form does not improve, address **LPHC**.

If you see...

- Excessive Anterior Pelvic Tilt
- Arms Fall Forward

Then

Perform **Hands on Hips** Modification

If form improves, program for **shoulder** complex, particularly the latissimus dorsi.

If form does not improve, address **core stability**.

If...

Client displays NO compensations

Next Assessment

Figure 9-4   CES Assessment Flow: overhead squat assessment

Starting Position

1. The individual stands with the feet hip-to-shoulder-width apart and pointed straight ahead and parallel. The foot and ankle complex should be in a neutral position. The assessment should be performed with the shoes off if possible to best view the foot and ankle complex.
2. Have the individual raise their arms overhead, extended and aligned with the torso.

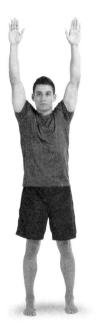
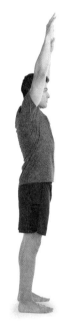
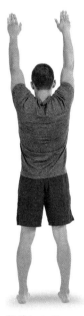

OHSA starting position—anterior view

OHSA starting position—lateral view

OHSA starting position—posterior view

Movement

1. Instruct the individual to squat to a depth that brings the femur parallel to the ground (roughly the height of a chair) and then return to the starting position. The squat depth can also be reduced if the client has discomfort with a deeper squat.
2. Have the client repeat the movement for five repetitions, observing from anterior, lateral, and posterior views (five repetitions for each viewpoint).

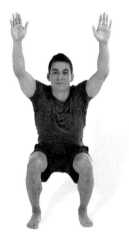
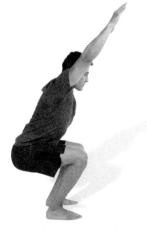
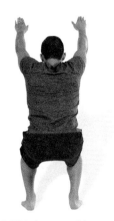

OHSA down position—anterior view

OHSA down position—lateral view

OHSA down position—posterior view

OBSERVATION

Each viewpoint will require focus on specific kinetic chain checkpoints. Some impairments may be seen from more than one viewpoint. For each, ideal performance of the OHSA exhibits the following:

- **Anterior**: View the feet, knees, and LPHC from the front. The feet and hips should remain in the sagittal plane with the knees tracking in line with the foot (second and third toes). The LPHC should not shift from side to side or rotate.
- **Lateral**: View the feet, ankles, knees, LPHC, shoulders, and head from the side. The heels should stay on the ground. The pelvis and spine should remain in a neutral posture. The torso should remain in parallel with the tibia while the arms stay in line with the torso. Head should remain neutral.
- **Posterior**: View the feet and ankles (if not wearing shoes) and shoulders from the back. The arch of the foot and calcaneus (i.e., heel) should remain in a neutral position. Shoulders/scapulae should be neutral.

From the *anterior view*, look for the following potential movement impairments:

- **Foot and ankle**: Feet turn out
- **Knee**: Valgus or varus
- **LPHC**: Asymmetric weight shift
- **Shoulder**: Scapular elevation

From the *lateral view*, look for the following potential movement impairments:

- **Foot and ankle**: Heel rise
- **Knee**: Knee dominance
- **LPHC**:
  - Excessive anterior pelvic tilt
  - Excessive posterior pelvic tilt
  - Excessive forward trunk lean
- **Shoulder**: Arms fall forward
- **Head and cervical spine**: Forward head

From the *posterior view*, look for the following potential movement impairments:

- **Foot and ankle**: Excessive foot pronation
- **LPHC**: Asymmetric weight shift
- **Shoulder**: Scapular elevation

When performing the assessment, record all findings on the **Overhead Squat Observational Findings** template. Then, refer to Table 9-2 to determine potential causes of these movement impairments that can be corrected using a focused corrective exercise program. It will be used for all three transitional movement assessments (overhead squat, split squat, and single-leg squat).

Each of the following movement impairments may be caused by, or associated with, other movement impairments due to the impact of each joint in the kinetic chain. Movement assessments reveal the group of possible overactive and underactive muscles that are related to a particular movement impairment. Mobility assessments in the next stage may further distinguish which particular muscles within a group are the primary contributors to that movement impairment; and if over- or underactivity is more responsible for the impairment. These refined observations lead the Corrective Exercise Specialist to the best exercise selections to address a given movement pattern or impairment.

OVERHEAD SQUAT OBSERVATIONAL FINDINGS

CHECKPOINT	VIEWPOINT	MOVEMENT IMPAIRMENT	RESULT
Foot and Ankle	**Anterior**	• Feet turn out	• Right • Left • Both
	Lateral	• Heel rise	• Right • Left • Both
	Posterior	• Excessive pronation	• Right • Left • Both
Knee	**Anterior**	• Valgus	• Right • Left • Both
		• Varus	• Right • Left • Both
	Lateral	• Knee dominance	• Right • Left • Both
LPHC	**Anterior or Posterior**	• Asymmetric weight shift	*Direction:* • Right • Left
	Lateral	• Excessive anterior pelvic tilt	• YES • NO
		• Excessive posterior pelvic tilt	• YES • NO
		• Excessive forward trunk lean	• YES • NO
Shoulders and Thoracic Spine	**Anterior or Posterior**	• Scapular elevation	• Right • Left • Both
	Lateral	• Arms fall forward	• Right • Left • Both
Head and Cervical Spine	**Lateral**	• Excessive cervical extension/forward head	• YES • NO

Mark *Right* or *Left* or *Both* based on which limb a movement impairment was observed at. For asymmetric weight shift, mark the direction in which the shift occurred.

MODIFICATIONS

Heels Elevated	Squat performance improves?	• YES • NO
Hands on Hips	Squat performance improves?	• YES • NO

Overhead squat observational findings

MODIFICATIONS TO THE OVERHEAD SQUAT ASSESSMENT

When certain movement impairments are observed during the OHSA, modifications to the assessment should be used to gain a clearer picture of the probable causes in other areas of the kinetic chain. These modifications include elevating the individual's heels and performing the squat with the hands on the hips (instead of overhead). Researchers have documented that these modifications will often improve an individual's performance on the OHSA (Richards et al., 2016).

In the context of the RI model, improvements in performance with the modifications help to better identify the root causes of impairments. Frequently, the root cause is found in other regions of the body than where the impairment was originally observed. Note that the heels-elevated modification is intended as a variation of dynamic postural assessment, not of workout or training technique.

HEELS ELEVATED

If a client exhibits movement impairments at the foot and ankle complex, knee, or LPHC, the root cause may usually be found at either the foot and ankle complex or the LPHC. For example, knee valgus may be an impairment due to a lack of ankle dorsiflexion or muscle imbalances at the hip, such as overactive adductors and underactive gluteals. Elevating the heels during a squat (**Figure 9-5**) places the ankle in plantar flexion, which decreases the extensibility required from the plantar flexor muscles (gastrocnemius, soleus), effectively providing "artificial" dorsiflexion. If knee valgus is related to ankle dorsiflexion restriction, elevating the heels will improve the alignment of the knee. If the knee valgus is not related to ankle dorsiflexion restriction, elevating the heels will not improve the alignment of the knee.

Excessive forward trunk lean is another compensation that may be related to foot and ankle or LPHC limitations. If ankle dorsiflexion restriction is present, the client may compensate at the LPHC to squat. However, the movement impairment may also be related to muscle imbalances at the LPHC, such as overactive hip flexors and underactive hip extensors. If the heels-elevated modification improves the squat, then the Corrective Exercise Specialist should focus on the foot and ankle complex. However, if the modification does not improve the squat, then the Corrective Exercise Specialist should perform additional assessment of the LPHC.

Elevating the heels also alters the client's center of gravity by allowing the individual to sit more upright. This is important because with less forward lean there will be more knee excursion and less hip flexion utilized during the squat. This places less emphasis on the LPHC.

This modification allows the Corrective Exercise Specialist to see the influence the ankle has on the individual's deviations (Richards et al., 2016). If an individual displays a movement impairment during the overhead squat that is improved after elevating the heels, then the Corrective Exercise Specialist can direct their corrective exercise plan toward improving ankle dorsiflexion. If the squat performance is not improved by elevating the heels, then the observed movement impairment is likely not related to dysfunction at the ankle.

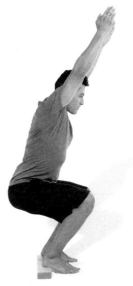

Figure 9-5 OHSA heels elevated

TRAINING TIP

Palm orientation: Palms may face each other or forward during the OHSA. Palm position may affect shoulder comfort and ROM while raising the arms overhead due to muscle tension differences with each position. Ultimately, palm orientation comes down to client and professional preference, but should remain consistent for subsequent assessments.

Footwear: Shoes may affect static and dynamic posture because they often place the ankle in a chronically plantar flexed position. It is important (provided facilities allow it) for clients to perform the OHSA without shoes and in their natural state.

HANDS ON HIPS

The RI model is again demonstrated in the upper body by using the hands-on-hips modification to the OHSA. With virtually every global muscular subsystem crossing the hip, when an excessive anterior pelvic tilt is observed during the OHSA, the root cause is typically in muscles either above or below the LPHC itself. In this specific case, an anterior pelvic tilt can either be caused by overactivity of the latissimus dorsi pulling up on the posterior hip or the hip flexor complex (rectus femoris or psoas) pulling down on the anterior hip.

Placing the hands on the hips directly removes the stretch placed on the latissimus dorsi and other shoulder extensors and requires less demand from the core stabilizers (**Figure 9-6**). This allows the Corrective Exercise Specialist to see the influence the upper body has on the individual's impairments (McMillian et al., 2016). If an individual's lumbar spine extends (excessive anterior pelvic tilt) during the OHSA, but the impairment is then corrected when performing the squat with the hands on the hips, then the primary region that most likely needs to be addressed is the latissimus dorsi. If the impairment still exists with the hands on the hips, then the primary regions that most likely need to be addressed are in the LPHC or lower extremities.

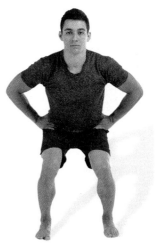

Figure 9-6 OHSA hands on hips

Single-Leg Squat Assessment

Seen as a progression to the OHSA, this transitional movement assessment also assesses dynamic posture, strength, balance, and overall neuromuscular control, only in a more-advanced, single-limb stance. Similar to the overhead squat, researchers have shown that observational screening during the single-leg squat (SLS) is a valid method to identify movement impairments, such as knee valgus (Mauntel et al., 2014; Räisänen et al., 2016; Ugalde et al., 2015). The single-leg squat assessment has also been shown to be a reliable and valid movement assessment for one or more professionals who administer the test (Garrick et al., 2018; Ressman et al., 2019) (see **Figure 9-7**).

This stance is the most challenging of the lower extremity transitional assessments due to the single-limb strength and balance required (Agresta et al., 2017; Gianola et al., 2017). Those that perform well during this test have been shown to have greater hip abductor strength and activation (Crossley et al., 2011; Garrick et al., 2018). This test should be used for clients who perform the OHSA with optimal form. Additionally, it is used to assess issues of trunk rotation (which typically do not present during the OHSA) or when considering the use of single-leg exercises with clients (to test their readiness for single-leg movements).

The SLS is also a good assessment of an individual's ability to balance, which is an important functional consideration for activities of daily living and exercise programming. It should be noted that this assessment should be avoided for clients who are at risk for falls and loss of balance or are recovering from a knee injury. It should be anticipated that clients complaining of knee pain will often display significant compensatory movement impairments at other joints when completing this assessment (Nakagawa et al., 2012a).

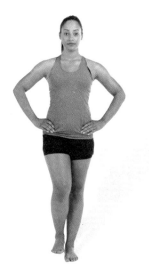

Single-leg squat assessment—
starting position

PROCEDURE

Starting Position

1. The individual should stand on one leg with the hands on the hips and eyes focused forward.
2. The stance foot should be pointed straight ahead and the foot, ankle, knee, and the LPHC should be in a neutral position.
3. The non-weight-bearing knee should be flexed with the foot next to, but not touching, the stance limb's calf.

Movement

1. Have the individual squat as deep as is comfortable and controllable, and return to the starting position.
2. Perform up to five repetitions per viewpoint, then repeat on the opposite leg. Perform at a comfortable pace without using momentum to bounce out of the bottom.

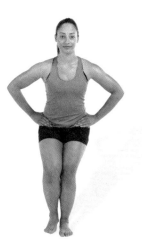

Single-leg squat assessment—
down position

OBSERVATION

Each viewpoint will require focus on specific kinetic chain checkpoints. For each, ideal performance of the single-leg squat is represented by the following:

- **Anterior**: View the feet, knees, and LPHC from the front. The feet and hips should remain in the sagittal plane with the knees tracking in line with the foot (second and third toes). The LPHC should remain level and not rotate or shift from side to side beyond what is needed to first obtain balance.

NASM CES Assessment Flow

1 Client Intake

2 Static Postural Assessment

3 Overhead Squat Assessment (OHSA) and Modified OHSA

4 **Single-Leg Squat and/or Split Squat Assessment**

4a Dynamic Assessments OPTIONAL

4b Loaded Assessments OPTIONAL

5 Mobility Assessments

6 Corrective Exercise Programming
INHIBIT • LENGTHEN
ACTIVATE • INTEGRATE

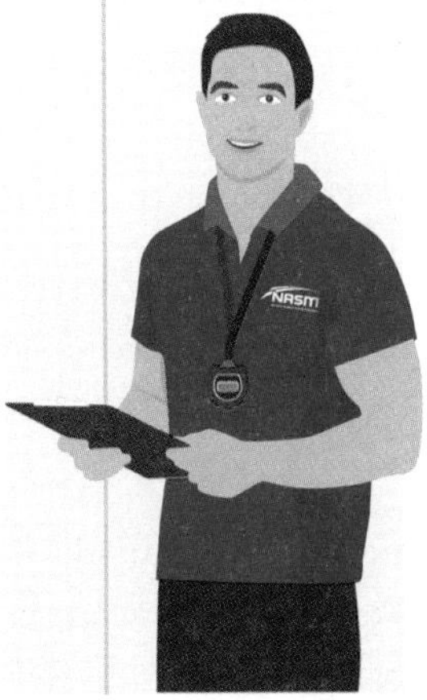

Single-Leg and/or Split Squat Assessment

Depending on client ability, safety, and goal

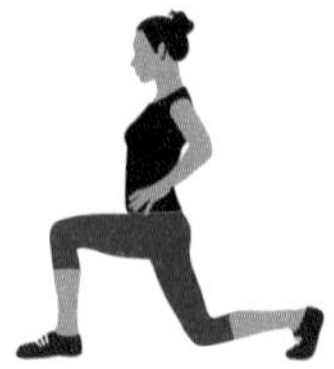

Perform single-leg squat assessment if client is able to safely do so. Otherwise, regress to split squat assessment, or move on to mobility assessments if it is unsafe to do either assessment.*

* If client has specific split-stance performance objectives both assessments may be useful.

Can client safely maintain single-leg positioning?

Yes → Perform Single-Leg Squat Assessment and note movement compensations

No → Split position OK → Perform Split Squat Assessment and note movement compensations

No → Split position unsafe

→ **Next Assessment**

Figure 9-7 CES Assessment Flow: single-leg squat and/or split squat assessment

- **Lateral**: View the feet, ankles, knees, and LPHC from the side. The heel should stay on the ground. The pelvis and spine should remain in a neutral posture. The torso should remain parallel with the tibia.
- **Posterior**: View the feet and ankles from the back. The arch of the foot and calcaneus should remain in a neutral position.

From the *anterior view*, look for the following potential movement impairments:

- **Knee**: Valgus or varus
- **LPHC**:
  - Asymmetric weight shift
  - Inward trunk rotation
  - Outward trunk rotation

From the *lateral view*, look for the following potential movement impairments:

- **Foot and ankle**: Heel rise
- **Knee**: dominance
- **LPHC**:
  - Excessive anterior pelvic tilt
  - Excessive posterior pelvic tilt
  - Excessive forward trunk lean

From the *posterior view*, look for the following potential movement impairments:

- **Foot and ankle**: Excessive foot pronation

When performing the assessment, record all findings on the **Single-Leg Squat Observational Findings** template. Then, refer to Table 9-2 to determine potential causes of these movement impairments and mobility assessment next steps.

SINGLE-LEG and/or SPLIT SQUAT OBSERVATIONAL FINDINGS

CHECKPOINT	VIEWPOINT	MOVEMENT IMPAIRMENT	RESULT
Foot and Ankle	Lateral	• Heel Rise	• Right • Left • Both
	Posterior	• Excessive pronation	• Right • Left • Both
Knee	Anterior	• Valgus	• Right • Left • Both
		• Varus	• Right • Left • Both
	Lateral	• Knee dominance	• Right • Left • Both
LPHC	Anterior	• Asymmetric weight shift	*Direction*: • Right • Left
		• Inward trunk rotation	• Right • Left • Both
		• Outward trunk rotation	• Right • Left • Both
	Lateral	• Excessive anterior pelvic tilt	• YES • NO
		• Excessive posterior pelvic tilt	• YES • NO
		• Excessive forward trunk lean	• YES • NO

Right/Left/Both refers to the stance or forward leg when the impairment occurs. Mark *Right* or *Left* or *Both* based on which limb a movement impairment was observed at. For asymmetric weight shift, mark the direction to which the shift occurs.

Single-leg squat observational findings

Split Squat Assessment

The split squat is used to assess dynamic posture, stability, and overall neuromuscular control while in a narrow stance. This movement mimics the stance required of a walking and running gait as well as many other activities of daily living (McMillian et al., 2016).

This assessment can be used in two ways. The first is as a regression to the single-leg squat. Many clients will not have the functional strength to complete a single-leg squat, so the split squat can be used as a regression to still refine observations of unilateral compensations seen during the OHSA. In that same light, the split squat can also help identify trunk rotation issues when a client is unable to perform a single-leg squat.

The split squat variation can also be used by the Corrective Exercise Specialist who wants to gain more information for programming decisions related to split-stance movements (e.g., walking lunges, split jumps, Olympic lifting, etc.). Although walking and step lunges are sometimes used as assessments, evidence suggests that a static split squat places less stress on the knee and may be safer for clients, especially those recovering from knee injury (Escamilla et al., 2010; Jalali et al., 2015). This movement is also effective in assessing an individual's balance and hip and knee extensor strength (Jönhagen et al., 2009). The client should first perform the split squat with one foot forward and the other foot back; then, they will switch foot position and perform the split squat again to isolate the opposite leg.

PROCEDURE

Starting Position

1. The individual stands in a narrow, split stance with the feet parallel (no wider than hip-width) and pointed straight ahead. The step length should be sufficient for the back knee to contact the ground behind the front foot.
2. Have the individual place their hands on the hips while standing in an upright position.

Movement

1. Instruct the individual to lower to a depth that brings their rear knee just above the ground without touching and return to the starting position. The front foot should remain planted on the ground while the rear foot heel is allowed to rise.
2. Repeat the movement for five repetitions, observing from each position (five reps per view). Perform at a comfortable pace without using momentum to bounce out of the bottom.

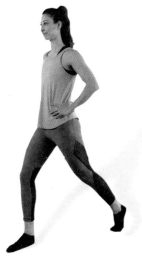

Split squat assessment—starting position

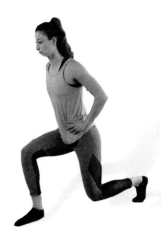

Split squat assessment—down position

Each viewpoint will require focus on specific kinetic chain checkpoints. For each, ideal performance of the split squat is represented by the following:

- **Anterior**: View the feet, knees, and LPHC from the front. The feet and hips should remain in the sagittal plane with the knees tracking in line with the foot (second and third toes). The LPHC should not shift from side to side or rotate.
- **Lateral**: View the feet, ankles, knees, and LPHC from the side. The front heel should stay on the ground and the front knee should not pass the toes. The pelvis and spine should remain in a neutral posture.
- **Posterior**: View the feet and ankles from the back. The arch of the foot and calcaneus should remain in a neutral position.

From the *anterior view*, look for the following potential movement impairments:

- **Knee**: Valgus or varus
- **LPHC**:
  - Asymmetric weight shift
  - Inward trunk rotation
  - Outward trunk rotation

From the *lateral view*, look for the following potential movement impairments:

- **Ankles**: Heel rise (front foot)
- **Knee**: Knee dominance (front knee)
- **LPHC**:
  - Excessive anterior pelvic tilt
  - Excessive posterior pelvic tilt

SINGLE-LEG and/or SPLIT SQUAT OBSERVATIONAL FINDINGS

CHECKPOINT	VIEWPOINT	MOVEMENT IMPAIRMENT	RESULT
Foot and Ankle	Lateral	• Heel Rise	• Right • Left • Both
	Posterior	• Excessive pronation	• Right • Left • Both
Knee	Anterior	• Valgus	• Right • Left • Both
	Anterior	• Varus	• Right • Left • Both
	Lateral	• Knee dominance	• Right • Left • Both
LPHC	Anterior	• Asymmetric weight shift	Direction: • Right • Left
		• Inward trunk rotation	• Right • Left • Both
		• Outward trunk rotation	• Right • Left • Both
	Lateral	• Excessive anterior pelvic tilt	• YES • NO
		• Excessive posterior pelvic tilt	• YES • NO
		• Excessive forward trunk lean	• YES • NO

Right/Left/Both refers to the stance or forward leg when the impairment occurs. Mark *Right* or *Left* or *Both* based on which limb a movement impairment was observed at. For asymmetric weight shift, mark the direction to which the shift occurs.

Split squat observational findings

From the *posterior view*, look for the following potential movement impairments:

- **Foot and ankle**: Excessive foot pronation

When performing the assessment, record all findings on the **Split Squat Observational Findings** template. Then, refer to Table 9-2 to determine potential causes of these movement impairments and the next steps for mobility assessment.

TRAINING TIP

Observing the Rear Foot During the Split Squat Assessment

In order to successfully demonstrate an in-line lunge, the trailing leg metatarsophalangeal (MTP) joints (i.e., the toes of the rear foot) must demonstrate ≥ 90 degrees of dorsiflexion (extension). In clients with a lack of MTP extension, the back foot may turn out to achieve a greater depth in the lunge. This is closely related to how a lack of dorsiflexion at the ankle can cause an excessive forward lean during the OHSA.

If a lack of ankle dorsiflexion has been identified, observation of the rear foot during a split squat can help pinpoint whether the issue is primarily above or below the ankle joint. If the rear foot does not turn out, then the Corrective Exercise Specialist can more reasonably assume that the lack of dorsiflexion is due to imbalances in the calf musculature.

However, if the rear foot turns out, then a lack of MTP extensibility (primarily the first MTP, or big toe) might also be a contributing factor. If this is seen, then the Corrective Exercise Specialist should include an assessment of first MTP joint range of motion during the mobility assessment process.

Loaded Movement Assessments

Loaded assessments, as the name suggests, are used to observe how a client maintains postural control under an external load. However, these assessments are not necessarily intended to be used as separate formal posture tests with clients. Rather, they can give the Corrective Exercise Specialist a framework by which to observe a client's posture as they perform common exercises during training sessions. The primary movements of pushing, pulling, overhead pressing, trunk rotation, squatting, hinging, split stance, and single-leg patterns should all be assessed over the course of a client's training sessions. Essentially, every workout with a client represents an opportunity for a Corrective Exercise Specialist to observe and evaluate a client's dynamic posture (see **Figure 9-8**).

That said, the following loaded movement assessments can still be optionally used on their own as a customized formal assessment to gain additional information about the client. They can also be used with clients who refuse, or are unable, to perform the transitional movement assessments. For such clients, Corrective Exercise Specialists can include the following formal loaded movement assessments in the client's workout. The common exercises used correlate to four of the body's primary movement patterns: squatting, pushing, pulling, and overhead pressing.

CRITICAL

Due to the increased risk of injury, loaded assessments should only be used after the client can perform the transitional assessments under control. The weight should also be carefully selected to impose an adequate challenge for the client while still ensuring their safety during the movement.

1   Client Intake

2   Static Postural
    Assessment

3   Overhead Squat
    Assessment
    (OHSA) and
    Modified OHSA

4   Single-Leg
    Squat and/or
    Split Squat
    Assessment

4a   Dynamic
     Assessments
     OPTIONAL

4b   **Loaded
     Assessments**
     OPTIONAL

5   Mobility
    Assessments

6   Corrective
    Exercise
    Programming
    INHIBIT · LENGTHEN
    ACTIVATE · INTEGRATE

Loaded Assessments (Optional)

Observe the primary movements patterns below during a client's first few workouts or as separate assessments for identifying kinetic chain compensation.

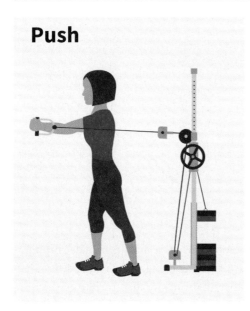

Push

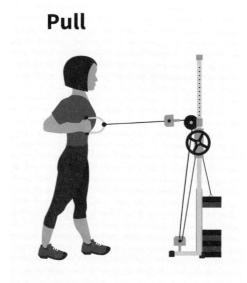

Pull

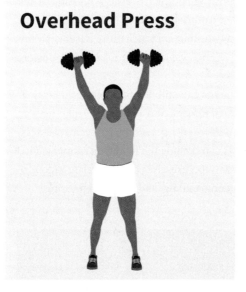

Overhead Press

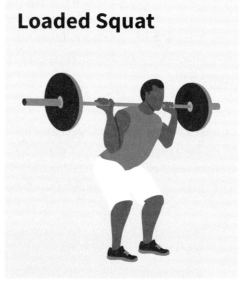

Loaded Squat

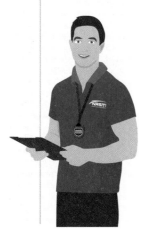

Figure 9-8   CES Assessment Flow: loaded assessments

Loaded Squat Assessment

The loaded squat assessment is designed to assess dynamic posture, core stability, and overall neuromuscular control while under external load. The loaded squat will allow the Corrective Exercise Specialist to observe how a client deals with external load and weight placement (e.g., front, back, or goblet), and how it influences their postural control (Glass & Albert, 2018; Richards et al., 2016). Furthermore, this can help determine which type of loaded squat a client might be ready to perform during workouts.

PROCEDURE

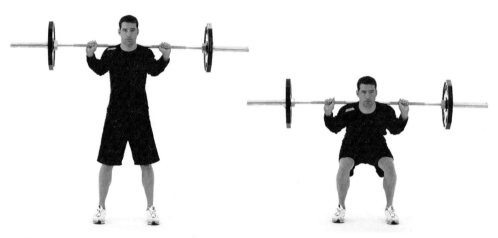

Loaded squat assessment

Starting Position

1. The individual stands with the feet hip-to-shoulder-width apart and pointed straight ahead. The foot and ankle complex should be in a neutral position. The assessment may be performed with the shoes off to better view the foot and ankle complex.
2. Choose a resistance that will challenge the client without exhausting them while executing the weight placement (front, back, goblet, etc.) that is desired for exercise programming.

Movement

1. Instruct the individual to squat to a depth of thighs parallel to the floor or normal chair height and return to the starting position.
2. The client will perform 15 total repetitions at a 2-0-2 (medium) tempo.
3. Repeat the movement for five repetitions, observing from each viewpoint (five reps per view). Increase or decrease repetition volume as needed to facilitate complete observation.

OBSERVATION

Each viewpoint will require focus on specific kinetic chain checkpoints. For each, ideal performance of the loaded squat is represented by the following:

- **Anterior**: View the feet, knees, and LPHC from the front. The feet and hips should remain in the sagittal plane with the knees tracking in line with the foot (second and third toes). The LPHC should not shift from side to side or rotate.

- **Lateral**: View the feet, ankles, knees, and LPHC from the side. The heels should stay on the ground and the knees should not pass the toes. The pelvis and spine should remain in a neutral posture. The torso should remain parallel with the tibia.
- **Posterior**: View the feet and ankles from the back. The arch of the foot and calcaneus should remain in a neutral position.

From the *anterior view*, look for the following potential movement impairments:

- **Foot and ankle**: Feet turn out
- **Knee**: Valgus or varus
- **LPHC**: Asymmetric weight shift

From the *lateral view*, look for the following potential movement impairments:

- **Foot and ankle**: Heel rise
- **Knee**: Knee dominance
- **LPHC**:
  - Excessive anterior pelvic tilt
  - Excessive posterior pelvic tilt
  - Excessive forward trunk lean

From the *posterior view*, look for the following potential movement impairments:

- **Foot and ankle**: Excessive foot pronation

When performing the assessment, record all findings on the **Loaded Squat Observational Findings** template. Then, refer to Table 9-2 to determine potential causes of these movement impairments and mobility next steps.

LOADED SQUAT OBSERVATIONAL FINDINGS

CHECKPOINT	VIEWPOINT	MOVEMENT IMPAIRMENT	RESULT
Foot and Ankle	Anterior	• Feet turn out	• Right • Left • Both
	Lateral	• Heel rise	• Right • Left • Both
	Posterior	• Excessive pronation	• Right • Left • Both
Knee	Anterior	• Valgus	• Right • Left • Both
		• Varus	• Right • Left • Both
	Lateral	• Knee dominance	• Right • Left • Both
LPHC	Anterior or Posterior	• Asymmetric weight shift	*Direction:* • Right • Left
	Lateral	• Excessive anterior pelvic tilt	• YES • NO
		• Excessive posterior pelvic tilt	• YES • NO
		• Excessive forward trunk lean	• YES • NO

Mark *Right* or *Left* or *Both* based on which limb a movement impairment was observed at. For asymmetric weight shift, mark the direction in which the shift occurred.

Loaded squat observational findings

Standing Push Assessment

The standing push assessment is a loaded assessment that assesses the performance of a horizontal pushing movement with both arms. The standing pushing assessment allows Corrective Exercise Specialists to observe scapular and shoulder mechanics, upper extremity muscle activation patterns, and the stability of the LPHC and cervical spine and head. Loaded push assessments are commonly used to measure the muscle forces produced by the body, biomechanical loads on the spine and joints, and the movement efficiency of the human movement system (de Looze et al., 2000; Knapik & Marras, 2009).

As previously stated, this type of assessment is intended to be used holistically any time a client is performing a push-type exercise; however, it can also be used with clients whose goals require a more detailed assessment of loaded dynamic posture. The Corrective Exercise Specialist should carefully evaluate all repetitions, because the client may begin with decent form and then begin to demonstrate movement impairments as they become fatigued during the assessment. This assessment is commonly performed using a cable machine or resistance band.

PROCEDURE

Starting Position

1. Instruct the client to stand with the abdomen drawn inward, feet in a split stance, and feet parallel with toes pointing forward.
2. Have the client hold a handle in each hand.

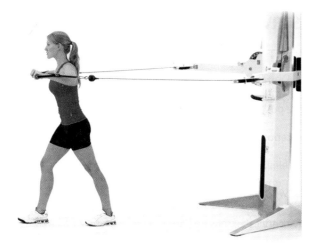
Loaded push assessment—start

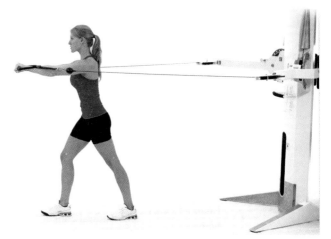
Loaded push assessment—finish

Movement

1. Choose a resistance that will challenge the client without exhausting them.
2. The client will perform 10 repetitions at a 2-0-2 (medium) tempo.
3. Instruct the client to perform five standing push repetitions (chest press).
4. The client then switches the feet and performs the push again for another five repetitions.

If the client is not able to perform a standing push movement in a narrow, split stance, use one of the following modifications:

- **Option 1**: The client stands in a wider split stance. This testing position still assesses the upper extremity and cervical spine and head, but it decreases the challenge to the LPHC and the individual's balance.

From the *lateral view*, look for the following potential movement impairments:

- **LPHC**:
  - Excessive anterior pelvic tilt
  - Excessive posterior pelvic tilt
  - Trunk rotation
- **Shoulder**: Scapular elevation
- **Cervical spine and head**: Excessive cervical extension/forward head

When performing the assessment, record all findings on the **Loaded Push and/or Pull Observational Findings** template. You can then refer to Table 9-2 to determine potential causes of these movement impairments and mobility next steps.

LOADED PUSH and/or PULL OBSERVATIONAL FINDINGS

CHECKPOINT	VIEWPOINT	MOVEMENT IMPAIRMENT	RESULT
		• Excessive anterior pelvic tilt	• YES • NO
LPHC	Lateral	• Excessive posterior pelvic tilt	• YES • NO
		• Trunk rotation	• YES • NO
Shoulders and Thoracic Spine	Lateral	• Scapular elevation	• YES • NO
		• Scapular winging (push assessment only)	• YES • NO
Head and Cervical Spine	Lateral	• Excessive cervical extension/forward head	• YES • NO

To observe *scapular winging* during the push assessment, view the client from a slight angle.

Loaded push and/or pull observational findings

Standing Overhead Dumbbell Press Assessment

The standing overhead dumbbell press assessment is a loaded assessment that informs the Corrective Exercise Specialist of a client's abilities and posture during vertical pushing movements in their exercise programming. As with other loaded assessments, it can be completed prior to a workout session as a separate assessment or as part of a workout session.

The standing overhead dumbbell press evaluates upper extremity strength and stability of the LPHC, scapula, and cervical spine and head in a manner that is similar to many sports (Saeterbakken & Fimland, 2012, 2013). The Corrective Exercise Specialist should carefully evaluate all repetitions, as the client may demonstrate movement impairments as they become fatigued during the assessment.

PROCEDURE

Starting Position

1. Instruct the individual to stand with their feet hip-to-shoulder-width apart and toes pointing forward.
2. Choose a dumbbell weight that will challenge the client without exhausting them.

3. The upper extremities should start at 90 degrees of horizontal abduction and 90 degrees of elbow flexion.

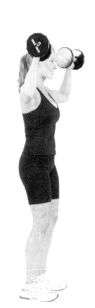

Standing overhead dumbbell press assessment—start

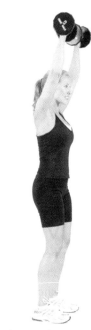

Standing overhead dumbbell assessment—finish

Movement

1. Instruct the individual to fully abduct the shoulders and extend the arms, pressing the dumbbells together overhead, and return to the starting position.
2. The client will perform 10 repetitions at a 2-0-2 (medium) tempo

OBSERVATION

The loaded overhead dumbbell press assessment is meant to be observed from the lateral view. Ideal performance of the loaded standing press assessment is represented by the following:

- **Lateral**: View the LPHC, shoulders, cervical spine, and head. The lumbar and cervical spine should remain neutral while the shoulders stay level. The arm should bisect the ears while pressing the dumbbells together overhead with full elbow extension.

From the *lateral view*, look for the following potential movement impairments:

- **LPHC**:
  - Excessive anterior pelvic tilt
  - Excessive posterior pelvic tilt
- **Shoulder**:
  - Scapular elevation
  - Arms fall forward
- **Cervical spine and head**: Excessive cervical extension/forward head

When performing the assessment, record all findings on the **Standing Overhead Dumbbell Press Observational Findings** template. Then, refer to Table 9-2 to determine potential causes of these movement impairments and mobility assessment next steps.

Because every kinetic chain checkpoint is in motion during the gait assessment, it can be helpful to take video recordings of the client from each viewpoint. This allows the Corrective Exercise Specialist to slow things down, pause, and replay to make sure nothing is overlooked.

PROCEDURE

Starting Position

1. The individual stands on a treadmill set at a 1-degree incline.

Movement

1. Instruct the individual to walk at a comfortable pace.

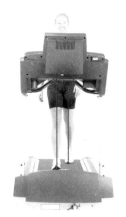 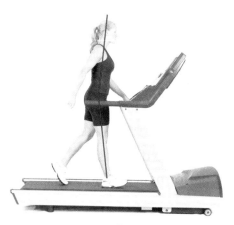 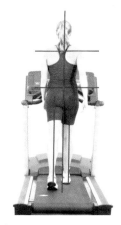

Gait assessment—anterior   Gait assessment—lateral   Gait assessment—posterior

OBSERVATION

The walking gait assessment is meant to be observed from all three viewpoints. Ideal walking gait exhibits the following:

- **Anterior**: View the feet, knees, and LPHC from the front. The feet should remain parallel and in the sagittal plane with the knees tracking in line with the foot (second and third toes). The LPHC should not shift from side to side or rotate.
- **Lateral**: View the LPHC from the side. The pelvis and spine should remain in a neutral posture.
- **Posterior**: View the feet and ankles from the back. The arch of the foot and calcaneus should remain in a neutral position with each step.

From the *anterior view*, look for the following potential movement impairments:

- **Foot and ankle**: Feet turn out
- **Knee**: Valgus or varus
- **LPHC**: Asymmetric weight shift

From the *lateral view*, look for the following potential movement impairments:

- **LPHC:**
  - Excessive anterior pelvic tilt
  - Excessive posterior pelvic tilt

From the *posterior view*, look for the following potential movement impairments:

- **Foot and ankle**: Excessive foot pronation

When performing the assessment, record all findings on the **Gait Assessment Observational Findings** template. Then, refer to Table 9-2 to determine potential causes of these movement impairments and mobility assessment next steps.

GAIT ASSESSMENT OBSERVATIONAL FINDINGS

CHECKPOINT	VIEWPOINT	MOVEMENT IMPAIRMENT	RESULT
Foot and Ankle	Anterior	• Feet turn out	• Right • Left • Both
	Posterior	• Excessive pronation	• Right • Left • Both
Knee	Anterior	• Valgus	• Right • Left • Both
		• Varus	• Right • Left • Both
LPHC	Anterior	• Asymmetric weight shift	*Direction*: • Right • Left
	Lateral	• Excessive anterior pelvic tilt	• YES • NO
		• Excessive posterior pelvic tilt	• YES • NO

Mark **Right** or **Left** or **Both** based on which limb a movement impairment was observed at. For asymmetric weight shift, mark the direction in which the shift occurred.

Gait assessment observational findings

TRAINING TIP

When to Avoid Dynamic Assessments

Although very helpful in uncovering movement deficiencies, dynamic movement assessments may not be appropriate for all populations. Subjective assessments, static posture, and transitional movement assessments are important to perform before dynamic assessments, because successful completion of those first steps are what qualifies the client to perform dynamic assessments.

For example, if an individual has difficulty performing the single-leg squat assessment, the depth jump assessment would not be appropriate for that individual. Or, if a client exhibits poor scapular stability during the pushing assessment, the Davies test should be avoided until that client can push under load with efficient form.

In those examples, the transitional movement assessments provide all of the answers necessary to begin developing a corrective exercise strategy. Then, as the client progresses, future reassessment periods can layer in the more complex, dynamic assessments to continue testing the client's abilities using higher demands.

Depth Jump Assessment

The depth jump assessment is a dynamic movement assessment for identifying movement impairments during jumping and landing tasks. This assessment is commonly used in clinical, rehabilitation, and sports performance settings. The depth jump assessment takes the client through essentially the same biomechanical movement pattern as the overhead squat, just progressed into an open chain, dynamic setting to observe the client in a more performance-focused scenario.

Along with postural assessments, this test has been shown to be a predictor of repeat ACL injuries in those who display knee valgus, knee dominance, and hip internal rotation (Paterno et al., 2010; Pollard et al., 2017). Research has shown that a well-designed corrective exercise program is effective at reducing movement impairments associated with jumping and landing tasks (DiStefano et al., 2009; Ford et al., 2011).

This assessment is considered a performance test and a maximal vertical jump should be encouraged in the explanation of the movement. However, the Corrective Exercise Specialist should maintain focus on movement quality and control during the assessment to aid in the development of a corrective exercise plan. Notation of whether a movement impairment occurs during the jumping or landing phases of the movement will allow the Corrective Exercise Specialist to focus on that aspect of the movement during corrective exercise programming.

TRAINING TIP

The client will be moving fast during the depth jump assessment, so it is highly recommended that the Corrective Exercise Specialist take video recordings of the client from each viewpoint. This allows the Corrective Exercise Specialist to slow things down, pause, and replay to ensure that movements are not overlooked.

PROCEDURE

Starting Position

1. The individual stands on a 12-inch box.
2. A target line is drawn on the floor 12 inches in front of the box.

Movement

1. The individual is instructed to hop off of the box and land with both feet just after the line.
2. Upon the initial landing, the client should quickly jump up for maximum height.
3. The client will then land a second time under control.
4. The number of repetitions may vary for each client depending on their ability to perform under fatigue. One to three repetitions per view are recommended as a starting point, following an opportunity to practice the movement after a demonstration.

TRAINING TIP

The client should be allowed one to two practice repetitions of the depth jump assessment before assessing the movement.

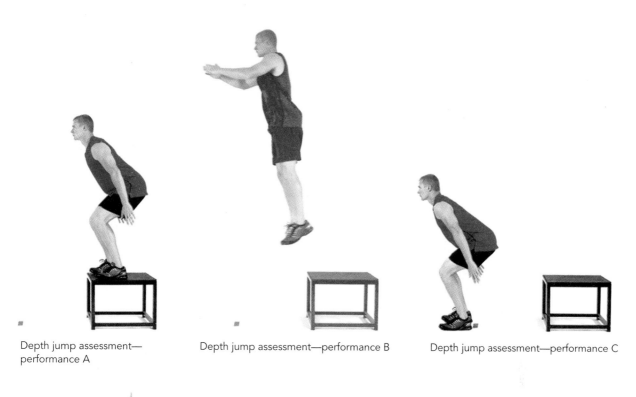

Depth jump assessment—performance A

Depth jump assessment—performance B

Depth jump assessment—performance C

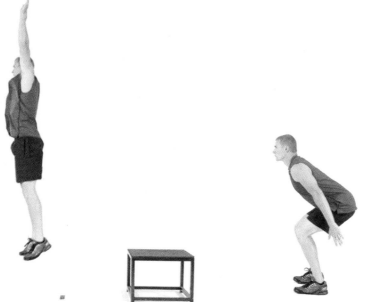

Depth jump assessment—performance D

Depth jump assessment—performance E

OBSERVATION

The depth jump should be observed from anterior and lateral views. Each viewpoint will require focus on specific kinetic chain checkpoints. For each, ideal performance of the depth jump is represented by the following:

- **Anterior**: View the feet, knees, and LPHC from the front. The feet and hips should remain in the sagittal plane with the knees tracking in line with the foot (second and third toes). Feet should be parallel and contact the ground simultaneously. The LPHC should not shift from side to side or rotate.

- **Lateral**: View the feet, ankles, knees, and LPHC from the side. The pelvis and spine should remain in a neutral posture. The torso should remain parallel with the tibia. The hips, knees, and ankles should move through an adequate range of motion for a soft landing.

From the *anterior view*, look for the following potential movement impairments:

- **Foot and ankle**:
  - Feet turn out
  - Excessive pronation
  - Asymmetric contact/landing
- **Knee**: Valgus or varus
- **LPHC**: Asymmetric weight shift

From the *lateral view*, look for the following potential movement impairments:

- **Knee**:
  - Knee dominance
  - Stiff landing
- **LPHC**:
  - Excessive anterior pelvic tilt
  - Excessive posterior pelvic tilt
  - Excessive forward trunk lean

Record all findings on the **Depth Jump Observational Findings** template. Then, refer to Table 9-2 to determine potential causes of these movement impairments and the next steps to refine the observations with mobility testing.

DEPTH JUMP OBSERVATIONAL FINDINGS

CHECKPOINT	VIEWPOINT	MOVEMENT IMPAIRMENT	RESULT
Foot and Ankle	Anterior	• Excessive pronation	• Right • Left • Both
		• Feet turn out	• Right • Left • Both
		• Asymmetric contact/landing	• Rt. first • Lt. first • NO
Knee	Anterior	• Valgus	• Right • Left • Both
		• Varus	• Right • Left • Both
	Lateral	• Knee dominance	• Right • Left • Both
		• Stiff landing	• YES • NO
LPHC	Anterior	• Asymmetric weight shift	*Direction*: • Right • Left
	Lateral	• Excessive anterior pelvic tilt	• YES • NO
		• Excessive posterior pelvic tilt	• YES • NO
		• Excessive forward trunk lean	• YES • NO

Mark *Right* or *Left* or *Both* based on which limb a movement impairment was observed at. For asymmetric weight shift, mark the direction in which the shift occurred.

Depth jump observational findings

Landing Versus Jumping

Although landing and jumping include the same joint motions, they involve opposite muscle actions. Landing involves deceleration of body weight against gravity via eccentric contractions, whereas jumping is accelerating via concentric contractions. When assessing jump performance, it is important to recognize that landing imposes higher load and greater difficulty than jumping. Thus, it may be more beneficial to observe impairments during landing versus jumping.

GETTING TECHNICAL

Researchers have documented that deeper hip and knee flexion angles decrease biomechanical stress on the knee (Tsai et al., 2017), allowing soft tissues, rather than joints, to absorb the forces of landing. During the depth jump assessment, the Corrective Exercise Specialist may notice that some clients may perform a *stiff landing* by not allowing their hips and knees to bend adequately (e.g., knees < 90 degrees). This may be due to issues such as, but not limited to, motor weakness, poor form, or a mobility deficit in the lower kinetic chain. Clients may also land with *asymmetric contact*, preferentially landing on one leg more than the other. This may also be due to motor weakness, poor form, mobility deficits, or prior injury (Paterno et al., 2011; Powell et al., 2018). In both situations, mobility testing of the lower extremity is warranted to pinpoint muscle imbalances.

Davies Test

The Davies test assessment is a dynamic movement assessment for identifying movement impairments during a repetitive, plyometric activity for the upper extremity. The Davies test requires upper extremity agility, strength and stabilization, and stability of the trunk and LPHC (Tucci et al., 2014). This assessment should only be used after the client can complete the standing push assessment with ease and after ensuring that they can safely begin upper extremity plyometric-style activities. The Davies test may not be suitable for individuals who lack shoulder stability, have current shoulder pain (Tucci et al., 2017), or lack the functional strength to perform a push-up.

This assessment is considered a performance test, and a maximal number of repetitions during the 15-second testing period should be encouraged in the explanation of the movement. However, the Corrective Exercise Specialist should maintain focus on movement quality and control during the assessment to aid in the development of a corrective exercise plan.

PROCEDURE

Starting Position

1. Place two pieces of tape on the floor 36 inches (approximately 90 centimters) apart.
2. Have the individual assume a push-up position with one hand on each piece of tape.

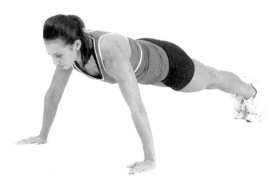

Upper extremity Davies test assessment position

Movement

1. Instruct the individual to quickly move the right hand to touch the left hand and then move the left hand to touch the right hand.
2. The individual's body weight should shift over the planted hand as they touch it with the floating hand, while maintaining postural control and minimizing unnecessary trunk motion (e.g., excessive rotation).
3. Perform alternating touching on each side for 15 seconds and record both the number of times a line is touched by both hands and movement impairments observed.
4. Perform for three trials.

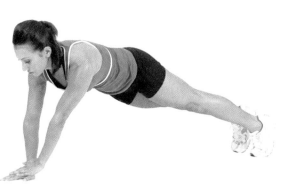

Davies test assessment—movement A

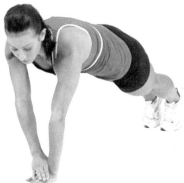

Davies test assessment—movement B

OBSERVATION

The Davies test should be observed from the lateral view. However, the Corrective Exercise Specialist should still be located anteriorly enough to the client to accurately count repetitions. Ideal performance of the Davies test is represented by the following:

- **Lateral**: View the LPHC, shoulders, cervical spine, and head from the side. The trunk should remain parallel to the ground with a neutral spine and stable scapulae.

 TRAINING TIP

Bringing in a third individual to help time and count repetitions of the Davies test can be extremely helpful. This will allow the fitness professional to focus attention on the client's form and performance while the helper handles the stopwatch and counting tasks.

From the *lateral view*, look for the following potential movement impairments:

- **LPHC**:
  - Excessive anterior pelvic tilt
  - Excessive posterior pelvic tilt
  - Excessive trunk movement
- **Shoulder**:
  - Scapular elevation
  - Scapular winging
- **Cervical spine and head**: Excessive cervical extension/forward head

When performing the assessment, record all findings on the **Davies Test Observational Findings** template. Then, refer to Table 9-2 to determine potential causes of these movement impairments and associated mobility assessments that will help refine the observations.

DAVIES TEST OBSERVATIONAL FINDINGS

CHECKPOINT	MOVEMENT IMPAIRMENT	RESULT
LPHC	• Excessive anterior pelvic tilt	• YES • NO
	• Excessive posterior pelvic tilt	• YES • NO
	• Excessive trunk movement	• YES • NO
Shoulders and Thoracic Spine	• Scapular elevation	• YES • NO
	• Scapular winging	• YES • NO
Head and Cervical Spine	• Excessive cervical extension/forward head	• YES • NO

TRIAL NUMBER	TIME	REPETITIONS (TOUCHES)
1	15 seconds	
2	15 seconds	
3	15 seconds	

Davies test observational findings

Assessment Implementation Options

Movement assessments are a key component in determining movement efficiency and potential risks for injury. These assessments, along with static posture and subsequent mobility assessments, are essential for designing a specific corrective exercise program to enhance functionality and overall performance, thus decreasing the risk for injury.

The primary movement assessment that the Corrective Exercise Specialist should perform with all clients is the overhead squat. This assessment provides the most information about a client's functional status in a relatively short time. The remaining upper- and lower-extremity loaded and dynamic assessments can be viewed as optional and performed if time allows and the client displays adequate ability to progress to more challenging assessments.

A second option to consider is that a comprehensive battery of the assessments covered in this chapter can become a client's entire first workout. From this first workout, the Corrective Exercise Specialist can then obtain optimal information about the individual's movement abilities. The client will think they are getting a workout, but the Corrective Exercise Specialist is obtaining valuable information about the client's structural integrity to help design and implement a corrective exercise program specific to their needs. However, it is important to remember that, depending on one's physical capabilities, not all assessments will be appropriate for all clients. The Corrective Exercise Specialist should only choose assessments that the client can perform safely.

Third, using movement assessments for promotional purposes could be a way for Corrective Exercise Specialists to build their client base. Offering 30- to 45-minute complimentary assessment sessions that take prospective clients through the assessment process can be a fantastic way to attract new members, sign new clients, and generate revenue.

SUMMARY

Movement assessments are the cornerstone of an integrated assessment process. All assessment sessions should begin with static postural assessments followed by transitional assessments. The overhead squat assessment should be the first assessment conducted for all clients followed by the split squat and single-leg squat assessments when the client is ready to perform them. Movement assessments challenge a client in a variety of stances, loads, and speeds, which correspond with activities of daily living and athletic movements.

If the client's functional movement capacity allows, the movement assessments can then be progressed to loaded and dynamic tests. Loaded assessments are used to determine if an individual can maintain proper posture under external load while assessing the upper and lower extremities. Ideally, every workout with a client should function as a loaded movement assessment, observing form and function any time they are squatting, pushing, pulling, or pressing overhead.

Dynamic movement assessments include a change in the base of support and often encourage fast movements or explosive jumping. The Corrective Exercise Specialist should only use dynamic assessments after improving movement impairments seen in the transitional assessments and ensuring the client can safely manage these advanced plyometric movements.

Each of the movement assessments is utilized to uncover movement impairments that may be altering the functional capacity of an individual or predisposing them to injury. With a thorough understanding of the human movement system and the use of the kinetic chain checkpoints to systematically detect impairment in joint motion, the underlying causes of a dysfunction can be addressed through the development of a comprehensive corrective exercise strategy.

Movement impairments are typically caused by overactive or underactive muscles leading to reduced joint range of motion and/or impaired motor control (or vice versa). The Corrective Exercise Specialist should always consider how movement impairments at one joint or region affect the functional movement of another region. After completing movement assessments and gaining an understanding of a client's muscle imbalances, targeted mobility assessments can be used to better pinpoint the source of dysfunction and inform a truly comprehensive evaluation of a client's structural and neuromuscular efficiency.

REFERENCES

Agresta, C., Church, C., Henley, J., Duer, T., & O'Brien, K. (2017). Single-leg squat performance in active adolescents aged 8–17 years. *Journal of Strength & Conditioning Research, 31*(5), 1187–1191.

Barton, C. J., Lack, S., Malliaras, P., & Morrissey, D. (2013). Gluteal muscle activity and patellofemoral pain syndrome: A systematic review. *British Journal of Sports Medicine, 47*(4), 207–214.

Birch, I., Raymond, L., Christou, A., Fernando, M. A., Harrison, N., & Paul, F. (2013). The identification of individuals by observational gait analysis using closed circuit television footage. *Science & Justice, 53*(3), 339–342. https://doi.org/10.1016/j.scijus.2013.04.005

Bolgla, L. A., Malone, T. R., Umberger, B. R., & Uhl, T. L. (2008). Hip strength and hip and knee kinematics during stair descent in females with and without patellofemoral pain syndrome. *Journal of Orthopedic and Sports Physical Therapy, 38*(1), 12–18.

Brunnekreef, J. J., van Uden, C. J. T., van Moorsel, S., & Kooloos, J. G. M. (2005). Reliability of videotaped observational gait analysis in patients with orthopedic impairments. *BMC Musculoskeletal Disorders, 6*(17). https://doi.org/10.1186/1471-2474-6-17

Crossley, K. M., Zhang, W. J., Schache, A. G., Bryant, A., & Cowan, S. M. (2011). Performance on the single-leg squat task indicates hip abductor muscle function. *American Journal of Sports Medicine, 39*(4), 866–873.

de Looze, M. P., van Greuningen, K., Rebel, J., Kingma, I., & Kuijer, P. P. (2000). Force direction and physical load in dynamic pushing and pulling. *Ergonomics, 43*(3), 377–390. https://doi.org/10.1080/001401300184477

DiStefano, L. J., Padua, D. A., DiStefano, M. J., & Marshall, S. W. (2009). Influence of age, sex, technique, and exercise program on movement patterns after an anterior cruciate ligament injury prevention in youth soccer players. *American Journal of Sports Medicine, 37*(3), 495–505.

dos Santos Bunn, P., de Paula Silva, G., & da Silva, E. B. (2018). Performance in the deep squat test and musculoskeletal injuries: A systematic review. *Fisioterapia em Movimento, 31*, 1–7. https://doi.org/10.1590/1980-5918.031.ao26

Escamilla, R. F., Zheng, N., Macleod, T. D., Imamura, R., Edwards, W. B., Hreljac, A., Fleisig, G., Wilk, K., Moorman, C., Paulos, L., & Andrews, J. R. (2010). Cruciate ligament forces between short-step and long-step forward lunge. *Medicine & Science in Sports & Exercise, 42*(10), 1932–1942. https://doi.org/10.1249/MSS.0b013e3181d966d4

Ford, K. R., Myer, G. D., Schmitt, L. C., Uhl, T. L., & Hewett, T. E. (2011). Preferential quadriceps activation in female athletes with incremental increases in landing intensity. *Journal of Applied Biomechanics, 27*(3), 215–222.

Garrick, L. E., Alexander, B. C., Schache, A. G., Pandy, M. G., Crossley, K. M., & Collins, N. J. (2018). Athletes rated as poor single-leg squat performers display measurable differences in single-leg squat biomechanics compared with good performers. *Journal of Sport Rehabilitation, 27*(6), 546–553. https://doi.org/10.1123/jsr.2016-0208

Gianola, S., Castellini, G., Stucovitz, E., Nardo, A., & Banfi, G. (2017). Single leg squat performance in physically and non-physically active individuals: A cross-sectional study. *BMC Musculoskeletal Disorders, 18*(1), 299. https://doi.org/10.1186/s12891-017-1660-8

Glass, S. C., & Albert, R. W. (2018). Compensatory muscle activation during unstable overhead squat using a water-filled training tube. *Journal of Strength and Conditioning Research, 32*(5), 1230–1237. https://doi.org/10.1519/jsc.0000000000002000

Greenberg, E., Dabbous, M., Leung, A., Marinaccio, G., Ruley, B., Karl, M., Dyke, J., Lawrence, T., & Ganley, T. J. (2019). Less than half of youth young athletes can achieve 90% limb symmetry on a battery of single leg hop tests. *Orthopaedic Journal of Sports Medicine, 7*(3 Suppl.), 1–3. https://doi.org/10.1177/2325967119S00052

Jalali, M., Farahmand, F., Mousavi, S. M., Golestanha, S. A., Rezaeian, T., Broujeni, S. S., Rahgozar, M., & Esfandiarpour, F. (2015). Fluoroscopic analysis of tibial translation in anterior cruciate ligament injured knees with and without bracing during forward lunge. *Iranian Journal of Radiology, 12*(3), e17832. https://doi.org/10.5812/iranjradiol.17832v2

Jönhagen, S., Ackermann, P., & Saartok, T. (2009). Forward lunge: A training study of eccentric exercises of the lower limbs. *Journal of Strength and Conditioning Research, 23*(3), 972–978. https://doi.org/10.1519/JSC.0b013e3181a00d98

Knapik, G. G., & Marras, W. S. (2009). Spine loading at different lumbar levels during pushing and pulling. *Ergonomics, 52*(1), 60–70. https://doi.org/10.1080/00140130802480828

Mauntel, T. C., Frank, B. S., Begalle, R. L., Blackburn, J. T., & Padua, D. A. (2014). Kinematic differences between those with and without medial knee displacement during a single-leg squat. *Journal of Applied Biomechanics, 30*(6), 707–712. https://doi.org/10.1123/jab.2014-0003

Mauntel, T. C., Post, E. G., Padua, D. A., & Bell, D. R. (2015). Sex differences during an overhead squat assessment. *Journal of Applied Biomechanics, 31*(4), 244–249.

McMillian, D. J., Rynders, Z. G., & Trudeau, T. R. (2016). Modifying the functional movement screen deep squat test: The effect of foot and arm positional variations. *Journal of Strength and Conditioning Research, 30*(4), 973–979. https://doi.org/10.1519/jsc.0000000000001190

Nakagawa, T. H., Moriya, É. T., Maciel, C. D., & Serrão, A. F. (2012a). Frontal plane biomechanics in males and females with and without patellofemoral pain. *Medicine & Science in Sports & Exercise, 44*(9), 1747–1755. https://doi.org/10.1249/MSS.0b013e318256903a.

Nakagawa, T. H., Moriya, É. T., Maciel, C. D., & Serrão, F. V. (2012b). Trunk, pelvis, hip, and knee kinematics, hip strength, and gluteal muscle activation during a single-leg squat in males and females with and without patellofemoral pain syndrome. *Journal of Orthopaedic & Sports Physical Therapy, 46*(2), 491–501. https://doi.org/10.2519/jospt.2012.3987

Paterno, M. V., Schmitt, L. C., Ford, K. R., Rauh, M. J., Myer, G. D., Huang, B., & Hewett, T. E. (2010). Biomechanical measures during landing and postural stability predict second anterior cruciate ligament injury after anterior cruciate ligament reconstruction and return to sport. *American Journal of Sports Medicine, 38*(10), 1968–1978. https://doi.org/10.1177/0363546510376053

Paterno, M. V., Schmitt, L. C., Ford, K. R., Rauh, M. J., Myer, G. D., & Hewett, T. E. (2011). Effects of sex on compensatory landing strategies upon return to sport after anterior cruciate ligament reconstruction. *Journal of Orthopaedic & Sports Physical Therapy, 41*(8), 553–559. https://doi.org/10.2519/jospt.2011.3591

Pollard, C. D., Sigward, S. M., & Powers, C. M. (2017). ACL injury prevention training results in modification of hip and knee mechanics during a drop-landing task. *Orthopaedic Journal of Sports Medicine, 5*(9), 1–7.

Post, E. G., Olson, M., Trigsted, S., Hetzel, S., & Bell, D. R. (2017). The reliability and discriminative ability of the overhead squat test for observational screening of medial knee displacement. *Journal of Sport Rehabilitation, 26*(1). https://doi.org/10.1123/jsr.2015-0178

Powell, H. C., Silbernagel, K. G., Brorsson, A., Tranberg, R., & Willy, R. W. (2018). Individuals post Achilles tendon rupture exhibit asymmetrical knee and ankle kinetics and loading rates during a drop countermovement jump. *Journal of Orthopaedic & Sports Physical Therapy, 48*(1), 34–43. https://doi.org/10.2519/jospt.2018.7684

Powers, C. M. (2010). The influence of abnormal hip mechanics on knee injury: A biomechanical perspective. *Journal of Orthopaedic & Sports Physical Therapy, 40*(2), 42–51.

Rabin, A., & Kozol, Z. (2017). Utility of the overhead squat and forward arm squat in screening for limited ankle dorsiflexion. *Journal of Strength and Conditioning Research, 31*(5), 1251–1258. https://doi.org/10.1519/jsc.0000000000001580

Räisänen, A., Pasanen, K., Krosshaug, T., Avela, J., Perttunen, J., & Parkkari, J. (2016). Single-leg squat as a tool to evaluate young athletes' frontal plane knee control. *Clinical Journal of Sport Medicine, 26*(6), 478–482.

Ressman, J., Grooten, W. J. A., Rasmussen, B. E., & Grooten, W. J. A. (2019). Visual assessment of movement quality in the single leg squat test: A review and meta-analysis of inter-rater and intrarater reliability. *BMJ Open Sport and Exercise Medicine, 5*(1), e000541.

Richards, J., Selfe, J., Sinclair, J., May, K., & Thomas, G. (2016). The effect of different decline angles on the biomechanics of double limb squats and the implications to clinical and training practice. *Journal of Human Kinetics, 52*, 125–138. https://doi.org/10.1515/hukin-2015-0200

Saeterbakken, A. H., & Fimland, M. S. (2012). Muscle activity of the core during bilateral, unilateral, seated and standing resistance exercise. *European Journal of Applied Physiology, 112*(5), 1671–1678. https://doi.org/10.1007/s00421-011-2141-7

Saeterbakken, A. H., & Fimland, M. S. (2013). Effects of body position and loading modality on muscle activity and strength in shoulder press. *Journal of Strength and Conditioning Research, 27*(7), 1824–1831. https://doi.org/10.1519/JSC.0b013e318276b873

Souza, R. B., & Powers, C. M. (2009). Differences in hip kinematics, muscle strength, and muscle activation between subjects with and without patellofemoral pain. *Journal of Orthopedic & Sports Physical Therapy, 39*(1), 12–19. https://doi.org/10.2519/jospt.2009.2885

Sueki, D. G., Cleland, J. A., & Wainner, R. S. (2013). A regional interdependence model of musculoskeletal dysfunction: Research, mechanisms, and clinical implications. *Journal of Manual and Manipulative Therapy, 21*(2), 90–102. https://doi.org/10.1179/2042618612Y.0000000027

Tas, S., Guneri, S., Kaymak, B., & Erden, Z. (2015). A comparison of results of 3-dimensional gait analysis and observational gait analysis in patients with knee osteoarthritis. *Acta Orthopaedica et Traumatologica Turcica, 49*(2), 151–159. https://doi.org/10.3944/aott.2015.14.0158

Tsai, L. C., Ko, Y. A., Hammond, K. E., Xerogeanes, J. W., Warren, G. L., & Powers, C. M. (2017). Increasing hip and knee flexion during a drop-jump task reduces tibiofemoral shear and compressive forces: Implications for ACL injury prevention training. *Journal of Sports Sciences, 35*(24), 2405–2411. https://doi.org/10.1080/02640414.2016.1271138

Tucci, H. T., Felicio, L. R., McQuade, K. J., Bevilaqua-Grossi, D., Camarini, P. M., & Oliveira, A. S. (2017). Biomechanical analysis of the closed kinetic chain upper-extremity stability test. *Journal of Sport Rehabilitation, 26*(1), 42–50. https://doi.org/10.1123/jsr.2015-0071

Tucci, H. T., Martins, J., Sposito, G. C., Camarini, P. M., & de Oliveira, A. S. (2014). Closed kinetic chain upper extremity stability test (CKCUES test): A reliability study in persons with and without shoulder impingement syndrome. *BMC Musculoskeletal Disorders, 15*(1), 1–9. https://doi.org/10.1186/1471-2474-15-1

Ugalde, V., Brockman, C., Bailowitz, Z., & Pollard, C. D. (2015). Single leg squat test and its relationship to dynamic knee valgus and injury risk screening. *PM & R, 7*(3), 229–235; quiz 235. https://doi.org/10.1016/j.pmrj.2014.08.361

Vidal, A. D., Nakajima, M., Wu, W. F. W., & Becker, J. (2018). Movement screens: Are we measuring movement dysfunction or movement skill? *International Journal of Sports Science & Coaching, 13*(5), 771–778. https://doi.org/10.1177/2F1747954118760225

Warner, M. B., Wilson, D. A., Herrington, L., Dixon, S., Power, C., Jones, R., Heller, M. O., Carden, P., & Lewis, C. L. (2019). A systematic review of the discriminating biomechanical parameters during the single leg squat. *Physical Therapy in Sport, 36*, 78–91. https://doi.org/10.1016/j.ptsp.2019.01.007

CHAPTER 10

Mobility Assessments

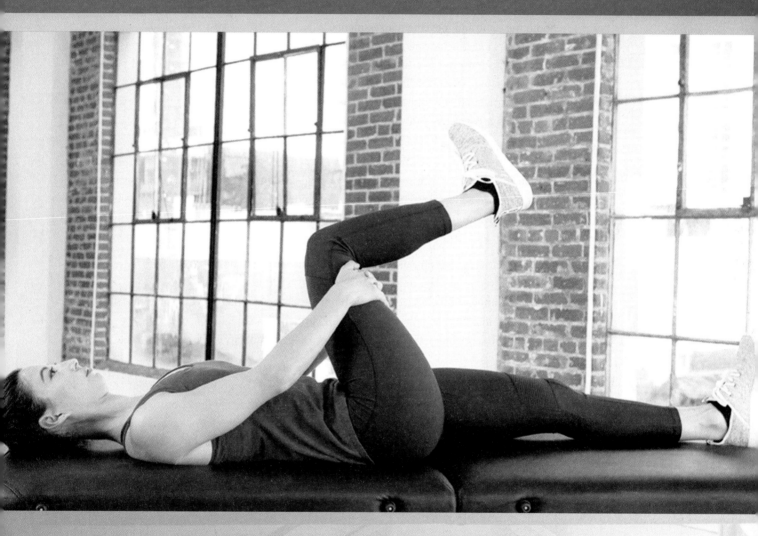

Learning Objectives

After reading this content, students should be able to demonstrate the following objectives:

- **Explain** the importance of achieving optimal flexibility and range of motion in human movement.

- **Explain** how the integrated function of the muscular, skeletal, and nervous systems collectively influences flexibility and the ability to move through a full range of motion.

- **Identify** common flexibility and joint range of motion assessments.

- **Explain** how to perform selected flexibility and range of motion assessments.

Introduction

Optimal human movement requires adequate mobility, which is dependent on a combination of adequate soft tissue extensibility and joint **range of motion (ROM)**. **Flexibility** is defined as the normal extensibility of all soft tissues (i.e., muscle length) that allow the full range of motion of a joint. However, **mobility** represents more than just flexibility. It accounts for the entire available range of motion at a joint as well as the body's neuromuscular control during motion (i.e., muscle length and state of neural activation). For this reason, targeted mobility assessments of the major body segments should be used to focus and confirm the observations made during both the static and movement assessments.

Factors affecting normal mobility include posture, pattern overload movements (e.g., computer work and repetitive lifting), joint structure, age, pain, injury, gender, and psychosocial influences (e.g., stress; Cuellar & Lanman, 2017; Fares et al., 2017; Page et al., 2010). The ability to identify altered mobility and correlate to a movement dysfunction is vital in developing safe and effective corrective strategies for clients.

The Mobility Assessment

Recall that in earlier assessment stages a particular kinetic chain movement impairment will have both overactive/shortened and underactive/lengthened muscles noted as possible contributing factors. Mobility assessments provide the Corrective Exercise Specialist with additional clues when answering the following questions:

1. Do overactive/shortened or underactive/lengthened muscles contribute more to the observed movement impairment?
2. Among the overactive/shortened muscles listed, are there specific ones that play a more prominent role in the movement impairment?
3. Is the corrective exercise program improving the mobility of the client or athlete over time?

Oftentimes, an observed movement impairment may result from flexibility limitations (due to overactive/shortened muscles or shortened soft tissue) or poor neuromuscular control (due to underactive/lengthened muscles). Mobility assessment helps direct exercise programming toward flexibility or strengthening strategies for that impairment. For example, if a movement impairment is observed during static and movement assessment stages, but mobility assessments do not show a flexibility (ROM) limitation at the relevant kinetic chain checkpoint, then it is more likely that poor neuromuscular control and underactive/lengthened muscles are the potential culprit; that is, muscle underactivity on one side of the joint contributes more to the impairment than overactivity on the other. The Corrective Exercise Specialist may then focus their program design on isolated strengthening and movement pattern integration for those muscles. This will also assist in avoiding unnecessary stretching techniques for muscles that already have adequate extensibility.

When observing the mobility of the kinetic chain, just as with both static posture and movement impairments, the Regional Interdependence (RI) model should always be considered. With mobility testing, the Corrective Exercise Specialist will look at specific joint motions that help determine if an area of dysfunction is affecting other regions above or below (Sueki et al., 2013). Mobility assessments used in the corrective exercise process have been determined to be reliable assessments for the spine (Giesche et al., 2019; Hirsch et al., 2014; Schafer et al., 2018), upper extremity (Luria et al., 2015; Terwee et al., 2005), and lower extremities (Holm et al., 2000; Rachkidi et al., 2009).

At a minimum, regular mobility assessment will serve as feedback regarding the effectiveness of the Corrective Exercise Specialist's programming for their client. Regular reassessment

---

Range of motion (ROM)

The amount of motion available at a specific joint.

Flexibility

The present state or ability of a joint to move through a range of motion.

Mobility

The entire available range of motion at a joint and the body's neuromuscular control of that motion.

of the particular kinetic chain checkpoints that commonly experience mobility restrictions will assist in the continual improvement of the client's workouts and movement quality.

GETTING TECHNICAL

Ensuring Reliability

When conducting assessments, it is important to be consistent with every client, especially if the tests are used as repeated measures over time by one or more professionals. In research and statistics, this is called test-retest reliability. The assessments used throughout the corrective exercise process have been chosen in part due to their ability to accurately measure the client over repeated sessions (Koo & Li, 2016).

The Scientific Rationale for Mobility Testing

Flexibility deficits can be caused by shortened contractile tissue (i.e., skeletal muscle) and changes in noncontractile tissue (e.g., tendons, ligaments), a common problem in the active population that can affect mobility (Behm et al., 2016). Several variables that may contribute to flexibility deficits include metabolic factors (Chang et al., 2015; Tojima et al., 2016), psychological factors (e.g., limbic system overactivity; Bhimani & Carney-Anderson, 2017; Bhimani et al., 2017), preexisting injury (Fasuyi et al., 2017; Jandre et al., 2015), neuromuscular factors (Bonser et al., 2017; Castellote-Caballero et al., 2013; Mills et al., 2015; Sharma et al., 2016), and myofascial dysfunction (e.g., trigger points; Quinn et al., 2016). If a mobility assessment reveals restricted motion by the client, then the Corrective Exercise Specialist should consider that contracted soft tissue or muscles may be present.

UPPER BODY MOBILITY TESTING

For the cervical and thoracic regions, if the static assessment reveals a postural distortion and/or the movement assessment reveals movement impairments, then a mobility assessment of the shoulders, head and neck, or cervicothoracic spine should be performed. Shortened cervical extensors, flexors, and rotators can cause mobility deficits for specific motions. Flexion, extension, rotation, and lateral flexion can be assessed by having the client actively move through the motions, which have been shown to be reliable when observed by one or more professionals (Jonsson & Rasmussen-Barr, 2018; Rondoni et al., 2017).

For the shoulder girdle and glenohumeral joint, a shortened pectoralis major and minor and latissimus dorsi often contribute to impairments during the overhead squat assessment (OHSA). The client may demonstrate an excessive anterior pelvic tilt and arms falling forward. A shortened pectoralis minor can often be found in Janda's upper crossed syndrome and can be assessed with scapular retraction (pectoralis minor test; Page et al., 2010). Decreased latissimus dorsi flexibility can be assessed with shoulder flexion (lat length test). Flexibility tests for the pectorals and latissimus dorsi have been shown to be reliable when conducted by one professional observing or using a tape measure or goniometer (Dawood et al., 2018; Rosa et al., 2016; Struyf et al., 2014; Weber et al., 2016).

Decreased glenohumeral internal and external rotation can also contribute to the arms falling forward during the OHSA or may limit upper extremity motions during basic functional activities (e.g., lifting a box above the head or throwing a ball). Shortened rotator cuff muscles, pectoralis major and minor, teres major, and latissimus dorsi can contribute to the impaired ROM. Flexibility of internal and external rotation can be assessed by having the client actively move through the motions, which has shown to be reliable when observed by one or more professionals or measured with a goniometer (Kolber & Hanney, 2012; Piotte et al., 2007).

For the elbow, forearm, and wrist, shortened muscles can affect overall upper extremity function, and vice versa. Shortening of the elbow and wrist flexors and extensors can be a cause of impairment. Flexibility testing can be assessed by having the client actively move through all the motions, which has been shown to be reliable when observed by one or more professionals or measured with a goniometer (Cools et al., 2014; Pourahmadi et al., 2017; van Rijn et al., 2018). The upper body mobility assessment section will provide a more detailed testing procedure and listing of potentially shortened muscles related to each movement.

LOWER BODY MOBILITY TESTING

Shortened soft tissue or muscles of the lumbo-pelvic-hip complex (LPHC), knee joint, and ankle joint commonly contribute to impairments seen in the OHSA. Clients may demonstrate an excessive forward trunk lean, excessive anterior and posterior pelvic tilt, asymmetric weight shift, knee valgus, feet turning out, and ankle/foot pronation.

For the LPHC, iliopsoas, rectus femoris, and tensor fascia latae (TFL)/IT band complex, flexibility can be tested with supine hip and knee extension (modified Thomas test). The test is reliable when performed by one or more professionals using pass–fail criteria (Peeler & Anderson, 2008b). Hip adductor (adductor magnus, adductor brevis, adductor longus, gracilis, and pectineus) flexibility can be tested using hip abduction and external rotation (adductor flexibility test). The test is reliable when performed by one professional, but reliability with two or more professionals has not been reported by researchers (Cejudo et al., 2015).

For the knee joint, flexibility of the quadriceps can be tested using prone knee flexion (Duncan-Ely test). This test is reliable when performed by one or more professionals using pass–fail criteria or using a goniometer to measure joint ROM (Peeler & Anderson, 2008a). Hamstring flexibility can also be tested using the active knee extension test (AKE), which is reliable when performed by one or more professionals (Hamid et al., 2013; Malliaropoulos et al., 2015; Neto et al., 2015; Reurink et al., 2013).

For the ankle joint, flexibility of the gastrocnemius and soleus can be tested with weight-bearing ankle dorsiflexion (weight-bearing lunge test), which is reliable when performed by one or more professionals (Baumbach et al., 2016; Munteanu et al., 2009; Powden et al., 2015). The lower body mobility assessment section will provide a more detailed testing procedure and listing of potentially shortened muscles related to each movement.

Active motion

The amount of motion obtained solely through voluntary contraction.

Passive motion

The amount of motion observed without any assistance from an external force.

⚠ **CRITICAL**

Mobility assessments are a combination of **active** and **passive motions** performed by the client while being observed by the Corrective Exercise Specialist. Full, pain-free motion is considered *normal* mobility. Restricted motion is considered a mobility issue, which may be caused by a flexibility deficit. Shortened (overactive) muscles and soft tissues are a common cause of decreased flexibility, which can affect mobility. These variables will be considered for each motion detailed in subsequent sections.

Mobility Assessment Procedures

Whereas static and movement assessments help identify muscles that are *potentially* over- or underactive, mobility assessments are used to confirm those findings and further pinpoint the areas in need of attention by the Corrective Exercise Specialist (**Figure 10-1**). The tests used to assess joint mobility are performed in a more stable position than the movement assessments, requiring less neuromotor control from the client. Thus, the findings can help provide

Mobility Assessments

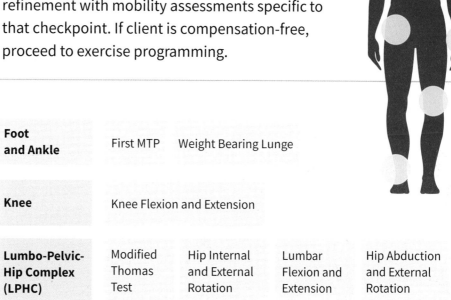

Any movement impairments present in kinetic chain checkpoints in previous assessments warrant further refinement with mobility assessments specific to that checkpoint. If client is compensation-free, proceed to exercise programming.

1   Client Intake

2   Static Postural Assessment

3   Overhead Squat Assessment (OHSA) and Modified OHSA

4   Single-Leg Squat and/or Split Squat Assessment

4a   Dynamic Assessments   OPTIONAL

4b   Loaded Assessments   OPTIONAL

5   Mobility Assessments

6   Corrective Exercise Programming   INHIBIT · LENGTHEN   ACTIVATE · INTEGRATE

Foot and Ankle	First MTP	Weight Bearing Lunge		
Knee	Knee Flexion and Extension			
Lumbo-Pelvic-Hip Complex (LPHC)	Modified Thomas Test	Hip Internal and External Rotation	Lumbar Flexion and Extension	Hip Abduction and External Rotation
Shoulders and Thoracic Spine	Thoracic Extension	Thoracic Rotation	Shoulder Flexion and Extension	Shoulder Internal and External Rotation Pectoralis Minor
Head and Cervical Spine	Cervical Flexion and Extension	Cervical Lateral Flexion	Cervical Rotation	

If shoulder and T-spine restriction present:

Elbow and Wrist	Elbow Flexion and Extension	Wrist Flexion and Extension

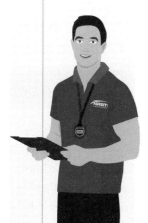

Figure 10-1   CES Assessment Flow: mobility assessments

information for whether a movement impairment is due to joint mobility restriction or neuromuscular control deficits. Again, mobility assessment answers the question, "Is a movement impairment primarily due to overactive/shortened muscles or underactive/lengthened muscles?" See **Figure 10-2**.

OBSERVATIONAL FINDINGS

MOBILITY ASSESSMENT	MOBILITY RESTRICTED?	IF YES – OVERACTIVE/SHORTENED MUSCLES
	Yes No	
	Yes No	
	Yes No	
	Yes No	
	Yes No	
	Yes No	
	Yes No	
	Yes No	
	Yes No	

Choose appropriate mobility assessments based on the movement impairments observed during the OHSA, Modified OHSA, and any additional transitional, loaded, and dynamic movement assessments. The suggested mobility assessments listed on the assessment solutions table are a starting point that should be narrowed down. The Corrective Exercise Specialist may also choose mobility assessments for the purpose of reassessment at their discretion.

Additional Notes

_____

_____

_____

Figure 10-2   Mobility assessment observations

Mobility restriction

The inability to move a joint through what should be its full range of motion.

A **mobility restriction** is the inability to move a joint through what should be its full ROM. If a client has restricted mobility, it means that overactive/shortened muscles and soft tissues on the side contralateral (opposite) to the observed restricted movement are responsible for reducing how far that joint can continue to move. Keeping the principle of force-couples in mind, this means, for example, that if a joint has restrictions in flexion, then overactive/shortened extensor muscles are restricting the ROM; or, if rotation of a segment to the right is restricted, then the muscles on the left side of the joint are overactive/shortened and are restricting the motion.

If the client can achieve what has been determined to be full ROM, mobility of that joint is identified as normal.

Consider a client who compensates with knee valgus during a given movement assessment and the hip adductors are identified as potentially overactive/short and the abductors identified as potentially underactive/lengthened. For someone with this movement impairment, much of the time the mobility assessment will show a restriction in hip abduction (the opposite motion of adduction), which confirms the overactivity of the adductors. But, if the client displays knee valgus yet has normal ROM in the lower extremity during mobility assessment, then it is more likely that the movement impairment is due to underactive/lengthened hip abductor muscles (i.e., neuromuscular control deficit) rather than adductor muscles that need improved flexibility.

HELPFUL HINT

The following is a helpful example that illustrates how mobility assessments refine programming.

Knee valgus observed → hip adductors potentially overactive/shortened → assess adductor mobility by observing abduction (the opposite motion)
→ if restricted → overactive/shortened hip adductors contribute to knee valgus → program inhibition and lengthening of the hip adductors
→ if mobility is normal → underactive/lengthened hip abductors contribute to knee valgus → program isolated strengthening of the hip abductors

The mobility assessments should be approached within the context of global movement patterns at the five kinetic chain checkpoints. In other words, a client only needs more specific mobility testing of a joint if the static and movement assessments (including the modified OHSA) identify a restriction. If the client does not demonstrate any static malalignments or movement impairments at a kinetic chain checkpoint, specific mobility testing for that checkpoint is not necessary. For example, if a client has a movement impairment at the shoulders but has normal lower extremity dynamic posture, only upper extremity mobility assessments should be performed with that client.

TRAINING TIP

Mobility assessments highlight different active and passive movements, normal motion values, specific landmarks, and potential flexibility deficits (Norkin & White, 2016). One traditional method of assessing those values is goniometry, which is a joint angle measurement technique that allied health professionals use to quantify joint ROM. While some Corrective Exercise Specialists may choose to use measurement devices, such as a goniometer, many may not have access to them. For ease of use and interpretation by all Corrective Exercise Specialists, NASM recommends performing mobility assessments based on observable landmarks on the body.

The assessments presented here allow the client to perform the movement themselves. Mobility of the observed joint will then simply be a binary determination of either *normal* or *restricted*. Restricted motion is determined by either an inability to move through a full ROM or a movement compensation during execution (e.g., forward foot flattens or turns out during the ankle dorsiflexion mobility assessment). Overactive/shortened muscles are associated with each restricted motion identified.

Foot and Ankle Screening

Clients who demonstrate the feet turning out, excessive pronation, knee valgus, or excessive forward trunk lean during the OHSA may reveal mobility restrictions at the foot and ankle complex. Additional testing for the ankle may help to identify specific limitations, thus allowing

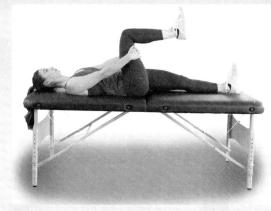

Active knee extension test—start

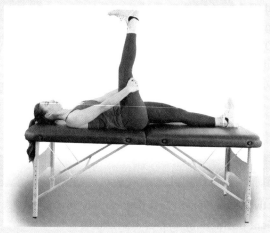

Active knee extension test—finish

Active Knee Extension Test

Client Position: Lying supine on a table

Type of motion: Active

Target motion: The client holds the test leg in 90 degrees of hip flexion and knee flexion. The pelvis should not posteriorly rotate or lumbar spine flatten. The client actively extends the knee while keeping the hip stable. The client's other leg is straight and relaxed on the table.

Verbal instructions: "Lift your right thigh to 90 degrees and hold your leg with your hands behind your knee, then actively straighten your knee as far as you can. Repeat on your left side."

Assessment:

- **Normal mobility:** The client can extend the knee nearly or completely straight without compensation.

- **Restricted knee extension:** The client is unable to extend their knee to the desired ROM or displays compensations such as the test thigh moving into extension (back toward the table) or movement in the opposite leg.

  - **Overactive/shortened:** Hamstrings complex

*Hamid et al., 2013; Malliaropoulos et al., 2015; Neto et al., 2015; Reurink et al., 2013

 TRAINING TIP

Remember that some muscle groups have a significant influence on the hip and knee. For example, the rectus femoris is classified as a two-joint muscle because it crosses both the hip and knee. Thus, it has an influence on both hip and knee function and ROM. For this reason, a comprehensive strategy for knee impairment should also include hip mobility tests (Earl-Boehm et al., 2018).

Lumbo-Pelvic-Hip Complex Screening

If static malalignments or movement impairments are observed at the LPHC or knee, mobility testing of the trunk is warranted. Clients who demonstrate excessive anterior or posterior pelvic tilt, asymmetric weight shift, knee valgus or varus, or excessive forward lean of the trunk during the OHSA may reveal mobility restrictions in the LPHC region of the body. Mobility testing

Elbow and Wrist Screening	Description
	Wrist Flexion and Extension *(continued)* ■ **Restricted flexion:** The client is unable to reach target mobility benchmark or displays compensation such as accessory motion in the fingers and elbows. • **Overactive/shortened:** Wrist extensors (extensor carpi radialis longus, extensor carpi radialis brevis, and extensor carpi ulnaris) ■ **Restricted extension:** The client is unable to reach target mobility benchmark or displays compensation such as accessory motion in the fingers and elbows. • **Overactive/shortened:** Wrist flexors (flexor carpi radialis, flexor carpi ulnaris, and palmaris longus)

Cervicothoracic Mobility

If static malalignments are observed above the hip, or movement compensations are observed at the shoulders or head/neck, a cervicothoracic mobility assessment should be performed. Clients who demonstrate a forward head posture, scapular elevation, or arms falling forward during the OHSA may reveal flexibility and ROM limitations in the upper body. Additional testing for the cervical and thoracic (cervicothoracic) regions may help to identify specific limitations, thus allowing the Corrective Exercise Specialist to create a more individualized upper body corrective exercise program for each client. To best explore cervicothoracic flexibility and ROM, the Corrective Exercise Specialist should begin with cervical tests and then proceed down to the thoracic spine.

HELPFUL HINT

The Corrective Exercise Specialist is encouraged to clearly provide instructions for the desired motion. For ease of interpretation, each mobility assessment will illustrate a standard, normal ROM value described by observable landmarks on the body and a rough visual estimate of rotation angles. Individuals with a ROM restriction will not be able to move through a full, pain-free ROM at the affected joint without compensation. Mobility of the observed joint can then be labeled as either *normal* or *restricted*.

Cervical Spine Screening	Description

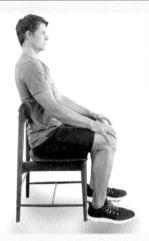

Start

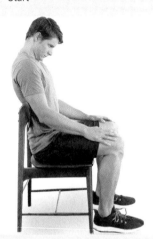

Cervical flexion

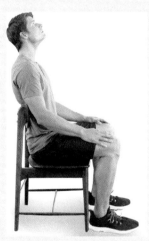

Cervical extension

Cervical Flexion and Extension

Client position: Standing or seated

Type of motion: Active

Target motions: The client is seated and bends their neck toward their chest (flexion) and up toward the ceiling (extension).

Verbal instruction: "Bring your chin down to your sternum and then look up toward the ceiling as far as you can while keeping your mouth closed."

Assessment:

- **Normal mobility:**
  - **Flexion:** The chin touches the sternum without compensation.
  - **Extension:** The face is roughly parallel to the horizon without compensation.
- **Restricted flexion:** The client is unable to reach the target mobility benchmark or displays compensations such as movement through the shoulders or cervical rotation.
  - **Overactive/shortened:** Erector spinae, deep cervical extensors, and upper trapezius
- **Restricted extension:** The client is unable to reach the target mobility benchmark or displays compensations such as movement through the shoulders or cervical rotation.
  - **Overactive/shortened:** Sternocleidomastoid and deep cervical flexors

Cervical Spine Screening	Description
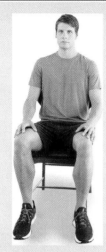 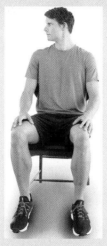 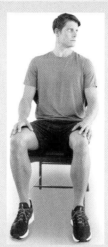 Cervical rotation—start Cervical rotation—movement 1 Cervical rotation—movement 2	**Cervical Rotation** **Client position:** Standing or seated **Type of motion:** Active **Target motions:** The client is seated and turns their neck to look over their right and left shoulder. **Verbal instruction:** "Look over your right then left shoulder as far as you comfortably can." **Assessment:** ■ **Normal mobility:** The nose aligns anywhere from over the clavicle to the tip of the shoulder without compensation. ■ **Restricted rotation:** The client is unable to reach the target mobility benchmark or displays compensations such as movement through the shoulders or cervical extension, flexion, or lateral flexion. ● **Overactive/shortened:** Sternocleidomastoid and scalenes on the side opposite of the observed restriction
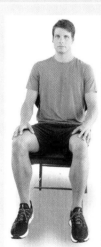 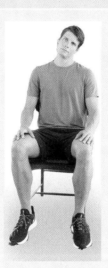 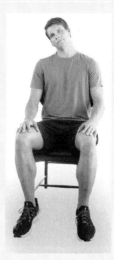 Cervical lateral flexion—start Cervical lateral flexion—movement 1 Cervical lateral flexion—movement 2	**Cervical Side Bending (Lateral Flexion)** **Client position:** Standing or seated **Type of motion:** Active **Target motions:** The client is seated and side bends (lateral flexion) to the right and left as far as possible without compensation. **Verbal instruction:** "Bring your ear toward your right shoulder then to the left as far as you comfortably can." **Assessment:** ■ **Normal mobility:** The head can tilt to roughly a 45-degree angle on each side without compensation. ■ **Restricted side bending:** The client is unable to reach the target mobility benchmark or displays compensations such as cervical rotation. ● **Overactive/shortened:** Sternocleidomastoid, scalenes, and erector spinae on the side opposite of the observed restriction

When assessing joint mobility, always keep the concept of force-couples in mind. For a joint to achieve its full available ROM and function optimally, muscles on all sides need to be in balance with the correct length-tension relationships. So, when mobility is restricted in one direction, it means muscles on the opposite side (contralateral) of the observed restriction are overactive/shortened and limiting how far that joint can continue to move. For example, if someone has restricted mobility when rotating their head to the left, that means that the muscles on the right side of the neck are holding that ROM back, and vice versa. This notion can be applied to the movement of every joint in the body.

THORACIC SPINE

Thoracic Spine Screening	Description
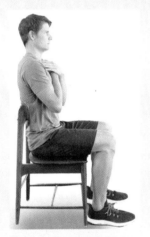 Thoracic extension—start 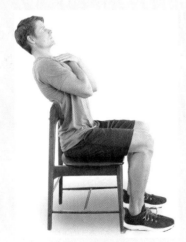 Thoracic extension—finish	**Thoracic Extension** **Client position:** Seated on a standard low-backed chair with hands and arms crossed over the chest, and lumbar and cervical spines neutral throughout. The chair back should end just beneath the client's shoulder blades. **Type of motion:** Active **Target motions:** The client arches their mid back over the chair as far as comfortably possible. **Verbal instruction:** "Cross your arms over your chest. While keeping your ribs and low back in place and neck in line with the torso, lean your mid back over the chair as far as you can without tipping the chair." **Assessment:** ■ **Normal mobility:** The upper back and head tilt backwards where the tops of the shoulders extend past the chair back (roughly 25 degrees of thoracic extension), and the sternum is nearly parallel to the horizon without compensation. ■ **Restricted thoracic extension:** The client is unable to reach target mobility benchmark or displays compensations such as cervical extension, ribs flaring, or lumbar extension. ● **Overactive/shortened:** Rectus abdominis, internal oblique, and external oblique

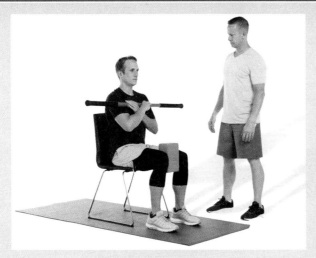

Seated thoracic rotation—start

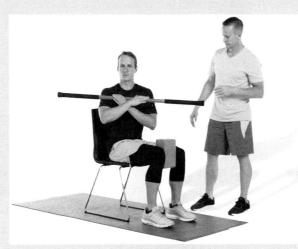

Seated thoracic rotation—movement 1

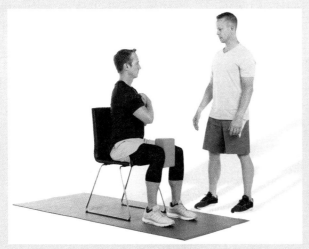

Seated thoracic rotation—movement 2

Seated Thoracic Rotation

Client position: Seated with hands crossed in front of body or crossed with holding a stick or dowel rod. Place a medicine ball or foam roller between the knees to stabilize the lower body. Ensure the shoulder blades are retracted and depressed.

Type of motion: Active

Target motions: The client squeezes the ball or roller between the knees to lock the hips in place and the client maintains a neutral cervical spine. The client then rotates the upper body to each side as far as possible.

Verbal instruction: "Hold the stick to your chest under crossed arms. Squeeze the roller between the knees, look forward, and keep your nose in line with the sternum. Rotate your trunk to the right as far as you can. Then, rotate to the left."

Assessment:

- **Normal mobility:** The sternum (or stick) rotates roughly 45 degrees from the starting position to each side without compensation.

- **Restricted thoracic rotation:** The client is unable to reach the target mobility benchmark or displays compensations such as lateral flexion of the spine, leaning forward or backward, and shoulder protraction.

  - **Overactive/shortened:** Rectus abdominis, internal oblique, external oblique, and erector spinae on the side opposite of the restriction

If the client demonstrates a specific, noticeable restriction of mobility, then it is recommended to inhibit and lengthen (phases 1 and 2 of the Corrective Exercise Continuum) muscles identified as potentially overactive/shortened. However, if a client demonstrates normal mobility in these tests, then emphasis should be placed on activating muscles that were identified as potentially underactive/lengthened during the previous static and movement assessments.

SUMMARY

The mobility assessment allows the Corrective Exercise Specialist to take a more comprehensive look at potential flexibility restrictions. This assessment stage is meant to refine the observations made during static and movement assessments, focus the corrective exercise program, and provide a way to monitor program effectiveness via continual reassessment. Essentially, when a static malalignment or a movement impairment is identified at a kinetic chain checkpoint in previous assessments, a targeted mobility assessment should be performed at that checkpoint to determine if the impairment is primarily a result of overactive or underactive musculature. When a mobility restriction is uncovered, it means there are overactive/shortened muscles on one side of the affected joint that are limiting how far that joint can continue to move. Conversely, if no mobility restrictions are found, but impairments were noted during movement assessments, that means the movement impairment is primarily due to neuromuscular control deficits in the muscles identified as probably underactive/lengthened.

The mobility assessments chosen for use in the corrective exercise process have the best evidence and are commonly used by Corrective Exercise Specialists. NASM recommends using observable body landmarks for ease of interpretation. Other tests and measures do exist but may not have good supporting evidence or require specialized equipment and training. Once a client's static posture, movement, and mobility have been assessed, the next step is to begin applying the Corrective Exercise Continuum during workouts, inhibiting and lengthening muscles identified as overactive/shortened in phases 1 and 2, activating muscles that are underactive/lengthened in phase 3, and then integrating those corrective phases into functional movement patterns with phase 4.

REFERENCES

Baumbach, S. F., Braunstein, M., Seeliger, F., Borgmann, L., Böcker, W., & Polzer, H. (2016). Ankle dorsiflexion: What is normal? Development of a decision pathway for diagnosing impaired ankle dorsiflexion and M. gastrocnemius tightness. *Archives of Orthopaedic and Trauma Surgery, 136*(9), 1203–1211. https://doi.org/10.1007/s00402-016-2513-x

Behm, D. G., Blazevich, A. J., Kay, A. D., & McHugh, M. (2016). Acute effects of muscle stretching on physical performance, range of motion, and injury incidence in healthy active individuals: A systematic review. *Applied Physiology, Nutrition, and Metabolism, 41*(1), 1–11. https://doi.org/10.1139/apnm-2015-0235

Bhimani, R., & Carney-Anderson, L. (2017). Lived experiences of muscle tightness symptoms from patients' perspectives. *Journal of Neuroscience Nursing, 49*(5), 280–285. https://doi.org/10.1097/jnn.0000000000000302

Bhimani, R. H., Gaugler, J. E., & Skay, C. (2017). Understanding symptom experiences of muscle tightness from patients' and clinicians' perspectives. *Journal of Clinical Nursing, 26*(13–14), 1927–1938. https://doi.org/10.1111/jocn.13506

Bonser, R. J., Hancock, C. L., Hansberger, B. L., Loutsch, R. A., Stanford, E. K., Zeigel, A. K., Baker, R. T., May, J., Nasypany, A., & Cheatham, S. (2017). Changes in hamstring range of motion after neurodynamic sciatic sliders: A critically appraised topic. *Journal of Sport Rehabilitation, 26*(4), 311–315. https://doi.org/10.1123/jsr.2015-0166

Caravaggi, P., Pataky, T., Goulermas, J. Y., Savage, R., & Crompton, R. (2009). A dynamic model of the windlass mechanism of the foot: Evidence for early stance phase preloading of the plantar aponeurosis. *Journal of Experimental Biology, 212*(Pt 15), 2491–2499. https://doi.org/10.1242/jeb.025767

Castellote-Caballero, Y., Valenza, M. C., Martín-Martín, L., Cabrera-Martos, I., Puentedura, E. J., & Fernández-de-Las-Peñas, C. (2013). Effects of a neurodynamic sliding technique on hamstring flexibility in healthy male soccer players. A pilot study. *Physical Therapy in Sport, 14*(3), 156–162. https://doi.org/10.1016/j.ptsp.2012.07.004

Cejudo, A., Ayala, F., De Baranda, P. S., & Santonja, F. (2015). Reliability of two methods of clinical examination of the flexibility of the hip adductor muscles. *International Journal of Sports Physical Therapy, 10*(7), 976–983.

Chang, K. V., Hung, C. Y., Li, C. M., Lin, Y. H., Wang, T. G., Tsai, K. S., & Han, D. S. (2015). Reduced flexibility associated with metabolic syndrome in community-dwelling elders. *PLoS One, 10*(1), e0117167. https://doi.org/10.1371/journal.pone.0117167

Çinar-Medeni, Ö., Atalay Guzel, N., & Basar, S. (2016). Mild hallux valgus angle affects single-limb postural stability in asymptomatic subjects. *Journal of Back and Musculoskeletal Rehabilitation, 29*(1), 117–121. https://doi.org/10.3233/bmr-150606

Cools, A. M., De Wilde, L., Van Tongel, A., Ceyssens, C., Ryckewaert, R., & Cambier, D. C. (2014). Measuring shoulder external and internal rotation strength and range of motion: Comprehensive intra-rater and inter-rater reliability study of several testing protocols. *Journal of Shoulder and Elbow Surgery, 23*(10), 1454–1461. https://doi.org/10.1016/j.jse.2014.01.006

Cuellar, J. M., & Lanman, T. H. (2017). "Text neck": An epidemic of the modern era of cell phones? *The Spine Journal, 17*(6), 901–902. https://doi.org/10.1016/j.spinee.2017.03.009

Cusack, J., Shtofmakher, G., Kilfoil, R. L., Jr., & Vu, S. (2014). Improved step length symmetry and decreased low back pain with the use of a rocking-soled shoe in a patient with unilateral hallux rigidus. *BMJ Case Reports, 2014.* https://doi.org/10.1136/bcr-2014-206408

Dawood, M., Van, R. A. J., Bekker, P. J., & Korkie, E. (2018). Inter- and intra-rater reliability of a technique assessing the length of the latissimus dorsi muscle. *South African Journal of Physiotherapy, 74*(1), 1–7.

Earl-Boehm, J. E., Bolgla, L. A., Emory, C., Hamstra-Wright, K. L., Tarima, S., & Ferber, R. (2018). Treatment success of hip and core or knee strengthening for patellofemoral pain: Development of clinical prediction rules. *Journal of Athletic Training, 53*(6), 545–552. https://doi.org/10.4085/1062-6050-510-16

Fares, J., Fares, M. Y., & Fares, Y. (2017). Musculoskeletal neck pain in children and adolescents: Risk factors and complications. *Surgical Neurology International, 8*, 72. https://doi.org/10.4103/sni.sni_445_16

Fasuyi, F. O., Fabunmi, A. A., & Adegoke, B. O. A. (2017). Hamstring muscle length and pelvic tilt range among individuals with and without low back pain. *Journal of Bodywork and Movement Therapies, 21*(2), 246–250. https://doi.org/10.1016/j.jbmt.2016.06.002

Ferber, R., Kendall, K. D., & McElroy, L. (2010). Normative and critical criteria for iliotibial band and iliopsoas muscle flexibility. *Journal of Athletic Training, 45*(4), 344–348.

Giesche, F., Krause, F., Niederer, D., Wilke, J., Engeroff, T., Vogt, L., & Banzer, W. (2019). Visual and instrumental diagnostics using

chromokinegraphics: Reliability and validity for low back pain stratification. *Journal of Back and Musculoskeletal Rehabilitation, 32*(2), 345–353. https://doi.org/10.3233/bmr-181203

Hamid, M. S., Ali, M. R., & Yusof, A. (2013). Interrater and intrarater reliability of the active knee extension (AKE) test among healthy adults. *Journal of Physical Therapy Science, 25*(8), 957–961. https://doi.org/10.1589/jpts.25.957

Harvey, D. (1998). Assessment of the flexibility of elite athletes using the modified Thomas test. *British Journal of Sports Medicine, 32*(1), 68–70. https://doi.org/10.1136/bjsm.32.1.68

Hirsch, B. P., Webb, M. L., Bohl, D. D., Fu, M., Buerba, R. A., Gruskay, J. A., & Grauer, J. N. (2014). Improving visual estimates of cervical spine range of motion. *American Journal of Orthopedics, 43*(11), E261–E265.

Holm, I., Bolstad, B., Lütken, T., Ervik, A., Røkkum, M., & Steen, H. (2000). Reliability of goniometric measurements and visual estimates of hip ROM in patients with osteoarthrosis. *Physiotherapy Research International, 5*(4), 241–248.

Jandre Reis, F. J., & Macedo, A. R. (2015). Influence of hamstring tightness in pelvic, lumbar and trunk range of motion in low back pain and asymptomatic volunteers during forward bending. *Asian Spine Journal, 9*(4), 535–540. https://doi.org/10.4184/asj.2015.9.4.535

Jonsson, A., & Rasmussen-Barr, E. (2018). Intra- and inter-rater reliability of movement and palpation tests in patients with neck pain: A systematic review. *Physiotherapy Theory and Practice, 34*(3), 165–180. https://doi.org/10.1080/09593985.2017.1390806

Kolber, M. J., & Hanney, W. J. (2012). The reliability and concurrent validity of shoulder mobility measurements using a digital inclinometer and goniometer: A technical report. *International Journal of Sports Physical Therapy, 7*(3), 306–313.

Koo, T. K., & Li, M. Y. (2016). A guideline of selecting and reporting intraclass correlation coefficients for reliability research. *Journal of Chiropractic Medicine, 15*(2), 155–163. https://doi.org/10.1016/j.jcm.2016.02.012

Luria, S., Apt, E., Kandel, L., Bdolah-Abram, T., & Zinger, G. (2015). Visual estimation of pro-supination angle is superior to wrist or elbow angles. *The Physician and Sportsmedicine, 43*(2), 155–160. https://doi.org/10.1080/00913847.2015.1037230

Malliaropoulos, N., Kakoura, L., Tsitas, K., Christodoulou, D., Siozos, A., Malliaras, P., & Maffulli, N. (2015). Active knee range of motion assessment in elite track and field athletes: Normative values. *Muscle, Ligaments and Tendons Journal, 5*(3), 203–207. https://doi.org/10.11138/mltj/2015.5.3.203

Mills, M., Frank, B., Goto, S., Blackburn, T., Cates, S., Clark, M., Aguilar, A., Fava, N., & Padua, D. (2015). Effect of restricted hip flexor muscle length on hip extensor muscle activity and lower extremity biomechanics in college-aged female soccer players. *International Journal of Sports Physical Therapy, 10*(7), 946–954.

Munteanu, S. E., Strawhorn, A. B., Landorf, K. B., Bird, A. R., & Murley, G. S. (2009). A weightbearing technique for the measurement of ankle joint dorsiflexion with the knee extended is reliable. *Journal of Science and Medicine in Sport, 12*(1), 54–59. https://doi.org/10.1016/j.jsams.2007.06.009

Neto, T., Jacobsohn, L., Carita, A. I., & Oliveira, R. (2015). Reliability of the active-knee-extension and straight-leg-raise tests in subjects with flexibility deficits. *Journal of Sport Rehabilitation, 24*(4). https://doi.org/10-1123/jsr.2014-0220

Norkin, C. C., & White, D. J. (2016). *Measurement of joint motion: A guide to goniometry* (5th ed.). F.A. Davis.

Page, P., Frank, C. C., & Lardner, R. (2010). *Assessment and treatment of muscle imbalance: The Janda approach.* Human Kinetics.

Peeler, J., & Anderson, J. E. (2008a). Reliability of the Ely's test for assessing rectus femoris muscle flexibility and joint range of motion. *Journal of Orthopaedic Research, 26*(6), 793–799. https://doi.org/10.1002/jor.20556

Peeler, J. D., & Anderson, J. E. (2008b). Reliability limits of the modified Thomas test for assessing rectus femoris muscle flexibility about the knee joint. *Journal of Athletic Training, 43*(5), 470–476. https://doi.org/10.4085/1062-6050-43.5.470

Piotte, F., Gravel, D., Nadeau, S., Moffet, H., & Bédard, C. (2007). Reliability of arthrometric measurement of shoulder lateral rotation movement in healthy subjects. *Physiotherapy Theory and Practice, 23*(3), 169–178. https://doi.org/10.1080/09593980701209121

Pourahmadi, M. R., Ebrahimi Takamjani, I., Sarrafzadeh, J., Bahramian, M., Mohseni-Bandpei, M. A., Rajabzadeh, F., & Taghipour, M. (2017). Reliability and concurrent validity of a new iPhone® goniometric application for measuring active wrist range of motion: A cross-sectional study in asymptomatic subjects. *Journal of Anatomy, 230*(3), 484–495. https://doi.org/10.1111/joa.12568

Powden, C. J., Hoch, J. M., & Hoch, M. C. (2015). Reliability and minimal detectable change of the weight-bearing lunge test: A systematic review. *Manual Therapy, 20*(4), 524–532. https://doi.org/10.1016/j.math.2015.01.004

Quinn, S. L., Olivier, B., & Wood, W. A. (2016). The short-term effects of trigger point therapy, stretching and medicine ball exercises on accuracy and back swing hip turn in elite, male golfers: A randomised controlled trial. *Physical Therapy in Sport, 22*, 16–22. https://doi.org/10.1016/j.ptsp.2016.04.002

Rachkidi, R., Ghanem, I., Kalouche, I., El Hage, S., Dagher, F., & Kharrat, K. (2009). Is visual estimation of passive range of motion in the pediatric lower limb valid and reliable? *BMC Musculoskeletal Disorders, 10*, 126. https://doi.org/10.1186/1471-2474-10-126

Reurink, G., Goudswaard, G. J., Oomen, H. G., Moen, M. H., Tol, J. L., Verhaar, J. A., & Weir, A. (2013). Reliability of the active and passive knee extension test in acute hamstring injuries. *The American Journal of Sports Medicine, 41*(8), 1757–1761. https://doi.org/10.1177/0363546513490650

Rondoni, A., Rossettini, G., Ristori, D., Gallo, F., Strobe, M., Giaretta, F., Battistin, A., & Testa, M. (2017). Intrarater and inter-rater reliability of active cervical range of motion in patients with nonspecific neck pain measured with technological and common use devices: A systematic review with meta-regression. *Journal of Manipulative and Physiological Therapeutics, 40*(8), 597–608. https://doi.org/10.1016/j.jmpt.2017.07.002

Rosa, D. P., Borstad, J. D., Pires, E. D., & Camargo, P. R. (2016). Reliability of measuring pectoralis minor muscle resting length in subjects with and without signs of shoulder impingement. *Brazilian Journal of Physical Therapy, 20*(2), 176–183. https://doi.org/10.1590/bjpt-rbf.2014.0146

Schäfer, A., Lüdtke, K., Breuel, F., Gerloff, N., Knust, M., Kollitsch, C., Laukart, A., Matej, L., Müller, A., Schöttker-Königer, T., & Hall, T. (2018). Validity of eyeball estimation for range of motion during the cervical flexion rotation test compared to an ultrasound-based movement analysis system. *Physiotherapy Theory and Practice, 34*(8), 622–628. https://doi.org/10.1080/09593985.2017.1423523

Sharma, S., Balthillaya, G., Rao, R., & Mani, R. (2016). Short-term effectiveness of neural sliders and neural tensioners as an adjunct to static stretching of hamstrings on knee extension angle in healthy individuals: A randomized controlled trial. *Physical Therapy in Sport, 17*, 30–37. https://doi.org/10.1016/j.ptsp.2015.03.003

Struyf, F., Meeus, M., Fransen, E., Roussel, N., Jansen, N., Truijen, S., & Nijs, J. (2014). Interrater and intrarater reliability of the pectoralis minor muscle length measurement in subjects with and without shoulder impingement symptoms. *Manual Therapy, 19*(4), 294–298. https://doi.org/10.1016/j.math.2014.04.005

Sueki, D. G., Cleland, J. A., & Wainner, R. S. (2013). A regional interdependence model of musculoskeletal dysfunction: Research, mechanisms, and clinical implications. *Journal of Manual & Manipulative Therapy, 21*(2), 90–102. https://doi.org/10.1179/2042618612y.0000000027

Terwee, C. B., de Winter, A. F., Scholten, R. J., Jans, M. P., Devillé, W., van Schaardenburg, D., & Bouter, L. M. (2005). Interobserver reproducibility of the visual estimation of range of motion of the shoulder. *Archives of Physical Medicine and Rehabilitation, 86*(7), 1356–1361.

Tojima, M., Noma, K., & Torii, S. (2016). Changes in serum creatine kinase, leg muscle tightness, and delayed onset muscle soreness after a full marathon race. *Journal of Sports Medicine and Physical Fitness, 56*(6), 782–788.

van Rijn, S. F., Zwerus, E. L., Koenraadt, K. L., Jacobs, W. C., van den Bekerom, M. P., & Eygendaal, D. (2018). The reliability and validity of goniometric elbow measurements in adults: A systematic review of the literature. *Shoulder & Elbow, 10*(4), 274–284. https://doi.org/10.1177/1758573218774326

Weber, C., Enzler, M., Wieser, K., & Swanenburg, J. (2016). Validation of the pectoralis minor length test: A novel approach. *Musculoskeletal Science & Practice, 22*, 50–55. https://doi.org/10.1016/j.math.2015.09.015

SECTION 4

Programming Strategies

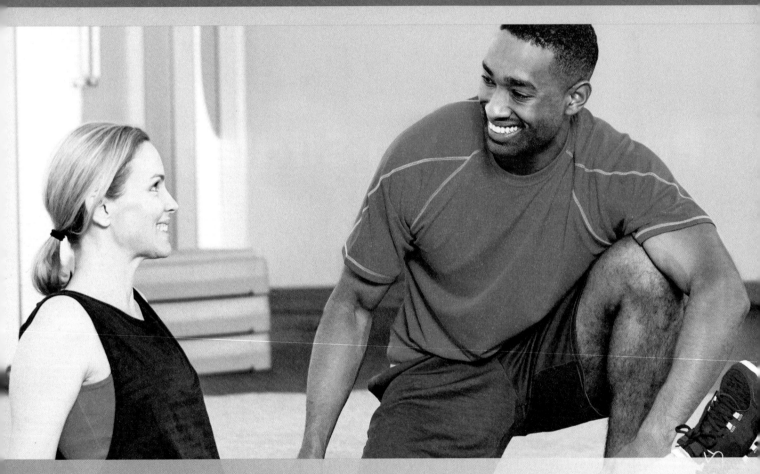

CHAPTER 11

Corrective Strategies for the Foot and Ankle

Learning Objectives

After reading this content, students should be able to demonstrate the following objectives:

- **Explain** basic functional anatomy of the foot and ankle complex.
- **Identify** the mechanisms for common foot and ankle injuries.
- **Describe** the influence of altered foot and ankle movement on the kinetic chain.
- **Determine** appropriate systematic assessment strategies for the foot and ankle.
- **Select** appropriate corrective exercise strategies for the foot and ankle.

Introduction

Human movement is a complex balance of sensory stimulation, neuromuscular control, and biomechanical stabilization. All closed-chain human movement begins with the relationship between the foot and the ground. This region of the body represents the platform from which an individual's base of support is derived and is the only contact point between the body and the ground. The foot must withstand a high amount of repetitive stress in the form of ground reaction forces with each step taken.

As the Regional Interdependence (RI) model shows, the body functions as an interconnected chain (kinetic chain), and compensation or impairment in one region of the body may lead to impairments in other areas of the body (Rath et al., 2016; Riskowski et al., 2013). This concept is particularly highlighted with the foot and ankle complex, where dysfunction will have a direct impact on overall lower extremity motion. This chapter will review the basic functional anatomy of the foot and ankle complex, its relationship with other segments of the body during movement, and corrective strategies to help improve foot and ankle movement impairment.

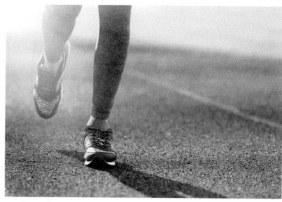

© Africa Studio/Shutterstock

Review of Foot and Ankle Functional Anatomy

The foot and ankle structure is complex with great potential for influence on the rest of the human movement system (HMS). Because this is a review of foot and ankle anatomy, not all anatomical structures will be covered in detail; however, the most important structures associated with lower extremity compensation patterns will be discussed. If advanced foot and ankle education is desired, professionals should explore these options as they grow within their career.

Bones and Joints

The foot and ankle complex can be broken down into three main regions: the rearfoot, the midfoot, and the forefoot. The rearfoot has a direct influence on distal structures (such as the mid- and forefoot) and proximal structures (such as the knee and hip). **Figure 11-1** demonstrates the rearfoot as the junction between the leg and foot. The rearfoot is composed of the two lower leg bones (tibia and fibula), two foot bones (talus and calcaneus), and two joints (talocrural or ankle joint and subtalar joint). Of the two lower leg bones, the tibia is the larger weight-bearing bone. The tibia is in direct contact with the first foot bone, the talus. The talus is in direct contact with the calcaneus, and the calcaneus is in direct contact with the ground. During dynamic movement, it is this relationship between the ground, calcaneus, talus, and tibia that transmits ground reaction forces as potential energy up the lower extremity through the knee and femur to the pelvis.

TALOCRURAL (ANKLE) JOINT

The first joint of the rearfoot, formed by the tibia, fibula, and talus, is the talocrural, or ankle, joint (**Figure 11-2**). During open-chain movement, the ankle joint is typically associated with sagittal plane dorsiflexion and plantar flexion. During open-chain movement, dorsiflexion is characterized by the top of the foot (dorsal surface) moving closer to the anterior tibia. During closed-chain dorsiflexion, the foot is in contact with the ground, so the anterior tibia

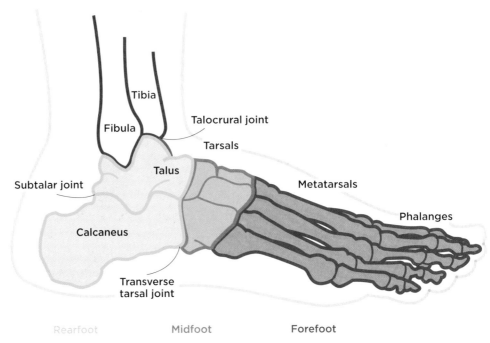

Figure 11-1 Foot and ankle structure

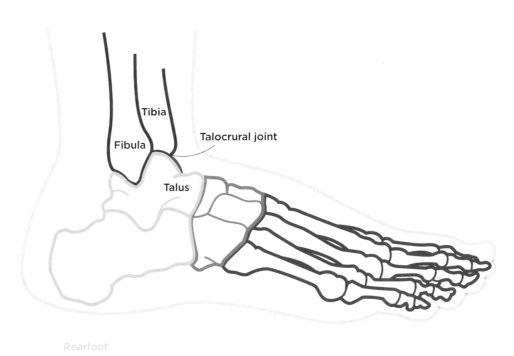

Figure 11-2 Talocrural (ankle) joint

approximates the dorsal aspect of the foot. Closed-chain dorsiflexion is necessary during the descent of a squat as the knee translates anteriorly (**Figure 11-3**). During open-chain movement, plantar flexion occurs when the bottom of the foot (plantar surface) moves closer to the posterior tibia. During closed-chain plantar flexion, the foot is again in contact with the ground and the approximation of the plantar aspect of the foot is less obvious. In the ascent of a squat, as the

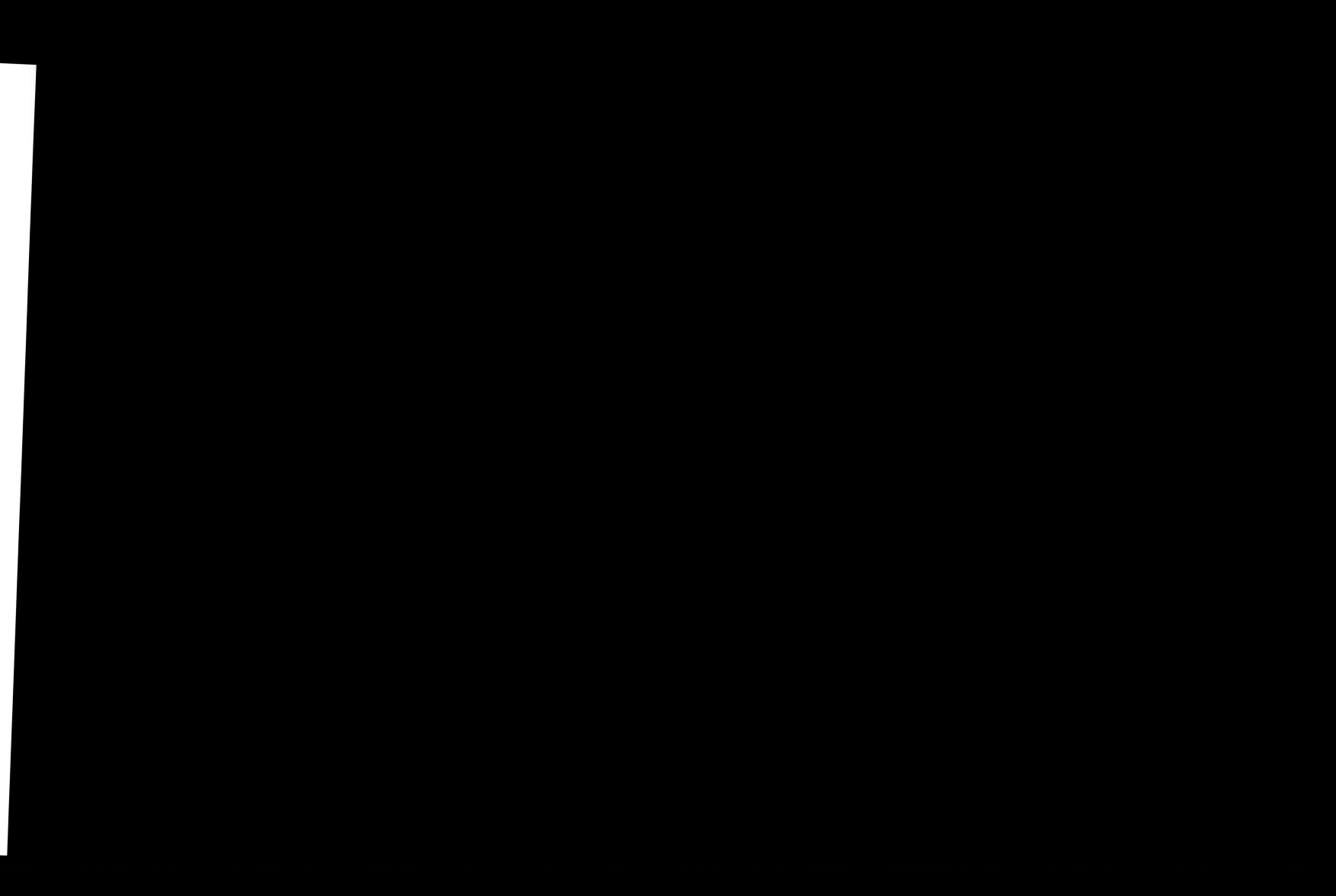

Every action of the ankle joint influences the STJ and vice versa. It is this relationship between the ankle joint and the STJ that is associated with compensation patterns observed in the foot and ankle complex.

Dorsiflexion at the ankle joint is associated with STJ eversion. Thus, during the loading or impact phase, the ankle is dorsiflexed and the STJ is everted or unlocked. This enhances the foot and ankle's ability to efficiently absorb impact forces.

Conversely, plantar flexion at the ankle joint is associated with STJ inversion. Thus, during the unloading or push-off phase, as the ankle plantar flexes, the STJ inverts or locks. This position creates a rigid lever, enhancing the ability to effectively toe off during movement.

TIBIAL ROTATION

The final step in understanding rearfoot function and influences in movement compensation is to appreciate the influence the rearfoot has on the tibia in the transverse plane. Due to the relationship between the talus and the tibia, during closed-chain movement, every action of the STJ and ankle joint will have an influence on the tibia or lower leg.

During closed-chain movement, each frontal plane motion of the STJ creates a transverse plane rotation through the leg. Transverse plane motions of the tibia are internal and external rotation, which are associated with force absorption and force production, respectively. From a coupled perspective, tibial internal rotation is associated with ankle dorsiflexion and STJ eversion. Collectively, these motions enhance the foot, ankle, and lower leg's ability to effectively absorb impact forces. Compensations often are observed here because individuals frequently lack control of the force absorption phase. While the coupling of tibial internal rotation, ankle dorsiflexion, and eversion is normal, the lack of control over that motion is when impairments are observed (i.e., too much motion occurring too soon). Conversely, tibial external rotation is associated with ankle plantar flexion and STJ inversion. Collectively, these motions enhance the ability of the foot, ankle, and lower leg to effectively produce force during movement.

PRONATION AND SUPINATION

Recognize that, due to coupling of the ankle joint and STJ, the motion of the rearfoot is triplanar. Thus, movement always occurs in the three planes and is referred to as pronation and supination. **Pronation** is the associated movements of ankle dorsiflexion (sagittal), foot abduction (transverse), and eversion (frontal). Pronation occurs most frequently during deceleration (i.e., eccentric muscle action) and presents an unlocked rearfoot that is best for force absorption, such as when lowering into a squat position. **Supination** is the associated movements of ankle

Pronation

A triplanar movement that is associated with force reduction.

Supination

A triplanar motion that is associated with force production.

 HELPFUL HINT

Triplanar Motion of the Rearfoot

Dorsiflexion + Foot abduction + Eversion = Pronation = Unlocked rearfoot = Force absorption
Plantar flexion + Foot adduction + Inversion = Supination = Locked rearfoot = Force production

Remember that figures displaying motions such as eversion or plantar flexion show them in isolation and at obvious end-ranges. When joint motions combine to produce movement in real life, especially at the foot and ankle complex, they are subtle in appearance and should still move within the proper ranges of kinetic chain alignment. *Excessive* pronation or supination is considered compensatory movement.

plantar flexion, foot adduction, and inversion. Supination occurs most frequently during acceleration (i.e., concentric muscle action) and presents a locked rearfoot that is best for force production, such as when rising from a squat or toeing off in a jump.

Recognize that pronation and supination occur during motion such as when squatting, walking, and running. However, in static observations, it is more common to use the terms pes planus and pes cavus. **Pes planus** is characterized by a flattened medial arch during weight bearing (**Figure 11-8**). Conversely, **pes cavus** is characterized by a high medial arch during weight bearing (**Figure 11-9**). These terms are important for describing impairment during the static assessments.

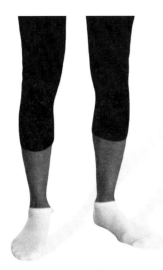

Figure 11-8   Pes planus

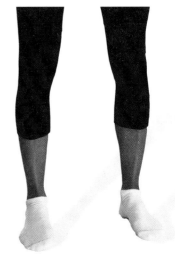

Figure 11-9   Pes cavus

Muscles

The two main types of muscles in the foot and ankle are extrinsic and intrinsic muscles. **Extrinsic muscles** originate in the lower leg and insert in the foot via tendons, whereas **intrinsic muscles** both originate and insert in the foot. Their relationship to each other is important in movement, with the intrinsic muscles thought of as the stabilizers and the extrinsic muscles being more the mobilizers.

When it comes to understanding optimal foot function and compensation patterns, the focus is on six main extrinsic muscles. These muscles can be divided into two groups based on their action on the rearfoot, namely to the subtalar joint and tibial rotations. During closed-chain movement, such as walking or squatting, certain muscles create **subtalar inversion** and contribute to **supination of the foot** during concentric acceleration, whereas others create **subtalar eversion** and contribute to **pronation of the foot** during eccentric deceleration (**Table 11-1**).

TABLE 11-1 Key Extrinsic Muscles of the Foot and Ankle Complex	
Invertors	**Evertors**
■ Anterior tibialis	■ Fibularis (peroneus) brevis
■ Posterior tibialis	■ Fibularis (peroneus) longus
■ Soleus	■ Gastrocnemius

The three invertors play an important role in maintaining a stable and locked position from the rearfoot all the way up into the hip during force production (e.g., the concentric unloading phase of gait), whereas the three evertors play a role in unlocking the foot and hip to allow for deceleration and the absorption of impact forces (e.g., the eccentric loading phase of gait). The invertor and evertor muscles work together with every step to help maintain alignment of the ankle, like two hands on a steering wheel.

Altered Foot and Ankle Movement

The ankle is the most commonly injured joint in both sports and daily life. Several studies have found that control at the hip is vital for maintaining control at the ankle (Emery et al., 2007). Proximal factors, such as lumbo-pelvic-hip complex (LPHC) muscle weakness, particularly in the frontal and transverse planes, have been found to contribute to altered lower extremity alignment, leading to increased foot pronation (**Figure 11-10**). If the hip lacks dynamic stability in the frontal and transverse planes during functional weight-bearing activities, the femur may adduct and internally rotate, whereas the tibia may externally rotate and the foot may go into excessive pronation. These static malalignments (altered length-tension relationships and joint arthrokinematics), abnormal muscle activation patterns, and dynamic malalignments

Subtalar eversion

Occurs when the bottom of the heel (inferior calcaneus) swings laterally.

Pronation of the foot

A multiplanar, synchronized joint motion that occurs with eccentric muscle function; the combination of subtalar eversion, dorsiflexion, and abduction.

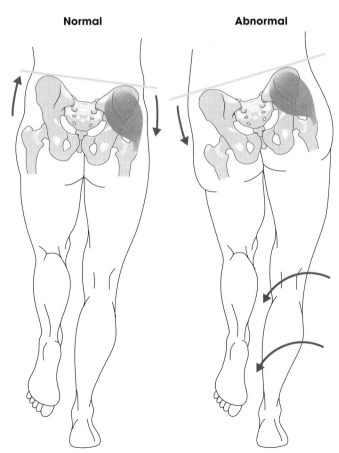

Normal   **Abnormal**

Figure 11-10 Effects of weak LPHC on the lower extremity

can alter neuromuscular control and can lead to plantar fasciitis, patellofemoral pain, IT-band tendonitis, and increased risk of anterior cruciate ligament (ACL) tears (Chou, 2014; Riskowski et al., 2013).

Static Malalignments

Common static malalignments of the foot and ankle include pes planus of the foot, which may result from overactivity of the fibularis muscles (peroneals) and lateral gastrocnemius, underactivity of the anterior and posterior tibialis, and decreased joint motion of the first metatarsophalangeal (MTP) joint and talus (decreased posterior glide). Posterior glide, a normal feature of ankle mobility, is the small rearward movement of the talus when the ankle dorsiflexes. It is hypothesized that decreased posterior glide of the talus can decrease dorsiflexion at the ankle. Statically, these clients may appear in a slightly plantar flexed position at the ankle when standing. Some studies have found decreased posterior glide of the talus in subjects with a history of lateral ankle sprains. Other studies have found a more rapid restoration of dorsiflexion and normalization of gait in patients with ankle sprains who were treated with manual posterior glide of the talus (Lewit, 2010; Riskowski et al., 2013). It is important to note that subtalar mobilization to improve glide is often a manual technique performed by licensed professionals.

Abnormal Muscle Activation Patterns

Postural sway

A measure of postural stability and control, often while standing. Refers to the amount of reflexive movement made by an individual around their center of gravity to remain balanced.

Subjects with unilateral chronic ankle sprains have been found to have weaker ipsilateral hip abduction strength and increased multiplanar **postural sway** (Cornwall & Murrell, 1991; Lentell et al., 1995). Subjects with increased postural sway have also been found to have up to seven times more ankle sprains than those subjects with better postural sway scores (McGuine et al., 2000; Tropp et al., 1985) Furthermore, fatigue in the knee and hip musculature (sagittal and frontal planes) creates even greater postural sway (Gribble & Hertel, 2004a, 2004b). Cerny (1984) found that weakness and decreased postural stability in the stabilizing muscles of the LPHC, such as the gluteus medius, may produce deviations in subtalar joint motion during gait. Foot placement depends on hip abduction and adduction moments generated during the swing phase of gait, and subsequent subtalar joint inversion may occur in response to medial foot placement errors secondary to overactivity of the hip adductors (Herzog et al., 2019). This has led to the determination through research that proximal stability and strength deficits at the hip can lead to ankle injuries (Chou, 2014; Emery et al., 2007; Michaud, 2011).

Dynamic Malalignment

Excessive pronation of the foot during weight-bearing activity has been shown to cause altered alignment of the tibia, femur, and pelvic girdle that can lead to internal rotation stresses at the lower extremity and pelvis, which may lead to increased strain on soft tissues (Achilles tendon, plantar fascia, patellar tendon, IT-band, etc.) and compressive forces on the joints (subtalar joint, patellofemoral joint, tibiofemoral joint, iliofemoral joint, and sacroiliac joint) that can become symptomatic. LPHC alignment has been shown by Khamis and Yizhar (2007) to be directly affected by bilateral excessive pronation of the feet. Excessive pronation of the feet induces an anterior pelvic tilt of the LPHC. The addition of 2 to 3 degrees of foot pronation led to a 20–30% increase in pelvic malalignment while standing and a 50–75% increase in anterior pelvic tilt during walking. Because anterior pelvic tilt has been correlated with increased lumbar curvature, the change in foot alignment might also influence lumbar spine position. Furthermore, an

(as might occur from a unilateral ankle sprain) may cause
nd lumbar alignment, which might increase symptoms or
aud, 2011).

le Dysfunction
onal
nce Model

n have a significant negative effect throughout the entire
le affects the proximal structures through disruption of the
le, tibia, femur, and hip. The motion of the STJ influences
ich directly impacts the knee and is closely associated with
2019). Additionally, decreased dorsiflexion during a squat
valgus and increased quadriceps activation, which is con-
se with patellofemoral pain (Macrum et al., 2012). Further,
ed hip strength as compared to those with a normal arch
ndicated in many impairments observed in the LPHC and

indicated that, while the disruption of the coupling is clear,
ss well known. For example, hip abductor weakness could
ng femoral and tibial internal rotation. However, excessive
bial and femoral internal rotation, resulting in chronically

g closed-chain dynamic movement, there is an associated
bility. From a mechanical or joint-coupling perspective,
rotation, femoral adduction, and a knee valgus alignment.
cle imbalances and inhibition are often associated with the
dering the overpronated foot with associated knee valgus,
muscles that keep the foot and knee in a neutral position,
and posterior tibialis) and hip external rotators (gluteus
prolonged overpronation of the foot and valgus position
associated with overactivity of the lateral gastrocnemius,
nsor fascia latae (TFL).

an oversupinated foot is one that demonstrates increased
closed-chain dynamic movements. Plantar flexion and in-
al rotation, which leads to foot, ankle, and hip tightness, as
en considering the oversupinated foot, mobilization is key
yofascial rolling (SMR) and stretching to the plantar foot,
tors (gluteus medius and gluteus maximus) are key. True
dition requiring healthcare evaluation before proceeding
g.

Although oversupination and pes cavus are rarer static and dynamic observations, the C⟦
still encounter them. It is common for an untrained individual to suspect pes cavus if they
position. Thus, it is vital to also observe the foot in a loaded position. True pes cavus cou
neurological disorder and should be further investigated. Oversupination is characterized
(i.e., the medial arch does not lower during the squat) or by a medial arch that rises durin
shifts weight to the lateral portion of the foot). Oversupination is often due to rigidity in t
Exercise Specialist is reminded to stay within their scope and not diagnose. A proposed
mobilization of the plantar surface via myofascial techniques once the client has been cl⟦

Assessment Results f⟦
and Ankle

Performing lower extremity assessments barefoot provides
ankle complex function. For some clients, the assessments c
the influence footwear has on movement patterns or if a fac

Identification of movement impairment is achieved th
cess (i.e., CES Assessment Flow), which includes static pos
ments. The integrated assessment process allows the Cor
mobility restrictions, muscle imbalance, and faulty moven
identified, the corrective exercise strategy can be develop⟦

TABLE 11-2 Foot and Ankle Assessment Results

Assessment(s)	Res⟦
Static posture	Fee⟦
	Low⟦
	(pla⟦
	Pes⟦
	Pes⟦
	Pes⟦
Transitional and loaded movement	Exce⟦
	Fee⟦
	Hee⟦
	Exce⟦
	Squ⟦
Dynamic movement	Exce⟦
	Fee⟦
Mobility	Limi⟦
Ankle dorsiflexion (weight-bearing lunge test)	Limi⟦
First MTP extension	

assessment results that warrant the implementation of a corrective strategy for the foot and ankle complex.

Static Foot and Ankle Posture

During static postural assessment, Corrective Exercise Specialists will compare their client's posture to the postural archetypes described by Janda's postural distortion syndromes, Kendall's spinal postures, and pes planus distortion syndrome. A key postural impairment that relates to the ankle is pes planus distortion syndrome, which is characterized by flat feet with knee valgus (**Figure 11-11**). This position of the knee can place excessive stress on the muscles and connective tissue associated with the ankle joint during dynamic movement.

Another postural impairment that needs to be considered is ankle plantar flexion, which is typically observed with knee hyperextension (i.e., the lower leg is posteriorly displaced). The positions of the knee and ankle are commonly observed in Janda's postural syndromes. The lower extremity joint positions may be influenced by the LPHC position or an ankle mobility deficit, which can be determined with more specific movement (modified OHSA) and mobility testing.

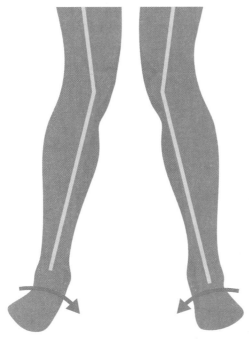

Figure 11-11   Pes planus distortion syndrome

 CHECK IT OUT

Orthotics

Certain foot postures, such as overpronation, may benefit from an orthotic, or shoe insert, that is designed to cushion or realign the foot and ankle complex into a neutral position. Orthotics may be over the counter, which typically offer moderate control, or custom molded, which are specific to an individual's foot type and potential biomechanical imbalances.

Custom orthotics, which are made by a medical professional, may be soft, semi-rigid, or rigid and often include modifications to the heel and arch to better provide support and control to the individual's foot type (Gross, 1995).

Transitional Movement Assessments

Based on the collective information obtained from the static postural assessment, the Corrective Exercise Specialist will have a high-level estimation of which muscles might be overactive/shortened and which ones are underactive/lengthened. As with static posture, the RI model highlights that an observed movement impairment at the foot and ankle could very well be due to muscle imbalances at the LPHC. Often, clients will have relatively impairment-free static posture; however, when in motion, active muscle imbalances may come to light that cannot be seen during static assessment.

OVERHEAD SQUAT ASSESSMENT

Because a squat requires optimal ankle mobility, many of the common movement impairments observed in an OHSA will be associated with a lack of ankle dorsiflexion. Excessive pronation is often observed with knee valgus and sometimes a heel lift on descent. Pronation and knee valgus may be due to insufficient sagittal plane mobility within the ankle joint, causing the feet to compensate by turning out. When the foot is turned out, this allows the client to bypass a restricted ankle joint. The feet may also turn out when there is a case of an overactive calf complex (**Figure 11-12**).

The compensation of heel rise may be seen when the client presents with an overactive/shortened calf complex, structurally short Achilles tendon, and/or a high-arched foot (**Figure 11-13**). The movement impairment of excessive forward trunk lean may be frequently observed in the place of the heels rising off the ground. In this compensation, the individual is not able to fully move through the ankle joint (cannot sufficiently dorsiflex) and uses relative flexibility to still accomplish the squat movement by bending over more at the hip (**Figure 11-14**).

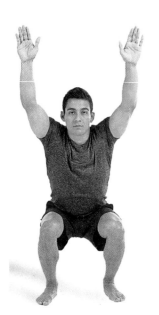

Figure 11-12   Feet turning out

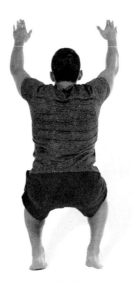

Figure 11-13   Heel rise

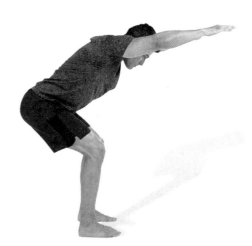

Figure 11-14   Excessive forward trunk lean

Based on the collective information obtained from the assessment, the Corrective Exercise Specialist can begin to identify potential muscle imbalances and joint range of motion (ROM) deficiencies to address. It is likely that poor performance on the transitional movement assessment is attributable to multiple factors at multiple joints. Several kinetic chain checkpoints may need to be addressed with targeted mobility assessments.

are associated with reduced
airments of feet turning out,
d modification can be used
kle complex or other areas,
reates a lack of dorsiflexion

nts seen during the OHSA,
gittal plane mobility in the
ensibility (i.e., a lack of dor-
HSA performance, then the
at the LPHC is likely to be
example, may be the source

nal assessment to perform,
s necessary (**Figures 11-15**
evident when squatting on
n performing the SLSA are

g squat: heel rise

rformance goals for ac-
ed to evaluate unilateral
on the ground provides
at may not have been as

Clients who demonstrate p
be progressed to using load
challenge to the musculatu
joints.

The loaded squat is high
at this point of physical rea
might be related to the und
can maintain optimal foot a
and ankle complex mobility
squat assessment, activatio
program. It is important to
used to confirm or rule out

Dynamic Mo

Dynamic movement assess
deficiencies exist while per
ing a gait assessment, obser
pronation. Like the OHSA

The phase of gait where
the foot is all the way behi
incidence of impairments
mobility is required. Impa
The most common gait ir
rotation. Like the transitio
are the same and can valid

Another, more advanc
depth jump may reveal n
the high eccentric deceler
for advanced clients with
that individuals who have
not need to perform the d
would certainly repeat du
ments lacking proper kin

Mobility Ass

If the client demonstrate
sessment, movement asse
be performed to better
Exercise Continuum. Lin
ROM) and limited exten
pacts throughout the ent

The Corrective Exerc
OHSA modification. If t
dysfunction at the foot
relevant mobility assessn
tive exercise program.

Corrective Strategy for the Foot and Ankle

The CES Assessment Flow will reveal movement compensation patterns that may warrant the implementation of corrective programming for the foot and ankle complex, with the most common one being overpronation. Once the static, movement, and mobility assessments have been performed and impairments have been identified, the corrective exercise strategy can be developed using NASM's Corrective Exercise Continuum. Prevention and rehabilitation programs have proved effective at decreasing the incidence of foot and ankle injuries in physically active individuals and improving ankle function (Hale et al., 2007). Most programs also incorporate proprioceptive or balance training with or without functional movements daily or multiple times per week.

Table 11-3, while not exhaustive, provides a list of common exercises and techniques when programming for this region. Specific exercise selection will depend on the client's individual results, needs, and abilities.

TABLE 11-3 Common Corrective Exercise Programming Selections for the Foot and Ankle

Phase	Modality	Muscle(s)/Exercise	Acute Training Variables
Inhibit	Self-myofascial rolling	Biceps femoris (short head) Fibularis complex (peroneals) Gastrocnemius Quadriceps Soleus TFL	Hold areas of discomfort for 30 to 60 seconds Perform four to six repetitions of active joint movement
Lengthen	Static stretching or neuromuscular stretching	Biceps femoris (short head) Gastrocnemius Quadriceps Soleus TFL	Static: 30-second hold Neuromuscular: 7- to 10-second isometric contraction, 30-second static hold
Activate	Isolated strengthening	Anterior tibialis Gluteus medius Medial hamstrings Posterior tibialis Short foot (intrinsic muscles)	10 to 15 reps with 4-second eccentric contraction, 2-second isometric contraction at end-range, and 1-second concentric contraction
Integrate*	Integrated dynamic movement	Lunge to balance progressions Single-leg balance reach Single-leg squat Step-up to balance	10 to 15 reps under control

*NOTE: Progress and regress as needed to match client ability, work capacity, and needs.

Common Exercise Selections for the Foot and Ankle

Exercises used for foot and ankle corrective strategies look to improve commonly observed movement impairments such as feet turn out, heel rise, and excessive pronation (aka overpronation). Oftentimes, multiple movement impairments occur together (such as excessive pronation and feet turn out) and may benefit from exercises that address both, based on the integrated assessment process. As such, the Corrective Exercise Specialist may create a program that efficiently addresses multiple impairments.

INHIBIT: SELF-MYOFASCIAL ROLLING

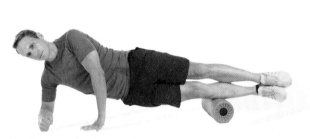

Fibularis complex (peroneals)

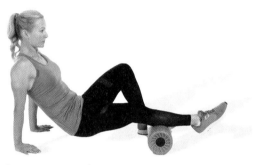

Gastrocnemius/soleus

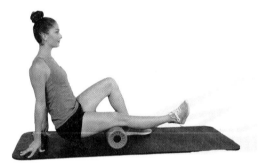

Biceps femoris

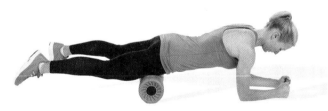

Quadriceps

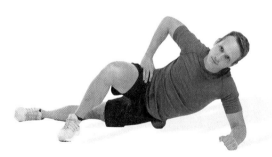

Tensor fascia latae

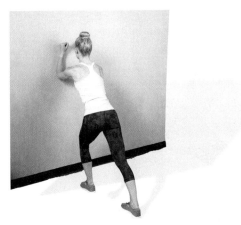

Static gastrocnemius stretch

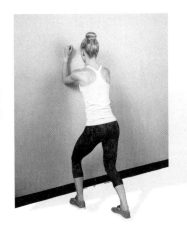

Static soleus stretch

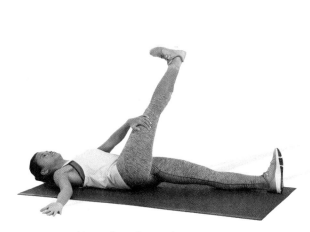

Static supine biceps femoris stretch

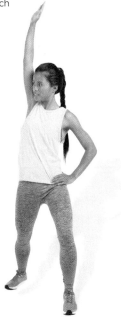

Static tensor fascia latae stretch

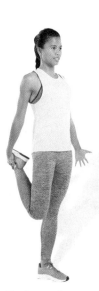

Static standing quadriceps stretch

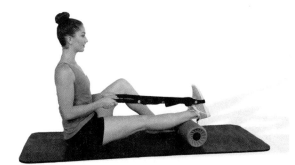

Self-NMS gastrocnemius/soleus

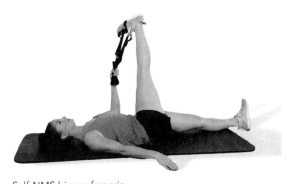

Self-NMS biceps femoris

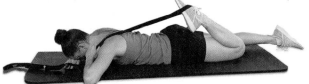

Self-NMS prone quadriceps

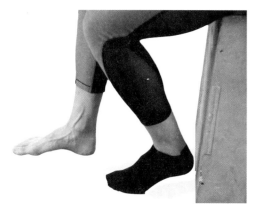

Short foot—start

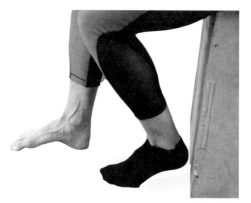

Short foot—finish

 TRAINING TIP

The short foot exercise is intended to activate and strengthen the intrinsic muscles of the foot by actively forming the longitudinal arch (Jung et al., 2011). Perform the short foot exercise by first placing the foot flat on the floor. Then, lift the arch of the foot while pulling the ball of the foot closer to the calcaneus. This movement should be performed with the toes relaxed. Exercise may be performed seated or standing in a partial-lunge/split-stance for increased difficulty.

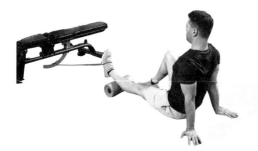

Anterior tibialis—start

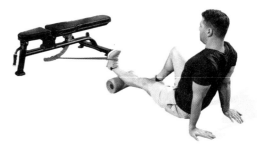

Anterior tibialis—finish

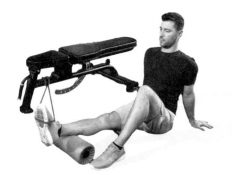

Posterior tibialis—start

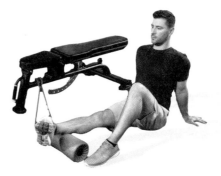

Posterior tibialis—finish

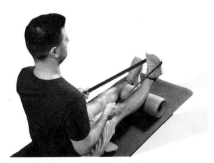

Medial gastrocnemius—start

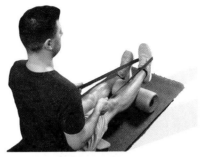

Medial gastrocnemius—finish

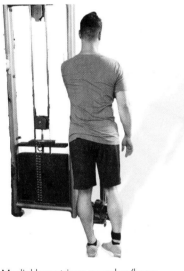

Medial hamstrings complex (knee flexion)—start

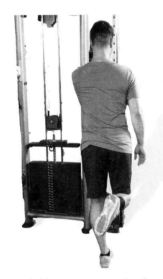

Medial hamstrings complex (knee flexion)—finish

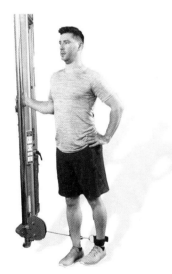

Gluteus medius—start

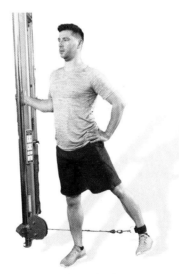

Gluteus medius—finish

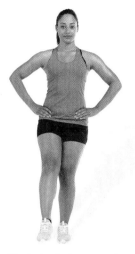

Single-leg balance reach—sagittal plane

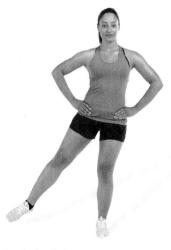

Single-leg balance reach—frontal plane

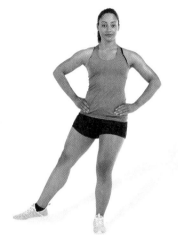

Single-leg balance reach—transverse plane

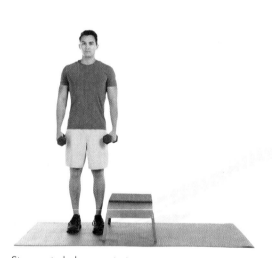

Step-up to balance—start

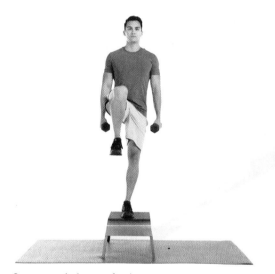

Step-up to balance—finish

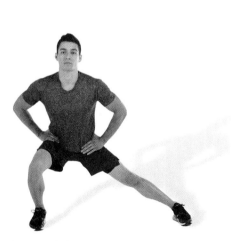

Lunge to balance—start

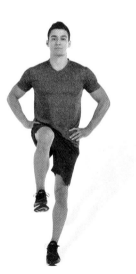

Lunge to balance—finish

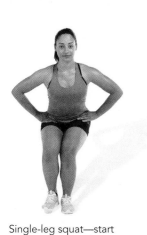

Single-leg squat—start

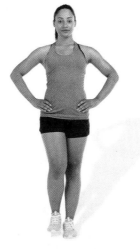

Single-leg squat—finish

Feet Turn Out

The Corrective Exercise Specialist should be selective regarding the techniques recommended to each client. To improve client adherence, it is recommended that the Corrective Exercise Specialist employ as few exercises as are effective in each phase of the continuum. The broad objectives of the program are to improve ideal dorsiflexion and improve the body's ability to control tibial rotation. When applied systematically, the Corrective Exercise Continuum contributes to efficient neuromuscular control and proper alignment of the foot and ankle complex during movement.

Recall that if the heels-elevated modification improved the squat, then only corrective strategies for the lower leg may be necessary.

PHASE 1: INHIBIT

Key regions to inhibit include the soleus, lateral gastrocnemius, biceps femoris, and possibly the TFL. Reducing tension in these tissues will facilitate extensibility, allowing appropriate levels of ideal dorsiflexion and tibial positioning to be achieved.

PHASE 2: LENGTHEN

Key lengthening exercises via static or neuromuscular stretches would include the soleus and gastrocnemius and biceps femoris. Reduction of tissue resistance to stretch allows these target areas to lengthen properly during movement, contributing to proper mechanics at the foot and ankle, tibia, and the rest of the lower extremity.

PHASE 3: ACTIVATE

Key activation exercises include the calf raise to target the medial gastrocnemius and knee flexion with tibial internal rotation to target the medial hamstrings. The objective of the selected activation exercises is to improve the intramuscular coordination of tissues considered underactive based on the integrated assessment process. Specific to the foot and ankle, these muscles will be responsible for concentrically creating greater tibial internal rotation and eccentrically decelerating tibial external rotation during movement patterns.

PHASE 4: INTEGRATE

An integration progression process could first include uniplanar exercises (sagittal plane) and then progress to multiplanar exercises (frontal and transverse). Exercises can begin as more transitional (moving with no change in the base of support such as a single-leg balance reach) to more dynamic exercises (movement with a change in the base of support such as a step-up to balance, to a lunge to balance, to a single-leg squat). The intermuscular coordination and movement pattern reeducation achieved by foot and ankle integration encourages neuromuscular control of the foot and ankle complex in multiple planes of motion. The foot and ankle should move with appropriate levels of dorsiflexion, plantar flexion, inversion, eversion, and control over tibial rotation. Focus should be placed on knee and foot and ankle alignment throughout dynamic exercises.

Table 11-4 is a sample program a client may use to improve the feet turn out movement impairment.

TABLE 11-4 Sample Corrective Exercise Program for the Foot and Ankle: Feet Turn Out

Phase	Modality	Muscle(s)/Exercise	Acute Training Variables
Inhibit	Myofascial rolling	Biceps femoris Gastrocnemius/soleus	Hold areas of discomfort for 30 to 60 seconds Perform four to six repetitions of active joint movement 90 to 120 seconds per muscle group
Lengthen	Static stretching	Biceps femoris (short head) Gastrocnemius	30-second hold
Activate	Isolated strengthening	Medial gastrocnemius Medial hamstrings	10 to 15 reps with 4-second eccentric contraction, 2-second isometric contraction at end-range, and 1-second concentric contraction
Integrate*	Integrated dynamic movement	Sagittal lunge to balance	10 to 15 reps under control

*NOTE: Progress and regress as needed to match client ability, work capacity, and needs.

Overpronation

The Corrective Exercise Specialist should be selective regarding the techniques recommended to each client. To improve client adherence, it is recommended that the Corrective Exercise Specialist employ as few exercises as are effective in each phase of the continuum. The broad objectives of the program are to improve ideal dorsiflexion and to improve the body's ability to decelerate excessive pronation (i.e., exhibit controlled pronation). Additionally, because knee valgus and overpronation often occur together, muscles that decelerate knee valgus (e.g., gluteus maximus and gluteus medius) should be considered for activation, based on the assessment process. When applied systematically, the Corrective Exercise Continuum contributes to efficient neuromuscular control and proper alignment of the foot and ankle complex during movement.

Recall that if the heels-elevated modification improved the squat, then only corrective strategies for the lower leg may be necessary.

PHASE 1: INHIBIT

Key regions to inhibit include the soleus and lateral gastrocnemius, fibularis complex (peroneals), and TFL. Reducing tension in these tissues will facilitate extensibility, allowing appropriate levels of ideal dorsiflexion and tibial positioning to be achieved.

Key lengthening exercises via static or neuromuscular stretches would include the soleus and gastrocnemius and TFL. Reduction of tissue resistance to stretch allows these target areas to lengthen properly during movement, contributing to proper mechanics at the foot and ankle, tibia, and the rest of the lower extremity.

PHASE 3: ACTIVATE

Key activation exercises include the short foot exercise and targeting the anterior tibialis, posterior tibialis, and gluteus medius. The objective of the selected activation exercises is to improve the intramuscular coordination of tissues considered underactive based on the integrated assessment process. Specific to the foot and ankle, these muscles will be responsible for concentrically creating greater dorsiflexion and eccentrically decelerating plantar flexion and knee valgus during movement patterns.

PHASE 4: INTEGRATE

An integration progression process could first include uniplanar exercises (sagittal plane) and then progress to multiplanar exercises (frontal and transverse). Exercises can begin as more transitional (moving with no change in the base of support such as a single-leg balance reach) to more dynamic exercises (movement with a change in the base of support such as a step-up to balance, to a lunge to balance, to a single-leg squat). The intermuscular coordination and movement pattern reeducation achieved by foot and ankle integration encourages neuromuscular control of the foot and ankle complex in multiple planes of motion. The foot and ankle should move with appropriate levels of dorsiflexion, plantar flexion, inversion, eversion, and control over tibial rotation. Focus should be placed on the proper alignment of the foot and ankle, knee, and hip throughout lower body exercise progressions.

Table 11-5 is a sample program a client may use to improve overpronation.

TABLE 11-5 Sample Corrective Exercise Program for the Foot and Ankle: Overpronation

Phase	Modality	Muscle(s)/Exercise	Acute Training Variables
Inhibit	Myofascial rolling	Fibularis complex (peroneals) Gastrocnemius/soleus TFL	Hold areas of discomfort for 30 to 60 seconds Perform four to six repetitions of active joint movement 90 to 120 seconds per muscle group
Lengthen	Static stretching	Gastrocnemius/soleus TFL	30-second hold
Activate	Isolated strengthening	Anterior tibialis Gluteus medius Short foot	10 to 15 reps with 4-second eccentric contraction, 2-second isometric contraction at end-range, and 1-second concentric contraction
Integrate*	Integrated dynamic movement	Step-up to balance	10 to 15 reps under control

*NOTE: Progress and regress as needed to match client ability, work capacity, and needs.

Heel Rise

The Corrective Exercise Specialist should be selective regarding the techniques recommended to each client. To improve client adherence, it is recommended that the Corrective Exercise Specialist employ as few exercises as are effective in each phase of the continuum. The broad objectives of the program are to improve ideal dorsiflexion and the extensibility of the quadriceps as deemed necessary during the assessment process. Heel rise may occur to create forward translation of the tibia in the absence of optimal knee extensor flexibility (i.e., knee flexion during descent is limited). The Corrective Exercise Specialist should rule out any issues around movement competency before assuming heel rise is based in muscle imbalance. That is, a client may simply not realize they should allow their hips to move back as their knees move forward. When applied systematically, the Corrective Exercise Continuum contributes to efficient neuromuscular control and proper alignment of the foot and ankle complex during movement.

PHASE 1: INHIBIT

Key regions to inhibit include the gastrocnemius/soleus complex and quadriceps. Reducing tension in these tissues will facilitate extensibility, allowing appropriate levels of ideal dorsiflexion and tibial positioning to be achieved.

PHASE 2: LENGTHEN

Key lengthening exercises via static or neuromuscular stretches would include the quadriceps and gastrocnemius/soleus complex (with focus on the soleus). Reduction of tissue resistance to stretch allows these target areas to lengthen properly during movement, contributing to proper mechanics at the foot and ankle, tibia, and rest of the lower extremity.

PHASE 3: ACTIVATE

Key activation exercises include the anterior tibialis. The objective of the selected activation exercises is to improve the intramuscular coordination of tissues considered underactive based on the integrated assessment process. Specific to the foot and ankle, these muscles will be responsible for concentrically creating greater dorsiflexion during movement patterns.

PHASE 4: INTEGRATE

An integration progression process could first include uniplanar exercises (sagittal plane) and then progress to multiplanar exercises (frontal and transverse). Exercises can begin as more transitional (moving with no change in the base of support such as a single-leg balance reach) to more dynamic exercises (movement with a change in the base of support such as a step-up to balance, to a lunge to balance, to a single-leg squat). The intermuscular coordination and movement pattern reeducation achieved by foot and ankle integration encourages neuromuscular control of the foot and ankle complex in multiple planes of motion. The foot and ankle should move with appropriate levels of dorsiflexion, plantar flexion, inversion, eversion, and control over tibial rotation.

Table 11-6 is a sample program a client may use to improve heel rise.

TABLE 11-6 Sample Corrective Exercise Program for the Foot and Ankle: Heel Rise

Phase	Modality	Muscle(s)/Exercise	Acute Training Variables
Inhibit	Myofascial rolling	Gastrocnemius/soleus Quadriceps	Hold areas of discomfort for 30 to 60 seconds Perform four to six repetitions of active joint movement 90 to 120 seconds per muscle group
Lengthen	Static stretching	Quadriceps Soleus	30-second hold
Activate	Isolated strengthening	Anterior tibialis	10 to 15 reps with 4-second eccentric contraction, 2-second isometric contraction at end-range, and 1-second concentric contraction
Integrate*	Integrated dynamic movement	Single-leg squat	10 to 15 reps under control

*NOTE: Progress and regress as needed to match client ability, work capacity, and needs.

Common Issues Associated with the Foot and Ankle

Due to the daily repetitive stress placed on the foot and ankle complex, these structures are uniquely susceptible to overuse and impact-related injury. The following are four of the most common foot and ankle injuries that may be encountered in a fitness and movement setting as well as how each can functionally influence the client's programming. This section is not intended to guide the Corrective Exercise Specialist to diagnose or rehabilitate any foot and/or ankle injury, but rather to understand their relationship to movement and the management required in a client presenting with each injury. A client who presents with any of the following or other pathology of the foot and ankle complex requires clearance and professional consultation with a qualified healthcare provider.

 CRITICAL

This section is intended to provide general information about specific medical conditions for the foot and ankle complex. The information provided should not be used to diagnose any medical condition. The fitness professional should refer to the appropriate medical professional if a client needs a diagnosis of a potential medical condition. This will ensure client safety and proper scope of practice.

Plantar Fasciitis

The plantar fascia is a thick, fibrous band of connective tissue that runs from the calcaneus toward the base of each digit. As the plantar fascia travels across the bottom of the foot, it fans out into three bands of tissue designed to provide dynamic support to the medial longitudinal arch of the foot (Hedrick, 1996). With each step a person takes, the plantar fascia lengthens and recoils to transfer the potential energy from ground reaction forces. In the case where a client lacks sufficient elasticity or stretch within the plantar fascia, the tissue can start to micro-tear during dynamic movement. These micro-tears are associated with pain and inflammation, leading to the classic presentation of plantar fasciitis.

An inflamed and irritated plantar fascia can be very painful (**Figure 11-17**). Plantar fasciitis presents as pain for the first step in the morning or after a period of rest (poststatic dyskinesia) or as pain in the plantar heel after periods of prolonged standing or ambulation (Irving et al., 2006). Risk factors for plantar fasciitis include limited mobility in the plantar fascia and Achilles tendon (Hedrick, 1996), excessive impact forces (overuse), an everted foot type (Patel & DiGiovanni, 2011), increased body mass index in a nonathletic population, and insufficient ankle mobility. Decreased plantar flexor and Achilles tendon length limit optimal ankle joint motion, resulting in excessive pronation compensations. Excessive pronation may increase the risk of plantar fasciitis because the plantar fascia has been exposed to excessive traction forces through the excessive and repeated stretching of the tissue during gait (Bolgla & Malone, 2004). Therefore, individuals who demonstrate feet turn out (foot abduction), excessive pronation, or excessive forward trunk lean in the OHSA may be at increased risk of plantar fasciitis.

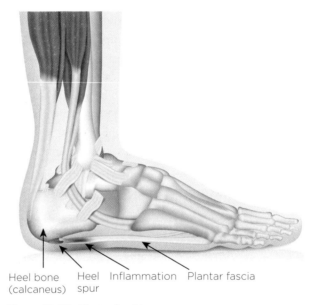

Heel bone   Heel   Inflammation   Plantar fascia
(calcaneus)   spur

Figure 11-17   Plantar fasciitis
© Medicalstocks/Shutterstock

In a client with active plantar fasciitis, it is important to avoid any impact-related activities and/or exercises that place excessive stress to the plantar foot and ankle mobility. The Corrective Exercise Specialist should instead focus on increasing foot and ankle mobility through myofascial release of the plantar foot and posterior muscle group (soleus and gastrocnemius).

Achilles Tendinopathy

Formed by the soleus and gastrocnemius tendon fibers, the Achilles tendon is the largest and strongest tendon in the human body. Running along the posterior lower leg toward the calcaneus, the Achilles tendon rotates on itself toward its insertion. This tendon rotation reduces friction between individual muscle fibers, allowing for increased energy transfer (Pekala et al., 2017). This powerful tendon provides most of the elastic recoil and energy return during dynamic movement.

Achilles **tendinopathy**, formerly known as Achilles tendinitis, is a common overuse injury that should be considered along a continuum. Reactive tendinopathy, tendon disrepair, and degenerative tendinopathy allow for a more accurate appreciation for the progressive nature of many tendon injuries (Cook & Purdam, 2009). One of the greatest risk factors for Achilles tendinopathy is limited ankle mobility or a tight Achilles tendon. Therefore, individuals who demonstrate feet turn out (foot abduction), excessive pronation, or excessive forward trunk lean in the OHSA may be at increased risk of Achilles tendinopathy.

Achilles tendinopathy presents as pain either at the Achilles tendon insertion onto the calcaneus or as pain along the middle of the tendon (**Figure 11-18**). Achilles tendon pain that is more insertional (on the calcaneus) is associated with uncontrolled absorption of impact forces, whereas the mid-tendon pain is associated with insufficient elasticity during dynamic movement and a subsequent micro-tearing (Chimenti et al., 2017; Cook & Purdam, 2009).

Tendinopathy

A broad term encompassing pain, swelling, and impaired performance occurring in and around tendons in response to overuse; commonly associated with the Achilles tendon.

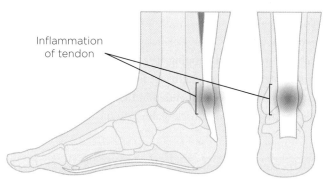

Figure 11-18 Achilles tendinopathy
© Aksanaku/Shutterstock

Similar to the client with plantar fasciitis, the Corrective Exercise Specialist should avoid any impact-related activities and/or exercises that place excessive stress on the Achilles tendon and ankle mobility (Irving et al., 2006). The focus is on increasing foot and ankle mobility through myofascial release of the plantar foot and posterior muscle group (soleus and gastrocnemius). Eccentric training is also one of the most effective ways to reduce the symptoms and stress to the Achilles tendon. Research has shown that high-volume eccentrics, such as a negative heel raise, are gold-standard exercises for the prevention and management of Achilles tendinopathy (O'Neill et al., 2015).

Medial Tibial Stress Syndrome

Medial tibial stress syndrome (MTSS) (**Figure 11-19**), also known as shin splints (Moen et al., 2009), is an overuse injury thought to be associated with the improper loading of impact forces and a more rigid foot type (Hubbard et al., 2009). Impact forces, which are perceived by the body as vibrations, are absorbed or dampened through a stiffening response within the myofascial system. This stiffening response of the lower leg muscles is a necessary component to proper absorption of impact forces because it creates a splinting effect in the surrounding lower

Medial tibial stress syndrome (MTSS)

Pain in the front of the tibia caused by an overload to the tibia and the associated musculature.

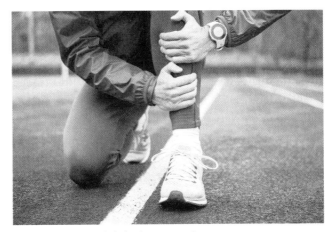

Figure 11-19 Medial tibial stress syndrome
© Luckyraccoon/Shutterstock

leg muscles. This splinting effect protects the bones from excessive vibrations and also prevents bending of the tibia on foot strike.

Individuals with MTSS complain of pain and tenderness along the lower third of the medial tibia, especially during dynamic movement such as running and jumping (Sommer & Vallentyne, 1995). Neglected MTSS can increase the risk of tibial stress fractures due to the persistent stress to the tibia. Risk factors for MTSS include improper footwear, overpronation, rigid foot type (supinated), gluteal weakness, and delayed stabilization on impact.

For the client experiencing MTSS, the Corrective Exercise Specialist should avoid impact-related activities such as running and jumping. The focus is on ensuring proper foot mobilization, building increased intrinsic foot strength and foot-to-core integration, which can enhance gluteal strength. Orthotics may be recommended in the client with an overpronated foot type, as this can help optimize the timing of muscle stabilization.

 CHECK IT OUT

Bone Adaptation and Stress Fractures
Stress fracture is the clinical term used to denote bone failure in fatigue. Stress fractures do not occur from a single traumatic event; rather, they are the product of repetitive submaximal loading (Hughes et al., 2017).

This stress to the bone can be considered mechanical stimuli that trigger bone formation and a repair process. Bone deposition through osteoblastic activity can occur on all surfaces of bone but is most common along the diaphysis of long bones. Deposition on the periosteal surface provides the greatest mechanical advantage (Hughes et al., 2017).

When the fatigue of an untrained and trained limb was assessed, the untrained limb fractured after an average of 15,000 cycles compared to the trained limb, which failed after an average of 1.5 million cycles. This 100-fold increase in fatigue resistance after a 5-week loading regimen demonstrates the potential importance of adaptive bone formation with progressive physical training (Hughes et al., 2017).

Ankle sprain

An injury to the ankle ligaments in which small tears occur in the ligaments.

Ankle Sprains and Chronic Ankle Instability

Ankle sprains are among the most commonly reported sports-related injuries (Herzog et al., 2019), accounting for over 50% of basketball injuries (Fong et al., 2007). Although ankle sprains can occur to both the medial and lateral aspect of the ankle joint, due to the increased inversion moment of the ankle, 73% of ankle sprains occur to the lateral aspect of the joint (Raghava

Patel, A., & DiGiovanni, B. (2011, Jan.). Association between plantar fasciitis and isolated contracture of the gastrocnemius. *Foot & Ankle International, 32*(1), 5–8.

Pekala, P. A., Henry, B. M., Ochała, A., Kopacz, P., Tatoń, G., Młyniec, A., Walocha, J. A., & Tomaszewski, K. A. (2017). The twisted structure of the Achilles tendon unraveled: A detailed quantitative and qualitative anatomical investigation. *Scandinavian Journal of Medicine & Science in Sports, 27*(12), 1705–1715. https://doi.org/10.1111/sms.12835

Raghava Neelapala, Y. V., Bhat, V. S., Almeida, S. & Molly, K. (2016). Relationship between gluteal muscle strength and balance in individuals with chronic ankle instability. *Physiotherapy Practice and Research, 38*(1), 1–5. https://doi.org/10.3233/PPR-160083

Rath, M. E., Stearne, D. J., Walker, C. R., & Cox, J. C. (2016). Effect of foot type on knee valgus, ground reaction force, and hip muscle activation in female soccer players. *Journal of Sports Medicine and Physical Fitness, 56*(5), 546–553.

Riskowski, J. L., Dufour, A. B., Hagedorn, T. J., Hillstrom, H. J., Casey, V. A., & Hannan, M. T. (2013). Associations of foot posture and function to lower extremity pain: Results from a population-based foot study. *Arthritis Care & Research, 65*(11), 1804–1812. https://doi.org/10.1002/acr.22049

Sommer, H. M., & Vallentyne, S. W. (1995). Effect of foot posture on the incidence of medial tibial stress syndrome. *Medicine & Science in Sports & Exercise, 27*(6), 800–804.

Tropp, H., Askling, C., & Gillquist, J. (1985). Prevention of ankle sprains. *American Journal of Sports Medicine, 13,* 259–262.

Tsai, L. C., Ko, Y. A., Hammond, K. E., Xerogeanes, J. W., Warren, G. L., & Powers, C. M. (2017). Increasing hip and knee flexion during a drop-jump task reduces tibiofemoral shear and compressive forces: Implications for ACL injury prevention training. *Journal of Sports Sciences, 35*(24), 2405–2411. https://doi.org/10.1080/02640414.2016.1271138

Zahran, S. S., Aly, S. M., & Zaky, L. A. (2017). Effects of bilateral flexible flatfoot on trunk and hip muscles' torque. *International Journal of Therapy and Rehabilitation, 24*(1), 7–14. https://doi.org/10.12968/ijtr.2017.24.1.7

CHAPTER 12

Corrective Strategies for the Knee

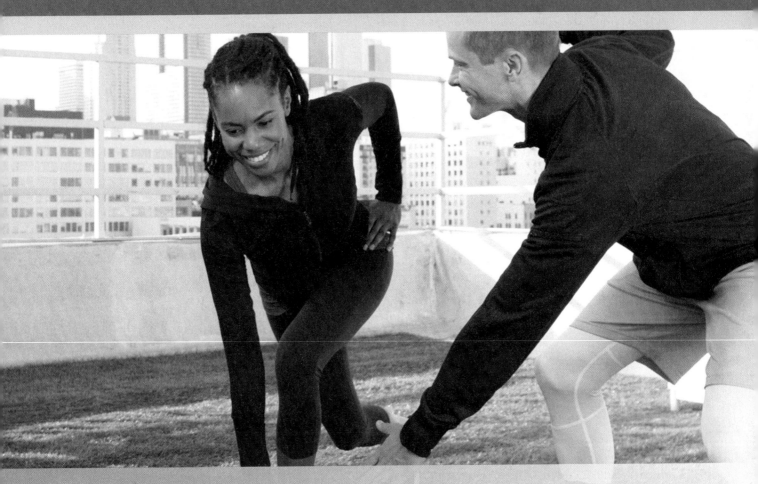

Learning Objectives

After reading this content, students should be able to demonstrate the following objectives:

- **Explain** basic functional anatomy of the knee.
- **Identify** the mechanisms for common knee injuries.
- **Describe** the influence of altered knee movement on the kinetic chain.
- **Determine** appropriate systematic assessment strategies for the knee.
- **Select** appropriate corrective exercise strategies for the knee.

Introduction

Injuries involving the lower extremity account for more than 66% of all injuries (Hootman et al., 2002). The knee is one of the most commonly injured regions of the body. Located between the foot and ankle complex below, and the hip complex above, the knee is susceptible to injuries resulting from lower kinetic chain impairments. One of the most severe injuries related to the knee is a rupture of the anterior cruciate ligament (ACL). Over 70% of ACL ruptures occur during single-foot contact in physical activity secondary to uncontrolled lower extremity biomechanics (Carlson et al., 2016). Other common injuries that can result from kinetic chain impairments include **patellar tendinopathy**, **patellofemoral pain syndrome**, and **iliotibial (IT) band syndrome**. To reduce the potential risk of these injuries from occurring, and to allow for individuals to maintain healthy and physically active lifestyles, it is important to understand the anatomy and most appropriate corrective exercise strategies for the knee as it relates to the Regional Interdependence (RI) model.

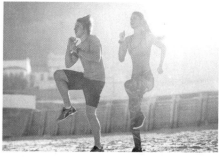
© Daxiao Productions/Shutterstock

Review of Knee Functional Anatomy

The knee is a part of a kinetic chain that is greatly affected by the linked segments from the proximal and distal joints. The foot and ankle and the lumbo-pelvic-hip complex (LPHC) play a major role in knee impairment because the structures that help to form the ankle and hip joints also make up the knee joint. This region is a prime example of how alterations in other joints within the human movement system (HMS) can dramatically affect the movement and increase the stress and injury capacity of another joint. Because this is to be a review of knee anatomy, not all anatomical structures will be covered in detail. This section will provide a general review of the most pertinent structures.

Bones and Joints

The knee joint is a synovial joint composed of two articulations: the tibiofemoral joint and the patellofemoral joint. The tibia and femur make up the tibiofemoral joint, and the patella and femur make up the patellofemoral joint (**Figure 12-1**) (Moore et al., 2014). The fibula is also noted because it is the attachment site of the biceps femoris, which crosses and affects the knee. Although the knee is primarily intended to flex and extend, it is capable of additional motion due to its architecture to allow reaction in frontal and transverse planes (Floyd, 2017; Komdeur et al., 2002). This includes internal and external rotation; valgus and varus; and rolling, sliding, and spinning. However, when improperly stabilized these motions become more prominent and can lead to injury. Corrective exercise methodologies look to minimize and control unwanted motions at the knee through neuromuscular control and stabilization of the joint (**Figure 12-2**).

The tibiofemoral joint is one of the most complex joints of the body (Kazemi et al., 2013). The **screw-home mechanism** is a primary example of this complexity. In an open-chain position, as the knee extends during the last 30 degrees, the tibia will externally rotate on the femur to lock the knee into extension, making the ligaments taut (Floyd, 2017). In a closed-chain position, such as in a squat, the femur will internally rotate on the tibia (Kim et al., 2015), given that the foot is fixated on the ground. Dysfunctions or compensations in the areas above and below the knee joint could alter the biomechanical forces at play in the screw-home mechanism.

Patellar tendinopathy

Often associated with jumper's knee; commonly an overuse injury affecting the patellar tendon, resulting in anterior knee pain.

Patellofemoral pain syndrome

A musculoskeletal condition in which a client experiences pain behind and around the patella with running, squatting, jumping, or other physical activity.

Iliotibial (IT) band syndrome

Often associated with runner's knee; usually an overuse injury where the iliotibial band rubs on the femur, resulting in lateral knee pain.

Screw-home mechanism

External tibial rotation on the femur in open-chain exercises and femoral internal rotation in closed-chain exercises, resulting in the knee "locking-out."

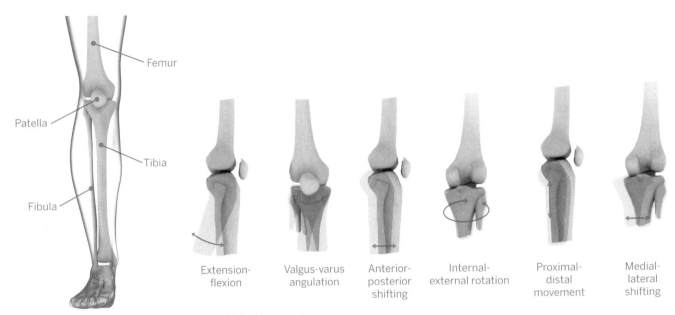

Figure 12-1 Bones of the knee

Femur
Patella
Tibia
Fibula

Figure 12-2 Knee motions

Extension-flexion | Valgus-varus angulation | Anterior-posterior shifting | Internal-external rotation | Proximal-distal movement | Medial-lateral shifting

The patellofemoral articulation is formed by the patella and the femur (Moore et al., 2014). This articulation, along with the quadriceps muscle group, is often referred to as the **extensor mechanism** because motion at this joint aids in knee extension. As the quadricep muscles join superiorly, they pass over the patella, forming the patellar tendon (Kenney et al., 2019). This region is highly susceptible to overuse injuries. As individuals squat, jump, land, run, and walk, the quadricep muscles eccentrically contract, increasing the amount pressure and pull on the patellofemoral articulation (Flandry & Hommel, 2011).

Proximally, the femur and the pelvis make up the iliofemoral joint and the sacrum and pelvis make up the sacroiliac joint (**Figure 12-3**) (Moore et al., 2014). Collectively, these structures anchor the proximal myofascial tissues. These bones and joints are of importance in corrective exercise because they will also have a functional effect on the knee. Distally, the tibia and fibula help form the talocrural (ankle) joint (**Figure 12-4**) (Moore et al., 2014). Collectively, these structures anchor the

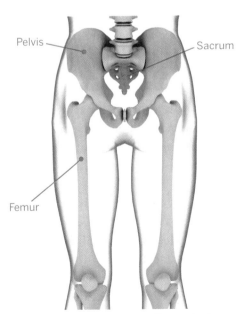

Pelvis
Sacrum
Femur

Figure 12-3 Proximal bones affecting the knee

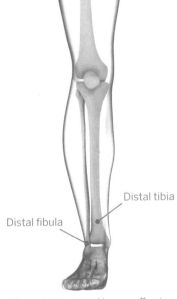

Distal tibia
Distal fibula

Figure 12-4 Distal bones affecting the knee

distal myofascial tissues of the knee. These bones and joints are of importance in corrective exercise because they also have a functional effect on the arthrokinematics of the knee.

Muscles

Several muscles in the LPHC and lower leg have functions that may be related to the knee (**Table 12-1**) (Floyd, 2017; Moore et al., 2014). For example, weakness of the hip external rotators and gluteus medius and maximus could cause overactivation of the tensor fascia latae (TFL), adductor complex, vastus lateralis, and gastrocnemius muscles. As frontal plane stability decreases because of weakness in the LPHC, the TFL and adductors become synergistically dominant, ultimately resulting in the femur internally rotating and the tibia externally rotating, creating a knee valgus compensation. Secondary to this knee valgus compensation, the vastus lateralis, given its lateral orientation and attachment to the patella, will cause the patella to track laterally and delay the activation of the vastus medialis obliquus (VMO) and, as a result, become overactive (Cowan et al., 2002). Finally, the gastrocnemius, due to tibial external rotation, also may become overactive. It is important to restore muscle balance and maintain normal range of motion (ROM) and strength to ensure that joints are operating optimally.

TABLE 12-1   Key Muscles Associated with the Knee

- Adductor complex
- Gastrocnemius/soleus
- Gluteus maximus and medius
- Medial and lateral hamstrings complexes
- Quadriceps
- Tensor fascia latae (TFL)/IT-band

Altered Knee Movement

The knee is the most commonly injured joint by adolescent athletes. An epidemiological report of nearly 10 years of knee injuries in the United States presented to emergency departments revealed that those 15 to 24 years of age had the highest injury rate. Knee injuries were reported to account for 60% of high school sports–related surgeries, and female athletes were reported to be four to six times more likely to sustain a major knee injury. The most common diagnoses were strains and sprains (42.1%), with individuals 65 years and older sustaining a higher proportion of injury due to stairs, ramps, landings, and floors (42.0%), compared to all other age groups (Gage et al., 2012).

The multidirectional forces imposed on the knee joint during physical activity explain the types of severe knee injuries, including ruptures of the ACL. Those same forces also contribute to clients who may complain of patellofemoral joint pain (PFP). Therefore, not surprisingly, two of the more common diagnoses resulting from physical activity (especially in sports) are PFP and ACL sprains or tears. Most knee injuries occur during noncontact deceleration in the frontal and transverse planes. It has also been shown that static malalignments, abnormal muscle activation patterns, and dynamic malalignments alter neuromuscular control and can lead to PFP, ACL injury, and IT-band tendinitis (Brown et al., 2014; Gage et al., 2012; Weiss & Whatman, 2015).

GETTING TECHNICAL

The hamstrings complex plays a critical role in lower extremity biomechanics. At the LPHC and the knee, the hamstrings provide essential concentric, eccentric, and isometric actions. **Table 12-2** provides an overview of the complexity of this double-joint muscle group.

TABLE 12-2 Intricacy of the Hamstrings Complex

Muscle Action	Knee	Hip	LPHC
Concentric	Flexion ■ Biceps femoris (short and long head) ■ Semimembranosus ■ Semitendinosus Tibial internal rotation ■ Semimembranosus ■ Semitendinosus Tibial external rotation ■ Biceps femoris (short and long head)	Extension ■ Biceps femoris (long head) ■ Semimembranosus ■ Semitendinosus	
Eccentric	Decelerates extension ■ Biceps femoris (short and long head) ■ Semimembranosus ■ Semitendinosus Decelerates tibial internal rotation ■ Biceps femoris (short and long head) Decelerates tibial external rotation ■ Semimembranosus ■ Semitendinosus	Decelerates flexion ■ Biceps femoris (long head)	
Isometric	Stabilizes the knee ■ Biceps femoris (short and long head) ■ Semimembranosus ■ Semitendinosus		Stabilizes the LPHC ■ Biceps femoris (long head) ■ Semimembranosus ■ Semitendinosus

Static Malalignments

Static malalignments can lead to increased PFP and knee injury. Common static malalignments include pes planus distortion syndrome, increased Q-angle (in one anatomical study Huberti and Hayes [1984] found a 10-degree shift in Q-angle increased patellofemoral contact forces by 45%) (**Figure 12-5**); excessive anterior pelvic tilt; and decreased flexibility of the quadriceps, hamstrings complex, and iliotibial band (Sahrmann, 2001; Thomée et al., 1995).

Abnormal Muscle Activation Patterns

Abnormal muscle activation patterns can lead to PFP, ACL injury, and other knee injuries. Abnormal contraction intensity and onset timing of the VMO and vastus lateralis have been demonstrated in subjects with PFP. Research by Ireland et al. (2003) demonstrated 26% less hip abduction strength and 36% less hip external rotator strength in subjects with PFP, leading to increased femoral adduction and internal rotation. Almeida et al. (2016) and Santos et al. (2015) also found decreased hip abduction strength in subjects with PFP. Mucha et al. (2017) determined that long-distance runners with IT-band syndrome had reduced hip abduction strength on the affected leg and observed that their symptoms were alleviated with a successful return to running after undergoing a hip abductor strengthening program. Baker et al. (2018) found that hip abductor weakness influenced greater knee valgus (femoral adduction or internal rotation and tibial external rotation) during the stance phase of running. Research has demonstrated that individuals with decreased hip external rotation strength have increased vertical ground reaction forces during landing, which is a potential predictor of PFP and ACL injury (Dierks et al., 2008). Research has also demonstrated increased adductor activity and decreased dorsiflexion in subjects demonstrating increased dynamic knee valgus and decreased neuromuscular control of core musculature (Heinert et al., 2008; Page et al., 2010).

Dynamic Malalignment

Dynamic malalignments may occur during movement as a result of poor neuromuscular control and dynamic stability of the trunk and lower extremities. Static malalignments (altered length-tension relationships and altered joint mobility) and abnormal muscle activation patterns (altered force-couple relationships) of the LPHC compromise dynamic stability of the lower extremity and result in dynamic malalignments in the lower extremity. This dynamic malalignment (multisegmental HMS impairment) has consistently been described as a combination of contralateral pelvic drop, femoral adduction and internal rotation, tibial external rotation, and excessive foot and ankle pronation. Some researchers have documented that an increase in knee valgus angle may increase biomechanical loads on the ACL (Ishida et al., 2014; Shin et al., 2011; Teng et al., 2017). This multisegmental dynamic malalignment (movement impairment syndrome) has been shown to alter force production, proprioception, coordination, and landing mechanics. Deficits in neuromuscular control of the LPHC may lead to uncontrolled trunk displacement during functional movements, which, in turn, may place the lower extremity in a valgus position, increase knee abduction motion and torque (femoral adduction or internal rotation and tibial external rotation occurring during knee flexion), and result in increased patellofemoral contact pressure, knee ligament strain, and ACL injury (Levine et al., 2012; Page et al., 2010).

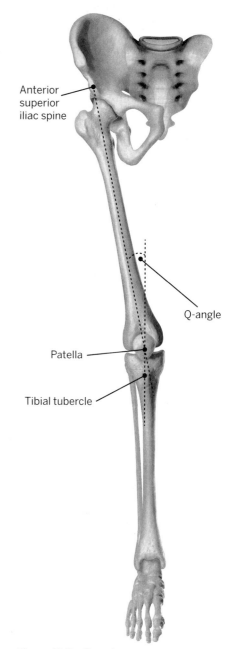

Anterior superior iliac spine

Q-angle

Patella

Tibial tubercle

Figure 12-5   Q-angle

Knee Dysfunction and the Regional Interdependence Model

The knee, as discussed previously, is greatly affected by other regions of the body, both superiorly and inferiorly. The foot and ankle complex requires a great deal of mobility and stability due to its anatomical makeup. Superiorly, the hip joint, a ball-and-socket joint, requires a great amount of mobility and stability (Sueki et al., 2013). The hinged knee joint, located in the middle of two highly mobile joints, requires relatively less multiplanar mobility and stability (Floyd, 2017). As such, restriction in motion, altered joint kinematics, and/or a limitation in stability/strength associated with either the foot and ankle complex or the LPHC can result in musculoskeletal pain at the knee. For example, PFP syndrome has been associated with muscular weakness in the LPHC, specifically the hip abductors and lateral rotators (Sueki et al., 2013). Similarly, regional interdependence research related to foot, ankle, and knee function has highlighted the importance of foot and ankle posture and stability in correlation to PFP syndrome (Molgaard et al., 2011; Nunes et al., 2019). During movement assessments, as the foot overpronates, the foot externally rotates and/or everts during movement, and tibial external rotation, femoral adduction, and hip internal rotation increase (Buldt et al., 2013). This compensatory movement will result in a knee valgus position, leading to limited neuromuscular control in the hip complex. Conversely, if the foot oversupinates, this may lead to a tightness of the lateral gastrocnemius/soleus complex, creating tibial external rotation caused by tightness of the biceps femoris, weakness of the adductor musculature, and tightness of the piriformis (Buldt et al., 2013). This will create a knee varus compensatory movement and has the potential to influence the mobility and stability at the hip. In either scenario, knee valgus or knee varus, altered chain reactions potentially influence pain and discomfort at the knee as well as other regional segments above and below. Specific corrective exercise programs addressing soft tissue restriction and neuromuscular stability and strength in the foot, ankle, and hip complexes may encourage proper knee alignment and reduce the risk of injury.

TRAINING TIP

Although the knee is directly affected by the joints above and below it, the Corrective Exercise Specialist should also be cognizant of knee positioning during athletic and performance movements. Special attention should be given to knee kinematics during exercise and functional activities such as cutting, jumping, and landing. This is especially true for single-leg activities. For example, if a client is performing a box step-up to balance exercise, verbal instruction should include, "Keep your knee in line with your second and third toe as you straighten the knee and hip." For single-leg squat exercises, the knee should remain in line with the midfoot throughout the entire exercise. Failure to maintain proper mechanics could have a direct effect on foot, ankle, and hip motion and strength.

Assessment Results for the Knee

Limiting the risk of lower extremity injuries begins with an integrated assessment process followed by targeted corrective exercise strategies. Compensatory static and dynamic posture of the knee is highly influenced by the mobility of both the hip and the foot and ankle complex. For that reason, information obtained from all three steps in the assessment process needs to be considered to identify potential impairments at the knee and properly address their root causes. Common findings indicating potential dysfunction at the knee are summarized in **Table 12-3**.

TABLE 12-3 Knee Assessment Results	
Assessment	**Results**
Static posture	Knee hyperextension Knee valgus Knee varus
Transitional and loaded movement	Knee dominance Knee valgus Knee varus
Dynamic movement	Knee dominance Knee valgus Knee varus
Mobility Modified Thomas test, active knee flexion test, active knee extension test, hip abduction and external rotation, weight-bearing lunge test, passive hip internal rotation, seated hip internal and external rotation	Limited ankle dorsiflexion ROM Limited hip abduction ROM Limited hip adduction ROM Limited hip extension ROM Limited hip external rotation ROM Limited hip internal rotation ROM Limited knee extension ROM Limited knee flexion ROM

Static Posture

During static postural assessment, Corrective Exercise Specialists will compare their client's posture to the postural archetypes described by Janda's postural distortion syndromes, Kendall's spinal postures, and pes planus distortion syndrome. Although the knee is the main focus of this chapter's corrective programming, fitness professionals should look at the kinetic chain check points above (e.g., LPHC) and below (e.g., foot and ankle) to determine their influence on the knee.

Typically, clients who exhibit an anterior pelvic tilt, as seen in Janda's lower crossed syndrome and most of Kendall's postures, will see some form of muscle imbalance affecting the lower extremity as well. Additionally, dysfunction at the ankle, as seen in pes planus distortion syndrome, can cause static postural malalignments at the knee. Pes planus distortion syndrome is characterized as possessing flat feet with knee valgus (**Figure 12-6**). This position of the knee can place excessive stress on the muscles and connective tissue associated with the knee joint during dynamic movement.

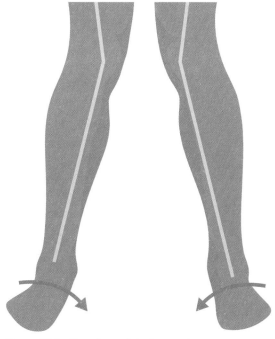

Figure 12-6 Pes planus distortion syndrome

Transitional Movement Assessments

Based on the collective information obtained from the static postural assessment, the fitness professional will have a high-level estimation of which muscles might be overactive/shortened and which ones are underactive/lengthened. As with static posture, the RI model highlights that an observed movement impairment at the knee could very well be due to muscle imbalances at the LPHC or the foot and ankle. Clients who have relatively impairment-free static posture may display muscle imbalances when in motion.

OVERHEAD SQUAT ASSESSMENT

When performing the overhead squat assessment (OHSA), the key movement impairments at the knee include knee valgus (**Figure 12-7**), knee varus (**Figure 12-8**), and knee dominance (**Figure 12-9**). However, both knee varus and knee dominance are relatively rare. Due to common activities of daily living in the greater population—specifically, wearing dress shoes and spending long hours in seated positions—knee valgus will be the typical movement impairment seen at the knee.

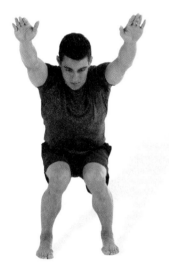

Figure 12-7   Knee valgus

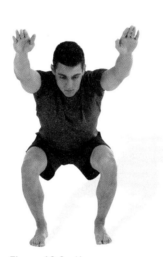

Figure 12-8   Knee varus

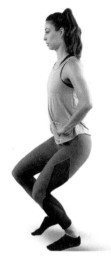

Figure 12-9   Knee dominance

Since many of the muscles that interact directly with the knees also attach near the hips and ankles, imbalances at either of those kinetic chain checkpoints may be the probable cause for a client's knees to be tracking incorrectly in the frontal plane. Knee valgus and knee varus are rarely true "knee issues," because the knee is primarily intended to operate in the sagittal plane (with small transverse plane arthrokinematics related to the screw-home mechanism).

Sometimes, knees falling inward is a secondary movement compensation caused by the feet turning out in response to the underlying foot and ankle impairment of excessive pronation. Other times, overactive/shortened adductor and femoral internal rotator muscles (all muscles that primarily interact between the femur and the hip and are also typically overactive/shortened in people with an anterior pelvic tilt) cause the knee to collapse inward as a consequence of the femur internally rotating too much. Conversely, when femoral external rotators and hip abductors are overactive/shortened, the knees will be pulled outward into the varus position during the OHSA.

The knee dominance movement impairment is observed at the knee and hip. In this situation, a client will squat with a far more upright posture above the hip (i.e., the opposite of an excessive forward lean) and increased anterior translation of the knee (i.e., the knee juts forward). Overactivity and shortening of the adductor magnus and piriformis (if derived more from the LPHC) creates a more upright posture at the hip. The combined overactivity/shortening of the soleus and quadriceps may contribute to excessive knee flexion and a possible heel rise as the body attempts to move the tibia forward during the descent of a squat pattern. Clients and athletes with underactive/lengthened gluteal muscles may also develop overactive quadriceps in an attempt to compensate for a loss of triple extension force production (Mills et al., 2015). These factors combined with underactivity of the core stabilizers contribute to the appearance of knee dominance.

HEELS-ELEVATED MODIFICATION

As noted earlier, the knee is often at the mercy of the joints above and below because it falls between the hips and the ankle. Many compensations observed at the knee may be due to reduced plantar flexor and Achilles tendon length. The heels-elevated modification can be used to pinpoint the source of the impairment to either the foot and ankle or the hip.

If elevated heels improve the alignment of the knee during the OHSA, then the root cause of the impairment is likely due to the lack of ankle dorsiflexion. However, if elevating the heels does not improve the squat, then musculature at the hips may be involved in the impairments, such as overactive adductors and underactive gluteals.

SINGLE-LEG SQUAT

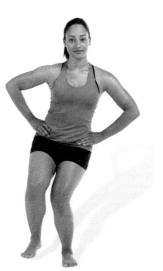

The single-leg squat assessment (SLSA) is also an important transitional assessment to perform to assess potential movement impairments at the knee joint. For individuals who can perform the SLSA, it might provide a deeper look into the functioning of the knee, especially for conditioned clients or athletes who know how to "fake" optimal form for the OHSA. Having to squat on one leg may show dysfunction not evident when squatting on two feet. The key compensation to observe when performing the SLSA is knee valgus (**Figure 12-10**); however, knee varus or knee dominance is seen in some individuals with overactive femoral external rotators.

Figure 12-10 Single-leg squat: knee valgus

SPLIT-SQUAT MODIFICATION

The split-squat modification can be used with individuals who have trouble performing the SLSA. Additionally, assessing a split stance squat can be beneficial to predict knee dysfunction that may translate over to dynamic movements like walking and running. Just like with the SLSA, the key impairment at the knee to look for is valgus; however, varus or knee dominance may be seen in some individuals.

LOADED MOVEMENT ASSESSMENT

Clients who demonstrate proper static and dynamic posture under body weight alone can be progressed to using loaded variants of primary movement patterns. This provides more challenge to the musculature and can help draw attention to any remaining imbalance at the joints.

The loaded squat is highly beneficial for observing knee movement in individuals at this point of physical readiness. Movement impairments that surface during a loaded squat might be related to the underactivity of key LPHC or foot and ankle muscles. For example, if a client can maintain optimal knee tracking during the OHSA and SLSA, but then demonstrates knee valgus during a loaded squat assessment, hip abductor musculature activation (e.g., gluteus medius) can be prioritized in the client's program. It is important to remember, however, that targeted mobility assessment should be used to confirm or deny observations made during transitional assessments.

Dynamic Movement Assessments

When performing the depth jump assessment with more-advanced clients, observe them from the anterior view to identify knee position on ground strike and throughout the eccentric phase of landing. Most impairments will be observed during deceleration. The most common depth jump compensation is knee valgus (Pollard et al., 2017); however, knee varus or knee dominance will be seen in some.

If performing this assessment, the Corrective Exercise Specialist has identified that the client already has adequate transitional movement (i.e., they have relatively compensation-free movement during the OHSA), and thus few to no short/overactive muscles. Many times compensations seen during the depth jump may reflect underactivity in the muscles, such as the gluteus maximus, gluteus medius, and core stabilizers. This supports the notion that most impairments will be seen on the landing, when muscles have to eccentrically decelerate the body.

If an individual is not ready to perform the depth jump assessment, but still has goals related to dynamic activities (e.g., obstacle course race), a basic gait analysis can also be performed to see their movement profile during a real-life activity. When observing gait for knee impairments, look at the client from the anterior viewpoint to see if their knee tracks medially (valgus) or laterally (varus) in the frontal plane.

Mobility Assessments

If the client demonstrates impairments related to the knee in the static postural assessment, movement assessments, or both, mobility assessments should be performed to better pinpoint the muscle imbalances to be corrected with the Corrective Exercise Continuum. That is, if knee valgus, varus, or dominance is observed, mobility of the knee and surrounding structures should be individually assessed. Overactivity in the hip flexors (modified Thomas test), quadriceps (modified Thomas test, active knee flexion test), hamstrings (active knee extension test), adductors (hip abduction and external rotation test), and abductors (modified Thomas test) can be assessed. Additionally, overactivity in hip external rotators (passive hip internal rotation, seated hip internal rotation), hip internal rotators (seated hip external rotation), and gastrocnemius/soleus (weight-bearing lunge test) may be confirmed using mobility assessments. The Corrective Exercise Specialist should consider that many of the muscles just mentioned cross both the hip and the knee, and thus both kinetic chain checkpoints need to be considered in the mobility assessment.

The Corrective Exercise Specialist needs to also consider the findings of the heels-elevated modification of the OHSA when deciding which mobility assessments to employ.

Corrective Strategies for the Knee

The integrated assessment process will reveal movement compensation patterns that warrant the implementation of corrective programming for the knee, with the most common one being knee valgus. Once the static, movement, and mobility assessments have been performed and impairments have been identified, the corrective exercise strategy can be developed using the NASM Corrective Exercise Continuum. Most programs that address lower extremity movement quality also incorporate proprioceptive or balance training, with or without functional movements, multiple times per week.

Table 12-4, while not exhaustive, provides a list of common exercise and technique selections when programming for this region. Specific exercise selection will depend on the client's individual results, needs, and abilities.

Phase	Modality	Muscle(s)/Exercise	Acute Training Variables
TABLE 12-4 Common Corrective Programming Selections for the Knee			
Inhibit	Self-myofascial rolling	Adductor complex Biceps femoris Fibularis complex (peroneals) Gastrocnemius Piriformis Quadriceps Soleus TFL	Hold areas of discomfort for 30 to 60 seconds Perform four to six repetitions of active joint movement
Lengthen	Static or neuromuscular stretching (NMS)	Adductor complex (for valgus) Biceps femoris Gastrocnemius Hip flexor complex Piriformis Quadriceps Soleus TFL	Static: 30-second hold NMS: 7- to 10-second isometric contraction, 30-second static hold
Activate	Isolated strengthening	Adductor complex (for varus) Anterior tibialis Core stabilizers Gluteus maximus Gluteus medius Medial hamstrings Posterior tibialis	10 to 15 reps with 4-second eccentric contraction, 2-second isometric contraction at end-range, and 1-second concentric contraction
Integrate*	Integrated dynamic movement	Lateral tube walking Lunge to balance progressions Single-leg squat Squat with medicine ball between knees (for varus) Squat with mini-band around knees (for valgus) Step-up to balance Wall jump	10 to 15 reps under control

*NOTE: Progress and regress as needed to match client ability, work capacity, and needs.

Common Exercise Selections for the Knee

The goal for exercises used for knee corrective strategies is to improve commonly observed movement impairments such as knee valgus, varus, and dominance. Oftentimes, multiple movement impairments across the kinetic chain occur together (such as feet turn out and knee valgus) and may benefit from exercises that address both, based on the integrated assessment process. For example, inhibition and lengthening of the short head of the biceps femoris may improve both impairments. As such, the Corrective Exercise Specialist may create a program that efficiently addresses multiple movement impairments.

INHIBIT: SELF-MYOFASCIAL ROLLING

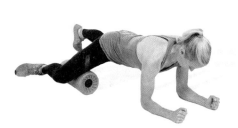

Adductor complex

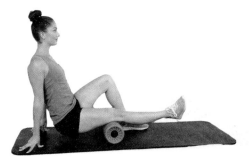

Biceps femoris

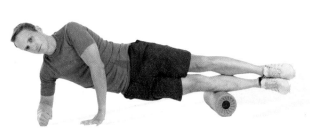

Fibularis complex (peroneals)

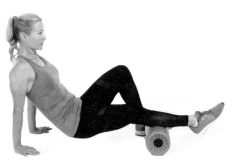

Gastrocnemius/soleus

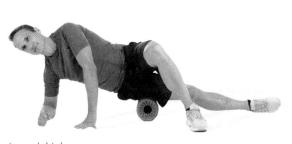

Lateral thigh

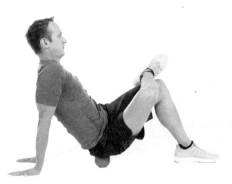

Piriformis

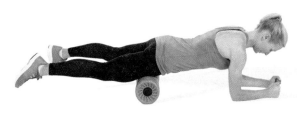

Quadriceps

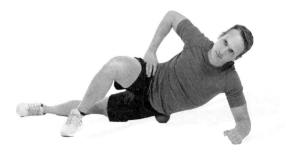

Tensor fascia latae

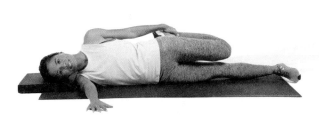

Static side-lying quadriceps stretch

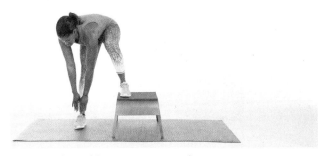

Static standing adductor magnus stretch

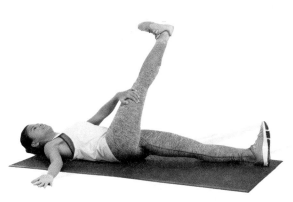

Static supine biceps femoris stretch

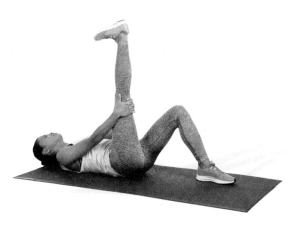

Static supine hamstrings stretch

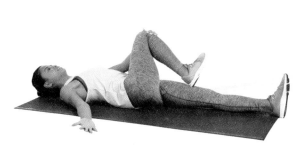

Static piriformis stretch

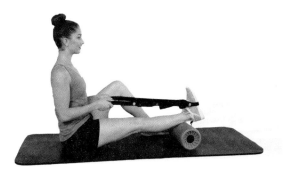

Self NMS gastrocnemius/soleus

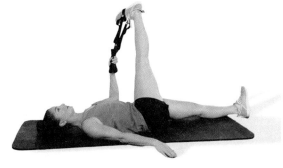

Self NMS biceps femoris

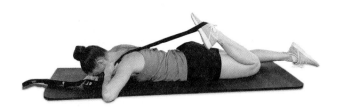

Self NMS prone quadriceps

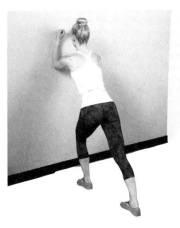

Static gastrocnemius stretch

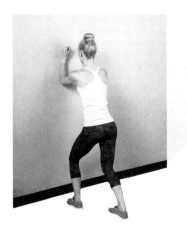

Static soleus stretch

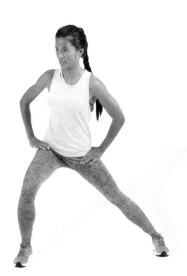

Static standing adductor stretch

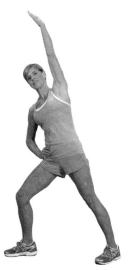

Static standing tensor fascia latae stretch

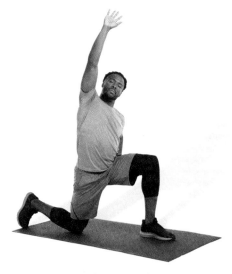

Static kneeling hip flexor stretch

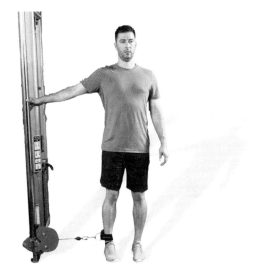

Adductors—start

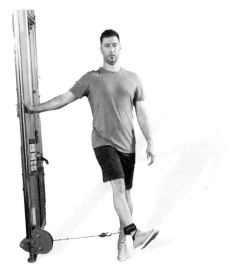

Adductors—finish

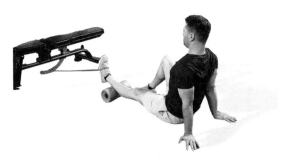

Anterior tibialis—start

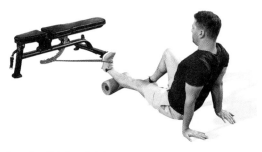

Anterior tibialis—finish

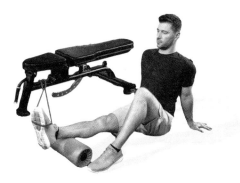

Posterior tibialis—start

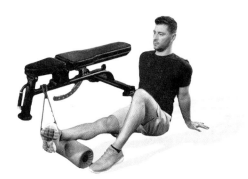

Posterior tibialis—finish

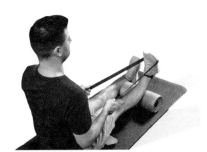

Medial gastrocnemius—start

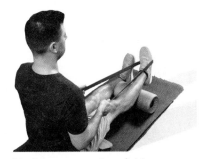

Medial gastrocnemius—finish

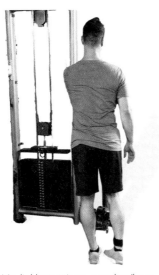

Medial hamstrings complex (knee flexion)—start

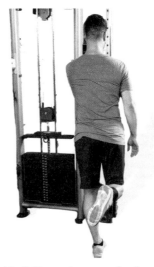

Medial hamstrings complex (knee flexion)—finish

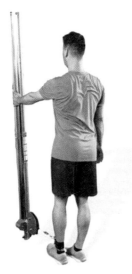

Gluteus maximus—start

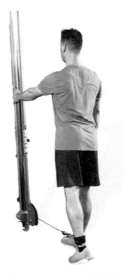

Gluteus maximus—finish

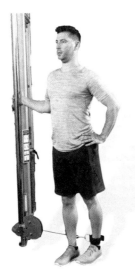

Gluteus medius—start

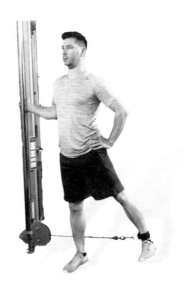

Gluteus medius—finish

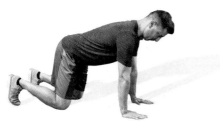

Quadruped opposite arm/leg raise—start

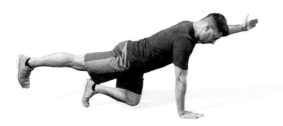

Quadruped opposite arm/leg raise—finish

INTEGRATE: DYNAMIC MOVEMENT PROGRESSIONS

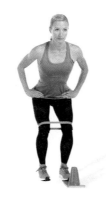

Lateral tube walking with mini-band around knees—start

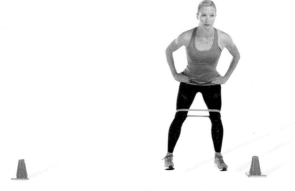

Lateral tube walking with mini-band around knees—finish

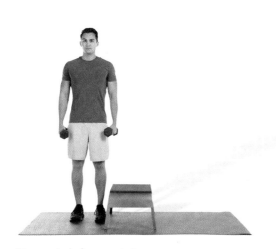

Step-up to balance—start

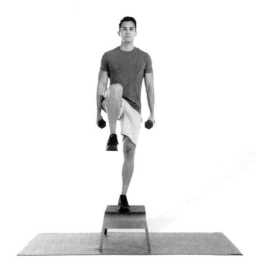

Step-up to balance—finish

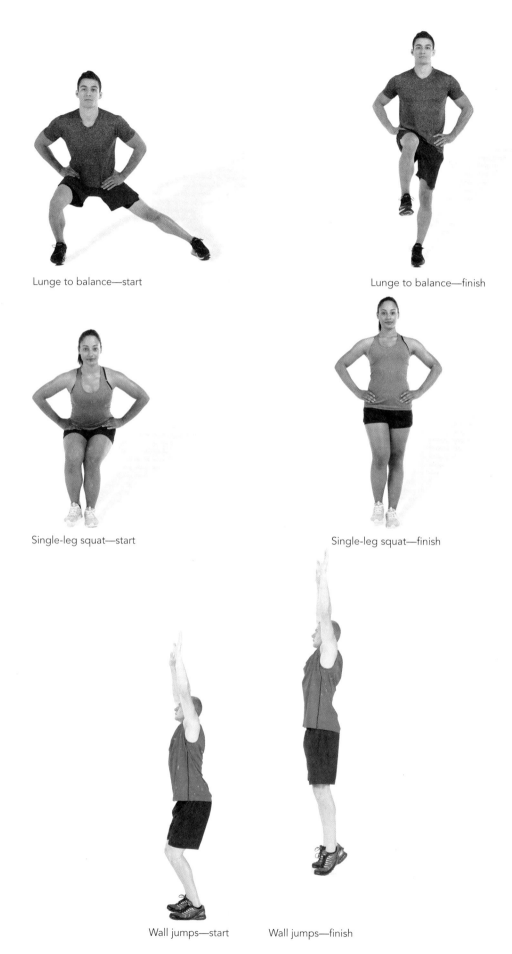

Lunge to balance—start

Lunge to balance—finish

Single-leg squat—start

Single-leg squat—finish

Wall jumps—start

Wall jumps—finish

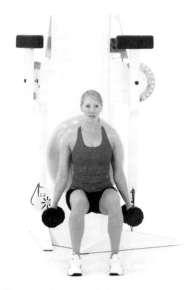

Supported squat—start

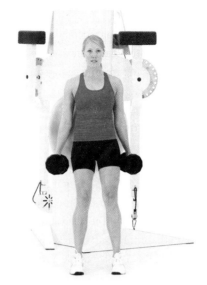

Supported squat—finish

Knee Valgus

The Corrective Exercise Specialist should be selective regarding the techniques recommended to each client. To improve client adherence, it is recommended that they employ as few exercises as are effective in each phase of the continuum. The programming objectives discussed here are commonly used for the compensation of knee valgus. The broad objectives of the program are to improve ideal mobility of the ankle, hip, and knee and the body's ability to decelerate and resist valgus forces. When applied systematically, the Corrective Exercise Continuum contributes to efficient neuromuscular control and proper alignment of the knee during movement.

Recall that if the heels-elevated modification improved the squat, then corrective strategies for the lower leg (the gastrocnemius/soleus complex in this case) may be warranted.

PHASE 1: INHIBIT

Key regions to inhibit via self-myofascial rolling include the gastrocnemius/soleus, adductor complex, TFL, and lateral thigh (emphasizing the vastus lateralis and/or short head of the biceps femoris).

PHASE 2: LENGTHEN

Key lengthening exercises via static and/or neuromuscular stretches would include the gastrocnemius/soleus, adductor complex, TFL, and biceps femoris.

PHASE 3: ACTIVATE

Key activation exercises include those involving the gluteus medius and gluteus maximus if the heels-elevated compensation did not improve the squat. Specific to the LPHC, these muscles will be responsible for concentrically creating greater hip abduction and external rotation and eccentrically decelerating hip adduction and internal rotation. If the heels-elevated modification did improve the squat, then the anterior and posterior tibialis should be included. The objective of the selected activation exercises is to improve the intramuscular coordination of tissues considered underactive based on the integrated assessment flow.

PHASE 4: INTEGRATE

An integration progression could first include uniplanar exercises (sagittal plane) and then progress to multiplanar exercises (frontal and transverse). Exercises can begin as more transitional, such as moving with no change in the base of support, as with a supported squat (e.g., ball squat with an elastic mini-band around the knees), and then progress to more dynamic exercises, such as movement with a change in the base of support (e.g., a lateral tube walk, to a step-up to balance, to a lunge to balance, to a single-leg squat). Further, integration exercises can be progressed to include increased rate of concentric force production and eccentric deceleration control with the inclusion of wall jumps, tuck jumps, 180-degree jumps, single-leg hops, and cutting maneuvers. Note that these advanced integration exercises should only be introduced if the client can control the positions. The Corrective Exercise Specialist should not advance the client too quickly. The knee should move with appropriate levels of flexion, extension, and control in the frontal and transverse planes.

Table 12-5 is a sample program a client may use to improve a knee valgus movement impairment.

TABLE 12-5 Sample Corrective Exercise Program for the Knee: Valgus

Phase	Modality	Muscle(s)/Exercise	Acute Training Variables
Inhibit	Self-myofascial rolling	Adductor complex Biceps femoris (short head) TFL	Hold areas of discomfort for 30 to 60 seconds Perform four to six repetitions of active joint movement 90 to 120 seconds per muscle group
Lengthen	Static stretching	Adductor complex Biceps femoris (short head) TFL	30-second hold
Activate	Isolated strengthening	Gluteus maximus Gluteus medius	10 to 15 reps with 4-second eccentric contraction, 2-second isometric contraction at end-range, and 1-second concentric contraction
Integrate*	Integrated dynamic movement	Supported squat with mini-band around knees Wall jump	10 to 15 reps under control

*NOTE: Progress and regress as needed to match client ability, work capacity, and needs.

 GETTING TECHNICAL

Core Activation and Lower Extremity Control

The Corrective Exercise Specialist may want to include exercises that target the LPHC, specifically the core stabilizers. Researchers have documented a link between LPHC muscle strength and lower extremity motor control (Bolgla et al., 2008; Nakagawa et al., 2012). A common exercise to consider could be the plank or any plank variation (e.g., plank with leg movements) to activate a greater amount of trunk muscles.

Knee Varus

The programming objectives discussed in this section are commonly used for the compensation of knee varus. The broad objectives of the program are to improve ideal mobility of the hip and knee and the body's ability to decelerate and resist varus forces. When applied systematically, the Corrective Exercise Continuum contributes to efficient neuromuscular control and proper alignment of the knee during movement.

Recall that if the heels-elevated modification improved the squat, then corrective strategies for the lower leg may be warranted.

PHASE 1: INHIBIT

Key regions to inhibit via foam rolling include the adductor magnus, piriformis, TFL, and biceps femoris (long head).

PHASE 2: LENGTHEN

Key lengthening exercises via static and/or neuromuscular stretches would include the adductor magnus, piriformis, TFL, and biceps femoris (long head).

PHASE 3: ACTIVATE

Key activation exercises include the adductor complex, medial hamstrings, and gluteus maximus. Specific to the LPHC, these muscles will be responsible for concentrically creating greater hip adduction and internal rotation and controlling hip abduction and external rotation. The objective of the selected activation exercises is to improve the intramuscular coordination of tissues considered underactive based on the integrated assessment process. While it is counter-intuitive that a hip external rotator (gluteus maximus) requires activation with a varus impairment, it is more likely that the gluteus maximus is underactive with a synergistically dominant piriformis in this situation. The Corrective Exercise Specialist should consider adding abdominal core exercises (e.g., quadruped opposite arm/leg raise) due to the interdependence of LPHC muscle strength and lower extremity motor control.

PHASE 4: INTEGRATE

An integration progression used for this compensation could be the same progression used for the compensation of knee valgus (uniplanar to multiplanar or transitional to dynamic). However, given that the knee is now demonstrating a varus position, a tool could be used to increase the activation of the adductors versus the abductors during movement. For example, during a supported squat, the Corrective Exercise Specialist could place a lightweight medicine ball between the client's knees. With this, the client will have to squeeze (i.e., activate the adductors) to hold the ball in position, thus improving overall knee alignment.

Table 12-6 is a sample program a client may use to improve a knee varus movement impairment.

Knee Dominance

The programming objectives discussed in this section are commonly used for the compensation of knee dominance. The broad objectives of the program are to improve ideal mobility of the hip and knee. When applied systematically, the Corrective Exercise Continuum contributes to efficient neuromuscular control and proper alignment of the knee during movement, specifically, the coordinated control of hip and knee motion during functional movements. Focus on the piriformis/adductor magnus versus quadriceps/soleus contribution will be determined by

TABLE 12-6 Sample Corrective Exercise Program for the Knee: Varus

Phase	Modality	Muscle(s)/Exercise	Acute Training Variables
Inhibit	Self-myofascial rolling	Adductor magnus Piriformis TFL	Hold areas of discomfort for 30 to 60 seconds Perform four to six repetitions of active joint movement 90 to 120 seconds per muscle group
Lengthen	Static stretching	Adductor magnus Piriformis TFL	30-second hold
Activate	Isolated strengthening	Adductors Gluteus maximus Medial hamstrings	10 to 15 reps with 4-second eccentric contraction, 2-second isometric contraction at end-range, and 1-second concentric contraction
Integrate*	Integrated dynamic movement	Supported squat with medicine ball between knees Wall jump	10 to 15 reps under control

*NOTE: Progress and regress as needed to match client ability, work capacity, and needs.

the corrective exercise assessment flow. Oftentimes when knee dominance is accompanied by a heel rise, the corrective exercise program can focus on the quadriceps/soleus. When LPHC impairment is present, the corrective exercise program for knee dominance can focus on the piriformis/adductor magnus combination.

Recall that if the heels-elevated modification improved the squat, then corrective strategies for the lower leg may be warranted.

PHASE 1: INHIBIT

Key regions to inhibit via foam rolling include the quadriceps and soleus and/or piriformis and adductor magnus.

PHASE 2: LENGTHEN

Key lengthening exercises via static and/or neuromuscular stretches may include the quadriceps, soleus, piriformis, and adductor magnus.

PHASE 3: ACTIVATE

Key activation exercises include the gluteus maximus and core stabilizers. The objective of the selected activation exercises is to improve the intramuscular coordination of tissues considered underactive based on the integrated assessment process. Specific to the LPHC, these muscles will be responsible for eccentrically decelerating hip flexion and knee extension and for stabilizing the LPHC. The Corrective Exercise Specialist should consider adding abdominal core exercises (e.g., planks) to the client's activation program.

An integration progression used for this movement impairment could be the same progression used for knee valgus and varus (uniplanar to multiplanar or transitional to dynamic). However, given that the knee is not necessarily demonstrating a valgus or varus movement, there is no need to emphasize abductors or adductors. Instead, the Corrective Exercise Specialist should encourage optimal alignment of the knee and coordinated movement with the hip and foot and ankle complex (i.e., a natural rhythm of triple flexion and extension) while executing smooth movement through a given range of motion.

Table 12-7 is a sample program a client may use to improve a knee dominance impairment.

TABLE 12-7	Sample Corrective Exercise Program for the Knee: Knee Dominance		
Phase	**Modality**	**Muscle(s)/Exercise**	**Acute Training Variables**
Inhibit	Self-myofascial rolling	Quadriceps Soleus	Hold areas of discomfort for 30 to 60 seconds Perform four to six repetitions of active joint movement 90 to 120 seconds per muscle group
Lengthen	Static stretching	Quadriceps Soleus	30-second hold
Activate	Isolated strengthening	Core stabilizers Gluteus maximus	10 to 15 reps with 4-second eccentric contraction, 2-second isometric contraction at end-range, and 1-second concentric contraction
Integrate*	Integrated dynamic movement	Squat pattern Wall jump	10 to 15 reps under control

*NOTE: Progress and regress as needed to match client ability, work capacity, and needs.

Common Issues Associated with the Knee

The hinged knee joint is highly susceptible to injury. Movement impairments related to the LPHC and the foot and ankle complex play a major role in common knee injuries. This section will provide a brief overview of some of the common knee injuries related to movement deficiencies, such as patellar tendinopathy, patellofemoral syndrome, iliotibial band syndrome, and **anterior cruciate ligament (ACL) injury**. Note that although this section discusses common injuries, fitness professionals are not trained or licensed to provide medical examinations or diagnoses. A Corrective Exercise Specialist's job is to evaluate movement and provide strategies for improving movement quality. Diagnosis or treatment of any of the following pathologies is outside the scope of practice. The presence of any of the following pathologies requires consultation with or referral to a qualified medical professional.

Anterior cruciate ligament (ACL) injury

One of the main knee ligaments; stabilizes the knee by stabilizing the anterior translation of the tibia relative to the femur. Injuries often take the form of over-stretching or tearing due to sudden lower extremity movements such as stops, changes of direction, rotation, etc.

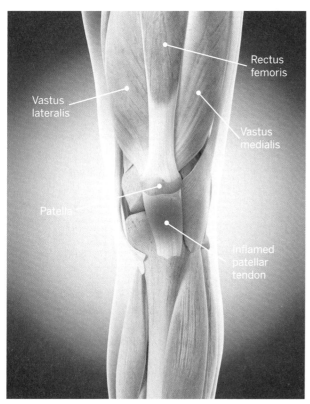

Figure 12-11 Patellar tendinopathy

Patellar Tendinopathy (Jumper's Knee)

The patellar tendon, originating on the base of the patella and inserting at the tibial tuberosity, is an essential anatomical component for knee kinematics (Moore et al., 2014). As has been noted, the patellofemoral articulation is often referred to as the extensor mechanism, and the patellar tendon provides the forces necessary to extend the knee in an open-chain position. As individuals perform daily living activities such as walking, squatting, stepping, and others, concentric, eccentric, and isometric forces act on the patellar tendon. With more advanced activities, such as running, jumping, cutting, and landing, forces acting on the extensor mechanism increase exponentially. Patellar tendinopathy is a common overuse injury and is characterized as pain at the base of the patella (**Figure 12-11**) (Figueroa et al., 2016). It occurs when an individual places repeated stress on the patellar tendon. Further, individuals with underactive gluteals may develop overactive quadriceps in an attempt to compensate for a loss of extensor force production (Mills et al., 2015). The increased activity of the quadriceps may add to the already cumulative forces being distributed through the patellar tendon.

The stress of patellar tendinopathy results in tiny tears in the tendon, which may cause inflammation, pain, and/or degenerative change in the tendon. Patellar tendinopathy is an injury common with, but not limited to, athletes, particularly those participating in jumping sports such as basketball, volleyball, football, and soccer (Everhart et al., 2017). Risk factors for patellar tendinopathy include the following:

- Knee valgus and varus
- An increased Q-angle
- Poor quadriceps and hamstrings complex flexibility
- Poor eccentric deceleration capabilities
- Overtraining and playing on hard surfaces (Everhart et al., 2017; Malliaras et al., 2015)

During transitional movement assessments (OHSA, SLSA, or split-squat), clients may present with various compensation patterns in the lower kinetic chain. Pain on or around the patellar tendon, especially when increasing knee flexion, may indicate some type of knee pathology. The fitness professional many need to modify or stop the assessment if knee pain is present. If a pathology is suspected, the client should be referred to a qualified medical professional.

Patellofemoral Syndrome

One of the most commonly accepted causes of patellofemoral syndrome (PFS) (**Figure 12-12**) is abnormal tracking of the patella within the femoral trochlea or patellar groove. When the patella is not properly aligned within the femoral trochlea, the stress per unit area on the patellar cartilage increases owing to a smaller contact area between the patella and the trochlea (Fulkerson, 2002). Abnormal tracking of the patella may be attributable to static (i.e., increased Q-angle) or dynamic lower extremity malalignment (i.e., increased femoral internal rotation, adduction, and knee valgus), altered muscle activation of surrounding knee musculature, decreased strength of the hip musculature, or various combinations (Bloomer & Durall, 2015; Powers et al., 2017; Rothermich et al., 2015). Similar to patellar tendinopathy, clients will present with pes planus distortion syndrome, excessive pronation, or heel rise. The SLSA will result in knee valgus or varus. Pain will be associated on the front aspect of the knee behind the patella. If the client is unable to complete the movement assessment process due to pain or swelling, the Corrective Exercise Specialist should refer the client to a medical professional for further evaluation.

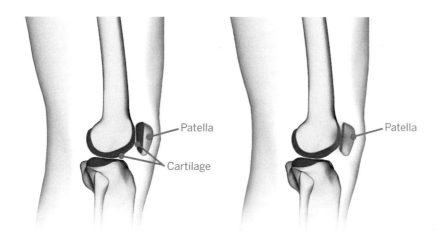

Normal knee   **Patellofemoral pain**

Figure 12-12   Patellofemoral syndrome

Iliotibial Band (IT-Band) Syndrome (Runner's Knee)

IT-band syndrome is the result of inflammation and irritation of the distal portion of the iliotibial tendon as it rubs against the lateral femoral condyle as well as compresses the fat pad underneath it (**Figure 12-13**), or less commonly, the greater trochanter of the hip, causing a greater trochanteric bursitis (Fairclough et al., 2006). Inflammation and irritation of the IT-band may occur because of a lack of flexibility of the TFL, which can result in an increase in tension on the IT-band during the stance phase of running.

IT-band syndrome is typically caused by overuse. The injury is most often reported in runners as a result of abnormal gait or running biomechanics, although other athletes (e.g., cyclists or tennis players) also may be affected. Weakness of muscle groups in the kinetic chain may also result in the development of IT-band syndrome. Weakness in the hip abductor muscles, such as the gluteus medius, may result in synergistic dominance of the TFL (increasing frontal plane instability; Aderem & Louw, 2015; Flato et al., 2017; Mucha et al., 2017; van der Worp et al., 2012). This, in turn, may lead to increased tension of the IT-band, and thus increased

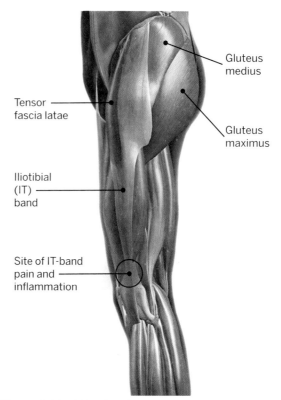

Gluteus
medius

Tensor
fascia latae

Gluteus
maximus

Iliotibial
(IT)
band

Site of IT-band
pain and
inflammation

Figure 12-13   IT-band syndrome

friction on the tissue, with inflammation being the end result. Clients presenting with knee valgus during the OHSA and SLSA or pes planus distortion syndrome may be more prone to IT-band irritability.

Anterior Cruciate Ligament (ACL) Injury

Beyond the common injuries indicated, which are more chronic in onset, one severe knee injury often occurring during physical activity is a rupture of the ACL. ACL injuries can affect both males and females of all ages, and it is estimated that more than 200,000 ACL injuries occur each year in the United States (Donnell-Fink et al., 2015). Many ACL injuries occur from indirect contact (such as changing direction and cutting) due to altered lower extremity neuromusculoskeletal control and the action of anterior forces, lateral forces, rotational forces, or a combination of all three forces on the knee (**Figure 12-14**) (Gagnier et al., 2013; Paterno et al., 2010; Weiss & Whatman, 2015). Proximal neuromusculoskeletal control deficits at the hip and trunk during landing are also potential contributing mechanisms to high-risk knee mechanics (Ford et al., 2006; Hewett et al., 2006). During movement assessments, the Corrective Exercise Specialist can play a significant role in identifying potential predisposing factors placing clients at an increased risk for an ACL injury. Researchers have demonstrated that ACL injuries can be reduced from 51% to 62% through the application of educational interventions and targeted neuromuscular training (Gagnier et al., 2013). To help reduce the risk of ACL injuries, the literature suggests that programming should focus on improving movement impairment, such as excessive knee valgus, knee rotation, hip adduction, and hip rotation; improving single-leg neuromuscular balance; and improving muscle strength (Huang et al., 2019). Many of these movement impairments can be identified during the OHSA and SLSA. Therefore, clients presenting with altered neuromuscular control such as knee valgus or varus during these assessments should be provided specific programming following the Corrective Exercise Continuum.

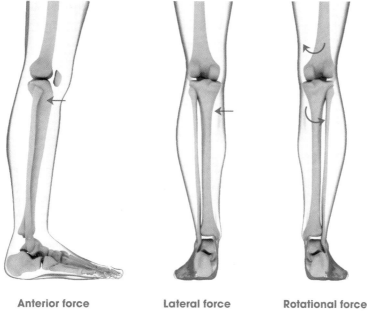

Anterior force   **Lateral force**   **Rotational force**

Figure 12-14 Anterior, lateral, and rotational forces

GETTING TECHNICAL

ACL Injury: Pre- and Postsurgical

In the unfortunate event a client sustains an ACL rupture, the Corrective Exercise Specialist, in coordination with a medical professional, can play a significant role in the recovery process both in pre- and postsurgical intervention. Presurgical intervention, also known as *prehabilitation*, is believed to set the foundation for the long postsurgical rehabilitation process. The main goals of a successful prehabilitation program are to reduce swelling, increase range of motion, and maintain strength in the lower extremity. Following the principles of regional interdependence and the kinetic chain, the Corrective Exercise Specialist can provide targeted inhibitory, lengthening, activation, and integration exercises for the foot and ankle complex and the LPHC.

After ACL surgical repair, a client will often present with limited range of motion secondary to pain and swelling and a loss of muscular strength and tone, especially in the quadriceps muscle group of the involved leg. The literature is inconsistent on appropriate return-to-play criteria, but many medical experts are following the trend of returning sooner not always being better, pushing for a more criteria-based protocol. The Corrective Exercise Specialist, as a member of the care and performance team for athletes and clients, can play a significant role in the recovery of an ACL surgical repair. Once the client or athlete has completed rehabilitation and been cleared by a medical professional, the Corrective Exercise Specialist can perform movement assessments, especially the OHSA and SLSA, to identify any potential movement impairments. Adequate programming to address those impairments can be implemented, thus limiting the risk of future lower-extremity injuries.

SUMMARY

Lower extremity injuries account for the majority of the total injuries in both college and high school athletes. The knee is one of the most commonly injured regions of the body (Brant et al., 2019; Fernandez et al., 2007). The knee is a part of the kinetic chain that is influenced by the linked segments from the proximal and distal joints. The Corrective Exercise Assessment Flow process evaluates distal and proximal kinetic chain segments relative to the knee and is informed by the RI model. On the basis of the collective information obtained from these assessments, overactive tissues and neuromuscular control deficits are identified for targeted exercise strategies. The outlined corrective exercise strategies for knee impairments provide Corrective Exercise Specialists with a systematic approach that can ultimately reduce the risk of knee and lower extremity injuries while improving performance measures.

REFERENCES

Aderem, J., & Louw, Q. A. (2015). Biomechanical risk factors associated with iliotibial band syndrome in runners: A systematic review. *BMC Musculoskeletal Disorders, 16*, 356. https://doi.org/10.1186/s12891-015-0808-7

Almeida, G. P. L., Silva, A. P. M. C. C., França, F. J. R., Magalhães, M. O., Burke, T. N., & Marques, A. P. (2016). Q-angle in patellofemoral pain: Relationship with dynamic knee valgus, hip abductor torque, pain and function. *Revista Brasileira de Ortopedia. English Edition, 51*(2), 181–186.

Baker, R. L., Souza, R. B., Rauh, M. J., Fredericson, M., & Rosenthal, M. D. (2018). Differences in knee and hip adduction and hip muscle activation in runners with and without iliotibial band syndrome. *PM&R, 10*(10), 1032–1039.

Bloomer, B. A., & Durall, C. J. (2015). Does the addition of hip strengthening to a knee-focused exercise program improve outcomes in patients with patellofemoral pain syndrome? *Journal of Sport Rehabilitation, 24*(4), 428–433. https://doi.org/10.1123/jsr.2014-0184

Bolgla, L., Malone, T., Umberger, B. R., & Uhl, T. L. (2008). Hip strength and hip and knee kinematics during stair descent in females with and without patellofemoral pain syndrome. *Journal of Orthopaedic & Sports Physical Therapy, 38*(1), 12–18. https://doi.org/10.2519/jospt.2008

Brant, J. A., Johnson, B., Brou, L., Comstock, R. D., & Vu, T. (2019). Rates and patterns of lower extremity sports injuries in all gender-comparable US high school sports. *Orthopaedic Journal of Sports Medicine, 7*(10). https://doi.org/10.1177/2325967119873059

Brown, S. R., Brughelli, M., & Hume, P. A. (2014). Knee mechanics during planned and unplanned sidestepping: A systematic review and meta-analysis. *Sports Medicine, 44*(11), 1573–1588. https://doi.org/10.1007/s40279-014-0225-3

Buldt, A. K., Murley, G. S., Butterworth, P., Levinger, P., Menz, H. B., & Landorf, K. B. (2013). The relationship between foot posture and lower limb kinematics during walking: A systematic review. *Gait & Posture, 38*(3), 363–372. https://doi.org/10.1016/j.gaitpost.2013.01.010

Carlson, V. R., Sheehan, F. T., & Boden, B. P. (2016). Video analysis of anterior cruciate ligament (ACL) injuries: A systematic review. *JBJS Review, 4*(11). https://doi.org/10.2106/jbjs.rvw.15.00116

Cowan, S. M., Bennell, K. L., Crossley, K. M., Hodges, P. W., & McConnell, J. (2002). Physical therapy alters recruitment of the vasti in patellofemoral pain syndrome. *Medicine & Science in Sports & Exercise, 34*(12), 1879–1885. https://doi.org/10.1249/01.MSS.0000038893.30443.CE

Dierks, T. A., Manal, K. T., Hamill, J., & Davis, I. S. (2008). Proximal and distal influences on hip and knee kinematics in runners with patellofemoral pain during a prolonged run. *Journal of Orthopaedic & Sports Physical Therapy, 38*(8), 448–456. https://doi.org/10.2519/jospt.2008.2490

Donnell-Fink, L. A., Klara, K., Collins, J. E., Yang, H. Y., Goczalk, M. G., Katz, J. N., & Losina, E. (2015). Effectiveness of knee injury and anterior cruciate ligament tear prevention programs: A meta-analysis. *PLoS One, 10*(12), e0144063. https://doi.org/10.1371/journal.pone.0144063

Everhart, J. S., Cole, D., Sojka, J. H., Higgins, J. D., Magnussen, R. A., Schmitt, L. C., & Flanigan, D. C. (2017). Treatment options for patellar tendinopathy: A systematic review. *Arthroscopy, 33*(4), 861–872. https://doi.org/10.1016/j.arthro.2016.11.007

Fairclough, J., Hayashi, K., Toumi, H., Lyons, K., Bydder, G., Phillips, N., Best, T. M., & Benjamin, M. (2006). The functional anatomy of the iliotibial band during flexion and extension of the knee: Implications for understanding iliotibial band syndrome. *Journal of Anatomy, 208*(3), 309–316. https://doi.org/10.1111/j.1469-7580.2006.00531.x

Fernandez, W. G., Yard, E. E., & Comstock, R. D. (2007). Epidemiology of lower extremity injuries among U.S. high school athletes. *Academic Emergency Medicine : Official Journal of the Society for Academic Emergency Medicine, 14*(7), 641–645.

Figueroa, D., Figueroa, F., & Calvo, R. (2016). Patellar tendinopathy: Diagnosis and treatment. *Journal of the American Academy of Orthopaedic Surgeons, 24*(12), e184–e192. https://doi.org/10.5435/jaaos-d-15-00703

Flandry, F., & Hommel, G. (2011). Normal anatomy and biomechanics of the knee. *Sports Medicine and Arthroscopy Review, 19*(2), 82–92. https://doi.org/10.1097/JSA.0b013e318210c0aa

Flato, R., Passanante, G. J., Skalski, M. R., Patel, D. B., White, E. A., & Matcuk, G. R., Jr. (2017). The iliotibial tract: Imaging, anatomy, injuries, and other pathology. *Skeletal Radiology, 46*(5), 605–622. https://doi.org/10.1007/s00256-017-2604-y

Floyd, R. T. (2017). *Manual of structural kinesiology* (20th ed.). McGraw-Hill Education.

Ford, K. R., Myer, G. D., Smith, R. L., Vianello, R. M., Seiwert, S. L., & Hewett, T. E. (2006). A comparison of dynamic coronal plane excursion between matched male and female athletes when performing single leg landings. *Clinical Biomechanics, 21*(1), 33–40. https://doi.org/10.1016/j.clinbiomech.2005.08.010

Fulkerson, J. P. (2002). Diagnosis and treatment of patients with patellofemoral pain. *American Journal of Sports Medicine, 30*(3), 447–456. https://doi.org/10.1177/03635465020300032501

Gage, B. E., McIlvain, N. M., Collins, C. L., Fields, S. K., & Comstock, R. D. (2012). Epidemiology of 6.6 million knee injuries presenting to United States emergency departments from 1999 through 2008. *Academic Emergency Medicine, 19*(4), 378–385. https//doi.org/10.1111/j.1553-2712.2012.01315.x

Gagnier, J. J., Morgenstern, H., & Chess, L. (2013). Interventions designed to prevent anterior cruciate ligament injuries in adolescents and adults: A systematic review and meta-analysis. *American Journal of Sports Medicine, 41*(8), 1952–1962. https//:doi.org/10.1177/0363546512458227

Heinert, B. L., Kernozek, T. W., Greany, J. F., & Fater, D. C. (2008). Hip abductor weakness and lower extremity kinematics during running. *Journal of Sport Rehabilitation, 17*(3), 243–256.

Hewett, T. E., Ford, K. R., Myer, G. D., Wanstrath, K., & Scheper, M. (2006). Gender differences in hip adduction motion and torque during a single-leg agility maneuver. *Journal of Orthopaedic Research, 24*(3), 416–421. https://doi.org/10.1002/jor.20056

Hootman, J. M., Macera, C. A., Ainsworth, B. E., Addy, C. L., Martin, M., & Blair, S. N. (2002). Epidemiology of musculoskeletal injuries among sedentary and physically active adults. *Medicine & Science in Sports & Exercise, 34*(5), 838–844. https://doi.org/10.1097/00005768-200205000-00017

Huberti, H. H., & Hayes, W. C. (1984). Patellofemoral contact pressures. The influence of q-angle and tendofemoral contact. *Journal of Bone and Joint Surgery. American Volume, 66*(5), 715–724.

Huang, Y. L., Jung, J., Mulligan, C. M. S., Oh, J., & Norcross, M. F. (2019). A majority of anterior cruciate ligament injuries can be prevented by injury prevention programs: A systematic review of randomized controlled trials and cluster-randomized controlled trials with meta-analysis. *American Journal of Sports Medicine,* 363546519870175. https://doi.org/10.1177/0363546519870175

Ireland, M. L., Willson, J. D., Ballantyne, B. T., & Davis, I. M. (2003). Hip strength in females with and without patellofemoral pain. *Journal of Orthopaedic and Sports Physical Therapy, 33*(11), 671–676. https://doi.org/10.2519/jospt.2003.33.11.671

Ishida, T., Yamanaka, M., Takeda, N., & Aoki, Y. (2014). Knee rotation associated with dynamic knee valgus and toe direction. *The Knee, 21*(2), 563–566. https://doi.org/10.1016/j.knee.2012.12.002

Kazemi, M., Dabiri, Y., & Li, L. P. (2013). Recent advances in computational mechanics of the human knee joint. *Computational and Mathematical Methods in Medicine, 2013,* 718423. https://doi.org/10.1155/2013/718423

Kenney, W. L., Wilmore, J. H., & Costill, D. L. (2019). *Physiology of sport and exercise* (7th ed.). Human Kinetics.

Kim, H. Y., Kim, K. J., Yang, D. S., Jeung, S. W., Choi, H. G., & Choy, W. S. (2015). Screw-home movement of the tibiofemoral joint during normal gait: Three-dimensional analysis. *Clinics in Orthopedic Surgery, 7*(3), 303–309. https://doi.org/10.4055/cios.2015.7.3.303

Komdeur, P., Pollo, F. E., & Jackson, R. W. (2002). Dynamic knee motion in anterior cruciate impairment: A report and case study. *Proceedings (Baylor University Medical Center), 15*(3), 257–259.

Levine, D., Richards, J., & Whittle, M. W. (2012). *Whittle's gait analysis* (5th ed.). Churchill Livingstone/Elsevier.

Malliaras, P., Cook, J., Purdam, C., & Rio, E. (2015). Patellar tendinopathy: Clinical diagnosis, load management, and advice for challenging case presentations. *Journal of Orthopaedic & Sports Physical Therapy, 45*(11), 887–898. https://doi.org/10.2519/jospt.2015.5987

Mills, M., Frank, B., Goto, S., Blackburn, T., Cates, S., Clark, M., Aguilar, A., Fava, N., & Padua, D. (2015). Effect of restricted hip flexor muscle length on hip extensor muscle activity and lower extremity biomechanics in college-aged female soccer players. *International Journal of Sports Physical Therapy, 10*(7), 946–954.

Molgaard, C., Rathleff, M. S., & Simonsen, O. (2011). Patellofemoral pain syndrome and its association with hip, ankle, and foot function in 16- to 18-year-old high school students: A single-blind case-control study. *Journal of the American Podiatric Medical Association, 101*(3), 215–222.

Moore, K. L., Dalley, A. F., & Agur, A. M. R. (2014). *Clinically oriented anatomy* (7th ed.). Lippincott, Williams, & Wilkins.

Mucha, M. D., Caldwell, W., Schlueter, E. L., Walters, C., & Hassen, A. (2017). Hip abductor strength and lower extremity running related injury in distance runners: A systematic review. *Journal of Science and Medicine in Sport, 20*(4), 349–355. https://doi.org/10.1016/j.jsams.2016.09.002

Nakagawa, T. H., Moriya, É. T., Maciel, C. D., & Serrão, A. F. (2012). Frontal plane biomechanics in males and females with and without patellofemoral pain. *Medicine & Science in Sports & Exercise, 44*(9), 1747–1755. https://doi.org/10.1249/MSS.0b013e318256903a

Nunes, G. S., Barton, C. J., & Viadanna Serrão, F. (2019). Females with patellofemoral pain have impaired impact absorption during a single-legged drop vertical jump. *Gait & Posture, 68,* 346–351. https://doi.org/10.1016/j.gaitpost.2018.12.013

Page, P., Frank, C. C., & Lardner, R. (2010). *Assessment and treatment of muscle imbalance: The Janda approach.* Human Kinetics.

Paterno, M. V., Schmitt, L. C., Ford, K. R., Rauh, M. J., Myer, G. D., Huang, B., & Hewett, T. E. (2010). Biomechanical measures during landing and postural stability predict second anterior cruciate ligament injury after anterior cruciate ligament reconstruction and return to sport. *American Journal of Sports Medicine, 38*(10), 1968–1978. https://doi.org/10.1177/0363546510376053

Pollard, C. D., Sigward, S. M., & Powers, C. M. (2017). ACL injury prevention training results in modification of hip and knee mechanics during a drop-landing task. *Orthopaedic Journal of Sports Medicine, 5*(9), 2325967117726267. https://doi.org/10.1177/2325967117726267

Powers, C. M., Witvrouw, E., Davis, I. S., & Crossley, K. M. (2017). Evidence-based framework for a pathomechanical model of patellofemoral pain: 2017 Patellofemoral Pain Consensus Statement from the 4th International Patellofemoral Pain Research Retreat, Manchester, UK: Part 3. *British Journal of Sports Medicine, 51*(24), 1713–1723. https://doi.org/10.1136/bjsports-2017-098717

Rothermich, M. A., Glaviano, N. R., Li, J., & Hart, J. M. (2015). Patellofemoral pain: Epidemiology, pathophysiology, and treatment options. *Clinics in Sports Medicine, 34*(2), 313–327. https://doi.org/10.1016/j.csm.2014.12.011

Sahrmann, S. A. (2001). *Diagnosis and treatment of movement impairment syndromes.* Mosby.

Santos, T. R., Oliveira, B. A., Ocarino, J. M., Holt, K. G., & Fonseca, S. T. (2015). Effectiveness of hip muscle strengthening in patellofemoral pain syndrome patients: A systematic review. *Brazilian Journal of Physical Therapy, 19*(3), 167–176. https://doi.org/10.1590/bjpt-rbf.2014.0089

Shin, C. S., Chaudhari, A. M., & Andriacchi, T. P. (2011). Valgus plus internal rotation moments increase anterior cruciate ligament strain more than either alone. *Medicine & Science in Sports & Exercise, 43*(8), 1484–1491. https://doi.org/10.1249/MSS.0b013e31820f8395

Sueki, D. G., Cleland, J. A., & Wainner, R. S. (2013). A regional interdependence model of musculoskeletal dysfunction: Research, mechanisms, and clinical implications. *Journal of Manual & Manipulative Therapy, 21*(2), 90–102. https://doi.org/10.1179/2042618612Y.0000000027

Teng, P. S. P., Kong, P. W., & Leong, K. F. (2017). Effects of foot rotation positions on knee valgus during single-leg drop landing: Implications for ACL injury risk reduction. *The Knee, 24*(3), 547–554. https://doi.org/10.1016/j.knee.2017.01.014

Thomée, R., Renström, P., Karlsson, J., & Grimby, G. (1995). Patellofemoral pain syndrome in young women: A clinical analysis of alignment, pain parameters, common symptoms, functional activity level. *Scandinavian Journal of Medicine & Science in Sports, 5*(4), 237–244.

van der Worp, M. P., van der Horst, N., de Wijer, A., Backx, F. J., & Nijhuis-van der Sanden, M. W. (2012). Iliotibial band syndrome in runners: A systematic review. *Sports Medicine, 42*(11), 969–992. https://doi.org/10.2165/11635400-000000000-00000

Weiss, K., & Whatman, C. (2015). Biomechanics associated with patellofemoral pain and ACL injuries in sports. *Sports Medicine, 45*(9), 1325–1337. https://doi.org/10.1007/s40279-015-0353-4

CHAPTER 13

Corrective Strategies for the Lumbo-Pelvic-Hip Complex

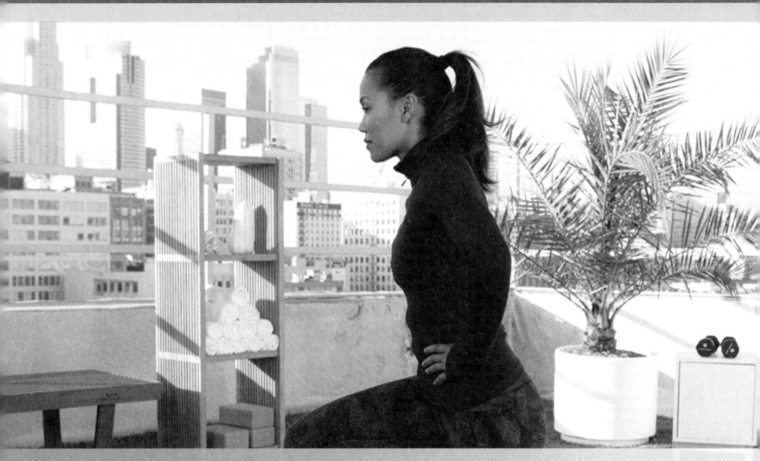

Learning Objectives

After reading this content, students should be able to demonstrate the following objectives:

- **Explain** the basic functional anatomy of the lumbo-pelvic-hip complex (LPHC).
- **Identify** the mechanisms for common LPHC injuries.
- **Describe** the influence of altered LPHC movement on the kinetic chain.
- **Determine** appropriate systematic assessment strategies for the LPHC.
- **Select** appropriate corrective exercise strategies for the LPHC.

Introduction

The lumbo-pelvic-hip complex (LPHC) is a region of the body that has a massive influence on the structures above and below it. The LPHC has more than 30 muscles that attach to the lumbar spine or pelvis (Cheatham & Kolber, 2016). Because of this, dysfunction of both the lower and upper extremities can lead to dysfunction of the LPHC, and vice versa, due to regional interdependence (Cheatham & Kreiswirth, 2014). The Corrective Exercise Specialist must understand differences in optimal movement patterns and dysfunctional movement patterns in daily living activities, exercise, and a number of structured assessments that provide avenues for objective and subjective feedback. Once dysfunctional movement(s) have been identified, it is the knowledge of functional anatomy that provides the foundation for successfully understanding and implementing NASM's Corrective Exercise Continuum. Understanding mechanisms of injury risk reduction will ensure that Corrective Exercise Specialists both optimize movement and refrain from unwittingly worsening movement impairments and pain.

Review of LPHC Functional Anatomy

The LPHC is complex, with great potential for influence on the rest of the human movement system (HMS). Because this is to be a review of LPHC anatomy, not all anatomical structures will be covered in detail. This section will provide a general review of the most pertinent structures.

Bones and Joints

In the LPHC region, the femur and the pelvis make up the iliofemoral joint and the pelvis and sacrum make up the sacroiliac joint. The lumbar spine and sacrum form the lumbosacral junction (**Figure 13-1**). Collectively, these structures anchor many of the major myofascial tissues that have a functional effect on the arthrokinematics of the structures above and below them.

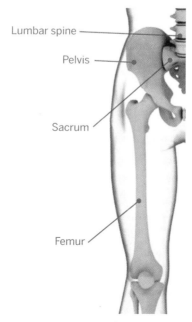

Lumbar spine

Pelvis

Sacrum

Femur

Figure 13-1   Bones of the LPHC

Above the LPHC are the thoracic and cervical spine, rib cage, scapula, humerus, and clavicle. These structures make up the thoracolumbar and cervicothoracic junctions of the spine, the scapulothoracic, glenohumeral, acromioclavicular (AC), and sternoclavicular (SC) joints (**Figure 13-2**).

Below the LPHC, the tibia and femur make up the tibiofemoral joint and the patella and femur make up the patellofemoral joint (**Figure 13-3**). The fibula is also noted because it is the attachment site of the biceps femoris, which originates from the pelvis.

The tibia, fibula, and talus help to form the talocrural (ankle) joint. Collectively, these structures anchor the myofascial tissues of the LPHC such as the biceps femoris, medial hamstrings complex, and rectus femoris. These bones and joints are of importance in corrective exercise because they will also have a functional effect on the arthrokinematics of the LPHC.

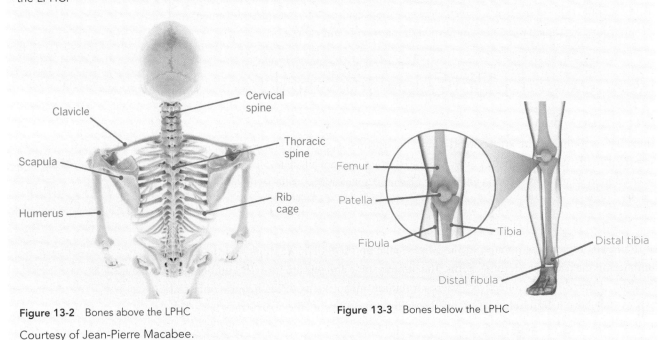

Figure 13-2   Bones above the LPHC

Courtesy of Jean-Pierre Macabee.

Figure 13-3   Bones below the LPHC

ILIOFEMORAL JOINT

The iliofemoral joint is where the femur attaches to the ilium (**Figure 13-4**). The acetabulum is the socket in the ilium where the femoral head connects and helps to deepen the socket. The iliofemoral joint is classified as a ball-and-socket joint with the ability to move in all three planes of motion (Cheatham & Kolber, 2016).

SACROILIAC JOINT

The sacrum is a triangular bone set between the left and right ilia, like a keystone. This is where the axial skeleton attaches to the pelvic girdle and the appendicular skeleton of the lower extremity. Little movement occurs at this joint, which is classified as a diarthrodial joint (Cheatham & Kolber, 2016).

LUMBOSACRAL JOINT

The lowest of the lumbar vertebrae, L5, has a caudal attachment to the sacrum. Where these two bones meet is known as the lumbosacral joint (**Figure 13-5**). This region of the body accepts incredible amounts of compressive forces, and therefore requires stability to support such forces.

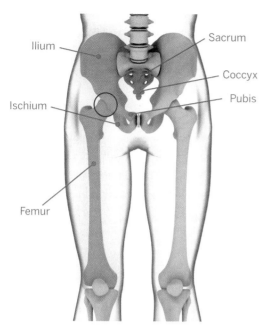

Figure 13-4 Iliofemoral joint

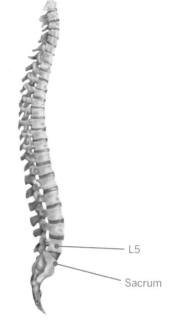

Figure 13-5 Lumbosacral joint

Muscles

A number of muscles in the upper and lower extremities may be related in function and have an effect on the LPHC (**Table 13-1**). Although not an exhaustive list, the following is a review of the major muscles that influence the LPHC.

TABLE 13-1 Key Muscles Associated with the LPHC	
■ Abdominal core complex	■ Hamstrings complex
■ Adductor complex	■ Hip flexors (psoas, rectus femoris)
■ Erector spinae	■ Intrinsic core stabilizers
■ Gastrocnemius/soleus	■ Latissimus dorsi
■ Gluteus maximus and medius	■ Tensor fascia latae (TFL)/IT-band

Altered LPHC Movement

Although Corrective Exercise Specialists do not treat pain or injury, discussing the relationship between a segment of the kinetic chain and its relevant injuries sheds light on mechanisms of dysfunction. LPHC impairment has numerous effects on the overall movement quality of the kinetic chain. Low-back pain (LBP) in particular is one of the most common global health problems and creates a substantial personal, community, and financial burden. Although occurrences are well known in adults, the prevalence of LBP in children and adolescents is growing and is becoming a public health concern (Calvo-Muñoz et al., 2013). Previous studies have found a high incidence of LBP in sports. For example, 85% of male gymnasts, 80% of weightlifters, 69% of wrestlers, 58% of soccer players, 50% of tennis players, 30% of golfers, and 60% to 80% of the general population were reported to have LBP (Daniels et al., 2011). Individuals who have LBP are significantly more likely to have additional low-back injuries, which can predispose the individual to future osteoarthritis and long-term disability. It has been demonstrated that static malalignments (altered length-tension relationships or altered joint arthrokinematics), abnormal muscle activation patterns (altered force-couple relationships), and dynamic malalignments (movement system impairments) can lead to LBP (Calvo-Muñoz et al., 2013; Cibulka et al., 1998; Daniels et al., 2011).

Static Malalignments

Optimal muscle performance is determined by the posture (length-tension) of the LPHC during functional activities. If the neutral lordotic curve of the lumbar spine is not maintained (i.e., low back excessively arches, low back rounds, or trunk excessively leans forward), the activation and the relative moment arm of the muscle fibers decrease. Vertebral disc injuries occur when the outer fibrous structure of the disc (annulus fibrosis) fails, allowing the internal contents of the disc (nucleus pulposus) to be extruded and irritate nerves exiting the intervertebral foramen (Cibulka et al., 1998; Neumann et al., 2016).

ABNORMAL MUSCLE ACTIVATION PATTERNS

Because LPHC musculature plays a critical role in stabilizing this complex, insufficiency of any of the musculature may induce biomechanical dysfunction and altered force-couple relationships. Subjects with LBP demonstrate impaired postural control, delayed muscle relaxation, and abnormal muscle recruitment patterns; notably, the transverse abdominis and multifidus activation is diminished in patients with LBP (Emami et al., 2018). A similar delay in activation of the internal oblique, multifidus, and gluteus maximus was observed on the symptomatic side of individuals with sacroiliac joint pain. Some studies have demonstrated that multifidus atrophy was present in clients even in the absence of continued LBP (Hodges et al., 2006). Further, other studies have demonstrated that trunk extensor strength was correlated with LBP in collegiate wrestlers (Iwai et al., 2004). More studies have indicated that a bilateral imbalance in isometric strength of the hip extensors was related to the development of LBP (Arab et al., 2019). The loads, forces, and movements that occur about the lumbar spine are controlled by a considerable number of ligaments and muscles. The ligaments that surround the spine limit intersegmental motion, maintaining the integrity of the lumbar spine. These ligaments may fail when proper motion cannot be created, proper posture cannot be maintained, or excessive motion cannot be resisted by the surrounding musculature (Floyd, 2017). Therefore, decreasing the ability of local and global stabilizing muscles to produce adequate force can lead to ligamentous injury (Page et al., 2010).

DYNAMIC MALALIGNMENT

Decreased abdominal core neuromuscular control may contribute to increased valgus positioning of the lower extremity, which can lead to increased risk of knee injuries (Almeida et al., 2016). Several studies have demonstrated that training of the trunk and hip musculature may increase the control of hip adduction and internal rotation during functional activities and prevent dynamic malalignments and the potential injuries that arise from this impaired movement pattern (Araujo et al., 2017; Baldon et al., 2015; Cronstrom et al., 2016; Tsai et al., 2017).

LPHC Dysfunction and the Regional Interdependence Model

Dysfunction at the LPHC can have a negative effect on the kinetic chain. The LPHC allows for movement in and through the three cardinal planes of motion and serves as a vital locus of stability and force transmission between the upper and lower kinetic chains. The LPHC influences body regions above and below, making it a vital component of functional interdependence of other areas (Sueki et al., 2013). The dynamic and interconnected nature of the HMS means that internal and external forces provide both direct and indirect influence throughout the kinetic chain through multiple tissues (Neumann et al., 2016). The following sections discuss common influences of the LPHC on issues above and below.

Influences Above the LPHC

Moving above the LPHC, common injuries are often seen in the cervical spine (Parfrey et al., 2014) and cervicothoracic region (Caneiro et al., 2010). The ability to recruit shoulder musculature (Mısırlıoğlu et al., 2018), anterior translation of the humeral head (Joseph et al., 2014), and even the elbow (Laudner et al., 2019) are all related to LPHC dysfunction. Respiration has also been shown to be negatively affected by altered LPHC positioning (Hwang & Kim, 2018). Core stabilization training has shown to increase thickness of the diaphragm and improve LPHC stability (Dülger et al., 2018). The function of the appendicular skeleton relies greatly on the attachments, force transmissions, stabilization, and interplay of multiple factors regarding neuromotor control of the muscles, the LPHC, and the axial skeleton.

Influences Below the LPHC

Moving below the LPHC toward the knee, evidence indicates that weakness in the abdominal core, or LPHC muscles, is a significant risk factor for lower extremity overuse injuries (De Blaiser et al., 2019). Common injuries at the knee associated with the LPHC include patellar tendinopathy (jumper's knee; Silva et al., 2015), iliotibial band (IT-band) tendinitis (runner's knee; Mucha et al., 2017), patellofemoral pain syndrome (Foroughi et al., 2019), and anterior cruciate ligament (ACL) tears (Myer et al., 2012). The ability to stabilize the LPHC has been shown to decrease hip flexion, adduction, and rotation while minimizing knee valgus and subtalar joint movement during dynamic single-leg landing mechanics (Fatahi et al., 2019). Dynamic postural control, core muscle strength, and core muscle endurance are all significant risk factors for the development of overuse injuries in the lower extremity (De Blaiser et al., 2019). Additionally, voluntary recruitment of the transverse abdominis and internal obliques increased maximum voluntary contraction of the hip muscles during corrective hip strengthening exercises (Tsang et al., 2018). This suggests a coactivation of the deep abdominal musculature and hip musculature.

At the foot and ankle, common injuries that are related to LPHC dysfunction include plantar fasciitis (McClinton et al., 2018), Achilles tendinopathy (Habets et al., 2017), and medial tibial stress syndrome (Winkelmann et al., 2016). The fitness professional must remember to stay within their scope of practice when working with clients with these conditions and not attempt to treat the pain. The focus should be on providing assessments that lead to identification of imbalance, weakness, and dysfunction. With this information, Corrective Exercise Specialists can provide exercises that address shortened and overactive muscles as well as lengthened, and potentially underactive muscles, and start to create better balance, stability, and movement.

Applying the concept of regional interdependence practically, if the ankle is restricted and unable to move during the descent of a squat, the hip will be required to move more (relative flexibility; Fuglsang et al., 2017). If there is a lack of sagittal plane dorsiflexion at the ankle due to an overactive gastrocnemius and soleus, the LPHC will be forced to increase forward flexion to alter the body's center of gravity to maintain balance (**Figure 13-6**). Increasing range of motion (ROM) at the ankle allows for the trunk to be more upright and minimizes shearing forces in the trunk and may serve as a preventive strategy for future back injuries/problems (Fuglsang et al., 2017).

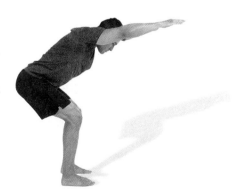

Figure 13-6 Excessive forward trunk lean

Assessment Results for the LPHC

The LPHC is perhaps the most regionally interdependent region in the body. Dysfunction at the ankles and knees below, as well as the thoracic region above, very often have their root causes related to positioning of the hip. For example, excessive anterior or posterior tilting of the pelvis creates direct responses in the position of the lumbar spine, extending or flexing it, respectively. Oftentimes, correcting a client's hip positioning back to neutral will improve impairments seen at the ankles, knees, and thoracic region of the back. **Table 13-2** provides a summary of the common assessment findings indicating potential dysfunction at the LPHC.

TABLE 13-2 LPHC Assessment Results	
Assessment	**Results**
Static posture	Hips extended
	Hips flexed
	Anterior pelvic tilt
	Posterior pelvic tilt
	Excessive lumbar lordosis
	Reduced lumbar lordosis (flattened lumbar spine)
Transitional and loaded movement	Asymmetric weight shift
	Excessive anterior pelvic tilt
	Excessive posterior pelvic tilt
	Excessive forward trunk lean
	Inward trunk rotation (single-leg and split squat)
	Outward trunk rotation (single-leg and split squat)
	Squat improves with hands on hips (address latissimus dorsi)
	Squat does not improve with hands on hips (address core stabilizers)
	Squat does not improve with heels elevated
Dynamic movement	Asymmetric weight shift
	Excessive anterior pelvic tilt
	Excessive posterior pelvic tilt
	Excessive forward trunk lean
	Excessive trunk motion (Davies test)
Mobility assessment Active knee extension, active knee flexion, ankle dorsiflexion, hip abduction and external rotation, seated hip internal and external rotation, lumbar flexion and extension, modified Thomas test, shoulder flexion	Limited knee flexion or extension ROM
	Limited lumbar flexion or extension ROM
	Limited hip abduction or adduction ROM
	Limited hip extension ROM
	Limited hip internal or external rotation ROM
	Limited dorsiflexion ROM
	Limited shoulder flexion ROM

Static LPHC Posture

During static postural assessment, Corrective Exercise Specialists will compare their client's posture to the postural archetypes described by Janda's postural distortion syndromes, Kendall's spinal postures, and pes planus distortion syndrome. Although the LPHC is the focus of this chapter's corrective programming, Corrective Exercise Specialists should look at the kinetic chain checkpoints above (e.g., shoulders, neck, and head) and below (e.g., knee, foot, and ankle) to determine their influence on the LPHC.

Static postural assessment shines a spotlight on the Regional Interdependence (RI) model because every one of the identified postural distortion patterns contains some form of incorrect alignment at the LPHC. Lower crossed and layered crossed syndromes both contain an anterior tilt of the pelvis with excessive lumbar lordosis, as do Kendall's lordotic and kyphosis-lordosis postures (**Figure 13-7**).

Conversely, sway-back and flat-back postures both have a posterior pelvic tilt, as do some individuals who align to Janda's upper crossed syndrome, where rounding of the upper back can be responded to at the lumbar spine with increased flexion that visually flattens out the low back (**Figure 13-8**). Additionally, pes planus distortion syndrome has the hallmark static malalignment of an anteriorly tilted pelvis.

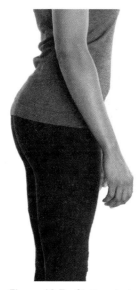

Figure 13-7 Static anterior pelvic tilt with excessive lordosis

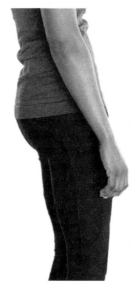

Figure 13-8 Static posterior pelvic tilt with lumbar flattening

Transitional Movement Assessments

Based on the collective information obtained from the static postural assessment, the Corrective Exercise Specialist will have a high-level estimation of which muscles might be overactive/shortened and which ones are underactive/lengthened. Occasionally, clients might have relatively impairment-free static posture; however, when in motion, active muscle imbalances may come to light. With essentially all movement having some interaction with the LPHC, the transitional movement assessments provide objective information from which to design effective corrective exercise programs.

OVERHEAD SQUAT ASSESSMENT

Many of the common movement impairments observed during the overhead squat assessment (OHSA) will be associated with LPHC dysfunction, because the squat movement requires optimal hip mobility. Similar to the postural distortion patterns used for static assessment, movement impairments observed at the hip may be caused by dysfunction of LPHC structures (e.g., muscles of the hip) or by dysfunction of distal segments of the body. The primary movement impairments observed at the hip include excessive anterior pelvic tilt, excessive posterior pelvic tilt, excessive forward trunk lean, and an asymmetric weight shift.

Focusing on the structures of the LPHC, an anterior pelvic tilt may be linked with overactive/shortened hip flexors and underactive abdominal muscles (**Figure 13-9**), whereas a posterior pelvic tilt (**Figure 13-10**) is associated with overactive/shortened hip extensors (e.g., hamstrings, adductor magnus) and underactivity of the hip flexors, spinal extensors, and latissimus dorsi. It is worth noting, that overactivity/shortening of the gluteus maximus is rare in the greater population due to most modern careers requiring extended periods of time seated at a computer or behind the wheel of a vehicle.

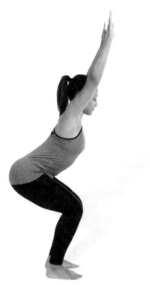

Figure 13-9   Anterior pelvic tilt

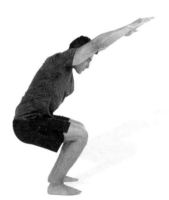

Figure 13-10   Posterior pelvic tilt

Excessive forward lean of the trunk (**Figure 13-11**) and an asymmetric weight shift (**Figure 13-12**) are typically associated with dysfunction located outside of the LPHC. Although excessive forward lean can be caused by an overactive/shortened rectus abdominis in some rare cases, it is much more frequently a relative flexibility response to overactive/shortened calf

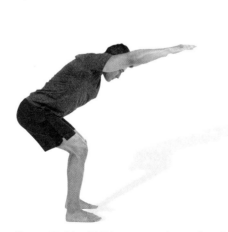

Figure 13-11   OHSA: excessive forward trunk lean

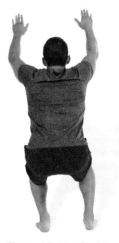

Figure 13-12   OHSA: asymmetric weight shift

muscles that make for limited dorsiflexion ROM. The squat movement requires efficient triple flexion of the lower extremity, and when the ankle cannot dorsiflex as much as it should, the body responds by flexing more at the hip instead, causing the entire trunk to fall forward.

Asymmetric weight shift is similar, in that it can be caused by dysfunction of muscles attached to the LPHC (e.g., adductors, TFL) or dysfunction at distal locations on the body (e.g., calf muscles). While pelvic tilt is indicative of muscle imbalance in the sagittal plane (i.e., anterior and posterior muscle imbalance), an asymmetric weight shift represents a frontal plane dysfunction, where muscles on the left and right side of the body are out of balance, specifically in the lower extremity.

OHSA HEELS-ELEVATED MODIFICATION

The purpose of the heels-elevated modification is to determine the influence the ankle has on the rest of the kinetic chain. Compensations at the LPHC may be related to a lack of ankle dorsiflexion. For example, if a client demonstrates an excessive forward trunk lean, it might be caused by short/overactive hip flexors or abdominal muscles or by a lack of ankle dorsiflexion resulting from reduced plantar flexor and Achilles tendon length. If the heels-elevated modification corrects the excessive forward trunk lean, then the root cause is likely a lack of ankle dorsiflexion. If elevating the heels does not improve the excessive forward trunk lean, then there is most likely a combination of overactivity in anterior LPHC muscles with underactivity of posterior muscles that hold the torso upright.

Elevating the heels places the ankle in a more plantar flexed position, thus reducing the influence of the foot and ankle complex on the squat movement (**Figure 13-13**). For individuals with a lack of dorsiflexion ROM, beginning their squat in a state of plantar flexion creates a greater available dorsiflexion ROM than when starting with a neutral ankle position, meaning that less relative flexibility needs to occur at the hip to accomplish the triple flexion needed for the squat movement. If elevating the heels does not improve OHSA performance, then this is an indication that observed movement impairments are related to muscle imbalances in the LPHC.

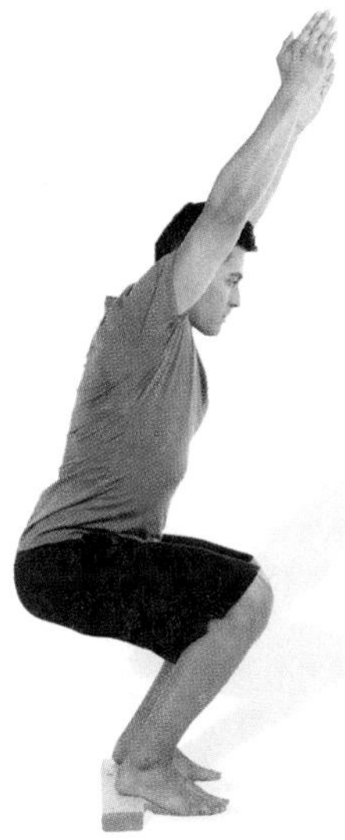

Figure 13-13 Heels-elevated OHSA

HANDS-ON-HIPS MODIFICATION

In situations where an individual has an anterior pelvic tilt (excessive lumbar lordosis), the movement impairment might be caused by a short and overactive hip flexor complex or latissimus dorsi. The anterior pelvic tilt might also be a consequence of limited thoracic extension. To identify whether the movement impairment is coming from the thoracic spine (above) or the LPHC (below), the hands-on-hips modification to the OHSA should be used.

Placing the hands on the hips reduces tension in the latissimus dorsi to allow more ROM throughout the trunk and reduces the extension moment of the thoracic spine. If the anterior pelvic tilt is improved with the hands on the hips (**Figure 13-14**), then mobility restrictions above the hip might be responsible for the lumbar lordosis. For these individuals, protocols to correct arms falling forward should help improve their lumbar dynamic posture as well. If the hands on the hips does not correct the excessive lumbar lordosis, then it is most likely primarily due to the muscle activity (or inactivity) contributing to an anterior pelvic tilt.

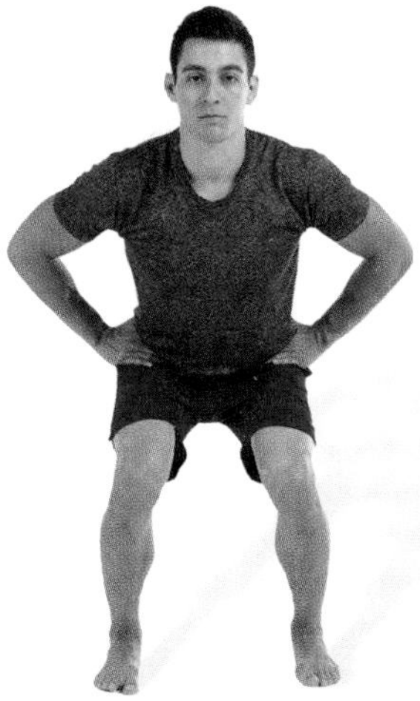

Figure 13-14 Hands-on-hips OHSA

SINGLE-LEG SQUAT ASSESSMENT

The single-leg squat assessment (SLSA) is also an important transitional movement assessment to perform to observe potential compensations at the LPHC. For individuals who can perform the SLSA, it might provide a deeper look into the functioning of the LPHC. Having to squat on one leg may show dysfunction not evident when squatting on two feet, because the reduced base of support increases the demand for frontal and transverse plane stability. The key compensations to look for when performing the SLSA are an asymmetric weight shift (**Figure 13-15**) and inward or outward trunk rotation (**Figures 13-16** and **13-17**).

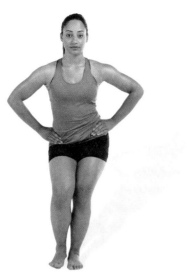

Figure 13-15A SLSA: asymmetric weight shift A

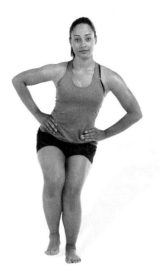

Figure 13-15B SLSA: asymmetric weight shift B

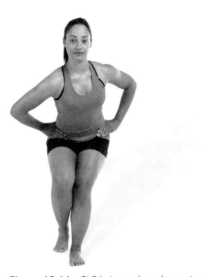

Figure 13-16 SLSA: inward trunk rotation

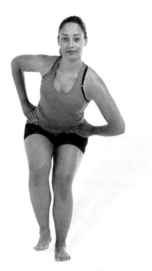

Figure 13-17 SLSA: outward trunk rotation

SPLIT-SQUAT MODIFICATION

If the SLSA is difficult for the client, the split-squat modification can be used. The narrow stance with both feet on the ground provides more stability but still provides more insight into unilateral compensations that may have been observed during the OHSA. Just like with the SLSA, key compensations to observe at the LPHC include asymmetric weight shift, inward and outward trunk rotation, and excessive anterior or posterior pelvic tilt.

LOADED MOVEMENT ASSESSMENT

Clients who demonstrate proper static and dynamic posture under body weight alone can be progressed to using loaded variants of primary movement patterns. This provides more challenge to the musculature and can help draw attention to any remaining imbalance at the joints.

The loaded squat is highly beneficial for observing LPHC movement in individuals at this point of physical readiness. Movement impairments that surface during a loaded squat might be related to the underactivity of key LPHC muscles. For example, if a client can maintain a neutral pelvis during the OHSA and SLSA, but then demonstrates an anterior tilt during a loaded squat assessment, hip extensor musculature activation (e.g., gluteus maximus) can be prioritized in the client's program. It is important to remember, however, that targeted mobility testing should be used to confirm or deny observations made during transitional assessments.

 TRAINING TIP

The squat is not the only loaded primary movement pattern that can demonstrate LPHC impairment. Any time someone is pushing, pulling, overhead pressing, rotating, or hinging, the muscles of the LPHC are at work to help stabilize the trunk and protect the spine. Always keep an eye out for excessive anterior or posterior tilting of the pelvis while coaching and cueing all exercises in a client's workout, especially those that are closed-chain and transfer forces through the LPHC.

Dynamic Movement Assessments

Dynamic movement assessments can help Corrective Exercise Specialists see how LPHC movement impairments influence functional movement patterns. Because the positions of the pelvis and lumbar spine influence the movement of all structures above and below the LPHC, choosing to perform dynamic assessments can be beneficial for clients with athletic performance goals. The depth jump assessment can be used, similar to how loaded assessments are used, in place of the OHSA after clients demonstrate sufficient strength and neuromuscular control with the transitional movement assessments. Because clients further along in their corrective programs have fewer flexibility deficits remaining, the eccentric landing focus of the depth jump can preferentially identify muscles that lack neuromuscular activation and control. In both the depth jump and gait assessments, the same pelvic tilt and asymmetric weight shift impairments seen in transitional assessments are also observed. In the Davies test, maintaining the stability and control of the trunk during performance is an indicator of LPHC movement quality. Impairments such as anterior tilting (hips sagging toward the floor) or posterior tilting (hips rounding toward the ceiling) of the pelvis or excessive trunk motion may be observed during testing.

Mobility Assessments

If the client demonstrates impairments related to the LPHC in the static posture assessment, movement assessments, or both, mobility assessments for the LPHC should be performed to better pinpoint the muscle imbalances to be corrected with the Corrective Exercise Continuum. For example, if a client aligns with one or more of the static postural distortion patterns (e.g., Janda's syndromes and Kendall's postures) and then demonstrates an anterior or posterior pelvic tilt, then lumbar flexion and extension tests, knee flexion and extension, hip abduction and external rotation, and the modified Thomas test may be assessed to pinpoint which muscles affecting LPHC movement warrant corrective programming.

Recall that if the client "passes" the mobility assessments, then the most likely cause of the observed movement impairment is underactivity of select muscles.

Corrective Strategies for the LPHC

The integrated assessment process will reveal movement compensation patterns that may warrant the implementation of corrective programming for the LPHC. Once the static, movement, and mobility assessments have been performed and impairments have been identified, the corrective exercise strategy can be developed using the NASM Corrective Exercise Continuum. Most programs also incorporate proprioceptive or balance training with or without functional movements on a daily basis or multiple times per week. See **Table 13-3**.

TABLE 13-3 Common Corrective Exercise Programming Selections for the LPHC

Phase	Modality	Muscle(s)/Exercise	Acute Training Variables
Inhibit	Self-myofascial rolling	Adductor complex Adductor magnus Biceps femoris Gastrocnemius/soleus Hamstrings complex Latissimus dorsi Piriformis Rectus femoris TFL	Hold areas of discomfort for 30 to 60 seconds Perform four to six repetitions of active joint movement
Lengthen	Static stretching or neuromuscular stretching	Abdominal complex Adductor complex Adductor magnus Biceps femoris Gastrocnemius/soleus Hamstrings complex Hip flexor complex Piriformis Spinal extensor complex TFL	Static: 30-second hold Neuromuscular stretching: 7- to 10-second isometric contraction 30-second static hold
Activate	Isolated strengthening	Adductor complex Anterior tibialis Core stabilizers Gluteus maximus Gluteus medius Hamstrings complex Hip flexor complex Latissimus dorsi Rectus abdominis Spinal extensor complex	10 to 15 reps with 4-second eccentric contraction, 2-second isometric contraction at end-range, and 1-second concentric contraction
Integrate*	Integrated dynamic movement	Ball wall squat with overhead press Cable squat to row Lateral tube walking Lunge to overhead press Step-up to overhead cable press	10 to 15 reps under control

*NOTE: Progress and regress as needed to match client ability, work capacity, and needs.

Common Exercise Selections for the LPHC

Exercises used for LPHC corrective strategies look to improve commonly observed movement impairments such as excessive anterior or posterior pelvic tilt, asymmetric weight shift, and excessive forward trunk lean. Oftentimes, multiple movement impairments occur together (such as excessive forward trunk lean and posterior pelvic tilt) and may benefit from exercises that address both, based on the integrated assessment process. As such, the Corrective Exercise Specialist may create a program that efficiently addresses multiple impairments. For example, programming for local core stabilizer and gluteal activation may positively influence more than one impairment observed in the client. While not an exhaustive list, the following are some exercises that may be used when creating corrective programs to address LPHC movement quality.

INHIBIT: SELF-MYOFASCIAL ROLLING

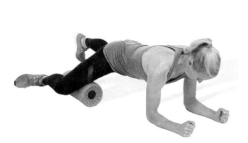

Adductor complex

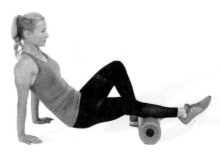

Gastrocnemius/soleus

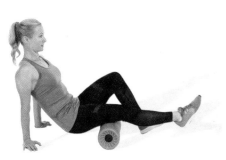

Hamstrings complex

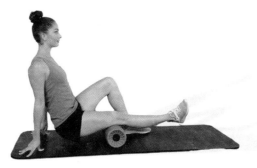

Biceps femoris

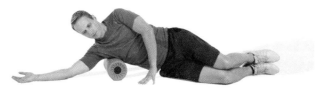

Latissimus dorsi

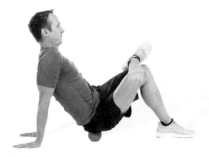

Piriformis

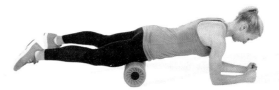

Rectus femoris

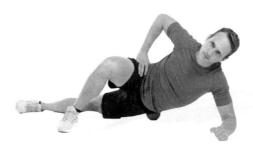

Tensor fascia latae

LENGTHEN: STATIC AND/OR NEUROMUSCULAR STRETCHING (NMS)

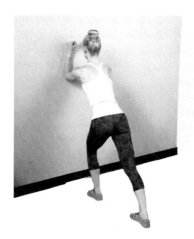

Static gastrocnemius stretch

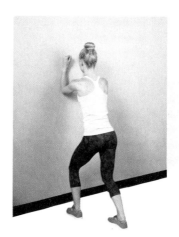

Static soleus stretch

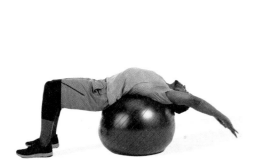

Static ball abdominal stretch

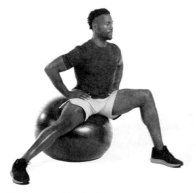

Static seated ball adductor stretch

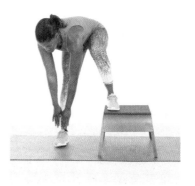

Static adductor magnus stretch

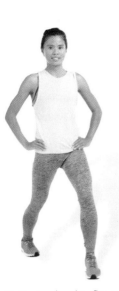

Static standing hip flexor stretch—start

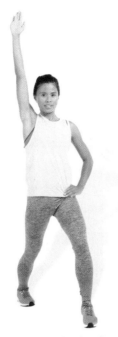

Static standing hip flexor stretch—movement

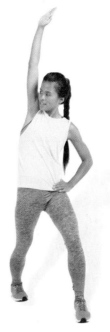

Static standing hip flexor stretch—finish

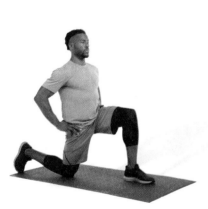

Static kneeling hip flexor stretch—start

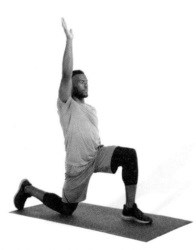

Static kneeling hip flexor stretch—movement

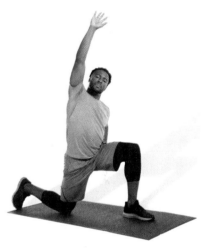

Static kneeling hip flexor stretch—finish

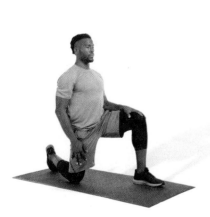

Static tensor fascia latae stretch—start

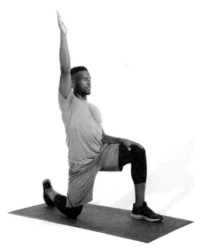

Static tensor fascia latae stretch—movement

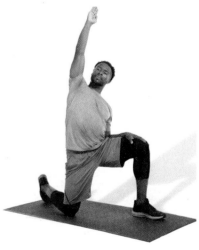

Static tensor fascia latae stretch—finish

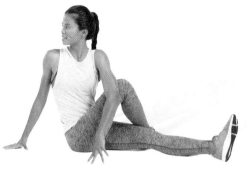

Static erector spinae (spinal extensors) stretch

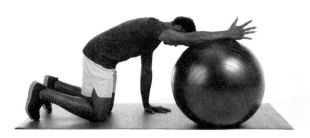

Static ball latissimus dorsi stretch

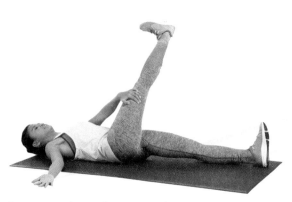

Static supine biceps femoris stretch

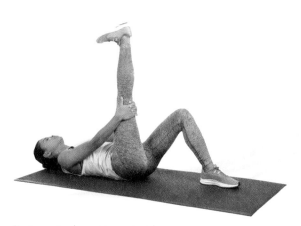

Static supine hamstrings stretch

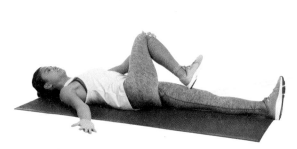

Static piriformis stretch

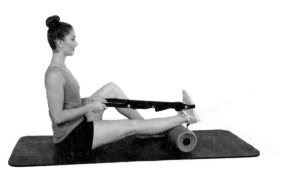

Self NMS gastrocnemius/soleus

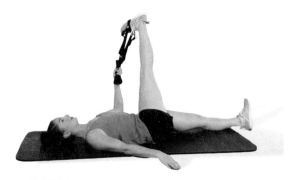

Self NMS biceps femoris

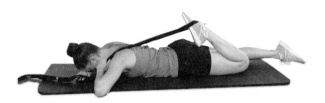

Self NMS prone quadriceps

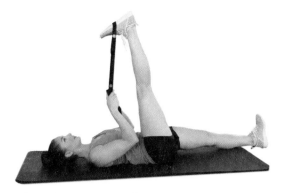

Self NMS hamstrings complex

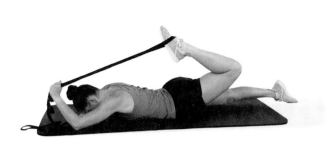

Self NMS hip flexor complex

ACTIVATE: ISOLATED STRENGTHENING

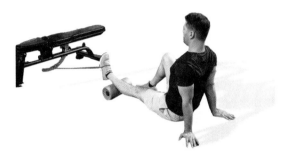

Anterior tibialis—start

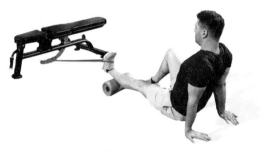

Anterior tibialis—finish

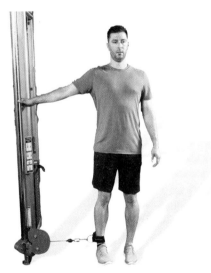

Adductors—start

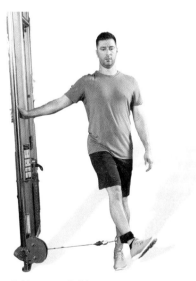

Adductors—finish

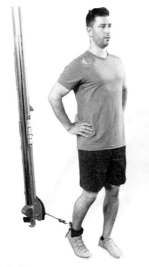

Hip flexors—start

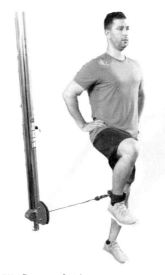

Hip flexors—finish

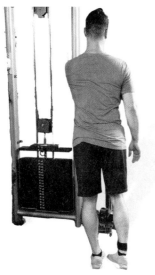

Medial hamstrings complex—start

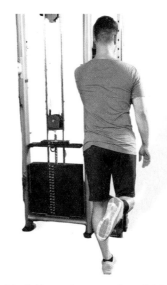

Medial hamstrings complex—finish

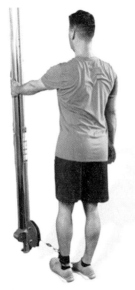

Gluteus maximus—start

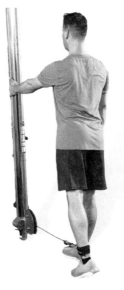

Gluteus maximus—finish

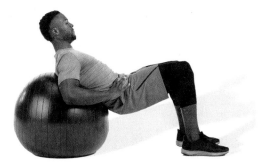

Ball bridge—start

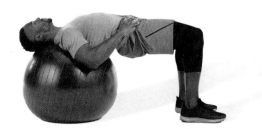

Ball bridge—finish

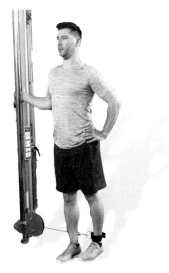

Gluteus medius—start

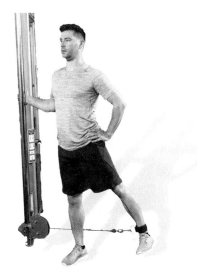

Gluteus medius—finish

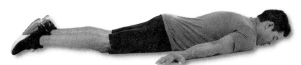

Floor cobra (emphasizing erector spinae)—start

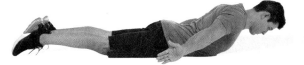

Floor cobra (emphasizing erector spinae)—finish

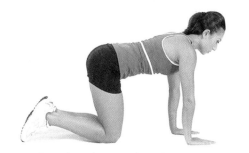

Quadruped arm/opposite leg raise—start

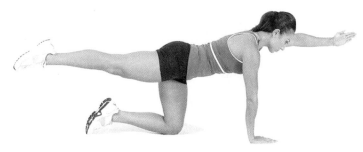

Quadruped arm/opposite leg raise—finish

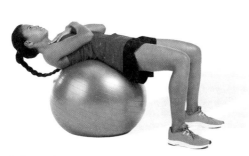

Ball crunch—start

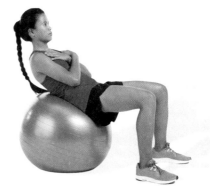

Ball crunch—finish

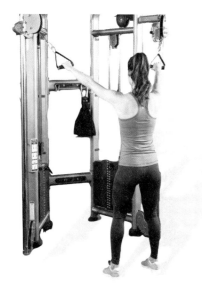

Standing cable lat pulldown—start

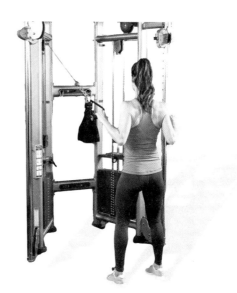

Standing cable lat pulldown—finish

INTEGRATE: DYNAMIC MOVEMENT PROGRESSIONS

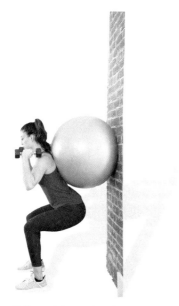

Ball squat to overhead press—start

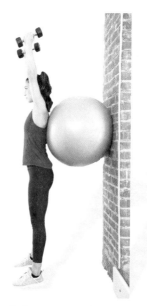

Ball squat to overhead press—finish

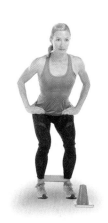
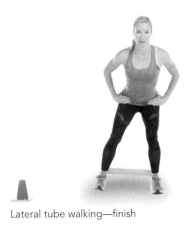

Lateral tube walking—start

Lateral tube walking—finish

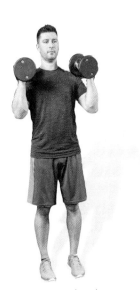
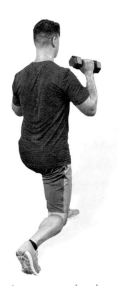
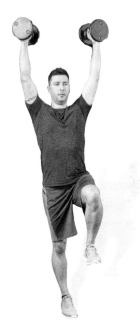

Lunge to overhead press—start

Lunge to overhead press—movement

Lunge to overhead press—finish

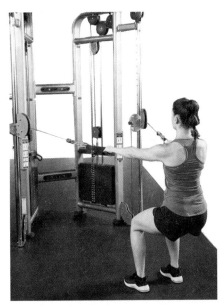
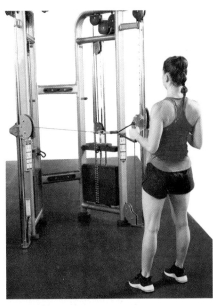

Squat to row—start

Squat to row—finish

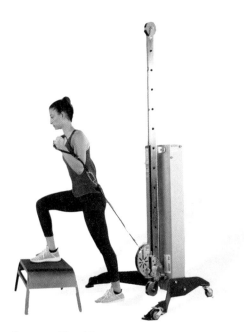

Step-up with cable press—start

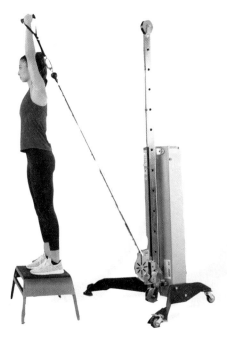

Step-up with cable press—finish

Excessive Forward Trunk Lean

The Corrective Exercise Specialist should be selective regarding the techniques recommended to each client. To improve client adherence, it is recommended that the Corrective Exercise Specialist employ as few exercises as are effective in each phase of the continuum. The following exercises are most used for the compensation of excessive forward trunk lean. The broad objectives of the program are to improve ideal dorsiflexion and hip extension as well as the body's ability to decelerate and control hip flexion. When applied systematically, the Corrective Exercise Continuum contributes to efficient neuromuscular control and proper alignment of the LPHC during movement.

Recall that if the heels-elevated modification improved the squat, then corrective strategies for the foot and ankle complex may take priority and have the most influence on movement quality.

PHASE 1: INHIBIT

Key regions to inhibit include the soleus, gastrocnemius, and hip flexor complex (rectus femoris and TFL). Reducing tension in these tissues will facilitate extensibility, allowing appropriate levels of ideal dorsiflexion and hip extension to be achieved.

PHASE 2: LENGTHEN

Key lengthening exercises via static and/or neuromuscular stretches include the gastrocnemius/soleus, hip flexor complex, and abdominal complex (particularly if lumbar flexion is concurrently observed). Reduction of tissue resistance to stretch allows these target areas to lengthen properly during movement, contributing to proper mechanics at the foot and ankle and LPHC.

PHASE 3: ACTIVATE

Key activation exercises via isolated strengthening exercises include the anterior tibialis, gluteus maximus, and intrinsic core stabilizers. The objective of the selected activation exercises is to improve the intramuscular coordination of tissues considered underactive based on the integrated assessment process. Muscles specific to the foot and ankle will be responsible for concentrically creating greater dorsiflexion. Muscles specific to the LPHC will be responsible for concentrically creating greater hip extension and spinal stability during movement patterns.

Select exercises appropriate to the ability and needs of the client (e.g., quadruped opposite arm/ leg raise vs. plank variations).

PHASE 4: INTEGRATE

An integration exercise could first include uniplanar exercises (sagittal plane) and then progress to multiplanar exercises (frontal and transverse). An appropriate exercise may be to begin with a ball squat. This exercise will help teach proper hip hinging while maintaining proper lumbo-pelvic control as well as providing additional dorsiflexion at the ankle by stepping slightly forward from the ball. Further, the pressure applied to the ball, initially, will assist in activating the muscles needed to maintain an upright torso. As the individual progresses, load may be added so the individual performs a ball squat to overhead press. Adding the overhead press component will place an additional challenge to the core. The individual can then progress to step-ups to overhead presses (sagittal, frontal, and transverse planes), then to lunges to overhead presses (sagittal, frontal, and transverse planes), and then to single-leg squats to overhead presses. See **Table 13-4** for program recommendations.

TABLE 13-4	Sample Corrective Exercise Program for the LPHC: Excessive Forward Trunk Lean		
Phase	**Modality**	**Muscle(s)/Exercise**	**Acute Training Variables**
Inhibit	Self-myofascial rolling	Gastrocnemius/soleus Rectus femoris TFL	Hold areas of discomfort for 30 to 60 seconds Perform four to six repetitions of active joint movement 90 to 120 seconds per muscle group
Lengthen	Static stretching	Abdominal complex Gastrocnemius/soleus Hip flexor complex	Static: 30-second hold
Activate	Isolated strengthening	Anterior tibialis Core stabilizers Gluteus maximus	10 to 15 reps with 4-second eccentric contraction, 2-second isometric contraction at end-range, and 1-second concentric contraction
Integrate*	Integrated dynamic movement	Ball wall squat with overhead press	10 to 15 reps under control

*NOTE: Progress and regress as needed to match client ability, work capacity, and needs.

Excessive Anterior Pelvic Tilt—Low Back Arches

The following exercises are most often used for the compensation of excessive anterior pelvic tilt. The broad objectives of the program are to improve hip extension and improve the body's ability to stabilize the LPHC. When applied systematically, the Corrective Exercise Continuum contributes to efficient neuromuscular control and proper alignment of the LPHC during movement.

Recall that if the heels-elevated modification improved the squat, then corrective strategies for the foot and ankle complex may be warranted as well. Or, if the hands-on-hips modification improved the squat, then corrective strategies for the shoulder, particularly the latissimus dorsi, may be warranted.

PHASE 1: INHIBIT

Key regions to inhibit via foam rolling include the anterior fibers of the adductor complex as well as the hip flexor complex (psoas, rectus femoris, and TFL), spinal extensors, and latissimus dorsi. Reducing tension in these tissues will facilitate extensibility, allowing appropriate levels of hip extension to be achieved.

PHASE 2: LENGTHEN

Key lengthening exercises via static and/or neuromuscular stretches include the hip flexor complex, spinal extensors, and latissimus dorsi. Reduction of tissue resistance to stretch allows these target areas to lengthen properly during movement, contributing to proper mechanics at the LPHC.

PHASE 3: ACTIVATE

Key activation exercises via isolated strengthening exercises include the gluteus maximus and abdominal complex. The objective of the selected activation exercises is to improve the intramuscular coordination of tissues considered underactive based on the integrated assessment process. Specific to the LPHC, these muscles will be responsible for concentrically creating greater hip extension and spinal stability during movement patterns.

PHASE 4: INTEGRATE

An integration exercise could first include uniplanar exercises (sagittal plane) and then progress to multiplanar exercises (frontal and transverse). An integration exercise implemented for this compensation could also be a ball squat to overhead press, using the same integrated progression that was provided for the excessive forward trunk lean programming. It is important to place the ball above the lumbar curve to prevent the individual from arching over the ball, thus potentially exacerbating the compensation. Squat to row progressions may also be useful to enforce proper coordination and activation of the posterior oblique subsystem. See **Table 13-5** for programming recommendations.

TABLE 13-5	Sample Corrective Exercise Program for the LPHC: Excessive Anterior Pelvic Tilt		
Phase	**Modality**	**Muscle(s)/Exercise**	**Acute Training Variables**
Inhibit	Self-myofascial rolling	Rectus femoris Latissimus dorsi TFL	Hold areas of discomfort for 30 to 60 seconds Perform four to six repetitions of active joint movement 90 to 120 seconds per muscle group
Lengthen	Static stretching	Hip flexor complex Latissimus dorsi Erector spinae	Static: 30-second hold
Activate	Isolated strengthening	Abdominal complex/core stabilizers Gluteus maximus	10 to 15 reps with 4-second eccentric contraction, 2-second isometric contraction at end-range, and 1-second concentric contraction
Integrate*	Integrated dynamic movement	Squat to row	10 to 15 reps under control

*NOTE: Progress and regress as needed to match client ability, work capacity, and needs.

Excessive Posterior Pelvic Tilt—Low Back Flattens

The following exercises are most commonly used for the compensation of excessive posterior pelvic tilt. The broad objectives of the program are to improve hip flexion and improve the body's ability to stabilize the LPHC. When applied systematically, the Corrective Exercise Continuum contributes to efficient neuromuscular control and proper alignment of the LPHC during movement.

Recall that if the heels-elevated modification improved the squat, then corrective strategies for the foot and ankle may be warranted.

PHASE 1: INHIBIT

Key regions to inhibit via foam rolling include the hamstrings complex, piriformis, and adductor magnus. Reducing tension in these tissues will facilitate extensibility, allowing appropriate levels of hip flexion to be achieved.

PHASE 2: LENGTHEN

Key lengthening exercises include the hamstrings complex, piriformis, abdominal complex (rectus abdominis and external obliques in particular), and adductor magnus. Reduction of tissue resistance to stretch allows these target areas to lengthen properly during movement, contributing to proper mechanics at the LPHC.

PHASE 3: ACTIVATE

Key activation exercises via isolated strengthening exercises include the gluteus maximus, hip flexors, and spinal extensors. The objective of the selected activation exercises is to improve the intramuscular coordination of tissues considered underactive based on the integrated assessment process. Specific to the LPHC, these muscles will be responsible for concentrically creating greater hip flexion and spinal stability during movement patterns. While it is counterintuitive to activate the gluteus maximus given an excessive posterior tilt, it is unlikely the gluteus maximus is truly overactive. It is more likely that the adductor magnus and piriformis are synergistically dominant while compensating for an underactive gluteus maximus, contributing to posterior tilting of the pelvis.

PHASE 4: INTEGRATE

An integration exercise could first include uniplanar exercises (sagittal plane) and then progress to multiplanar exercises (frontal and transverse). An integration exercise implemented for this compensation could also be a ball squat to overhead press, using the same integrated progression that was provided for the excessive forward trunk lean programming. Ensure that the ball is above the lumbar curve. Here, the goal is to encourage the individual to produce their own curve (i.e., neutral alignment) versus conforming to the shape of the ball. See **Table 13-6** for programming recommendations.

Asymmetric Weight Shift

The following exercises are most commonly used for the compensation of asymmetric weight shift. The broad objectives of the program are to address the asymmetries for improved movement and stabilization of the LPHC. When applied systematically, the Corrective Exercise Continuum contributes to efficient neuromuscular control and proper alignment of the LPHC during movement. An additional way to visualize the asymmetric weight shift is to view it as a holistic frontal plane control issue. The Corrective Exercise Specialist will then be addressing the efficiency of the lateral subsystem in particular as they create a program.

Recall that if the heels-elevated modification improved the squat, then corrective strategies for the foot and ankle complex may be warranted.

TABLE 13-6 Sample Corrective Exercise Program for the LPHC: Excessive Posterior Pelvic Tilt

Phase	Modality	Muscle(s)/Exercise	Acute Training Variables
Inhibit	Self-myofascial rolling	Adductor magnus Hamstrings complex Piriformis	Hold areas of discomfort for 30 to 60 seconds Perform four to six repetitions of active joint movement 90 to 120 seconds per muscle group
Lengthen	Static stretching	Abdominal complex Adductor magnus Hamstrings complex	Static: 30-second hold
Activate	Isolated strengthening	Erector spinae Gluteus maximus Hip flexors	10 to 15 reps with 4-second eccentric contraction, 2-second isometric contraction at end-range, and 1-second concentric contraction
Integrate*	Integrated dynamic movement	Ball wall squat with overhead press	10 to 15 reps under control

*NOTE: Progress and regress as needed to match client ability, work capacity, and needs.

PHASE 1: INHIBIT

Key regions to inhibit via foam rolling include the same-side (side toward shift) adductors and TFL and the opposite-side (side away from shift) piriformis and biceps femoris. The gastrocnemius and soleus can also play a major factor in this compensation. As the client descends into the squat, if one of the ankle joints lacks sagittal plane dorsiflexion, this forces the body to shift away from the restricted side and move to the side capable of greater motion. For example, if the left ankle is restricted, it can force the individual to the right to find that ROM. Reducing tension in these tissues will facilitate extensibility, allowing appropriate levels of mobility to be achieved.

MUSCLES TO BE INHIBITED
- Opposite-side biceps femoris
- Opposite-side gastrocnemius/soleus
- Opposite-side piriformis
- Same-side adductor complex
- Same-side TFL

PHASE 2: LENGTHEN

Key lengthening exercises via static and/or neuromuscular stretches include the same-side adductors and TFL and the opposite-side biceps femoris, gastrocnemius/soleus, and piriformis. Reduction of tissue resistance to stretch allows these target areas to lengthen properly during movement, contributing to proper mechanics at the LPHC.

MUSCLES TO BE LENGTHENED

- Opposite-side biceps femoris
- Opposite-side gastrocnemius/soleus
- Opposite-side piriformis
- Same-side adductor complex
- Same-side TFL

PHASE 3: ACTIVATE

Key activation exercises via isolated strengthening exercises include the same-side gluteus medius, the opposite-side adductor complex, and the core stabilizers. The objective of the selected activation exercises is to improve the intramuscular coordination of tissues considered underactive based on the integrated assessment process. Specific to the LPHC, these muscles will be responsible for concentrically creating greater hip and spinal stability and encourage symmetry during movement patterns.

MUSCLES TO BE ACTIVATED

- Core stabilizers
- Opposite-side adductor complex
- Same-side gluteus medius

PHASE 4: INTEGRATE

An integration exercise could first include uniplanar exercises (sagittal plane) and then progress to multiplanar exercises (frontal and transverse) with a focus on encouraging frontal plane control. An integration exercise that could be implemented for this compensation could be a step-up to overhead cable press, progressing to include multidirectional resistance. See **Table 13-7** for programming recommendations.

TABLE 13-7	Sample Corrective Exercise Program for the LPHC: Asymmetric Weight Shift		
Phase	**Modality**	**Muscle(s)/Exercise**	**Acute Training Variables**
Inhibit	Self-myofascial rolling	Adductors (same side) Biceps femoris (opposite side) Piriformis (opposite side) TFL (same side)	Hold areas of discomfort for 30 to 60 seconds Perform four to six repetitions of active joint movement 90 to 120 seconds per muscle group
Lengthen	Static stretching	Adductors (same side) Piriformis (opposite side) TFL (same side)	Static: 30-second hold
Activate	Isolated strengthening	Adductors (opposite side) Core stabilizers Gluteus medius (same side)	10 to 15 reps with 4-second eccentric contraction, 2-second isometric contraction at end-range, and 1-second concentric contraction
Integrate*	Integrated dynamic movement	Step-up to overhead cable press	10 to 15 reps under control

*NOTE: Progress and regress as needed to match client ability, work capacity, and needs.

Programming for Trunk Rotation

Sometimes during the single-leg squat, the torso may be seen to rotate inward or outward. Typically, this is due to underactive gluteus maximus and medius muscles paired with overactive hip internal or external rotator muscles in the stance leg. When an inward rotation is seen, the TFL and adductor complex (hip internal rotators) are likely overactive. When outward rotation is seen, the piriformis (a hip external rotator), posterior fibers of the adductor magnus, and biceps femoris are most likely overactive.

The probable overactive/underactive muscles for internal trunk rotation are essentially the same ones that also cause knee valgus. In fact, those two movement impairments are quite often seen together, and it can oftentimes be assumed that clients with noticeable knee valgus on the OHSA will also exhibit an internal trunk rotation during the SLSA. If an inward trunk rotation is seen on the SLSA, corrective protocols for knee valgus can be applied to whichever side of the body the rotation is seen (i.e., the stance leg being tested with the SLSA) to help remedy the excessive transverse plane movement.

An outward trunk rotation on the SLSA is more rarely seen, but can often be addressed by inhibiting the piriformis, activating the gluteus maximus and medius, and practicing proper form for two-leg and single-leg squat movement patterns (i.e., integration).

Common Issues Associated with the LPHC

Many of the common injuries associated with the LPHC include low-back pain, sacroiliac joint dysfunction, muscle strains, and pelvic floor dysfunction. However, the body is an interconnected chain, and compensation or movement impairment in the LPHC region can lead to dysfunctions in other areas of the body (Cheatham & Kreiswirth, 2014).

> ⚠️ **CRITICAL**
>
> This section is intended to provide general information about specific medical conditions for the LPHC. The information provided should not be used to diagnose any medical condition. The fitness professional should refer to the appropriate medical professional if a client needs a diagnosis of a potential medical condition. This will ensure client safety and proper scope of practice.

Low-Back Pain

The presence of low-back pain is significant in U.S. society, with up to 35% of individuals experiencing reduced activity due to chronic back conditions and approximately 7% of that number with back issues that persist for 6 months or more (U.S. Department of Health and Human Services, 2019). For clients in severe pain, it is paramount that the fitness professional refer them to a physician or medical professional. Low-back pain is, unfortunately, standard in our society. Low-back pain is very complex with several potential causes, which include, but are not limited to, muscle imbalances, decreased mobility, disc pathology, facet joint dysfunction, joint degeneration (spondylosis), and spinal instability (Cheatham & Kolber, 2016). The potential causes are commonly diagnosed by a medical professional who determines some type of management strategy that includes modification of activities, medications, referral to rehabilitation, and, at times, surgery.

The fitness professional can play a key role as part of the continuum of care for these clients. Often, these clients will return to the fitness setting after completing a rehabilitation program. The fitness professional can continue to work on related factors that can affect the client's low-back pain without working on the low back directly, which may include improving motor control, mobility, isolated LPHC strength, lifting and ergonomics, and client education. For example, there are numerous relationships between low-back pain and interventions that fitness professionals can provide. Poor passive hip extension (Roach et al., 2015), increased anterior pelvic tilt (Król et al., 2017), increased lumbar lordosis (Hosseinifar et al., 2017), limited LPHC stability (McGill, 2016; Mitra & Mande, 2019; Puntumetakul et al., 2018), weak gluteus maximus (Amabile et al., 2017), weak gluteus medius (Cooper et al., 2016), too much sitting (Brakenridge et al., 2018), awkward trunk postures (Nourollahi et al., 2018), altered motor control of LPHC musculature (Roshini & Leo Aseer, 2019), and pelvic floor dysfunction (Algudairi et al., 2019;

 GETTING TECHNICAL

Abdominal Bracing Versus Abdominal Hollowing

Much research supports the benefits of abdominal muscle activation techniques in those with low-back pain; namely, abdominal hollowing (or drawing in) and abdominal bracing.

Abdominal hollowing (or the draw-in maneuver) and abdominal bracing are both incorporated by therapists, trainers, and other exercise specialists to benefit persons with lumbar instability (Vaičienė et al., 2018). Professionals tend to pick one of these interventions while downplaying the validity and value of the other. Integrated training is based on implementing all evidence that works during the appropriate time with an understanding of how outcomes can be optimized for clients. The following is a brief review of the research surrounding abdominal hollowing and abdominal bracing to provide a better understanding of the evidence for their practical applications.

Studies suggest that isometric spinal stabilization training is superior to dynamic exercises at developing LPHC stiffness (Lee & McGill, 2015). Spinal stiffness is not the issue, however; the debate is whether abdominal hollowing or abdominal bracing is superior at creating stiffness and supporting the lumbar spine. Engagement of the transverse abdominis during abdominal bracing has shown to be highly effective at minimizing low-back pain (LBP) and increasing LPHC stability. Evidence shows that deep abdominal muscles are more activated with abdominal hollowing and surface muscles are more activated with abdominal bracing (Vaičienė et al., 2018). Hollowing has been shown to increase local spinal stabilizers (Kim & Oh, 2015; Lee et al., 2013, 2016; Suehiro et al., 2014) and LPHC stability while minimizing the facilitation of global muscle activity during exercise (Kahlaee et al., 2017; Suehiro et al., 2014). Abdominal hollowing was found superior to abdominal bracing for increasing LPHC stability and leg stiffness in hopping tasks (Dupeyron et al., 2013). Although it does seem that maintaining a neutral spine (Reeve & Dilley, 2009) and performing costodiaphragmatic (chest and belly) breathing is important to the optimization of muscle activation while performing abdominal hollowing (Ha et al., 2014), Maeo et al. (2013) note that abdominal bracing is one of the more effective techniques to activate the deep core musculature. During vertical jump landing, abdominal bracing has been shown to enhance pelvic stability, improve sensorimotor control and positioning of the lower extremity, and reduce biomechanical factors associated with ACL injury while protecting the lumbar spine (Haddas et al., 2016). Multiple data questions the efficacy of treating LBP solely using abdominal hollowing (Vasseljen et al., 2012; Wong et al., 2013). Monfort-Pañego et al. (2009) performed a literature synthesis on abdominal exercises using electromyographic (EMG) feedback and showed that biomechanical studies on spinal stability suggest that local and global muscles of the LPHC play a vital and harmonious role in achieving spinal stability. McGill (2016), arguably one of the top researchers on exercise and the spine, is not a proponent of abdominal hollowing and argues that the transverse abdominis should activate when abdominal bracing is done appropriately without the need to draw in the navel. He provides evidence that core stiffness is of more value when it comes to protecting the back (Lee & McGill, 2015).

So, which should a Corrective Exercise Specialist perform?

Evidence supporting both abdominal bracing and abdominal hollowing work to increase LPHC stabilization. We are not left with a debate on the efficacy of these two techniques but of application. Which application should we employ and when? In early stages of the training, cueing abdominal hollowing may be considered a good starting point to ensure transverse abdominis activation. However, abdominal bracing can be implemented immediately during core stabilization exercises to increase stiffness and minimize movement in the LPHC. The value of an integrated model is that professionals are not limited to just one technique but can implement any and all techniques that provide value and outcomes for their clients, which includes both abdominal hollowing and abdominal bracing.

Dufour et al., 2018) are all correlated with low-back pain. These are all factors that Corrective Exercise Specialists can address with their clients via exercises, cueing, and education. However, these strategies must be done within the fitness professional's scope of practice.

Intervertebral Disc Injury

The exact mechanism underlying injury to the intervertebral disc is unclear, but it is generally proposed that it is caused by a combination of motion with compressive loading. Increases in disc pressure and stress are influenced by the kinematics of the lumbar spine. Disc pressure increases with lumbar flexion and decreases in lordosis during the performance of activities. In addition, a combination of motions about the lumbar spine have been demonstrated to increase the strain placed on the discs and include flexion with lateral bending (Neumann et al., 2016). This combination of motions may generate an axial torque that some researchers have demonstrated to increase the initiation of disc herniation. Other researchers combined all these factors and were able to demonstrate that compression combined with bending and twisting moments about the disc contributed to earlier degeneration in compromised intervertebral discs. Pelvic asymmetry (iliac rotation asymmetry or sacroiliac joint asymmetry) has been shown to alter movement of the HMS in standing and sitting. Pelvic asymmetry alters static posture of the entire LPHC, which alters normal arthrokinematics (coupling movement of the spine; Sorensen et al., 2016). These changes in trunk kinematics were linked to nonspecific LBP (Jandre Reis & Macedo, 2015). It has also been demonstrated that hip rotation asymmetry, decreased hip internal rotation range of motion, is present in clients with sacroiliac joint dysfunction (Cibulka et al., 1998) (**Figure 13-18**).

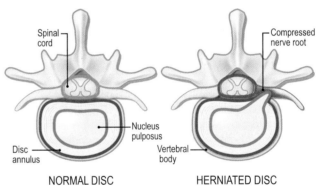

Figure 13-18 Intervertebral disc injury
© Designua/Shutterstock

Sacroiliac Joint Dysfunction

Sacroiliac joint pain describes symptoms that originate at the sacroiliac joint. Pain generated from the sacroiliac joint can refer pain to other parts of the hip and pelvis and, at times, down the leg (Kurosawa et al., 2017). The mechanical features associated with sacroiliac pain are controversial. Some evidence appears to suggest a small amount of movement, which occurs at the sacroiliac joint (Vleeming et al., 2012). However, it is not clear how movement influences symptoms. Unfortunately, a myriad of ligamentous, fascial, and muscular structures is present in the LPHC, with an extensive array of pain-generating nerve receptors (Cheatham & Kolber, 2016).

Mechanisms that may contribute to sacroiliac pain include, but are not limited to, LPHC muscle imbalances, neuromotor weakness, trauma, overuse, poor sitting posture, and pregnancy. This can make the identification of the specific area of pain difficult (Cheatham & Kolber, 2016). The fitness professional should consider that a client with history of sacroiliac joint pain may exhibit decreased motor control and performance with transitional movements, dynamic movements, and functional movements (Hungerford et al., 2003).

As with low-back pain, the fitness professional can play a key role as part of the continuum of care and performance for these clients. Often, these clients will return to the fitness setting after completing a rehabilitation program. The fitness professional can focus on enhancing stability and mobility around the LPHC. For stability, LPHC muscle stabilization exercises can benefit clients by helping to restore motor control and stability to the muscles that affect the sacroiliac joint (Pel et al., 2008; Wallden, 2014). For mobility, improving hip joint range of motion and enhancing flexibility of the hip flexors, quadriceps, adductor complex, and hamstrings complex may provide positive results for these clients (Cibulka et al., 1998; Kurosawa et al., 2017; Massoud Arab et al., 2011; Sadeghisani et al., 2015).

 GETTING TECHNICAL

The Corrective Exercise Specialist must be able to recognize the pain locations caused by low-back and/or sacroiliac joint dysfunction. Lumbar spine pain locations are often determined by which spinal level is affected. For example, if there is a disc herniation at the L5–S1 level, it will cause possible pain and neurological symptoms (e.g., numbness and tingling) down the leg into the foot. An injury at a higher spinal level (e.g., L1–L3) would produce symptoms in the LPHC. The lumbar spine pain referral locations are called dermatomes (Cheatham & Kolber, 2016) (**Figure 13-19**). Sacroiliac joint

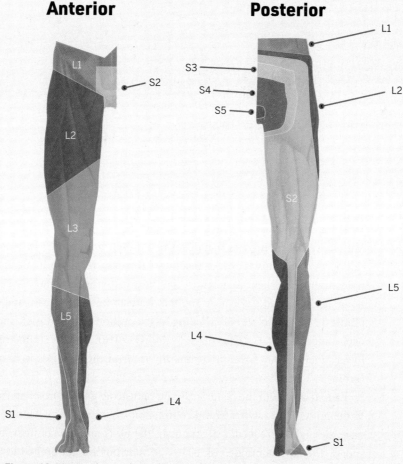

Figure 13-19 Lumbar and sacral vertebrae pain location

(continues)

pain primarily occurs around the posterior buttocks or sacroiliac region and can refer into the groin or down the posterior lateral leg to the knee in some individuals (**Figure 13-20**) (Cheatham & Kolber, 2016; Kurosawa et al., 2017).

Fitness professionals should be careful to stay within their scope of practice and not attempt to diagnose a potential lumbar or sacroiliac joint pathology. This information provides more in-depth information about these pathologies so the fitness professional can better recognize a potential safety issue and refer the client to a medical professional if needed.

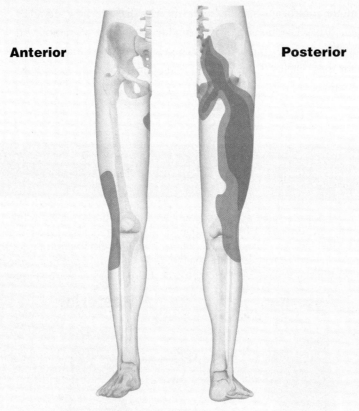

Figure 13-20 Sacroiliac joint pain location

Muscle Strains

Muscle strains are injuries that occur to a muscle and or muscle–tendon unit. Muscle strains can occur if the muscle works beyond its capacity, resulting in a tear of the muscle fibers. In mild strains, the client may report tightness or tension. In more severe cases, the client may report feeling a sudden tear or pop that leads to immediate pain and weakness in the muscle (**Table 13-8**) (Floyd, 2017). Swelling, discoloration (ecchymosis), and loss of function often occur after the injury (Cheatham & Kolber, 2016). Muscle strains related to the LPHC and lower kinetic chain extremity primarily occur in the quadriceps, hamstrings, and adductors (groin).

Muscle strains of the quadriceps and hamstring groups are often caused by a severe stretch to the muscle or a rapid, forceful contraction (e.g., sprinting). Among the two, the hamstrings have the highest frequency of strains in the body and are common in running and jumping sports. The most common risk factors include but are not limited to prior injury of the same

TABLE 13-8	Muscle Strain Classification
Grade	Description
Grade I (mild strain)	*Result:* Few muscle fibers damaged *Symptoms:* Mild or moderate pain *Functional ability:* Mild weakness or normal strength
Grade II (moderate strain)	*Result:* Greater number of muscle fibers involved *Symptoms:* Moderate or severe pain, mild swelling, and possible discoloration *Functional ability:* Noticeable weakness
Grade III (severe strain)	*Result:* Complete tear of muscle fibers *Symptoms:* Pop or ripping sensation and severe pain, swelling, and discoloration *Functional ability:* Loss of muscle function

Reproduced from Eckert, R. (2016). Transtheoretical model – Applications to personal training. *Personal Training Quarterly, 3,* 26.

muscle, age, poor flexibility, lower extremity muscle imbalance, improper warm-up, and training errors (Ahmad et al., 2013; Cheatham & Kolber, 2016).

Adductor or groin strains are common in sports such as soccer, ice hockey, and figure skating (Kerbel et al., 2018). These activities require explosive acceleration, deceleration, and change of direction. With injury, the client may report an initial pull of the groin muscles followed by intense pain and loss of function. The most common risk factors include, but are not limited to, prior injury, preseason training errors, core muscle weakness, and muscle imbalance between the adductors and abductors (Cheatham & Kolber, 2016; Kerbel et al., 2018).

SUMMARY

The LPHC operates as an integrated functional unit, enabling the entire kinetic chain to work synergistically to produce force, reduce force, and dynamically stabilize in multiple planes against changes in direction and force. In an efficient state, each structural component distributes weight, absorbs force, and transfers ground reaction forces. This integrated, interdependent system needs to be appropriately trained to enable it to function efficiently during dynamic activities. Because of the many muscles associated with the LPHC, dysfunction in this region can potentially lead to dysfunction in both the upper and lower extremities, and dysfunction in either the upper or lower extremities can lead to LPHC dysfunction. For this reason, it becomes a crucial region to assess and will most likely be a region that will need to be addressed in most individuals with movement deficits.

Ahmad, C. S., Redler, L. H., Ciccotti, M. G., Maffulli, N., Longo, U. G., & Bradley, J. (2013). Evaluation and management of hamstring injuries. *The American Journal of Sports Medicine, 41*(12), 2933–2947. https://doi.org/10.1177/0363546513487063

Algudairi, G., Aleisa, E., & Al-Badr, A. (2019). Prevalence of neuropathic pain and pelvic floor disorders among females seeking physical therapy for chronic low back pain. *Urology Annals, 11*(1), 20–26.

Almeida, G. P., Silva, A. P., Franca, F. J., Magalhães, M. O., Burke, T. N., & Marques, A. P. (2016). Relationship between frontal plane projection angle of the knee and hip and trunk strength in women with and without patellofemoral pain. *Journal of Back and Musculoskeletal Rehabilitation, 29*(2), 259–266. https://doi.org/10.3233/bmr-150622

Amabile, A. H., Bolte, J. H., & Richter, S. D. (2017). Atrophy of gluteus maximus among women with a history of chronic low back pain. *PLoS One, 12*(7), e0177008. https://doi.org/10.1371/journal.pone.0177008

Arab, A. M., Soleimanifar, M., & Nourbakhsh, M. R. (2019). Relationship between hip extensor strength and back extensor length in patients with low back pain: A cross-sectional study. *Journal of Manipulative and Physiological Therapeutics, 42*(2), 125–131. https://doi.org/10.1016/j.jmpt.2019.03.004

Araujo, V. L., Souza, T. R., Carvalhais, V. O. D. C., Cruz, A. C., & Fonseca, S. T. (2017). Effects of hip and trunk muscle strengthening on hip function and lower limb kinematics during step-down task. *Clinical Biomechanics, 44*, 28–35. https://doi.org/10.1016/j.clinbiomech.2017.02.012

Baldon, R., Piva, S. R., Scattone Silva, R., & Serrão, F. V. (2015). Evaluating eccentric hip torque and trunk endurance as mediators of changes in lower limb and trunk kinematics in response to functional stabilization training in women with patellofemoral pain. *American Journal of Sports Medicine, 43*(6), 1485–1493. https://doi.org/10.1177/0363546515574690

Brakenridge, C. L., Chong, Y. Y., Winkler, E. A. H., Hadgraft, N. T., Fjeldsoe, B. S., Johnston, V., Straker, L. M., Healy, G. N., & Clark, B. K. (2018). Evaluating short-term musculoskeletal pain changes in desk-based workers receiving a workplace sitting-reduction intervention. *International Journal of Environmental Research and Public Health, 15*(9), 1975. https://doi.org/10.3390/ijerph15091975

Calvo-Muñoz, I., Gómez-Conesa, A., & Sánchez-Meca, J. (2013). Prevalence of low back pain in children and adolescents: A meta-analysis. *BMC Pediatrics, 13*, 14. https://doi.org/10.1186/1471-2431-13-14

Caneiro, J. P., O'Sullivan, P., Burnett, A., Barach, A., O'Neil, D., Tveit, O., & Olafsdottir, K. (2010). The influence of different sitting postures on head/neck posture and muscle activity. *Manual Therapy, 15*(1), 54–60. https://doi.org/10.1016/j.math.2009.06.002

Cheatham, S. W., & Kolber, M. J. (2016). *Orthopedic management of the hip and pelvis.* Elsevier.

Cheatham, S. W., & Kreiswirth, E. M. (2014). The regional interdependence model: A clinical examination concept. *International Journal of Athletic Therapy & Training, 19*(3), 8–14. https://doi.org/10.1123/ijatt.2013-0113

Cibulka, M. T., Sinacore, D. R., Cromer, G. S., & Delitto, A. (1998). Unilateral hip rotation range of motion asymmetry in patients with sacroiliac joint regional pain. *Spine, 23*(9), 1009–1015. https://doi.org/10.1097/00007632-199805010-00009

Cooper, N. A., Scavo, K. M., Strickland, K. J., Tipayamongkol, N., Nicholson, J. D., Bewyer, D. C., & Sluka, K. A. (2016). Prevalence of gluteus medius weakness in people with chronic low back pain compared to healthy controls. *European Spine Journal, 25*(4), 1258–1265. https://doi.org/10.1007/s00586-015-4027-6

Cronstrom, A., Creaby, M. W., Nae, J., & Ageberg, E. (2016). Modifiable factors associated with knee abduction during weight-bearing activities: A systematic review and meta-analysis. *Sports Medicine, 46*(11), 1647–1662. https://doi.org/10.1007/s40279-016-0519-8

Daniels, J. M., Pontius, G., El-Amin, S., & Gabriel, K. (2011). Evaluation of low back pain in athletes. *Sports Health, 3*(4), 336–345. https://doi.org/10.1177/1941738111410861

De Blaiser, C., De Ridder, R., Willems, T., Vanden Bossche, L., Danneels, L., & Roosen, P. (2019). Impaired core stability as a risk factor for the development of lower extremity overuse injuries: A prospective cohort study. *American Journal of Sports Medicine, 47*(7), 1713–1721. https://doi.org/10.1177/0363546519837724

Dufour, S., Vandyken, B., Forget, M. J., & Vandyken, C. (2018). Association between lumbopelvic pain and pelvic floor dysfunction in women: A cross sectional study. *Musculoskeletal Science & Practice, 34*, 47–53.

Dülger, E., Bilgin, S., Bulut, E., İnal İnce, D., Köse, N., Türkmen, C., Çetin, H., & Karakaya, J. (2018). The effect of stabilization exercises on diaphragm muscle thickness and movement in women with low back pain. *Journal of Back and Musculoskeletal Rehabilitation, 31*(2), 323–329. https://doi.org/10.3233/BMR-169749

Dupeyron, A., Hertzog, M., Micallef, J. P., & Perrey, S. (2013). Does an abdominal strengthening program influence leg stiffness during hopping tasks? *Journal of Strength & Conditioning Research, 27*(8), 2129–2133. https://doi.org/10.1519/JSC.0b013e318278f0c7

Emami, F., Yoosefinejad, A. K., & Razeghi, M. (2018). Correlations between core muscle geometry, pain intensity, functional disability and postural balance in patients with nonspecific mechanical low back pain. *Medical Engineering & Physics, 60*, 39–46. https://doi.org/10.1016/j.medengphy.2018.07.006

Fatahi, F., Ghasemi, G., Karimi, M., & Beyranvand, R. (2019). The effect of eight weeks of core stability training on the lower extremity joints moment during single-leg drop landing. *Baltic Journal of Health & Physical Activity, 11*(1), 34–44. https://doi.org/10.29359/BJHPA.11.1.04

Floyd, R. T. (2017). *Manual of structural kinesiology* (20th ed.). McGraw-Hill Education.

Foroughi, F., Sobhani, S., Yoosefinejad, A. K., & Motealleh, A. (2019). Added value of isolated core postural control training on knee pain and function in women with patellofemoral pain syndrome: A randomized controlled trial. *Archives of Physical Medicine and Rehabilitation, 100*(2), 220–229. https://doi.org/10.1016/j.apmr.2018.08.180

Fuglsang, E. I., Telling, A. S., & Sárensen, H. (2017). Effect of ankle mobility and segment ratios on trunk lean in the barbell back squat. *Journal of Strength & Conditioning Research, 31*(11), 3024–3033. https://doi.org/10.1519/JSC.0000000000001872

Ha, S. M., Kwon, O. Y., Kim, S. J., & Choung, S. D. (2014). The importance of a normal breathing pattern for an effective abdominal-hollowing maneuver in healthy people: An experimental study. *Journal of Sport Rehabilitation, 23*(1), 12–17. https://doi.org/10.1123/jsr.2012-0059

Habets, B., Smits, H. W., Backx, F. J. G., van Cingel, R. E. H., & Huisstede, B. M. A. (2017). Hip muscle strength is decreased in middle-aged recreational male athletes with midportion Achilles tendinopathy: A cross-sectional study. *Physical Therapy in Sport, 25*, 55–61. https://doi.org/10.1016/j.ptsp.2016.09.008

Haddas, R., Hooper, T., James, C. R., & Sizer, P. S. (2016). Volitional spine stabilization during a drop vertical jump from different landing heights: Implications for anterior cruciate ligament injury. *Journal of Athletic Training, 51*(12), 1003–1012. https://doi.org/10.4085/1062-6050-51.12.18

Hodges, P., Holm, A. K., Hansson, T., & Holm, S. (2006). Rapid atrophy of the lumbar multifidus follows experimental disc or nerve root injury. *Spine, 31*(25), 2926–2933. https://doi.org/10.1097/01.brs.0000248453.51165.0b

Hosseinifar, M., Ghiasi, F., Akbari, A., & Ghorbani, M. (2017). The effect of stabilization exercises on lumbar lordosis in patients with low back pain. *Annals of Tropical Medicine & Public Health, 10*(6), 1779–1784. https://doi.org/10.4103/ATMPH.ATMPH_654_17

Hungerford, B., Gilleard, W., & Hodges, P. (2003). Evidence of altered lumbopelvic muscle recruitment in the presence of sacroiliac joint pain. *Spine, 28*(14), 1593–1600.

Hwang, Y. I., & Kim, K. S. (2018). Effects of pelvic tilt angles and forced vital capacity in healthy individuals. *Journal of Physical Therapy Science, 30*(1), 82–85. https://doi.org/10.1589/jpts.30.82

Iwai, K., Nakazato, K., Irie, K., Fujimoto, H., & Nakajima, H. (2004). Trunk muscle strength and disability level of low back pain in collegiate wrestlers. *Medicine & Science in Sports & Exercise, 36*(8), 1296–1300.

Jandre Reis, F. J., & Macedo, A. R. (2015). Influence of hamstring tightness in pelvic, lumbar and trunk range of motion in low back pain and asymptomatic volunteers during forward bending. *Asian Spine Journal, 9*(4), 535–540. https://doi.org/10.4184/asj.2015.9.4.535

Joseph, L. H., Hussain, R. I., Naicker, A. S., Htwe, O., Pirunsan, U., & Paungmali, A. (2014). Myofascial force transmission in sacroiliac joint dysfunction increases anterior translation of humeral head in contralateral glenohumeral joint. *Polish Annals of Medicine, 21*(2), 103–108. https://doi.org/10.1016/j.poamed.2014.07.007

Kahlaee, A. H., Ghamkhar, L., & Arab, A. M. (2017). Effect of the abdominal hollowing and bracing maneuvers on activity pattern of the lumbopelvic muscles during prone hip extension in subjects with or without chronic low back pain: A preliminary study. *Journal of Manipulative and Physiological Therapeutics, 40*(2), 106–117. https://doi.org/10.1016/j.jmpt.2016.10.009

Kerbel, Y. E., Smith, C. M., Prodromo, J. P., Nzeogu, M. I., & Mulcahey, M. K. (2018). Epidemiology of hip and groin injuries in collegiate athletes in the United States. *Orthopaedic Journal of Sports Medicine, 6*(5), 2325967118771676. https://doi.org/10.1177/2325967118771676

Kim, M.-H., & Oh, J.-S. (2015). Effects of performing an abdominal hollowing exercise on trunk muscle activity during curl-up exercise on an unstable surface. *Journal of Physical Therapy Science, 27*(2), 501–503. https://doi.org/10.1589/jpts.27.501

Król, A., Gleb, K., Polak, M., Szczygiel, E., & Wójcik, P. (2017). Relationship between mechanical factors and pelvic tilt in adults with and without low back pain. *Journal of Back and Musculoskeletal Rehabilitation, 30*(4), 699–705.

Kurosawa, D., Murakami, E., & Aizawa, T. (2017). Groin pain associated with sacroiliac joint dysfunction and lumbar disorders. *Clinical Neurology and Neurosurgery, 161*, 104–109. https://doi.org/10.1016/j.clineuro.2017.08.018

Laudner, K. G., Wong, R., & Meister, K. (2019). The influence of lumbopelvic control on shoulder and elbow kinetics in elite baseball pitchers. *Journal of Shoulder and Elbow Surgery, 28*(2), 330–334. https://doi.org/10.1016/j.jse.2018.07.015

Lee, A. Y., Baek, S. O., Cho, Y. W., Lim, T. H., Jones, R., & Ahn, S. A. (2016). Pelvic floor muscle contraction and abdominal hollowing during walking can selectively activate local trunk stabilizing muscles. *Journal of Back and Musculoskeletal Rehabilitation, 29*(4), 731–739.

Lee, A. Y., Kim, E. H., Cho, Y. W., Kwon, S. O., Son, S. M., & Ahn, S. H. (2013). Effects of abdominal hollowing during stair climbing on the activations of local trunk stabilizing muscles: A cross-sectional study. *Annals of Rehabilitation Medicine, 37*(6), 804–813. https://doi.org/10.5535/arm.2013.37.6.804

Lee, B. C., & McGill, S. M. (2015). Effect of long-term isometric training on core/torso stiffness. *Journal of Strength & Conditioning Research, 29*(6), 1515–1526. https://doi.org/10.1519/JSC.0000000000000740

Maeo, S., Takahashi, T., Takai, Y., & Kanehisa, H. (2013). Trunk muscle activities during abdominal bracing: Comparison among muscles and exercises. *Journal of Sports Science & Medicine, 12*(3), 467–474.

Massoud Arab, A., Reza Nourbakhsh, M., & Mohammadifar, A. (2011). The relationship between hamstring length and gluteal muscle strength in individuals with sacroiliac joint dysfunction. *Journal of Manual & Manipulative Therapy, 19*(1), 5–10. https://doi.org/10.1179/106698110X12804993426848

McClinton, S., Weber, C. F., & Heiderscheit, B. (2018). Low back pain and disability in individuals with plantar heel pain. *Foot, 34*, 18–22. https://doi:10.1016/j.foot.2017.09.003

McGill, S. (2016). *Low back disorders: Evidence-based prevention and rehabilitation* (3rd ed.). Human Kinetics.

Mitra, M., & Mande, M. (2019). Effectiveness of core stabilization training with pressure biofeedback in the management of mechanical low back pain in subjects between age group of 20–25 years. *Indian Journal of Physiotherapy & Occupational*

Therapy, 13(1), 82–87. https://doi.org/10.5958/0973
-5674.2019.00016.9

Mısırlıoğlu, T. Ö., Eren, İ., Canbulat, N., Çobanoğlu, E., Günerbüyük,
C., & Demirhan, M. (2018). Does a core stabilization exercise
program have a role on shoulder rehabilitation? A comparative
study in young females. *Turkish Journal of Physical Medicine
& Rehabilitation, 64*(4), 328–336. https://doi.org/10.5606/
tftrd.2018.1418

Monfort-Pañego, M., Vera-García, F. J., Sánchez-Zuriaga, D., &
Sarti-Martínez, M. A. (2009). Electromyographic studies
in abdominal exercises: A literature synthesis. *Journal of
Manipulative & Physiological Therapeutics, 32*(3), 232–244.
https://doi.org/10.1016/j.jmpt.2009.02.007

Mucha, M. D., Caldwell, W., Schlueter, E. L., Walters, C., & Hassen,
A. (2017). Hip abductor strength and lower extremity running
related injury in distance runners: A systematic review. *Journal of
Science and Medicine in Sport, 20*(4), 349–355. https://doi.org
/10.1016/j.jsams.2016.09.002

Myer, G. D., Ford, K. R., Brent, J. L., & Hewett, T. E. (2012). An
integrated approach to change the outcome part II: Targeted
neuromuscular training techniques to reduce identified
ACL injury risk factors. *Journal of Strength and Conditioning
Research, 26*(8), 2272–2292. https://doi.org/10.1519/JSC
.0b013e31825c2c7d

Neumann, D. A. (2016). *Kinesiology of the musculoskeletal system:
Foundations for rehabilitation* (3rd ed.). Elsevier.

Nourollahi, M., Afshari, D., & Dianat, I. (2018). Awkward trunk postures
and their relationship with low back pain in hospital nurses. *Work,
59*(3), 317–323. https://doi.org/10.3233/WOR-182683

Page, P., Frank, C. C., & Lardner, R. (2010). *Assessment and treatment of
muscle imbalance: The Janda approach.* Human Kinetics.

Parfrey, K., Gibbons, S. G. T., Drinkwater, E. J., & Behm, D. G. (2014).
Effect of head and limb orientation on trunk muscle activation
during abdominal hollowing in chronic low back pain. *BMC
Musculoskeletal Disorders, 15*(52). https://doi.org/10.1186
/1471-2474-15-52

Pel, J. J., Spoor, C. W., Pool-Goudzwaard, A. L., Hoek van Dijke, G. A., &
Snijders, C. J. (2008). Biomechanical analysis of reducing
sacroiliac joint shear load by optimization of pelvic muscle and
ligament forces. *Annals of Biomedical Engineering, 36*(3), 415–424.
https://doi.org/10.1007/s10439-007-9385-8

Puntumetakul, R., Chalermsan, R., Hlaing, S. S., Tapanya, W.,
Saiklang, P., & Boucaut, R. (2018). The effect of core stabilization
exercise on lumbar joint position sense in patients with subacute
non-specific low back pain: A randomized controlled trial. *Journal
of Physical Therapy Science, 30*(11), 1390–1396. https://doi
.org/10.1589/jpts.30.1390

Reeve, A., & Dilley, A. (2009). Effects of posture on the thickness of
transversus abdominis in pain-free subjects. *Manual Therapy,
14*(6), 679–684. https://doi.org/10.1016/j.math.2009.02.008

Roach, S. M., San Juan, J. G., Suprak, D. N., Lyda, M., Bies, A. J., &
Boydston, C. R. (2015). Passive hip range of motion is reduced in
active subjects with chronic low back pain compared to controls.
International Journal of Sports Physical Therapy, 10(1), 13–20.

Roshini, P. D., & Leo Aseer, P. A. (2019). Motor control training in
chronic low back pain. *Journal of Clinical and Diagnostic Research,
13*(4), YC01–YC05. https://doi.org/10.7860/JCDR/2019
/39618.12746

Sadeghisani, M., Manshadi, F. D., Kalantari, K. K., Rahimi, A.,
Namnik, N., Karimi, M. T., & Oskouei, A. E. (2015). Correlation
between hip rotation range-of-motion impairment and low back
pain. A literature review. *Ortopedia Traumatologica, Rehabilitacjal,
17*(5), 455–462. https://doi.org/10.5604/15093492.1186813

Silva, R. S., Ferreira, A. L. G., Nakagawa, T. H., Santos, J. E. M., &
Serrão, F. V. (2015). Rehabilitation of patellar tendinopathy using
hip extensor strengthening and landing-strategy modification:
Case report with 6-month follow-up. *Journal of Orthopaedic and
Sports Physical Therapy, 45*(11), 899–909.

Sorensen, C. J., Johnson, M. B., Norton, B. J., Callaghan, J. P., & Van
Dillen, L. R. (2016). Asymmetry of lumbopelvic movement
patterns during active hip abduction is a risk factor for low back
pain development during standing. *Human Movement Science, 50,*
38–46. https://doi.org/10.1016/j.humov.2016.10.003

Suehiro, T., Mizutani, M., Watanabe, S., Ishida, H., Kobara, K., &
Osaka, H. (2014). Comparison of spine motion and trunk muscle
activity between abdominal hollowing and abdominal bracing
maneuvers during prone hip extension. *Journal of Bodywork &
Movement Therapies, 18*(3), 482–488. https://doi.org/10.1016
/j.jbmt.2014.04.012

Sueki, D. G., Cleland, J. A., & Wainner, R. S. (2013). A regional
interdependence model of musculoskeletal dysfunction: Research,
mechanisms, and clinical implications. *Journal of Manual &
Manipulative Therapy, 21*(2), 90–102. https://doi.org/10.1179/2042
618612y.0000000027

Tsai, L. C., Ko, Y. A., Hammond, K. E., Xerogeanes, J. W., Warren, G. L., &
Powers, C. M. (2017). Increasing hip and knee flexion during
a drop-jump task reduces tibiofemoral shear and compressive
forces: Implications for ACL injury prevention training. *Journal
of Sports Sciences, 35*(24), 2405–2411. https://doi.org/10.1080
/02640414.2016.1271138

Tsang, S. M. H., Lam, A. H. M., Ng, M. H. L., Ng, K. W. K., Tsui, C. O. H., &
Yiu, B. (2018). Abdominal muscle recruitment and its effect on
the activity level of the hip and posterior thigh muscles during
therapeutic exercises of the hip joint. *Journal of Electromyography
and Kinesiology, 42,* 10–19. https://doi.org/10.1016/j.jelekin
.2018.06.005

U.S. Department of Health and Human Services. (2019). Arthritis,
osteoporosis, and chronic back conditions. *Healthy People 2020.*
Retrieved from https://www.healthypeople.gov/2020/data-search
/Search-the-Data#topic-area=3507

Vaičienė, G., Berškienė, K., Slapsinskaite, A., Mauricienė, V., & Razon,
S. (2018). Not only static: Stabilization manoeuvres in dynamic
exercises—a pilot study. *PLoS One, 13*(8), e0201017. https://doi
.org/10.1371/journal.pone.0201017

Vasseljen, O., Unsgaard-Tøndel, M., Westad, C., & Mork, P. J. (2012).
Effect of core stability exercises on feed-forward activation of
deep abdominal muscles in chronic low back pain. *Spine, 37*(13),
1101–1108. https://doi.org/10.1097/BRS.0b013e318241377c

Vleeming, A., Schuenke, M. D., Masi, A. T., Carreiro, J. E., Danneels, L., & Willard, F. H. (2012). The sacroiliac joint: An overview of its anatomy, function and potential clinical implications. *Journal of Anatomy, 221*(6), 537–567. https://doi.org/10.1111/j.1469-7580.2012.01564.x

Wallden, M. (2014). The middle crossed syndrome: New insights into core function. *Journal of Bodywork & Movement Therapies, 18*(4), 616–620. https://doi.org/10.1016/j.jbmt.2014.09.002

Winkelmann, Z. K., Anderson, D., Games, K. E., & Eberman, L. E. (2016). Risk factors for medial tibial stress syndrome in active individuals: An evidence-based review. *Journal of Athletic Training, 51*(12), 1049–1052. https://doi.org/10.4085/1062-6050-51.12.13

Wong, A. Y., Parent, E. C., Funabashi, M., Stanton, T. R., & Kawchuk, G. N. (2013). Do various baseline characteristics of transversus abdominis and lumbar multifidus predict clinical outcomes in nonspecific low back pain? A systematic review. *Pain, 154*(12), 2589–2602. https://doi.org/10.1016/j.pain.2013.07.010

CHAPTER 14

Corrective Strategies for the Thoracic Spine and Shoulder

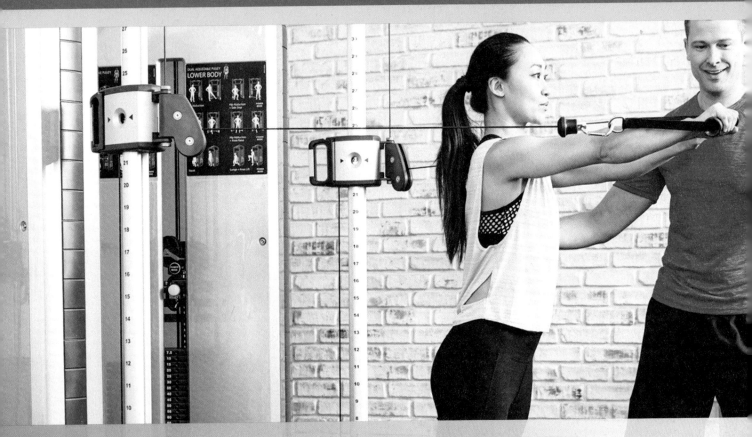

Learning Objectives

After reading this content, students should be able to demonstrate the following objectives:

- **Explain** the basic functional anatomy of the thoracic spine and shoulder.
- **Identify** the mechanisms for common thoracic spine and shoulder injuries.
- **Describe** the influence of altered thoracic spine and shoulder movement on the kinetic chain.
- **Determine** appropriate systematic assessment strategies for the thoracic spine and shoulder.
- **Select** appropriate corrective exercise strategies for the thoracic spine and shoulder.

Introduction

The thoracic spine and shoulder provide the upper body with a high level of mobility. Although the thoracic spine is not inherently mobile, optimal thoracic spine mobility combines with the scapula and shoulder to provide significant degrees of freedom. The shoulder is the most mobile joint in the body (Moore et al., 2014). This mobility provides the upper extremity with tremendous movement capabilities. The large amount of mobility allows for specialized actions like the baseball pitch or volleyball serve.

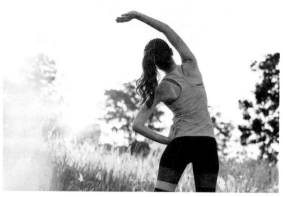

© GP PIXSTOCK/Shutterstock

The concept of regional interdependence is seen in the upper body as movement impairment in the hips and lumbar spine region that may directly affect the thoracic spine and shoulder (Sueki et al., 2013). This chapter will review the basic functional anatomy of the thoracic spine and shoulder, their relationship to other segments of the body, and corrective strategies to help improve thoracic spine and shoulder dysfunction.

Review of Thoracic Spine and Shoulder Functional Anatomy

The thoracic spine and shoulder are regions that are significantly affected by other regions of the kinetic chain. However, the thoracic spine and shoulder may also influence other aspects of the human movement system (HMS). Because this is to be a review of thoracic spine and shoulder anatomy, not all anatomical structures will be covered in detail. This section will provide a general review of the most pertinent structures.

Bones and Joints: Thoracic Spine

The thoracic spine runs from the base of the neck down to the abdomen and articulates with the rib cage (**Figure 14-1**). Due to the articulation with the rib cage, the thoracic spine is more

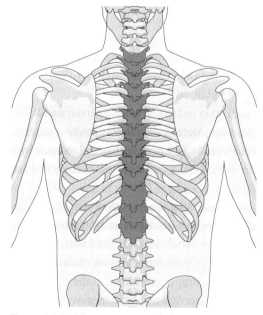

Figure 14-1   Thoracic spine and rib cage connections

Dynamic stabilization

Ability of the human movement system to control and minimize unwanted joint motions during movement.

the middle and inferior glenohumeral ligaments (**Figure 14-9**) (Bakhsh & Nicandri, 2018). The inferior ligament is divided into three sections: the anterior-inferior, axillary pouch, and posterior-inferior glenohumeral ligaments. Toward the end-ranges of glenohumeral motion, these ligaments tighten to limit motion and provide functional stability. These ligaments attach to the glenoid labrum and blend into the humeral head. The complex inferior glenohumeral ligament is the primary stabilizer against anterior translation of the humeral head. The anterior and posterior portions of this ligament help stabilize the joint by becoming taut in extreme ranges of internal and external rotation and often are injured with repetitive use in these positions. However, in the midranges of shoulder motion these ligaments are relatively lax and the joint must rely heavily on the musculature that surrounds the joint for **dynamic stability** (Allen et al., 2019).

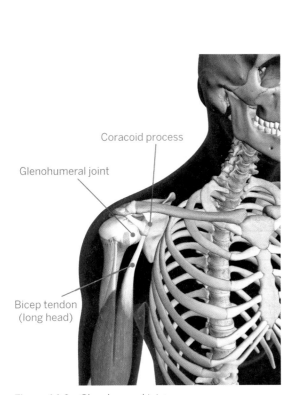

Figure 14-8   Glenohumeral joint

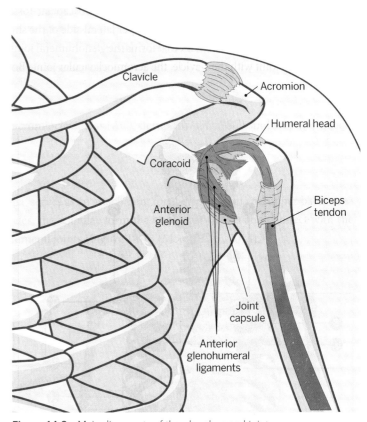

Figure 14-9   Major ligaments of the glenohumeral joint

 GETTING TECHNICAL

Behind-the-Neck Exercises

The close-packed position is when the joint surfaces are maximally aligned, which creates the greatest amount of mechanical stability. This position is achieved at 90 degrees of glenohumeral abduction and full external rotation (Floyd, 2017). In this position, most of the ligaments and a capsule surrounding the joint are taut. Performing exercises in this position increases a compressive and shear force applied to the joint and increases the risk for injury. To decrease stress on the joint and decrease the risk of injury, the joint should be placed in the loose-packed position. This is the position where the joint has the most extensibility in the capsule and ligaments (Floyd, 2017). For example, many people try to strengthen their latissimus dorsi and deltoids by performing behind-the-neck pulldowns or presses. This forces a person to place their shoulder into the closed-packed position (shoulder external rotation, abduction, and maximal elevation). However, a simple modification is to pull or press the load in front of the shoulder (front lat pulldowns or front shoulder presses), which avoids the closed-packed position and provides a safer alternative to avoid injuries in the future.

SCAPULOTHORACIC JOINT

The scapulothoracic joint is not a true joint but an articulation and is formed by the convex surface of the posterior thoracic cage and the concave surface of the anterior scapula (**Figure 14-10**) (Moore et al., 2014). The scapula is a flat bone with the gliding surfaces formed by the subscapularis and the serratus anterior (**Figure 14-11**). The scapulothoracic joint indirectly "attaches" to the axial skeleton through the acromioclavicular joint and the sternoclavicular joint (Moore et al., 2014). The scapulothoracic articulation allows shoulder movement beyond the 120 degrees of elevation provided by the glenohumeral joint. For every 2 degrees of glenohumeral elevation, there is 1 degree of scapulothoracic elevation (McClure et al., 2006; Timmons et al., 2012). The scapulothoracic joint also plays an important role in providing motion and shoulder girdle stability through the 17 muscles that attach to the scapula (Bakhsh & Nicandri, 2018). When these muscles function properly, they provide a stable base for the humerus to glide on and allow for an efficient transfer of force from the lower extremities and trunk. This is accomplished through force-couples of the upper, middle, and lower trapezius as well as the serratus anterior (**Figure 14-12**).

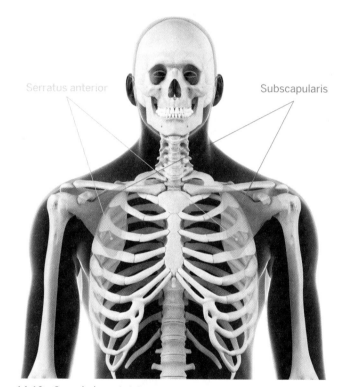

Serratus anterior   Subscapularis

Figure 14-10   Scapulothoracic joint

STERNOCLAVICULAR JOINT

The sternoclavicular joint is where the clavicle and sternum meet. It is the only bony connection of the scapula to the entire axial skeleton by way of the clavicle. The acromioclavicular joint and the sternoclavicular joint are at each end of the collarbone, connecting the shoulder girdle to the rest of the body. The scapula "floats" on top of the rib cage and is held in place by muscles and two small joints (Moore et al., 2014).

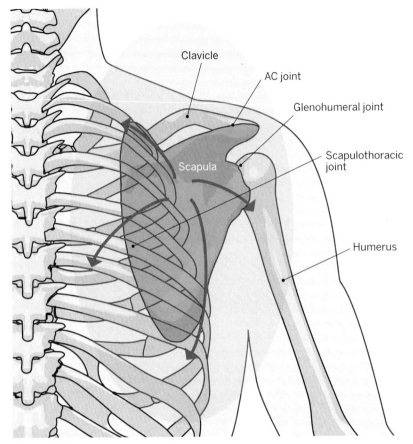

Figure 14-11 Scapulothoracic articulations

Clavicle

AC joint

Glenohumeral joint

Scapulothoracic joint

Humerus

Scapula

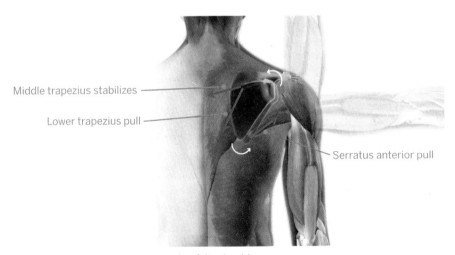

Figure 14-12 Force-couple example of the shoulder

Middle trapezius stabilizes

Lower trapezius pull

Serratus anterior pull

Muscles

Many muscles are associated with the shoulder joint (**Table 14-1**). The dynamic stability of the glenohumeral joint is dependent on the musculature that surrounds the joint, including the rotator cuff and the scapular stabilizers (Bakhsh & Nicandri, 2018). The rotator cuff is the primary steering mechanism of the glenohumeral joint. The rotator cuff is made up of the supraspinatus

TABLE 14-1 Key Muscles Associated with the Shoulder and Their Concentric Actions

Muscle	Concentric Action
Supraspinatus	Abduction
Subscapularis	Internal rotation
Infraspinatus	External rotation
Teres major	Internal rotation, adduction, and extension
Teres minor	External rotation
Anterior deltoid	Flexion and internal rotation
Lateral deltoid	Abduction
Posterior deltoid	Extension and external rotation
Pectoralis major	Flexion, horizontal adduction, and internal rotation
Pectoralis minor	Scapular protraction, forward translation over thoracic wall
Latissimus dorsi	Internal rotation, adduction, and extension
Rhomboids	Scapular retraction
Upper trapezius	Scapular elevation, cervical extension, lateral flexion, and rotation
Middle trapezius	Scapular retraction
Lower trapezius	Scapular depression
Serratus anterior	Scapular protraction
Levator scapulae	Scapular elevation and downward rotation, cervical extension, and lateral flexion

Data from Bakhsh, W., & Nicandri, G. (2018). Anatomy and physical examination of the shoulder. *Sports Medicine and Arthroscopy Review, 26*(3), e10–e22. https://doi.org/10.1097/jsa.0000000000000202

and subscapularis anteriorly, with the infraspinatus and teres minor posteriorly (**Figure 14-13**) (Floyd, 2017). The supraspinatus initiates the first 15 degrees of shoulder abduction followed by deltoid activation for the remainder of the arc of motion. The deltoid and supraspinatus work together in a force-couple to control the humeral head in the frontal plane. The main action of the subscapularis is stabilization of the humeral head from external rotation. Secondary actions are internal rotation and depression of the humeral head. The infraspinatus and teres minor prevent internal rotation of the shoulder. In addition, they decelerate the humerus during internal rotation, such as slowing the arm down during the pitching follow through. The subscapularis

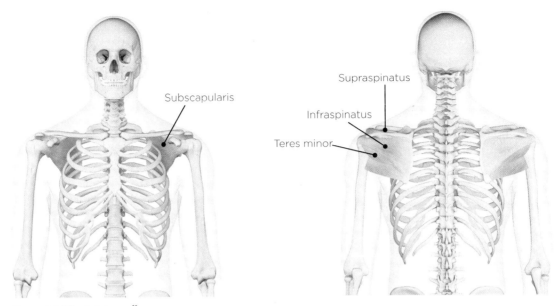

Figure 14-13 Rotator cuff

and posterior rotator cuff function together in a force-couple, controlling the humeral head in the transverse plane (Bakhsh & Nicandri, 2018).

The muscles of the scapula that do not cross the glenohumeral joint include the serratus anterior, pectoralis minor, trapezius, levator scapulae, and rhomboids (Moore et al., 2014). These five muscles all originate on the thoracic spine and rib cage and insert on the scapula and are responsible for controlling motion of the scapulae.

The effectiveness of these force-couples is reliant on the presence of optimal length-tension relationships between opposing muscles. Decreases in force production may lead to disruption in normal muscle synergies and lessen the ability of a force-couple to functionally control joint motion (Hamill & Knutzen, 2006). For example, tightness in the pectoralis minor, which inserts on the coracoid process of the scapula, will limit the effectiveness of the serratus anterior to upwardly rotate and posteriorly tilt the scapula. This alters the length-tension relationships of the rotator cuff, trapezius, and rhomboids, decreasing their ability to stabilize the glenohumeral joint (Kibler et al., 2006) and may negatively affect scapular movement due to poor length-tension relationships. Therefore, the pectoralis minor plays an important role in scapula malposition as it can pull the scapula into a more protracted and anteriorly tilted position (**Figure 14-14**) (Borstad, 2006; Borstad & Ludewig, 2005).

 HELPFUL HINT

The mnemonic **SITS** can be used to help remember the muscles that make up the rotator cuff. The four muscles that form the rotator cuff are the **s**upraspinatus, **i**nfraspinatus, **t**eres minor, and **s**ubscapularis (Moore et al., 2014). Each rotator cuff muscle performs a specific and important function for the shoulder joint.

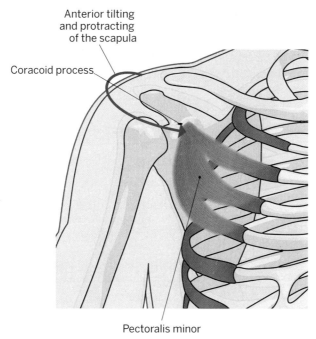

Anterior tilting
and protracting
of the scapula

Coracoid process

Pectoralis minor

Figure 14-14   Pectoralis minor and scapula malposition

Altered Thoracic Spine and Shoulder Movement

Having the ability to perform many movements about the shoulder can also lead to both acute and cumulative injuries (Bakhsh & Nicandri, 2018). Shoulder pain and dysfunction are highly prevalent musculoskeletal problems that often have multifactorial underlying pathologies and are associated with high societal cost. Self-reported prevalence of shoulder pain is estimated to be between 16% and 26% (Meislin et al., 2005; Mitchell et al., 2005; Villafañe et al., 2015). The four most common causes of shoulder pain described in the literature include rotator cuff disorders, glenohumeral disorders, acromioclavicular joint disease, and referred neck pain (Bau et al., 2017; Pillastrini et al., 2016). The Corrective Exercise Specialist can help reduce injury risk by first identifying postural and movement dysfunctions of the shoulder and thoracic spine and then addressing these dysfunctions with corrective strategies and integrated exercises to improve movement quality.

Static Malalignments

As mentioned previously, the human spine has natural curves forming an S-shape. Abnormalities of the spine, like **scoliosis** (**Figure 14-15**) can affect the body's ability to provide a sufficient articulating surface for the scapulae and alter normal muscle activity of the shoulder, upper extremity, neck, and lower back (Shakil et al., 2014). Muscle imbalances along the sides of the spine have been noted to have strength differences from side to side (Šarčević, 2010; Shakil et al., 2014). In the thoracic region, the middle and lower trapezius and the serratus anterior on the convex (inner angle) side of the curve appear to be weaker compared to the concave (outer angle) side. On the concave side, the rhomboids appear to be weaker compared to the convex side (Šarčević, 2010). Scoliosis can occur for a number of reasons, and a comprehensive discussion on the topic is beyond the scope of this chapter. The Corrective Exercise Specialist should note muscle imbalances and train appropriately by considering core stability training and unilateral training to attempt balance between the muscle groups. If undiagnosed

Scoliosis

Sideways curvature of the spine that occurs most often during the growth spurt just before puberty.

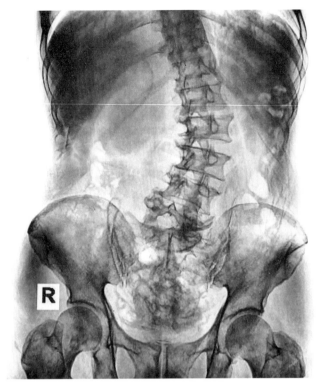

Figure 14-15 Scoliosis
© Tewan Banditrukkanka/Shutterstock

scoliosis is detected, comanagement with the clients' healthcare provider is necessary, especially in the developing adolescent.

Common symptoms associated with scoliosis include the following (Shakil et al., 2014):

- One shoulder blade that is higher than the other
- One shoulder blade that sticks out more than the other
- Uneven hips
- A rotating spine
- Problems breathing because of reduced area in the chest for lungs to expand
- Back pain

Normal anterior to posterior thoracic curvature is called a kyphosis or kyphotic curve and should be 20 to 40 degrees. When the curve is larger than 40 degrees, the individual is considered hyperkyphotic. **Hyperkyphosis** can occur in the thoracic spine for a number of reasons, but only the most common will be discussed here (Morita et al., 2014).

Postural kyphosis, or round back, is usually the result of poor posture. Previously, this condition was most common in adolescents and young adults, because they often slouch when standing and sitting, causing the spine to curve forward. Whether as a result of age-related changes or the increase of cell phone and computer use, people of all ages can experience this condition (Briggs et al., 2004, 2007). Many times, this posture will be evident with an increased lumbar lordosis, as in Janda's layered syndrome or Kendall's kyphosis-lordosis posture. Recall that in this posture the head is held forward, the neck is hyperextended, the thoracic spine is flexed more than usual (and, usually, the scapulae are protracted or rounded forward), the lumbar spine is hyperextended, the pelvis is tilted anteriorly, and the hip joints are somewhat flexed. Typically, the knees are slightly hyperextended and the ankles are slightly plantar flexed.

Some cases of hyperkyphosis are caused by degeneration, or wear and tear. Over time, the degenerative process can result in collapse of the intervertebral disc, changes in the shape of the vertebrae, and weakening of the ligaments that support the spine. This can result in the gradual development

Hyperkyphosis

A spinal disorder in which an excessive outward curve of the spine results in an abnormal rounding of the upper back.

of hyperkyphosis over many years. Once the hyperkyphosis begins to form, it gets worse because the imbalance of the forces continually increases the wear and tear (Singla & Veqar, 2017).

Regardless of the cause, hyperkyphosis in the thoracic spine causes positional changes in the joints and segments above, namely the scapulae, neck, and shoulder. This increased curve places the head into a forward head position and causes anterior rounding of the shoulders. These altered postures create range of motion and altered length-tension relationships, thus decreasing performance and placing the individual at a high risk of injury (Singla & Veqar, 2017). Hyperkyphosis will cause increases in multisegmental spinal loads and trunk muscle forces in upright and sitting positions. These factors are likely to accelerate degenerative processes in spinal motion segments and contribute to dysfunction of not only the thoracic spine but to the segments above (Briggs, van Dieen, et al., 2007).

Abnormal Muscle Activation Patterns

Rounded shoulders can be a result of poor posture, increased thoracic kyphosis, muscle weakness, muscle tightness, or any combination and can be classified as the Janda upper crossed syndrome. With this static observation, the back muscles of the neck and shoulders (upper trapezius and levator scapula) become overactive and strained (Borstad, 2006; Borstad & Ludewig, 2005). The muscles in the front of the chest (e.g., pectoralis minor) become shortened and overactive, as does the latissimus dorsi, which causes internal rotation of the humerus. As a result of these overactive muscles, the surrounding countermuscles become underactive and lengthened, contributing to poor length-tension relationships (Borstad, 2006; Borstad & Ludewig, 2005; Hébert et al., 2002).

Dynamic Malalignment

Dynamic movements such as throwing, hitting, and serving occur as the result of integrated, multisegmented, sequential joint motion and muscle activation. This system is referred to as the kinetic chain (Sciascia & Cromwell, 2012). Proper utilization of the kinetic chain allows maximal force to develop at the legs and hips through the core, which can then be efficiently transferred to the arm. For the tasks to be effective and efficient, the different body segments must have optimal amounts of joint flexibility and strength. When the body segments do not have the required flexibility or strength along the kinetic chain, increased load and stress may occur on the shoulder, elbow, and wrist joints, which can lead to dysfunction in other areas away from the dysfunctional segments. A Corrective Exercise Specialist should focus on identifying the cause(s) that led or contributed to movement impairments by using the CES Assessment Flow process. The Corrective Exercise Specialist then has the opportunity to identify these impairments and implement individualized exercise programs, which will attempt to maximize the health and movement quality of the shoulder girdle while simultaneously decreasing the risk of injury (Sciascia & Cromwell, 2012).

Thoracic Spine and Shoulder Dysfunction and the Regional Interdependence Model

Dysfunction of the thoracic spine can cause issues to joints and regions both above and below the area. These areas may include the scapulae, neck, shoulder, elbow, wrist, and lumbar spine, respectively. Increasing thoracic spine mobility has been shown to reduce discomfort and ROM in patients with neck and/or shoulder dysfunction (Bergman et al., 2004; Boyles et al., 2009;

Cleland et al., 2005, 2007, 2010; Cross et al., 2011; Mintken et al., 2010; Walser et al., 2009; Young et al., 2014). Therefore, a significant relationship may exist between the thoracic spine and surrounding regions. Although many of the studies included thrust manipulation by a licensed healthcare provider (physical therapist or chiropractor), improvements have also been seen by nonthrust mobilization (Dunning et al., 2012, 2016) and self-mobilization (Nakamaru et al., 2019). The Corrective Exercise Specialist can teach their clients myofascial rolling using foam rollers (and other mobility tools) to apply these studies' outcomes.

 CRITICAL

Fitness professionals must stay within their scope of practice. Manual therapy (using one's hands on a patient) should only be done by a licensed healthcare professional.

Influence Above the Shoulder and Thoracic Spine

Numerous studies have focused on the use of thoracic spine mobilization versus specific cervical spine therapy for treating individuals with neck dysfunction (Cleland et al., 2005, 2010; Cleland, Childs, et al., 2007). All of the studies utilizing multiple interventions combined with thoracic mobilization (multimodal approach) found improved function and decreased dysfunction (Cleland, Childs et al., 2007; Dunning et al., 2016; Fernández-de-las-Peñas et al., 2009; González-Iglesias, Fernández-de-las-Peñas, Cleland, Alburquerque-Sendin, et al., 2009; González-Iglesias, Fernández-de-las-Peñas, Cleland, Gutiérrez-Vega Mdel et al., 2009; Lau et al., 2011; Masaracchio et al., 2013). Five of the studies also found improved cervical spine range of motion after intervention (Dunning et al., 2012; Fernández-de-las-Peñas et al., 2009; Gonzalez-Iglesias, Fernández-de-las-Peñas, Cleland, Alburquerque-Sendin et al., 2009; González-Iglesias, Fernández-de-las-Peñas, Cleland, Gutiérrez-Vega Mdel et al., 2009; Lau et al., 2011) These findings would suggest that having good mobility of the thoracic spine is imperative to improving injury resistance and ROM to the regions above the thoracic spine.

Influences Related to the Shoulder and Thoracic Spine

Additional effects on the shoulder girdle after thoracic mobilization include increased middle trapezius activity in individuals with rotator cuff tendinopathy (Muth et al., 2012) and increased lower trapezius strength in asymptomatic individuals (Cleland et al., 2004). This improved muscle function after mobilization may provide support for mobilizing the thoracic spine using a foam roller (or other modality) prior to horizontal or vertical push/pull exercises.

There appears to be a relationship between shoulder dysfunction and reduced upper thoracic spine mobility (Haik et al., 2014; Norlander et al., 1997; Norlander & Nordgren, 1998; Sobel et al., 1996). Numerous studies have reported individuals complaining of shoulder dysfunction where more than 40% had associated mobility problems of the cervicothoracic spine and adjacent ribs (Sobel et al., 1996, 1997) and determined that the dysfunction in these adjacent areas may be a primary cause of some patients' shoulder dysfunction. A study by Crosbie et al. (2008) described the relationship between thoracic spine mobility and arm elevation. The study described how thoracic spine **hypomobility** may lead to impairment of shoulder mechanics. Ensuring good thoracic spine mobility may help improve shoulder performance via improved force-coupling and muscle activity.

Hypomobility

Decrease in normal movement and functionality of a joint, which affects range of motion.

Influence Below the Shoulder and Thoracic Spine

The lumbar spine has about 10 to 12 degrees cumulatively of rotation (Bible et al., 2010). The thoracic spine should contribute between 45 to 60 degrees of rotation (Johnson & Grindstaff, 2010). If the thoracic spine is not rotating well, the body will allow the lumbar spine to make up the difference in movement. Most lumbar spine injuries occur at L5/S1 and L4/L5. These lower lumbar vertebrae will move excessively to compensate for a lack of movement in the thoracic spine directly above. Excessive movement at these joints can cause early wear and tear, dysfunction, and pain (Cole & Grimshaw, 2016).

For example, the hips are like the speed limiter of a golf cart. The cart can have all the horsepower in the world, but if the limiter only allows a top speed of 25 miles per hour, it will never make use of its full capabilities. The same thing applies for a baseball pitcher. A person can have a lot of power in the legs, but if they have no range of motion in the hips, it makes transferring energy created from the lower body to the upper body impossible. The restricted mobility of the hip becomes the limiting factor of ground reaction force transfer to the upper extremities. Robb et al. (2010) found that poor hip range of motion adversely affected pitching biomechanics and ball velocity. Two of the key components to pitching velocity are hip range of motion and trunk rotation. This study demonstrated that by improving hip range of motion, trunk rotation also improves, allowing more opportunity for hip to shoulder separation, and therefore greater velocity. This study also showed good hip mobility increased stride length, which is an indication of more power from the lower body and perceived velocity to the hitter.

Assessment Results for the Shoulder and Thoracic Spine

Because of the extreme degrees of freedom of the shoulder joint, its limited contact surface, and its regional interdependence with the lumbo-pelvic-hip complex (LPHC) and cervical spine, key static positions and movement impairments can be used to identify shoulder dysfunction. **Table 14-2** presents a summary of the assessment process and common findings that warrant the use of corrective exercise at the shoulder kinetic chain checkpoint.

TABLE 14-2 Shoulder Assessment Results	
Assessment	**Results**
Static posture	Rounded shoulders Excessive thoracic kyphosis (hyperkyphosis) Shoulders elevated
Transitional and loaded movement	Arms fall forward Scapular elevation Scapular winging
Dynamic movement	Scapular elevation Scapular winging

(continues)

TABLE 14-2	Shoulder Assessment Results (*continued*)
Assessment	**Results**
Mobility	Limited shoulder flexion ROM
Shoulder flexion, shoulder extension, shoulder retraction, shoulder internal and external rotation, thoracic extension, seated thoracic rotation	Limited shoulder extension ROM
	Limited shoulder retraction ROM
	Limited shoulder internal rotation ROM
	Limited shoulder external rotation ROM
	Limited thoracic extension ROM
	Limited thoracic rotation ROM

Static Posture

The postural distortion patterns that determine potential shoulder and thoracic spine dysfunction include Janda's upper crossed and layered crossed syndromes, as well as Kendall's flat back, sway back, and kyphosis-lordosis postures (Kendall et al., 2005; Page et al., 2010). In all of them, the thoracic spine exhibits excessive kyphosis (upper back rounding). That rounding of the upper back is typically caused by a combination of overactivity of the latissimus dorsi and pectoralis minor muscles paired with underactivity of shoulder and scapular retractor muscles. This leads to forward-positioned shoulders that create the visual appearance of rounding of the upper back as the thoracic spine responds (**Figure 14-16**). The muscle imbalances responsible for this static posture are also the same ones that cause arms to fall forward during an overhead squat assessment (OHSA).

Upper Crossed Syndrome

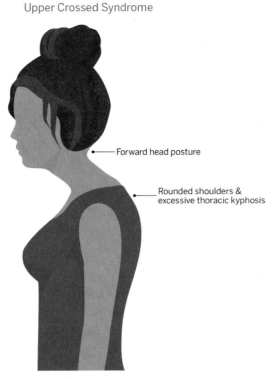

Forward head posture

Rounded shoulders & excessive thoracic kyphosis

Figure 14-16 Rounded back and shoulders

To demonstrate how shoulder position affects the posture of the spine, stand with neutral posture perpendicular to a mirror and round your shoulders and head forward. When doing so, you will notice the middle of the upper back comes into view, highlighting the tight-knit regional interdependence of the upper torso. Next, retract the shoulders and stand up straight. Now you should see the thoracic region move back into a neutral position and be blocked from view by the shoulders now that they are back in line with the ears and hips.

Transitional Movement Assessment

Based on the collective information obtained from the static postural assessment, the Corrective Exercise Specialist will have a high-level estimation of which muscles might be overactive/shortened and which ones might be underactive/lengthened. Occasionally, clients might have relatively impairment-free static posture; however, when in motion, active muscle imbalances may come to light. With essentially all movement having some influence on the thoracic spine and shoulder, the transitional movement assessments provide objective information from which to design effective corrective exercise programs.

OVERHEAD SQUAT ASSESSMENT

A squat with the arms overhead requires optimal glenohumeral mobility, thoracic extension, and shoulder girdle stability. Due to these factors, many common movement impairments associated with a lack of thoracic extension, glenohumeral flexion, and scapular muscle weakness can be observed in the OHSA. The movement impairment of arms fall forward is often observed when a client lacks optimal shoulder mobility. The lack of full shoulder flexion may be due to overactive pectoralis major/minor and latissimus dorsi muscles, which pull the shoulders forward and contribute to excessive thoracic kyphosis (**Figure 14-17**).

Sometimes, to compensate for a lack of glenohumeral flexion and thoracic extension, individuals may recruit upper trapezius and levator scapulae muscles to accomplish the arms overhead position, producing shoulder elevation as a means of relative flexibility. If this is difficult to observe during the OHSA, it may also be evaluated during a loaded pushing/pulling assessment.

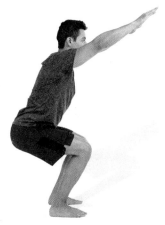

Figure 14-17 Arms fall forward

TRAINING TIP

Bending Elbows During the OHSA
Once again highlighting the Regional Interdependence (RI) model at work, the movement impairment of elbow flexion (i.e., the inability to fully straighten the arms overhead) may frequently be seen in clients whose arms also fall forward during the OHSA. A rounded shoulder posture is sometimes also associated with overactivity or shortening of the biceps brachii muscle. Corrective strategies for the elbow and wrist should be followed when this movement impairment is observed.

HANDS-ON-HIPS MODIFICATION

If an individual exhibits arms fall forward on the OHSA, limited thoracic extension above the lumbar spine may be a primary contributor. To help confirm this assumption, the hands-on-hips modification to the OHSA should be used.

Just as elevating the heels increases available dorsiflexion ROM by taking tension off the calf musculature, placing the hands on the hips reduces tension in the latissimus dorsi and creates more ROM throughout the trunk. If an excessive anterior pelvic tilt is improved with the hands on the hips, this indicates that mobility restrictions above the hip at the shoulder (likely due to an overactive latissimus dorsi) are more responsible for the excessive tilt than below. For these individuals, protocols to correct arms fall forward should help improve their lumbar dynamic posture. If placing the hands on the hips does not correct the excessive tilt, then the corrective program should focus on the LPHC. Remember that programming decisions should be made with a full set of assessment results.

LOADED MOVEMENT ASSESSMENTS

Clients who demonstrate proper static and dynamic posture under body weight alone can be progressed to using loaded variants of primary movement patterns. This provides more challenge to the musculature and can help draw attention to any remaining imbalance at the joints. While the OHSA does a good job of bringing sagittal plane movement impairments of the shoulder to light, other areas of shoulder dysfunction may be best observed during pushing and pulling tasks, provided the client is able to perform them. A standing cable machine press or pull is a suitable exercise to evaluate a horizontally loaded position.

During pushing and pulling, the optimal position of the scapulae and shoulders is a depressed and retracted state while still allowing for normal scapulothoracic rhythm where scapular protraction is not excessive. This posture extends the thoracic spine and allows for maximal protection and alignment of the torso from which the most efficient force can be generated. When there is a lack of thoracic extension ROM, upper trapezius and levator scapulae muscles can become dominant and cause the shoulder structures to migrate upward when they should otherwise be held down in place (**Figure 14-18**).

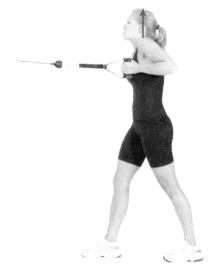

Figure 14-18 Pulling with shoulder elevation

Scapular winging will be best seen during pushing tasks and is typically due to underactivity of the serratus anterior and scapular stabilizers. The location of these muscles is sandwiched between the scapula and the posterior rib cage. When they are not properly recruited, the scapulae are not held as tightly against the rib cage as they should be and can externally rotate slightly in the transverse plane, causing them to look like small "wings" on the individual's back.

Another loaded movement pattern that may be utilized to assess the shoulder complex is the standing overhead dumbbell press, provided the client can safely perform the exercise. This primary movement pattern requires at least a foundational level of core stability and strength, as well as upper body mobility, stability, and strength to perform it safely. Any time an individual is pressing a load overhead, observe their shoulder and scapular mechanics for any impairments. Overhead presses also provide an opportunity to assess the corrective progress of the arms fall forward movement impairment.

It is important to remember that targeted mobility testing should be used to confirm or deny observations made during transitional assessments.

Dynamic Movement Assessments

The use of the Davies test introduces repetitive plyometric movements for the upper extremity, testing the stabilization and dynamic posture of the shoulder in a more complex situation than the OHSA and loaded primary movement patterns (**Figure 14-19**). When clients are ready for this assessment, they have already demonstrated relatively efficient form in all previous assessments, so compensations in the Davies test are typically due to deficits in muscular stability and strength rather than ROM deficits. This is an advanced technique, so the Corrective Exercise Specialist should make sure their clients have proper push-up and plank form, as well as adequate strength to remain in the high-plank push-up position for prolonged periods of time.

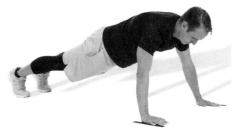

Figure 14-19A Upper extremity Davies assessment position

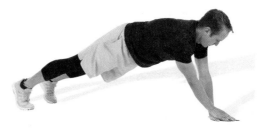

Figure 14-19B Davies assessment—movement A

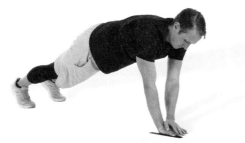

Figure 14-19C Davies assessment—movement B

Mobility Assessments

If the client demonstrates impairments related to the thoracic spine or shoulder in the static posture assessment, movement assessments, or both, mobility assessments for the thoracic spine or shoulder should be performed to better pinpoint the muscle imbalances requiring correction via the Corrective Exercise Continuum. Mobility of the shoulders and thoracic spine can be evaluated using tests for shoulder flexion (latissimus dorsi length) and extension, shoulder retraction (pectoralis minor length), shoulder internal and external rotation, thoracic extension, and thoracic rotation.

Flexibility of the shoulder extensor group, including the latissimus dorsi and pectorals, has a considerable influence on the positioning of the glenohumeral joint, as is demonstrated with the arms fall forward movement impairment. For most, internal rotation of the shoulders will not be limited due to the already-forward shoulder position many will present with; however, individuals with rounded shoulders will tend to have limited external rotation ROM.

Corrective Strategies for the Thoracic Spine and Shoulder

The integrated assessment process will reveal movement compensation patterns that may warrant the implementation of corrective programming for the thoracic spine and shoulder complex with the most common one being arms fall forward. Once the static, movement, and mobility assessments have been performed and impairments have been identified, the corrective exercise strategy can be developed using the NASM Corrective Exercise Continuum. Most programs can be performed daily or multiple times per week (see **Table 14-3**).

TABLE 14-3 Common Corrective Programming Selections for the Thoracic Spine and Shoulder			
Phase	**Modality**	**Muscle(s)/Exercise**	**Acute Training Variables**
Inhibit	Self-myofascial rolling	Biceps brachii Latissimus dorsi Levator scapulae Pectoralis major Pectoralis minor Thoracic spine Upper trapezius	Hold areas of discomfort for 30 to 60 seconds Perform four to six repetitions of active joint movement
Lengthen	Static or neuromuscular stretching (NMS)	Biceps brachii Latissimus dorsi Levator scapulae Pectoralis major Pectoralis minor Posterior capsule/deltoid Upper trapezius	Static: 30-second hold NMS: 7- to 10-second isometric contraction; 30-second hold
Activate	Isolated strengthening	Ball combo 1 Ball combo 2 Cobra Push-up plus Rotator cuff (resisted internal and external rotation) Scaption	10 to 15 reps with 4-second eccentric contraction, 2-second isometric contraction at end-range, and 1-second concentric contraction
Integrate*	Integrated dynamic movement	Pulling progressions Pushing progressions Single-leg RDL to PNF pattern Squat to row	10 to 15 reps under control

* NOTE: Progress and regress as needed to match client ability, work capacity, and needs.

Common Exercise Selections for the Thoracic Spine and Shoulder

Exercises used for thoracic spine and shoulder corrective strategies look to improve commonly observed movement impairments such as arms fall forward, scapular elevation, and scapular winging. Oftentimes, multiple movement impairments across the kinetic chain occur together (such as excessive kyphosis during static assessment and arms fall forward during the OHSA) and may benefit from exercises that address both, based on the integrated assessment process. For example, inhibition and lengthening of the pectorals may improve both impairments. As such, the Corrective Exercise Specialist may create a program that efficiently addresses multiple movement impairments.

INHIBIT: SELF-MYOFASCIAL ROLLING

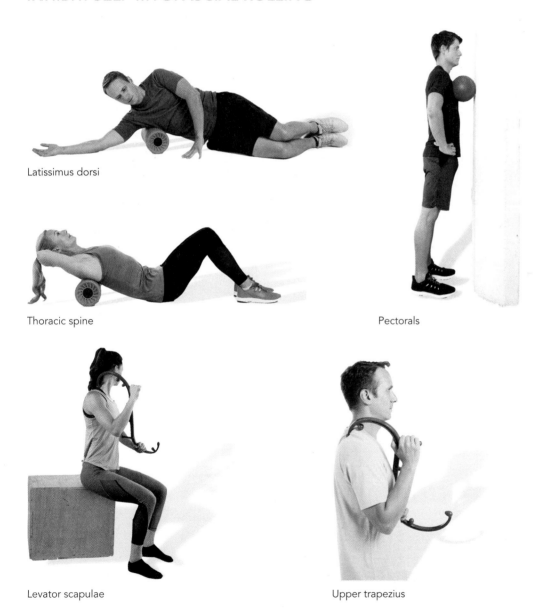

Latissimus dorsi

Thoracic spine

Pectorals

Levator scapulae

Upper trapezius

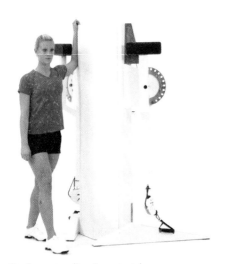

Static pectoralis minor stretch

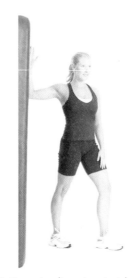

Static pectoralis major stretch

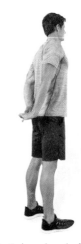

Static long head of biceps stretch

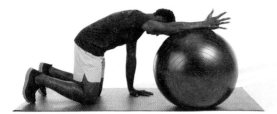

Static ball latissimus dorsi stretch

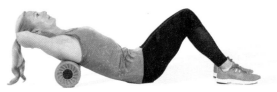

Thoracic spine extension on foam roller

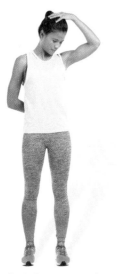

Static levator scapulae stretch

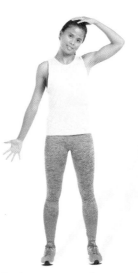

Static upper trapezius stretch

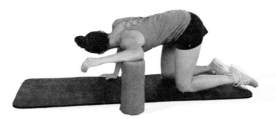

Self-NMS prone pectoral

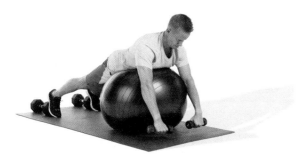

Ball combo 1—start

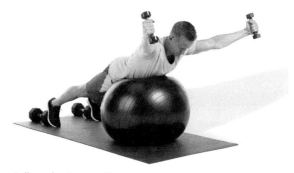

Ball combo 1—scaption

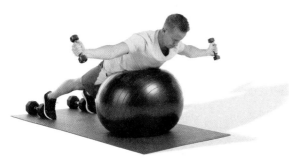

Ball combo 1—retraction

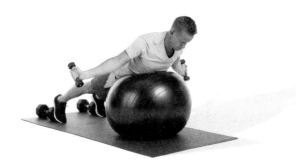

Ball combo 1—cobra (finish)

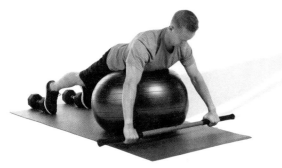

Ball combo 2 with dowel rod—start

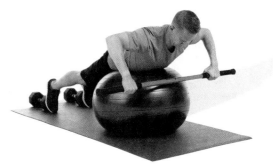

Ball combo 2 with dowel rod—row

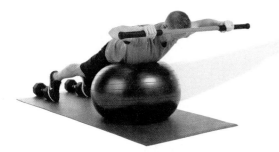

Ball combo 2 with dowel rod—rotate

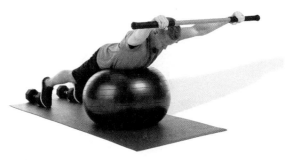

Ball combo 2 with dowel rod—press

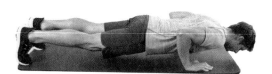

Push-up plus—start

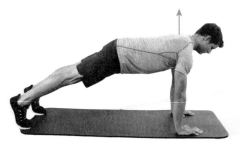

Push-up plus—finish

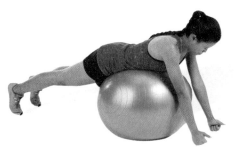

Ball cobra—start

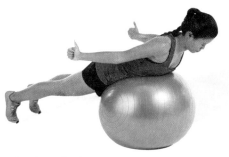

Ball cobra—finish

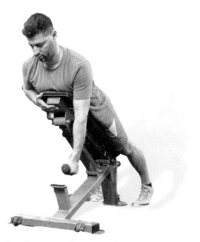

Single-arm incline scaption—start

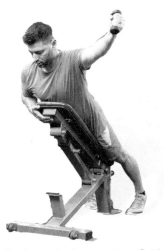

Single-arm incline scaption—finish

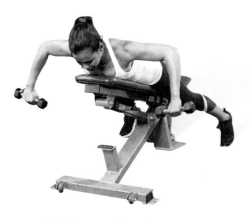

Prone shoulder external rotation—start

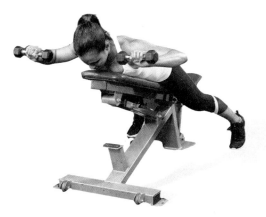

Prone shoulder external rotation—finish

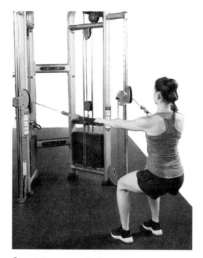

Squat to row—start

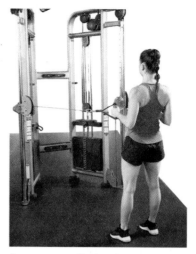

Squat to row—finish

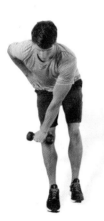

Single-leg Romanian deadlift with PNF
pattern—start

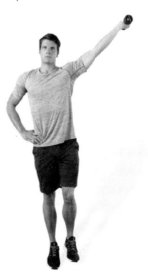

Single-leg Romanian deadlift with PNF
pattern—finish

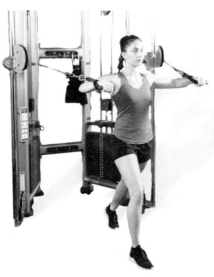

Standing cable chest press—start

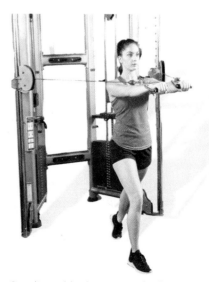

Standing cable chest press—finish

Arms Fall Forward

The Corrective Exercise Specialist should be selective regarding the techniques recommended to each client. To improve client adherence, it is recommended that the Corrective Exercise Specialist employ as few exercises as are effective in each phase of the continuum. Although not an exhaustive list of possibilities, the following exercises may be used for the compensation of arms fall forward. The broad objectives of the program are to improve ideal shoulder flexion and scapular stability. When applied systematically, the Corrective Exercise Continuum contributes to efficient neuromuscular control and proper alignment of the thoracic spine and shoulder girdle during movement.

PHASE 1: INHIBIT

Key regions to inhibit with foam rolling include the latissimus dorsi and pectorals. A small massage ball or medicine ball placed between the client and a wall are often more effective than using a roller on the pectorals. Self-myofascial rolling the thoracic spine is primarily done to reduce tension, reinforce scapular retraction, and improve thoracic extension.

PHASE 2: LENGTHEN

Key lengthening exercises with static stretches include the latissimus dorsi, pectorals, and thoracic extension over a foam roller.

PHASE 3: ACTIVATE

Key activation exercises with isolated strengthening exercises include the middle and lower trapezius, rhomboids, and rotator cuff (ball combo 2 with dowel rod is an effective exercise to engage rotator cuff external rotation). The ball combo 2 exercise can also be performed with dumbbells, as needed.

PHASE 4: INTEGRATE

An integration progression should be implemented first to emphasize scapular retraction and depression, such as a squat to row. Note that the sagittal plane row is largely dominated by the latissimus dorsi and that the latissimus dorsi are often overactive. Thus, the Corrective Exercise Specialist should place importance on form and scapular mechanics (**Table 14-4**).

TABLE 14-4	Sample Corrective Exercise Program for the Thoracic Spine and Shoulder: Arms Fall Forward		
Phase	**Modality**	**Muscle(s)/Exercise**	**Acute Training Variables**
Inhibit	Self-myofascial rolling	Latissimus dorsi Pectorals Thoracic spine	Hold areas of discomfort for 30 to 60 seconds Perform four to six repetitions of active joint movement 90 to 120 seconds per muscle group
Lengthen	Static stretching	Latissimus dorsi Pectorals	30-second hold
Activate	Isolated strengthening	Rhomboids Trapezius (middle and lower)	10 to 15 reps with 4-second eccentric contraction, 2-second isometric contraction at end-range, and 1-second concentric contraction
Integrate*	Integrated dynamic movement	Squat to row (transverse)	10 to 15 reps under control

* NOTE: Progress and regress as needed to match client ability, work capacity, and needs.

Progress by moving to alternating arms or using a transverse plane row (i.e., wide-grip row) rather than by increasing load. Additional progressions may include one-arm and eventually base-of-support changes.

Shoulder Elevation

If a body is correctly aligned, the shoulders will be at the same height and neutral (facing forward and slightly retracted). Uneven shoulders occur when one shoulder is higher than the other. This can be a slight or significant difference and may be due to several causes. If the shoulder is elevated both statically and dynamically, the Corrective Exercise Specialist should look for structural issues that may be contributing, such as scoliosis. Once this is ruled out by a qualified medical professional, correcting the observed muscular impairments will diminish or minimize the elevated shoulder presentation. The Corrective Exercise Specialist should be selective regarding the techniques recommended to each client. To improve client adherence, it is recommended that the Corrective Exercise Specialist employ as few exercises as are effective in each phase of the continuum. The following exercises are the ones most used for the compensation of shoulder elevation. Many times, the client may demonstrate a combination of shoulder elevation with forward head posture (FHP). The example program that follows is for shoulder elevation without FHP, for simplicity. The broad objectives of the program are to improve the position of the scapula. When applied systematically, the Corrective Exercise Continuum contributes to efficient neuromuscular control and proper alignment of the shoulder girdle during movement.

PHASE 1: INHIBIT

Key regions to inhibit with foam rolling and apparatus-assisted modalities include the pectoralis minor, thoracic spine, upper trapezius, and levator scapulae.

PHASE 2: LENGTHEN

Key lengthening exercises with static stretches include the pectoralis minor, upper trapezius, and levator scapulae. Reinforcing thoracic extensibility over a foam roller is also effective for shoulder elevation.

PHASE 3: ACTIVATE

Key activation exercises with isolated strengthening exercises include the ball cobra and ball scaption to reinforce scapulothoracic rhythm and downward rotation and depression of the scapula.

PHASE 4: INTEGRATE

An integration progression should be implemented first to emphasize scapular depression and cervical spine stability. An integration exercise that may be implemented includes a single-leg Romanian deadlift with PNF (proprioceptive neuromuscular facilitation) pattern. One additional integration exercise that can be implemented is a standing lat pulldown. During this exercise, it is vital to ensure the client is focusing on scapular retraction and depression first, and then humeral adduction. This movement may be progressed by reducing the base of support or performing with a single arm. **Table 14-5** provides a sample program to address shoulder elevation.

TABLE 14-5 Sample Corrective Exercise Program for the Thoracic Spine and Shoulder: Shoulder Elevation

Phase	Modality	Muscle(s)/Exercise	Acute Training Variables
Inhibit	Self-myofascial rolling	Levator scapulae Pectoralis minor Upper trapezius	Hold areas of discomfort for 30 to 60 seconds Perform four to six repetitions of active joint movement 90 to 120 seconds per muscle group
Lengthen	Static stretching	Levator scapulae Pectoralis minor Upper trapezius	30-second hold
Activate	Isolated strengthening	Lower trapezius Serratus anterior	10 to 15 reps with 4-second eccentric contraction, 2-second isometric contraction at end-range, and 1-second concentric contraction
Integrate*	Integrated dynamic movement	Single-leg RDL to PNF pattern	10 to 15 reps under control

* NOTE: Progress and regress as needed to match client ability, work capacity, and needs.

Scapular Winging

Scapular winging is an impairment that affects the shoulder blades. The scapulae usually rest flat against the back of the rib cage. Winging occurs when a shoulder blade "sticks out" or appears as if the medial portion of the scapula is coming off of the rib cage. The dysfunction can disrupt scapulohumeral rhythm, resulting in a loss of power and limited flexion and abduction of the upper extremity; it can also be a source of considerable pain (Martin & Fish, 2008).

PHASE 1: INHIBIT

Key regions to inhibit with foam rolling include the pectoralis minor, latissimus dorsi, upper trapezius, and thoracic spine.

PHASE 2: LENGTHEN

Key lengthening exercises with static stretches include the pectoralis minor, latissimus dorsi, and upper trapezius.

PHASE 3: ACTIVATE

Key activation exercises with isolated strengthening include the serratus anterior (e.g., push-up plus) and middle and lower trapezius (e.g., ball combo 1).

PHASE 4: INTEGRATE

An integration exercise that could also be implemented for this compensation might be a standing one-arm cable chest press (see **Table 14-6**).

TABLE 14-6 Sample Corrective Exercise Program for the Thoracic Spine and Shoulder: Scapular Winging

Phase	Modality	Muscle(s)/Exercise	Acute Training Variables
Inhibit	Self-myofascial rolling	Latissimus dorsi Pectoralis minor Upper trapezius	Hold areas of discomfort for 30-60 seconds Perform four to six repetitions of active joint movement 90 to 120 seconds per muscle group
Lengthen	Static stretching	Latissimus dorsi Pectoralis minor Upper trapezius	30-second hold
Activate	Isolated strengthening	Serratus anterior Trapezius (middle and lower)	10 to 15 reps with 4-second eccentric contraction, 2-second isometric contraction at end-range, and 1-second concentric contraction
Integrate*	Integrated dynamic movement	Standing one-arm cable chest press	10 to 15 reps under control

* NOTE: Progress and regress as needed to match client ability, work capacity, and needs.

Common Issues Associated with the Thoracic Spine and Shoulder

Primary care reports an annual incidence rate of at least 14.7 per 1,000 patients per year experiencing shoulder dysfunction (Smith et al., 2014). The athletic population experiences rates of injury of about 2.27 shoulder injuries per 10,000 athletic exposures at the high school level. Overall, shoulder injuries accounted for 8% of all injuries sustained at the high school level (Bonza et al., 2009). Olympic weightlifters and powerlifters can experience up to a 50% shoulder injury rate depending on experience level and age (Aasa et al., 2017). CrossFit® athletes experience injury rates to the shoulder that are comparable to Olympic weightlifting, rugby, football, gymnastics, or ice hockey (Klimek et al., 2018). In weightlifting, Olympic lifting, and CrossFit, risk factors for shoulder injuries include poor mobility and strength, lifting heavy loads overhead, quick and explosive movements like the snatch and jerk, and kipping pull-ups (Klimek et al., 2018). Corrective Exercise Specialists should identify these risk factors in both programming and individuals' capabilities in order to reduce incidence of shoulder injuries and improve performance.

Thoracic spine pain and dysfunction is less common than in other regions of the spine. One study of a Norwegian population found a 1-year estimate of thoracic spine pain prevalence of 13% compared with 43% and 44% for low-back and neck pain, respectively (Leboeuf-Yde et al., 2009). A different study found lifetime prevalence data for thoracic spine pain ranged from 3.7% to 77% (Briggs et al., 2009) with a higher incidence found in teenagers and women. Thoracic spine pain and dysfunction is often associated with pathologies such

Osteoporosis

Literally "porous bone"; a disease in which the density and quality of bone is reduced.

Osteoarthritis

The most common form of arthritis, affecting millions of people worldwide; occurs when the protective cartilage that cushions the ends of the bones wears down over time.

Scheuermann's disease

A developmental disorder of the spine that causes abnormal growth of usually the thoracic (upper back) vertebrae, but it can also be found in the lumbar vertebrae.

Ankylosing spondylitis

A form of arthritis that primarily affects the spine, although other joints can become involved; causes inflammation of the spinal joints (vertebrae) that can lead to severe chronic pain and discomfort.

Shoulder impingement

Occurs when the space between the bone on top of the shoulder (acromion) and the tendons of the rotator cuff rub against each other during arm elevation.

 GETTING TECHNICAL

Shoulder Injury Continuum

In 2009, Cook and Purdam proposed a continuum model of tendon pathology. The Cook and Purdam model describes the progression from a normal tendon to reactive tendinopathy, to tendon disrepair, and, ultimately, to degenerative tendinopathy. Reactive rotator cuff tendinopathy is an inflamed, overloaded tendon that causes pain on activity. The rotator cuff tendon is substantially overloaded and displays incomplete healing in the stage of tendon disrepair. The inflamed tendon may have degenerated to a small partial-thickness tear. Degenerative tendinopathy manifests in large partial- and full-thickness rotator cuff tears, as well as massive rotator cuff tears, that cannot heal (van Zuydam et al., 2015).

as **osteoporosis**, **osteoarthritis**, **Scheuermann's disease**, and **ankylosing spondylitis** (Briggs et al., 2009); however, this section will only discuss the most common thoracic pain dysfunctions.

The joints of the upper extremity are intimately linked in a functional chain. Function at one joint affects function at the others. For example, while reaching, a complex and synchronous control of movements at the shoulder, elbow, and wrist must occur (Liu et al., 2013). Amazingly, slight finger motions stimulate postural changes throughout the entire upper extremity (Caronni & Cavallari, 2009). This limb-wide activation occurs to provide stability proximally (shoulder) with the goal of counteracting torques created distally (elbow and wrist). Torques are created by two joint muscles crossing the wrist and elbow to stabilize the shoulder. Therefore, limitations at one joint in this system will affect movement at the other joints (Muth et al., 2012).

A Corrective Exercise Specialist's job is to evaluate movement and provide strategies for improving movement quality overall; diagnosis or treatment of any of the following pathologies is outside the scope of practice. The presence of any of the following pathologies requires consultation with or referral to a qualified medical professional.

 CRITICAL

This section is intended to provide general information about specific medical conditions of the thoracic spine and shoulder. The information provided should not be used to diagnose any medical condition. The fitness professional should refer to the appropriate medical professional if a client needs a diagnosis of a potential medical condition. This will ensure client safety and proper scope of practice.

Shoulder Impingement Syndrome (SIS)

Shoulder impingement refers to the findings of a positive physical examination that could be produced by a variety of subacromial pathologies, including subacromial bursitis, partial rotator cuff tears, biceps tendinitis, scapular dyskinesis, a tight posterior capsule, and postural abnormalities (Kuhn, 2009). Shoulder impingement syndrome (SIS) can be defined as compression of the rotator cuff and the subacromial bursa against the anteroinferior aspect of the acromion and the coracoacromial ligament, leading to pain and/or weakness around the shoulder joint, especially with overhead activity (Hughes et al., 2012).

Impingement is traditionally divided into external impingement and internal impingement groups, with the external impingement group being subdivided into primary and secondary subgroups. Primary external impingement implies abnormalities of the superior bony structures, leading to encroachment of the subacromial space from above. An abnormally shaped acromion is often the cause, but an acromial bony spur may occur in older age groups (Ogawa et al., 2005). Secondary external impingement refers to narrowing of the subacromial space by anterior tilt and excessive internal rotation of an unstable scapula. Weakness and inactivity of the scapular stabilizing muscles leads to an abnormal scapulohumeral rhythm (Hébert et al., 2002). Internal impingement often occurs due to repetitive microtrauma to the rotator cuff tendons (predominantly supraspinatus) in athletes who engage in throwing, racquet, or other overhead actions (Myers et al., 2006). Many times, surgical intervention is used to decompress the structures, but more recent literature is suggesting exercise is as, or more, effective than surgery without the increased risk of death (2% to 4% for general surgery; Dong et al., 2015; Hébert et al., 2002; Meislin et al., 2005; Michener et al., 2003; Muraki et al., 2017) (**Figure 14-20**).

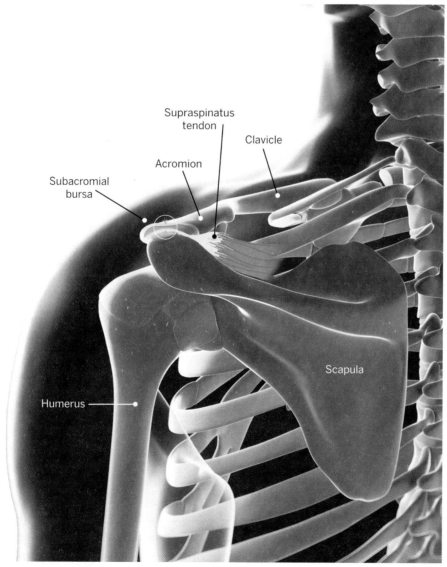

Figure 14-20 Shoulder impingement

Acromioclavicular Separation

An acromioclavicular joint separation, or AC separation, is a frequent injury among physically active people. The clavicle separates from the scapula. It is usually caused by a fall directly on the point of the shoulder or a hit to the AC joint in a contact sport like football or rugby (Deans et al., 2019) (**Figure 14-2 1**).

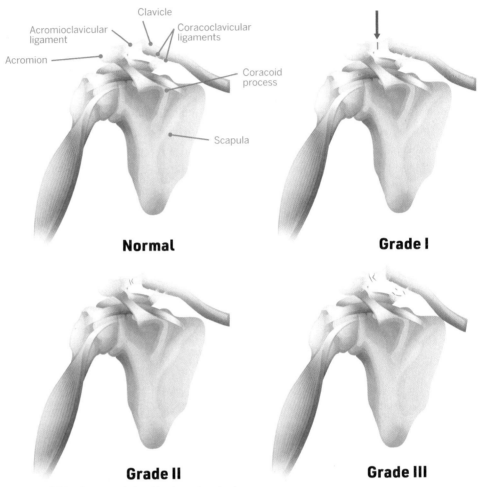

Normal

Grade I

Grade II

Grade III

Figure 14-21 Separated shoulder (anterior view)
© Alila Medical Media/Shutterstock

Rotator Cuff Strain

Rotator cuff **strains** or tears are caused by either overuse or an acute injury. The tendons that connect muscles to bones can overstretch (strain) or tear partially or completely (rupture). The rotator cuff can also strain or tear after a fall, a car accident, or another sudden injury. Tears to the rotator cuff can occur in a fitness setting while lifting too heavy of a load with an outstretched arm, ballistic movements like a kipping pull-up, or repetitive overhead lifting with poor form (Allen et al., 2019; Bartolozzi et al., 1994; Cibulas et al., 2019; Kibler et al., 2006; Kukkonen et al., 2015).

Biceps Tendinopathy

Biceps tendinopathy presents as pain and dysfunction of the tendon around the long head of the biceps muscle. Not usually found in isolation, it is usually caused by overuse, tendon impingement, shoulder joint instability, or trauma. Therefore, it coexists with other pathologies of the shoulder, including rotator cuff impingement syndrome, rotator cuff tears, labral tears, superior labrum from anterior to posterior (SLAP) lesions, and shoulder instability (Raney et al., 2017).

Frozen Shoulder and Osteoarthritis

In frozen shoulder, medically termed adhesive capsulitis, inflammation develops in the shoulder, causing pain and stiffness. As a frozen shoulder progresses, movement in the shoulder can be severely limited. The etiology of frozen shoulder is unknown, and it often self-resolves within 12 months (Hsu et al., 2011).

Osteoarthritis is the common wear-and-tear arthritis that occurs with aging. The shoulder is less often affected by osteoarthritis than the knee, but it can occur at the AC joint. It is aptly named *weightlifter's shoulder* due to the wear and tear from upper body pressing movements (Oh et al., 2011).

Shoulder Instability

Shoulder instability occurs when the head of the humerus is forced out of the shoulder socket and causes laxity in the structures that hold the humeral head in place. This can happen as a result of a sudden injury or from overuse. When the shoulder is loose and slips out of place repeatedly, it is called chronic shoulder instability.

The two most common types of labral injuries are SLAP tears and Bankart tears. SLAP tears occur at the front of the upper arm where the biceps tendon connects to the shoulder. Athletes most prone to this injury include baseball pitchers and volleyball players who engage in high-energy, quick-snap motions over the top of the shoulder. Bankart tears typically occur with shoulder dislocation in younger patients and occur when the head of the humerus either shifts anteriorly or posteriorly causing instability in either of those directions.

It is important to consider that the connections of the sacrum, pelvis, and spine to the arms, legs, and head are functionally interrelated through muscular, fascial, and ligamentous structures. Efficient body movement does not provide a solution for individual joints but orchestrates efficient reaction forces to integrate and stabilize the segments of the body. For example, focusing on singular anatomical structures to comprehend lumbopelvic pain, rather than considering the spine and pelvis as an integrated, interdependent, and dynamic biological structure might blind the observer to the larger picture (Vora et al., 2010). Because of this interconnectivity, the health and stability of the shoulder girdle are directly related to the ability of other segments to accept, distribute, and stabilize forces.

SUMMARY

The thoracic spine and shoulder girdle are prone to being affected by and, in turn, influencing many other parts of the kinetic chain. Given the vast amount of mobility, stability, and control required from this region of the body, even minor restrictions in mobility or strength deficits are likely to have a significant influence on overall movement quality. For this reason, it is vital to thoroughly assess clients and athletes using an integrated process such as the CES Assessment Flow. Shoulder stability, strength of underactive tissues, and extensibility of overactive tissues are to be prioritized. In this way, the efficiencies of the multiple joints of the shoulder girdle may be optimized, and injury resistance and client durability improved.

Aasa, U., Svartholm, I., Andersson, F., & Berglund, L. (2017). Injuries among weightlifters and powerlifters: A systematic review. *British Journal of Sports Medicine, 51*(4), 211–219. https://doi.org/10.1136/bjsports-2016-096037

Allen, H., Chan, B. Y., Davis, K. W., & Blankenbaker, D. G. (2019). Overuse injuries of the shoulder. *Radiologic Clinics of North America, 57*(5), 897–909. https://doi.org/10.1016/j.rcl.2019.03.003

Aspegren, D., Hyde, T., & Miller, M. (2007). Conservative treatment of a female collegiate volleyball player with costochondritis. *Journal of Manipulative and Physiological Therapeutics, 30*(4), 321–325.

Bakhsh, W., & Nicandri, G. (2018). Anatomy and physical examination of the shoulder. *Sports Medicine and Arthroscopy Review, 26*(3), e10–e22. https://doi.org/10.1097/jsa.0000000000000202

Bartolozzi, A., Andreychik, D., & Ahmad, S. (1994). Determinants of outcome in the treatment of rotator cuff disease. *Clinical Orthopaedics and Related Research, 308*, 90–97.

Bau, J. G., Chia, T., Wei, S. H., Li, Y. H., & Kuo, F. C. (2017). Correlations of neck/shoulder perfusion characteristics and pain symptoms of the female office workers with sedentary lifestyle. *PLoS One, 12*(1), e0169318. https://doi.org/10.1371/journal.pone.0169318

Bergman, G. J., Winters, J. C., Groenier, K. H., Pool, J. J. M., Meyboom-de Jong, B., Postema, K., & van der Heijden, G. J. (2004). Manipulative therapy in addition to usual medical care for patients with shoulder dysfunction and pain: A randomized, controlled trial. *Annals of Internal Medicine, 141*(6), 432–439.

Bible, J. E., Biswas, D., Miller, C. P., Whang, P. G., & Grauer, J. N. (2010). Normal functional range of motion of the lumbar spine during 15 activities of daily living. *Journal of Spinal Disorders & Techniques, 23*(2), 106–112.

Bogduk, N. (2016). Functional anatomy of the spine. *Handbook of Clinical Neurology, 136*, 675–688. https://doi.org/10.1016/b978-0-444-53486-6.00032-6

Bonza, J. E., Fields, S. K., Yard, E. E., & Dawn Comstock, R. (2009). Shoulder injuries among United States high school athletes during the 2005–2006 and 2006–2007 school years. *Journal of Athletic Training, 44*(1), 76–83. https://doi.org/10.4085/1062-6050-44.1.76

Borstad, J. D. (2006). Resting position variables at the shoulder: Evidence to support a posture-impairment association. *Physical Therapy, 86*(4), 549–557.

Borstad, J. D., & Ludewig, P. M. (2005). The effect of long versus short pectoralis minor resting length on scapular kinematics in healthy individuals. *Journal of Orthopaedic & Sports Physical Therapy, 35*(4), 227–238. https://doi.org/10.2519/jospt.2005.35.4.227

Boyles, R. E., Ritland, B. M., Miracle, B. M., Barclay, D. M., Faul, M. S., Moore, J. H., Koppenhaver, S. L., & Wainner, R. S. (2009). The short-term effects of thoracic spine thrust manipulation on patients with shoulder impingement syndrome. *Manual Therapy, 14*(4), 375–380.

Briggs, A., Straker, L., & Greig, A. (2004). Upper quadrant postural changes of school children in response to interaction with different information technologies. *Ergonomics, 47*(7), 790–819. https://doi.org/10.1080/00140130410001663569

Briggs, A. M., Bragge, P., Smith, A. J., Govil, D., & Straker, L. M. (2009). Prevalence and associated factors for thoracic spine pain in the adult working population: A literature review. *Journal of Occupational Health, 51*(3), 177–192. https://doi.org/10.1539/joh.k8007

Briggs, A. M., van Dieen, J. H., Wrigley, T. V., Greig, A. M., Phillips, B., Lo, S. K., & Bennell, K. L. (2007). Thoracic kyphosis affects spinal loads and trunk muscle force. *Physical Therapy, 87*(5), 595–607. https://doi.org/10.2522/ptj.20060119

Briggs, A. M., Wrigley, T. V., Tully, E. A., Adams, P. E., Greig, A. M., & Bennell, K. L. (2007). Radiographic measures of thoracic kyphosis in osteoporosis: Cobb and vertebral centroid angles. *Skeletal Radiology, 36*(8), 761–767. https://doi.org/10.1007/s00256-007-0284-8

Caronni, A., & Cavallari, P. (2009). Anticipatory postural adjustments stabilise the whole upper-limb prior to a gentle index finger tap. *Experimental Brain Research, 194*(1), 59–66.

Cibulas, A., Leyva, A., Cibulas, G., 2nd, Foss, M., Boron, A., Dennison, J., Gutterman, B., Kani, K., Porrino, J., Bancroft, L. W., & Scherer, K. (2019). Acute shoulder injury. *Radiologic Clinics of North America, 57*(5), 883–896. https://doi.org/10.1016/j.rcl.2019.03.004

Cleland, J. A., Childs, J. D., Fritz, J. M., Whitman, J. M., & Eberhart, S. L. (2007). Development of a clinical prediction rule for guiding treatment of a subgroup of patients with neck pain: Use of thoracic spine manipulation, exercise, and patient education. *Physical Therapy, 87*(1), 9–23.

Cleland, J. A., Childs, J. D., McRae, M., Palmer, J. A., & Stowell, T. (2005). Immediate effects of thoracic manipulation in patients with neck pain: A randomized clinical trial. *Manual Therapy, 10*(2), 127–135.

Cleland, J. A., Glynn, P., Whitman, J. M., Eberhart, S. L., MacDonald, C., & Childs, J. D. (2007). Short-term effects of thrust versus nonthrust mobilization/manipulation directed at the thoracic spine in patients with neck pain: A randomized clinical trial. *Physical Therapy, 87*(4), 431–440.

Cleland, J. A., Mintken, P. E., Carpenter, K., Fritz, J. M., Glynn, P., Whitman, J., & Childs, J. D. (2010). Examination of a clinical prediction rule to identify patients with neck pain likely to benefit from thoracic spine thrust manipulation and a general cervical range of motion exercise: Multi-center randomized clinical trial. *Physical Therapy, 90*(9), 1239–1250.

Cleland, J., Selleck, B., Stowell, T., Browne, L., Alberini, S., St. Cyr, H., & Caron, T. (2004). Short-term effects of thoracic manipulation on lower trapezius muscle strength. *Journal of Manual & Manipulative Therapy, 12*(2), 82–90.

Cole, M. H., & Grimshaw, P. N. (2016). The biomechanics of the modern golf swing: Implications for lower back injuries. *Sports Medicine, 46*(3), 339–351. https://doi.org/10.1007/s40279-015-0429-1

Cook, J. L., & Purdam, C. R. (2009). Is tendon pathology a continuum? A pathology model to explain the clinical presentation of load-induced tendinopathy. *British Journal of Sports Medicine, 43*(6), 409–416.

Crosbie, J., Kilbreath, S. L., Hollmann, L., & York, S. (2008). Scapulo-humeral rhythm and associated spinal motion. *Clinical Biomechanics, 23*(2), 184–192.

Cross, K. M., Kuenze, C., Grindstaff, T. L., & Hertel, J. (2011). Thoracic spine thrust manipulation improves pain, range of motion, and self-reported function in patients with mechanical neck pain: A systematic review. *Journal of Orthopaedic & Sports Physical Therapy, 41*(9), 633–642.

Deans, C. F., Gentile, J. M., & Tao, M. A. (2019). Acromioclavicular joint injuries in overhead athletes: A concise review of injury mechanisms, treatment options, and outcomes. *Current Reviews in Musculoskeletal Medicine, 12*(2), 80–86. https://doi.org/10.1007/s12178-019-09542-w

Dong, W., Goost, H., Lin, X. B., Burger, C., Paul, C., Wang, Z. L., Zhang, T.-Y., Jiang, Z.-C., Welle, K., & Kabir, K. (2015). Treatments for shoulder impingement syndrome: A PRISMA systematic review and network meta-analysis. *Medicine (Baltimore), 94*(10), e510.

Dunning, J. R., Butts, R., Mourad, F., Young, I., Fernández-de-Las Peñas, C., Hagins, M., Stanislawski, T., Donley, J., Buck, D., Hooks, T. R., & Cleland, J. A. (2016). Upper cervical and upper thoracic manipulation versus mobilization and exercise in patients with cervicogenic headache: A multi-center randomized clinical trial. *BMC Musculoskeletal Disorders, 17*, 64. https://doi.org/10.1186/s12891-016-0912-3

Dunning, J. R., Cleland, J. A., Waldrop, M. A., Arnot, C. F., Young, I. A., Turner, M., & Sigurdsson, G. (2012). Upper cervical and upper thoracic thrust manipulation versus nonthrust mobilization in patients with mechanical neck pain: A multicenter randomized clinical trial. *Journal of Orthopaedic & Sports Physical Therapy, 42*(1), 5–18.

Fernández-de-las-Peñas, C., Cleland, J. A., Huijbregts, P., Palomeque-del-Cerro, L., & González-Iglesias, J. (2009). Repeated applications of thoracic spine thrust manipulation do not lead to tolerance in patients presenting with acute mechanical neck pain: A secondary analysis. *Journal of Manual & Manipulative Therapy, 17*(3), 154–162.

Floyd, R. T. (2017). *Manual of structural kinesiology* (20th ed.). McGraw-Hill Education.

González-Iglesias, J., Fernández-de-las-Peñas, C., Cleland, J. A., Alburquerque-Sendín, F., Palomeque-del-Cerro, L., & Méndez-Sánchez, R. (2009). Inclusion of thoracic spine thrust manipulation into an electro-therapy/thermal program for the management of patients with acute mechanical neck pain: A randomized clinical trial. *Manual Therapy, 14*(3), 306–313.

González-Iglesias, J., Fernández-de-las-Peñas, C., Cleland, J. A., & Gutiérrez-Vega Mdel, R. (2009). Thoracic spine manipulation for the management of patients with neck pain: A randomized clinical trial. *Journal of Orthopaedic & Sports Physical Therapy, 39*(1), 20–27.

Haik, M. N., Alburquerque-Sendín, F., Silva, C. Z., Siqueira-Junior, A. L., Ribeiro, I. L., & Camargo, P. R. (2014). Scapular kinematics pre- and post-thoracic thrust manipulation in individuals with and without shoulder impingement symptoms: A randomized controlled study. *Journal of Orthopaedic & Sports Physical Therapy, 44*(7), 475–487.

Hamill, J., & Knutzen, K. (2006). *Biomechanical basis of human movement* (2nd ed.). Lippincott Williams & Wilkins.

Hébert, L. J., Moffet, H., McFadyen, B. J., & Dionne, C. E. (2002). Scapular behavior in shoulder impingement syndrome. *Archives of Physical Medicine and Rehabilitation, 83*(1), 60–69.

Hsu, J. E., Anakwenze, O. A., Warrender, W. J., & Abboud, J. A. (2011). Current review of adhesive capsulitis. *Journal of Shoulder and Elbow Surgery, 20*(3), 502–514. https://doi.org/10.1016/j.jse.2010.08.023

Hughes, P. C., Green, R. A., & Taylor, N. F. (2012). Measurement of subacromial impingement of the rotator cuff. *Journal of Science and Medicine in Sport, 15*(1), 2–7. https://doi.org/10.1016/j.jsams.2011.07.001

Johnson, K. D., & Grindstaff, T. L. (2010). Thoracic rotation measurement techniques: Clinical commentary. *North American Journal of Sports and Physical Therapy, 5*(4), 252–256.

Kendall, F. P., McCreary, E. K., Provance, P. G., McIntyre Rodgers, M., & Romani, W. A. (2005). *Muscles: Testing and function, with posture and pain* (5th ed.). Lippincott, Williams, & Wilkins.

Kibler, W. B., Sciascia, A., & Dome, D. (2006). Evaluation of apparent and absolute supraspinatus strength in patients with shoulder injury using the scapular retraction test. *American Journal of Sports Medicine, 34*(10), 1643–1647. https://doi.org/10.1177/0363546506288728

Klimek, C., Ashbeck, C., Brook, A. J., & Durall, C. (2018). Are injuries more common with CrossFit training than other forms of exercise? *Journal of Sport Rehabilitation, 27*(3), 295–299. https://doi.org/10.1123/jsr.2016-0040

Kuhn, J. E. (2009). Exercise in the treatment of rotator cuff impingement: A systematic review and a synthesized evidence-based rehabilitation protocol. *Journal of Shoulder and Elbow Surgery, 18*(1), 138–160. https://doi.org/10.1016/j.jse.2008.06.004

Kukkonen, J., Joukainen, A., Lehtinen, J., Mattila, K. T., Tuominen, E. K., Kauko, T., & Äärimaa, V. (2015). Treatment of nontraumatic rotator cuff tears: A randomized controlled trial with two years of clinical and imaging follow-up. *Journal of Bone and Joint Surgery (American Volume), 97*(21), 1729–1737. https://doi.org/10.2106/JBJS.N.01051

Lau, H. M., Wing Chiu, T. T., & Lam, T.-H. (2011). The effectiveness of thoracic manipulation on patients with chronic mechanical neck pain: A randomized controlled trial. *Manual Therapy, 16*(2), 141–147.

Leboeuf-Yde, C., Nielsen, J., Kyvik, K. O., Fejer, R., & Hartvigsen, J. (2009). Pain in the lumbar, thoracic or cervical regions: Do age and gender matter? A population-based study of 34,902 Danish twins 20–71 years of age. *BMC Musculoskeletal Disorders, 10*, 39. https://doi.org/10.1186/1471-2474-10-39

Liu, W., Whitall, J., & Kepple, T. M. (2013). Multi-joint coordination of functional arm reaching: Induced position analysis. *Journal of Applied Biomechanics, 29*(2), 235–240.

Martin, R. M., & Fish, D. E. (2008). Scapular winging: Anatomical review, diagnosis, and treatments. *Current Reviews in Musculoskeletal Medicine, 1*(1), 1–11. https://doi.org/10.1007/s12178-007-9000-5

Masaracchio, M., Cleland, J. A., Hellman, M., & Hagins, M. (2013). Short-term combined effects of thoracic spine thrust manipulation and cervical spine nonthrust manipulation in individuals with mechanical neck pain: A randomized clinical trial. *Journal of Orthopaedic & Sports Physical Therapy, 43*(3), 118–127. https://doi.org/10.2519/jospt.2013.4221

McClure, P. W., Michener, L. A., & Karduna, A. R. (2006). Shoulder function and 3-dimensional scapular kinematics in people with and without shoulder impingement syndrome. *Physical Therapy*, *86*(8), 1075–1090.

Meislin, R. J., Sperling, J. W., & Stitik, T. P. (2005). Persistent shoulder pain: Epidemiology, pathophysiology, and diagnosis. *American Journal of Orthopedics*, *34*(12 Suppl.), 5–9.

Michener, L. A., McClure, P. W., & Karduna, A. R. (2003). Anatomical and biomechanical mechanisms of subacromial impingement syndrome. *Clinical Biomechanics*, *18*(5), 369–379.

Mintken, P. E., Cleland, J. A., Carpenter, K. J., Bieniek, M. L., Keirns, M., & Whitman, J. M. (2010). Some factors predict successful short-term outcomes in individuals with shoulder pain receiving cervicothoracic manipulation: A single-arm trial. *Physical Therapy*, *90*(1), 26–42.

Mitchell, C., Adebajo, A., Hay, E., & Carr, A. (2005). Shoulder pain: Diagnosis and management in primary care. *BMJ*, *331*(7525), 1124–1128. https://doi.org/10.1136/bmj.331.7525.1124

Moore, K. L., Dalley, A. F., & Agur, A. M. R. (2014). *Clinically oriented anatomy* (7th ed.). Lippincott, Williams, & Wilkins.

Morita, D., Yukawa, Y., Nakashima, H., Ito, K., Yoshida, G., Machino, M., Kanbara, S., Iwase, T., & Kato, F. (2014). Range of motion of thoracic spine in sagittal plane. *European Spine Journal*, *23*(3), 673–678. https://doi.org/10.1007/s00586-013-3088-7

Muraki, T., Yamamoto, N., Sperling, J. W., Steinmann, S. P., Cofield, R. H., & An, K. N. (2017). The effect of scapular position on subacromial contact behavior: A cadaver study. *Journal of Shoulder and Elbow Surgery*, *26*(5), 861–869. https://doi.org/10.1016/j.jse.2016.10.009

Muth, S., Barbe, M. F., Lauer, R., & McClure, P. W. (2012). The effects of thoracic spine manipulation in subjects with signs of rotator cuff tendinopathy. *Journal of Orthopaedic & Sports Physical Therapy*, *42*(12), 1005–1016. https://doi.org/10.2519/jospt.2012.4142

Myers, J. B., Laudner, K. G., Pasquale, M. R., Bradley, J. P., & Lephart, S. M. (2006). Glenohumeral range of motion deficits and posterior shoulder tightness in throwers with pathologic internal impingement. *American Journal of Sports Medicine*, *34*(3), 385–391. https://doi.org/10.1177/0363546505281804

Nakamaru, K., Aizawa, J., Kawarada, K., Uemura, Y., Koyama, T., & Nitta, O. (2019). Immediate effects of thoracic spine self-mobilization in patients with mechanical neck pain: A randomized controlled trial. *Journal of Bodywork and Movement Therapies*, *23*(2), 417–424.

Norlander, S., Gustavsson, B. A., Lindell, J., & Nordgren, B. (1997). Reduced mobility in the cervico-thoracic motion segment—a risk factor for musculoskeletal neck-shoulder pain: A two-year prospective follow-up study. *Scandinavian Journal of Rehabilitation Medicine*, *29*(3), 167–174.

Norlander, S., & Nordgren, B. (1998). Clinical symptoms related to musculoskeletal neck-shoulder pain and mobility in the cervico-thoracic spine. *Scandinavian Journal of Rehabilitation Medicine*, *30*(4), 243–251.

Ogawa, K., Yoshida, A., Inokuchi, W., & Naniwa, T. (2005). Acromial spur: Relationship to aging and morphologic changes in the rotator cuff. *Journal of Shoulder and Elbow Surgery*, *14*(6), 591–598.

Oh, J. H., Chung, S. W., Oh, C. H., Kim, S. H., Park, S. J., Kim, K. W., Hyuk Park, J., Lee, S. B., & Lee, J. J. (2011). The prevalence of shoulder osteoarthritis in the elderly Korean population: Association with risk factors and function. *Journal of Shoulder and Elbow Surgery*, *20*(5), 756–763.

Page, P., Frank, C. C., & Lardner, R. (2010). *Assessment and treatment of muscle imbalance: The Janda approach*. Human Kinetics.

Pillastrini, P., Rocchi, G., Deserri, D., Foschi, P., Mardegan, M., Naldi, M. T., Villafañe, J. H., & Bertozzi, L. (2016). Effectiveness of neuromuscular taping on painful hemiplegic shoulder: A randomised clinical trial. *Disability and Rehabilitation*, *38*(16), 1603–1609. https://doi.org/10.3109/09638288.2015.1107631

Raney, E. B., Thankam, F. G., Dilisio, M. F., & Agrawal, D. K. (2017). Pain and the pathogenesis of biceps tendinopathy. *American Journal of Translational Research*, *9*(6), 2668–2683.

Robb, A. J., Fleisig, G., Wilk, K., Macrina, L., Bolt, B., & Pajaczkowski, J. (2010). Passive ranges of motion of the hips and their relationship with pitching biomechanics and ball velocity in professional baseball pitchers. *American Journal of Sports Medicine, 38*(12), 2487–2493.

Šarčević, Z. (2010). Scoliosis: Muscle imbalance and treatment. *British Journal of Sports Medicine*, *44*, i16.

Sciascia, A., & Cromwell, R. (2012). Kinetic chain rehabilitation: A theoretical framework. *Rehabilitation Research and Practice, 2012*, 853037–853037. https://doi.org/10.1155/2012/853037

Shakil, H., Iqbal, Z. A., & Al-Ghadir, A. H. (2014). Scoliosis: Review of types of curves, etiological theories and conservative treatment. *Journal of Back and Musculoskeletal Rehabilitation*, *27*(2), 111–115. https://doi.org/10.3233/bmr-130438

Singla, D., & Veqar, Z. (2017). Association between forward head, rounded shoulders, and increased thoracic kyphosis: A review of the literature. *Journal of Chiropractic Medicine*, *16*(3), 220–229. https://doi.org/10.1016/j.jcm.2017.03.004

Smith, E., Hoy, D. G., Cross, M., Vos, T., Naghavi, M., Buchbinder, R., Woolf, A. D., & March, L. (2014). The global burden of other musculoskeletal disorders: Estimates from the Global Burden of Disease 2010 study. *Annals of Rheumatic Diseases*, *73*(8), 1462–1469. https://doi.org/10.1136/annrheumdis-2013-204680

Sobel, J. S., Kremer, I., Winters, J. C., Arendzen, J. H., & de Jong, B. M. (1996). The influence of the mobility in the cervicothoracic spine and the upper ribs (shoulder girdle) on the mobility of the scapulohumeral joint. *Journal of Manipulative and Physiological Therapeutics*, *19*(7), 469–474.

Sobel, J. S., Winters, J. C., Groenier, K., Arendzen, J. H., & Meyboom de Jong, B. (1997). Physical examination of the cervical spine and shoulder girdle in patients with shoulder complaints. *Journal of Manipulative and Physiological Therapeutics*, *20*(4), 257–262.

Sueki, D. G., Cleland, J. A., & Wainner, R. S. (2013). A regional interdependence model of musculoskeletal dysfunction: Research, mechanisms, and clinical implications. *Journal of Manual & Manipulative Therapy*, *21*(2), 90–102. https://doi.org/10.1179/2042618612Y.0000000027

Timmons, M. K., Thigpen, C. A., Seitz, A. L., Karduna, A. R., Arnold, B. L., & Michener, L. A. (2012). Scapular kinematics and subacromial-impingement syndrome: A meta-analysis. *Journal of Sport Rehabilitation*, *21*(4), 354–370.

van Zuydam, J., Janse van Rensburg, D. C., Grant, C. C., Janse van Rensburg, A., & Patricios, J. (2015). Shouldering the blame for impingement: The rotator cuff continuum. *South African Family Practice, 57*(1), 34–38.

Villafañe, J. H., Valdes, K., Anselmi, F., Pirali, C., & Negrini, S. (2015). The diagnostic accuracy of five tests for diagnosing partial-thickness tears of the supraspinatus tendon: A cohort study. *Journal of Hand Therapy, 28*(3), 247–251; quiz 252. https://doi.org/10.1016/j.jht.2015.01.011

Vora, A. J., Doerr, K. D., & Wolfer, L. R. (2010). Functional anatomy and pathophysiology of axial low back pain: Disc, posterior elements, sacroiliac joint, and associated pain generators. *Physical Medicine and Rehabilitation Clinics of North America, 21*(4), 679–709. https://doi.org/10.1016/j.pmr.2010.07.005

Walser, R. F., Meserve, B. B., & Boucher, T. R. (2009). The effectiveness of thoracic spine manipulation for the management of musculoskeletal conditions: A systematic review and meta-analysis of randomized clinical trials. *Journal of Manual & Manipulative Therapy, 17*(4), 237–246.

Young, J. L., Walker, D., Snyder, S., & Daly, K. (2014). Thoracic manipulation versus mobilization in patients with mechanical neck pain: A systematic review. *Journal of Manual & Manipulative Therapy, 22*(3), 141–153.

CHAPTER 15

Corrective Strategies for the Wrist and Elbow

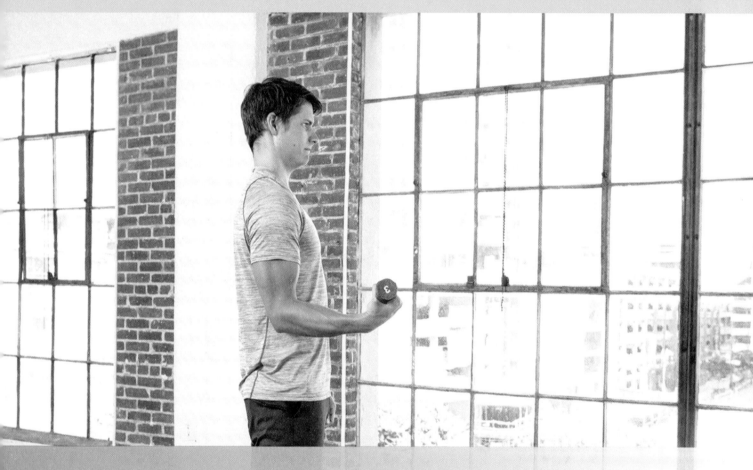

Learning Objectives

After reading this content, students should be able to demonstrate the following objectives:

- **Explain** the basic functional anatomy of the wrist and elbow.
- **Identify** the mechanisms for common wrist and elbow injuries.
- **Describe** the influence of altered wrist and elbow movement on the kinetic chain.
- **Determine** appropriate systematic assessment strategies for the wrist and elbow.
- **Select** appropriate corrective exercise strategies for the wrist and elbow.

Introduction

The elbow joint functions as a link between the shoulder and wrist, providing a large amount of stability and motion. The elbow joint is not a simple hinge joint; it also involves **forearm pronation** and **supination**. Pronation involves rotation of the forearm and hand so that the palm faces downward. Conversely, supination involves rotation of the forearm and hand so that the palm faces upward. **Force transmission** in the forearm is a complex interaction of the radius, ulna, and interosseous membrane. Forces at the wrist affect the transmission of force through the forearm to the elbow joint. During some activities, like a baseball pitch, the force generated by the large muscles of the lower extremity and trunk during the wind-up and stride phases are transferred to the ball through the shoulder and elbow (Chalmers et al., 2017). Numerous kinematic factors have been identified that increase shoulder and elbow torques, which are linked to increased risk for injury. Given the complexity and necessity of the wrist and hand, dysfunction can often be debilitating to normal activities of daily living.

These motions, stability, and force interactions are all capable due to the forearm's form and function. Regions above (i.e., shoulder and thoracic spine) directly affect optimal function at the elbow and wrist. Further, an event at the elbow joint affects the forearm and the wrist, and, conversely, injury or disease at the wrist joint can affect the elbow (Kijima & Viegas, 2009; Werner & An, 1994).

Review of Elbow and Wrist Functional Anatomy

The elbow and wrist are complex structures that, along with the shoulder, afford an almost limitless variety of movements for the upper extremity. The wrist allows the connection between the forearm and the hand, allowing force to be transferred from the rest of the body to the hand. Conversely, the wrist also allows force to be transferred from the hand to the rest of the body.

Bones and Joints

The elbow appears relatively simple as it is composed of only three bones. However, the wide variety of articulation points and movements available at the elbow make it a truly unique joint. The wrist is composed of many more bones, yet it does not have as wide a range of movement.

ELBOW

The three bones in the elbow are the humerus, ulna (pinky side), and radius (thumb side). The articulations between the humerus and ulna form the humeroulnar joint (Moore et al., 2013). The humeroulnar joint is a hinge joint that is primarily responsible for elbow flexion and extension. Thus, the humeroulnar joint specifically is often simply called the elbow joint, even with the presence of additional articulations. The articulations between the humerus and radius form the humeroradial joint between the capitulum of the humerus and radial head. The fossa of the radial head is shallow and articulates with the rounded eminence (bony projection) of the capitulum, affording a variety of motions at the humeroradial joint (Moore et al., 2013). Both flexion/extension and rotation are allowed, providing both sagittal and transverse plane (supination/pronation) motion at the elbow (Floyd, 2017). Additionally, the ulna and radius have an articulation at the elbow called the proximal radioulnar joint. The proximal radioulnar joint is composed of the head of the radius and the radial notch of the ulna. The radius is held in place by the radial annular ligament, which forms a collar around the joint (Moore et al., 2013). Forearm

Forearm pronation

Internal rotation of the forearm and hand so that the palm faces downward.

Forearm supination

External rotation of the forearm and hand so that the palm faces upward.

Force transmission

Muscle forces applied to the skeleton via pathways other than muscular origin and insertion.

pronation and supination occurs at the proximal radioulnar joint and is produced by the head of the radius rotating within the ligament. Because the humeroulnar joint is a hinge joint, and thus does not allow rotation, pronation involves the radius crossing over the stationary ulna, forming an *X*; the bones are parallel when supinated (**Figure 15-1**) (Floyd, 2017).

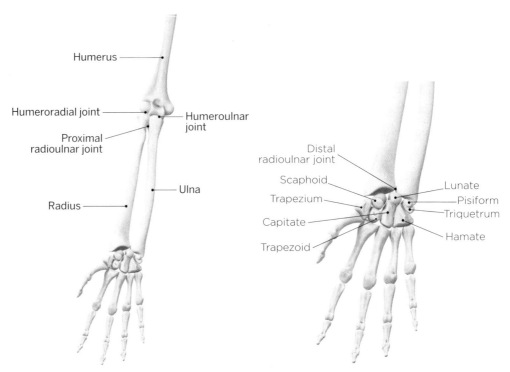

Figure 15-1 Humeroulnar and radioulnar joints   **Figure 15-2** Proximal wrist joint

WRIST

Acting as a hinge, the wrist articulates with the forearm and the bones of the hand. Together, the 37 bones in the wrist and hand allow the precise finger movements needed to perform many necessary tasks, such as typing, writing, and eating. Distally, the radius and ulna make the distal radioulnar joint, which interacts with the carpal bones. The carpus, or wrist, is composed of eight small bones arranged in two rows. The proximal row contains the scaphoid, lunate, triquetrum, and pisiform. This row interacts with the ulna and radius. The distal row contains the trapezium, trapezoid, capitate, and hamate. This row interacts with the five metacarpal bones of the hand (Moore et al., 2013). The majority of wrist flexion and extension and radial and ulnar deviation range of motion (ROM) derives from the proximal wrist joint, which is the site of most wrist flexion and extension, as well as radial and ulnar deviation (**Figure 15-2**) (Floyd, 2017).

HELPFUL HINT

Try this simple mnemonic to remember the carpal bones beginning on the proximal row, medial aspect (ulnar side): Please Take Larry Shopping. He's Come To Town.

Proximal row: Pisiform, triquetrum, lunate, scaphoid
Distal row: Hamate, capitate, trapezoid, trapezium

Muscles

Many muscles are associated with the elbow and wrist. Although not all muscles will be individually addressed in a corrective exercise program, **Table 15-1** provides a detailed list of the muscles, categorized by their actions.

TABLE 15-1 Key Muscles Associated with the Elbow and Wrist and Their Function	
Elbow flexion ■ Biceps brachii ■ Brachialis ■ Brachioradialis ■ Pronator teres (weak elbow flexor) Elbow extension ■ Triceps brachii Forearm pronation ■ Pronator quadratus ■ Pronator teres Forearm supination ■ Supinator (primary) ■ Biceps brachii (secondary) Wrist ulnar deviation ■ Extensor carpi ulnaris ■ Flexor carpi ulnaris Wrist radial deviation ■ Abductor pollicis longus ■ Extensor carpi radialis longus ■ Extensor carpi radialis brevis ■ Flexor carpi radialis	Wrist flexion ■ Flexor carpi radialis ■ Flexor carpus ulnaris ■ Palmaris longus Wrist extension ■ Extensor carpi radialis brevis ■ Extensor carpi radialis longus ■ Extensor carpi ulnaris ■ Extensor digiti minimi ■ Extensor digitorum ■ Extensor indicis ■ Extensor pollicis brevis ■ Extensor pollicis longus

Data from Floyd, R. T. (2017). *Manual of structural kinesiology* (20th ed.). New York, NY: McGraw-Hill Education.

Movement at the elbow (flexion, extension, supination, and pronation) is accomplished by seven muscles; an additional nine muscles cross the elbow to act on the hand and wrist. Elbow flexion is primarily accomplished by the brachialis and is assisted by the biceps brachii and brachioradialis (Floyd, 2017). The biceps brachii is a multiarticular muscle, crossing both the elbow and the shoulder. The biceps brachii often gets attention as it is the bulkiest of the elbow flexor group. However, the brachialis is considered the prime mover of elbow flexion because it generates more overall force (Saladin et al., 2015). Both the biceps brachii and the brachioradialis attach to the radius, which allows them to produce supination (Floyd, 2017). Interestingly, the position of the brachioradialis allows it to both supinate and pronate the forearm, depending on forearm position. It is important to recognize that these muscles cannot supinate the elbow when it is fully extended.

The prime mover of supination comes from the supinator muscle but the biceps brachii also assists with the movement. Unlike the biceps brachii, the supinator can produce supination whether the elbow is flexed or extended.

Pronation of the forearm is accomplished by the pronator quadratus and pronator teres muscles. These muscles tend to be very weak relative to the supination muscles.

 CHECK IT OUT

"Righty Tighty"
You've heard the saying "righty tighty, lefty loosey" when thinking about tightening a lid on a jar or loosening a screw. Most screws, lids, bolts, etc. tighten when turned clockwise because turning involves supination of the right arm. Most people are right-handed, and supination is more powerful than pronation because it is controlled by the supinator muscle and the large biceps brachii.

The elbow extensors include the long head and two shorter heads of the triceps brachii. The three heads of the triceps (long, lateral, and medial) all have different origins with the long head, crossing the shoulder and attaching to the scapula. Thus, in addition to elbow extension, the long head can also assist with shoulder extension (Floyd, 2017).

 TRAINING TIP

Workout programs often tout the benefits of positioning the arms in a certain position to help target certain parts of the triceps. This holds true due to the origin attachment points of the heads of the triceps. Shoulder position influences the length of the long head of the triceps and therefore alters its force production during elbow extension. Shoulder flexion increases the length of the long head, which decreases the amount of force it produces (refer back to length-tension relationships), thus potentially increasing the relative amount of force required by the lateral and medial head (Kholinne et al., 2018).

Lucas-Osma and Collazos-Castro (2009) found that the medial head of the triceps was primarily composed of type I fibers and motor units, the lateral head is primarily type II fibers and motor units, and the long head is a balanced mixture of both. Therefore, the medial head may be more involved in movements requiring fine motor skills, the lateral used in more powerful elbow extension movements, and the long head used a little for both and for those tasks requiring higher endurance. Thus, lifting heavier loads or moving more explosively may recruit more of the lateral head fibers, and lighter loads at a longer duration may recruit more of the medial head fibers. However, given that all triceps share a common insertion on the ulna, rotation of the forearm will not influence one head of the triceps over another.

All the muscles that influence the wrist begin in the forearm or even on the humerus. Given the total number of muscles influencing the hand and wrist, they will be discussed in groups as wrist extensors and wrist flexors. Due to the origin and location of the wrist extensors, they produce not only wrist extension, but also extension of the fingers. Similarly, the wrist flexors produce not only wrist flexion, but also flexion of the fingers (Floyd, 2017; Moore et al., 2013) (**Figures 15-3** and **15-4**). For wrist radial deviation, both the flexors and extensors on the radial (thumb side) work together to perform the movement. For wrist ulnar deviation, the flexors and extensors on the ulnar side (pinky finger side) work together to perform the movement (Floyd, 2017).

All muscles also have a stabilization and force reduction component. In many sports, both forearm flexors and extensors are exposed to heavy eccentric loads. In tennis, for example,

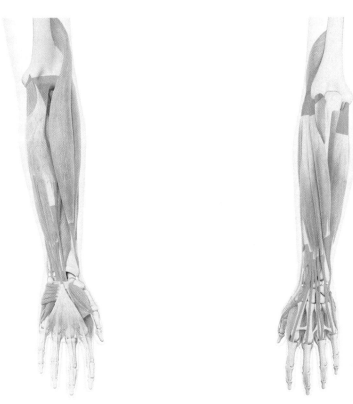

Figure 15-3 Structure of wrist musculature: wrist flexors (palmar surface)

Figure 15-4 Structure of wrist musculature: wrist extensors (dorsal surface)

athletes must forcefully decelerate the forward moving arm during an overhead serve. While much of this deceleration is derived from the shoulder musculature, the wrist extensors contribute a great deal. Conversely, in golf, the wrist flexors must act forcefully to prevent wrist extension when contact is made with the ball. Much dysfunction in the muscles of the forearm are likely attributed to these repetitive actions (**Figure 15-5**) (Chung & Lark, 2017).

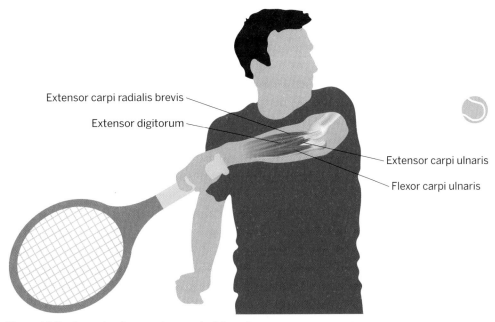

Extensor carpi radialis brevis

Extensor digitorum

Extensor carpi ulnaris

Flexor carpi ulnaris

Figure 15-5 Example of eccentric control of the wrist

Given that many of the movers of the wrist originate in the forearm and above the elbow, corrective exercise programs should work to optimize flexibility, allowing for stabilization of the elbow and wrist. In accordance with the Regional Interdependence (RI) model, it is common for dysfunction to be found below or above a symptomatic joint. Therefore, a more comprehensive analysis of the neck, shoulder, scapula, elbow, and wrist should be conducted with any upper extremity dysfunctional pattern, such as elbows bending on the overhead squat pattern (Sueki et al., 2013).

Altered Elbow and Wrist Movement

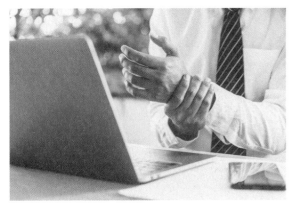
© Nopphon_1987/Shutterstock

Musculoskeletal injuries to the elbow, forearm, and wrist account for approximately one-third of all workday illnesses (Barr et al., 2004; Shiri & Viikari-Juntura, 2011). Between 1% and 3% of the U.S. population experiences elbow pain (Kane et al., 2014), and approximately 25% of all sports-related injuries involve the wrist and hand (Avery et al., 2016). Wrist pain is also becoming more common due to the prolonged repetitive movements and positions required for the typical worker (Huysman et al., 2012). Elbow and wrist pain are usually assessed and managed in primary care, and the incidence of lateral elbow pain in general practice is 4 to 7 per 1,000 people a year (Kane et al., 2014). The elbow and wrist are a functional extension of the shoulder. As such, the lower extremity, lumbar-pelvic-hip complex (LPHC), and shoulder all influence optimal function of this region.

Static Malalignments

Common static malalignments of the elbow may cause constant or chronic elbow flexion, which may result from overactivity of the biceps brachii and brachialis and underactivity of the triceps. This increased length of the triceps may also either affect or be affected by shoulder instability. Further, excessive elbow flexion has been shown to restrict wrist ROM (Murray et al., 2002).

A static malalignment for the wrist presents as chronic wrist extension or flexion. Chronic wrist extension is often seen in those who spend an excessive amount of time using a computer keyboard without wrist support. This malalignment may be due to tightness in the wrist extensors and is often linked to lateral elbow pain. However, those with chronic wrist flexion may perform repetitive activities requiring excessive gripping or carrying of heavy objects. This malalignment may be due to tightness in the wrist flexors and linked to medial elbow pain. Many conditions afflicting the wrist are considered overuse due to the repetitive positions of either flexion or extension. Thus, Parmelee-Peters and Earthorne (2005) stated that an emphasis should be placed on a neutral position when possible. Therefore, injury risk reduction strategies should aim to decrease exposure to repetitive tasks and limit extremes of elbow and wrist motion (Trudel et al., 2004).

Abnormal Muscle Activation Patterns

A number of studies have demonstrated that many individuals with elbow or wrist impairments have less-than-optimal stability and ROM, along with altered muscle activation patterns at the glenohumeral joint (Antony & Keir, 2010; Cantero-Téllez, Orza, et al., 2018; Lucado et al., 2010). Repeated wrist and elbow motion can lead to an overuse of the wrist extensors and to tendon injury (Herquelot et al., 2013). Overload due to repetitive forearm movements leads to changes in the shoulder complex (Lucado et al., 2010). Further, elbow dysfunction may arise because of changes in the shoulder complex and the compensatory actions caused by the overloaded forearm muscles (Lucado et al., 2010). The shoulder stabilizers that may be altered in some cases of elbow and wrist dysfunction are the serratus anterior, rhomboids, lower trapezius, and rotator cuff complex. Thus, improving serratus anterior and rotator cuff activation has been shown to decrease elbow dysfunction (Lee et al., 2018).

Further, those with wrist dysfunction may also have higher rates of shoulder impairment. Cantero-Téllez, Orza, et al. (2018) demonstrated that wrist immobilization resulted in increased shoulder pain. The authors highlighted that the compensatory movement from the loss of wrist motion was likely to blame. Additionally, research has shown altered muscle activation patterns with a redistribution of force in the shoulder musculature during gripping (Antony & Keir, 2010). Thus, in the case of altered recruitment patterns at the shoulder, an individual may demonstrate altered firing patterns along the entire upper extremity.

Dynamic Malalignment

Research has demonstrated that a lack of wrist and elbow movement can lead to alterations in shoulder girdle activation patterns as more movement proximally may be required to compensate for the reduced distal mobility (Antony & Keir, 2010; Cantero-Téllez, Orza, et al., 2018). These changes may lead to increased strain on the elbow musculature, tendons, and rotator cuff.

Elbow and Wrist Dysfunction and the Regional Interdependence Model

Proper elbow and wrist function are dependent on the proximal structures of the upper extremity. Proper mobility of the thoracic spine, scapular stability, and shoulder position can play a large role in dysfunction and injury at the elbow and wrist (Day et al., 2015). Length-tension relationships in the upper extremity may be compromised due to poor posture, repetitive activities, or immobilization in a cast or brace (Page, 2012), reducing optimal force production and leading to synergistic dominance. Recall Janda's upper crossed syndrome creating a shortening of the cervical extensors, pectoralis major/minor, and possibly the elbow flexor group. A shortened muscle can potentially limit full joint motion both at the involved joint and segments above and below (Page, 2012). For example, when trying to stabilize something overhead, a shortened pectoralis group (e.g., pectoralis minor) can cause rounded shoulders and limit full-shoulder flexion. One potential compensatory pattern is to demonstrate wrist hyperextension to balance the mass over the base of support. Changes in ROM at one joint can create faulty movement patterns, resulting in pain, guarding, overuse, or fatigue in joints either above or below (Borboni et al., 2017; Cantero-Téllez, Orza, et al., 2018; Cantero-Téllez, Valdes, et al., 2018; Cantero-Téllez, Villafañe, et al., 2018). This is commonly seen in overhead athletes such as baseball pitchers where mobility deficits or movement impairments at one joint in the upper kinetic chain (UKC) or lower kinetic chain (LKC) will affect related joints along the total kinetic chain during the throwing motion (Chalmers et al., 2017; Shimamura et al., 2015). Optimal joint positions should be enforced to improve muscle activity and force-couples. Therefore, ensuring proper neck, shoulder, and scapulae alignment during all exercise movements can help improve function at and below the region.

Influence on the Wrist

Because the joints of the upper extremity are linked in a functional chain in which the function at one joint affects function at the others, the shoulder and elbow can influence the wrist. For example, reaching requires complex and simultaneous control of movements at the shoulder, elbow, and wrist (Liu et al., 2013). Limitations at one joint in this system will affect movement at another joint during functional activity. Excessive elbow flexion due to biceps brachii shortening has been demonstrated to restrict wrist ROM (Murray et al., 2002). Having restricted wrist mobility due to shortened forearm/elbow flexors is an important consideration in sports, especially in overhead movements like the jerk and snatch, where heavy loads are overhead. Limited wrist motion can overstress the joint and cause dysfunction and/or injury. Similar limitations at the joints in the UKC can been seen in golfers, which can lead to forearm and wrist injuries (Zouzias et al., 2018).

The Corrective Exercise Specialist must understand that the function and health of the elbow, wrist, and shoulder girdle are closely linked. As demands on the upper extremity increase due to workload and/or sport, the Corrective Exercise Specialist must realize the potential for compensation, overuse, and possible injury in the wrist, elbow, head, neck, and shoulder. Optimizing upper body motion requires an understanding of their closely interrelated nature.

Assessment Results for the Elbow and Wrist

The elbow and wrist should be viewed as an extension of the shoulder and upper body. Essentially, any time dysfunction is seen at the shoulder, there is a probability that dysfunction at the elbow or wrist is contributing to it. For example, overactivity of the biceps brachii can contribute to rounded shoulder static posture and the arms fall forward movement impairment, because that muscle crosses the glenohumeral joint.

Furthermore, if a client's shoulders round or their arms rest in a bent position during the static postural assessment, if they have trouble straightening their arms overhead, or if the arms fall forward during the overhead squat assessment (OHSA) or a loaded overhead press, elbow and wrist mobility assessments should also be included in addition to the shoulder and thoracic spine mobility assessments. **Table 15-2** provides a summary of the assessment process and common findings that indicate potential dysfunction in the elbow and wrist.

TABLE 15-2	Elbow and Wrist Assessment Results
Assessment	**Results**
Static posture	Elbows rest in flexed position
	Wrists rest in non-neutral position
Transitional and loaded movement	Arms fall forward
	Arms do not straighten
	Wrists in non-neutral position
Mobility Elbow flexion and extension, wrist flexion and extension	Limited elbow flexion ROM
	Limited elbow extension ROM
	Limited wrist flexion ROM
	Limited wrist extension ROM

Static Posture

Corrective Exercise Specialists will see that there are no discussions of the elbow or wrist with Janda's syndromes and Kendall's spinal postures. However, due to concepts of regional interdependence, the muscles of the arm can have a significant effect on an individual's upper body static posture. If a client presents with rounded shoulders and excessive thoracic kyphosis (e.g., as with upper crossed syndrome and swayback postures), there is a strong chance that limited mobility of the elbow or wrist is a related factor.

Additionally, when observing static posture from a lateral view, the position of the elbows and wrists should also be noted. When standing with arms at the side, they should hang in a relatively straight line with the hips and legs, with the wrist in a straight, neutral position. If the elbow or wrist rests in a bent position, that is a sign that arm mobility assessments should be performed.

Transitional Movement Assessments

Similar to observing static posture, Corrective Exercise Specialists should also observe the elbow and wrist during transitional movement assessments. Specifically, OHSA and overhead press movements may reveal muscle imbalances that exist in the arms.

OVERHEAD SQUAT ASSESSMENT

Because placing the arms overhead requires full mobility in the upper body, shoulders, and elbows, many of the common compensations of the elbow and wrist can be identified in the OHSA. The most common movement impairments seen in the arms are the elbows not fully extending overhead and the wrists moving into a non-neutral position. The lack of elbow extension is often attributed to overactive/shortened biceps brachii and other elbow flexor muscles. Highlighting the regionally interdependent relationship of the upper extremity, in some cases, individuals may compensate with wrist hyperextension as a form of relative flexibility to accomplish fully extended elbows.

Muscle imbalances at the elbows and wrists may also be contributing to the arms falling forward on the OHSA even if a client is able to keep the elbows and wrists straight during the motion. The biceps brachii provide a divergent tension with the latissimus dorsi at the shoulder (both contributing to the complex force-couple at the glenohumeral joint); when the arms are fully extended overhead, both muscles are stretched into an elongated position. If one or both of the muscles are overactive/shortened, the arms can be pulled forward out of alignment with the ears as the individual lowers into the squat and additional tension is placed on the latissimus dorsi. When the arms fall forward during the OHSA, that is a sign to perform targeted mobility assessments of both the elbow and shoulder joints to determine where the primary cause of the mobility restriction may be located (i.e., biceps brachii, latissimus dorsi, or both).

Loaded Movement Assessment

Clients who demonstrate proper static and dynamic posture under body weight alone can be progressed to using loaded variants of primary movement patterns. This provides increased challenge to the musculature and can help draw attention to any remaining imbalance at the joints.

Although the OHSA provides a strong estimation of potential dysfunction in the arms, predictions of limited elbow and wrist ROM can also be made by observing a client during any pushing, pulling, or overhead pressing exercise, provided the client is able to perform them safely. Standing or seated overhead dumbbell press is a suitable exercise to further evaluate shoulder, elbow, and wrist position.

If an individual demonstrates a lack of full elbow extension and/or an inability to maintain the wrist in a neutral position at the end of a push or press movement, muscle imbalances are probable and targeted mobility testing of the elbow and wrist should be performed. Similar to the compensatory arm movement that can be seen during the OHSA, wrist hyperextension can be seen in some individuals at the end-range of a push or a press.

A loaded pull movement can help bring to light any overactivity/shortening of the wrist flexor musculature. At the end-range of the concentric phase of a pull, inward curling wrists are a signal to perform a wrist mobility assessment and potentially develop a corrective exercise protocol to help the individual better maintain neutral wrist positioning.

If a client can perform the OHSA with optimal form but then demonstrates compensations during the loaded variations, specific activation exercises can be prioritized in the client's program. It is important to remember, however, that targeted mobility testing should be used to confirm or deny observations made during movement assessments.

Mobility Assessments

If the client demonstrates impairments related to the elbow or wrist in the static postural assessment, movement assessments, or both, mobility assessments for the elbow or wrist should be performed to better pinpoint the muscle imbalances to be corrected with the Corrective Exercise Continuum. The elbow and wrist are a functional extension of the shoulder. Any time movement impairments are identified in the shoulder and thoracic spine, overactive/shortened arm musculature is also likely. Tests for elbow and wrist flexion and extension ROM should be performed when the arms fall forward movement impairment is observed, when a client has difficulty fully straightening their arms, or when they cannot keep their wrists in a straight neutral position during exercise.

Corrective Strategies for the Elbow and Wrist

The integrated assessment process will reveal movement compensation patterns that may warrant the implementation of corrective programming for the elbow and wrist, with the most common ones being elbow flexion and non-neutral wrist. Once the static, transitional, loaded, and mobility assessments have been performed and impairments have been identified, the corrective exercise strategy can be developed using the NASM Corrective Exercise Continuum. Most programs can be performed daily or multiple times per week (**Table 15-3**).

Common Exercise Selections for the Elbow and Wrist

Exercises used for elbow and wrist corrective strategies look to improve commonly observed movement impairments such as a non-neutral wrist or chronic elbow flexion. Oftentimes, multiple movement impairments occur together and may benefit from exercises that address more than one, based on the integrated assessment process.

INHIBIT: SELF-MYOFASCIAL ROLLING

To maintain client safety and due to the small surface area of the forearms and elbow flexors, self-applied pressure using the fingertips or a small massage ball is recommended over the use

TABLE 15-3 Common Corrective Programming Selections for the Elbow and Wrist

Phase	Modality	Muscle(s)/Exercise(s)	Acute Training Variables
Inhibit	Self-myofascial rolling (using fingertips or massage ball)	Biceps brachii Brachialis Wrist extensors Wrist flexors	Hold areas of discomfort for 30 to 60 seconds Perform four to six repetitions of active joint movement
Lengthen	Static stretching	Biceps brachii Wrist extensors Wrist flexors	30-second hold
Activate	Isolated strengthening	Elbow extension Wrist flexion or extension	10 to 15 reps with 4-second eccentric contraction, 2-second isometric contraction at end-range, and 1-second concentric contraction
Integrate*	Integrated dynamic movement	Inverted row Prone ball triceps extension with cobra Standing cable press Triceps extension progressions	10 to 15 reps under control

*NOTE: Progress and regress as needed to match client ability, work capacity, and needs.

of a foam roller. It is important to apply pressure only on muscle bellies and avoid the brachial artery, which is just medial to the biceps along the inner portion of the upper arm. The radial and ulnar arteries branch off from the brachial artery and run along the lateral and medial aspects of the forearm, respectively.

- Self-applied pressure to wrist extensors or flexors in the forearm
- Self-applied pressure to the biceps brachii or brachialis

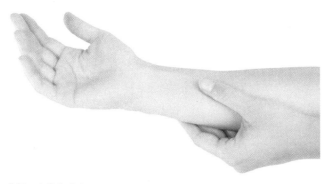

© Eskymaks/Shutterstock

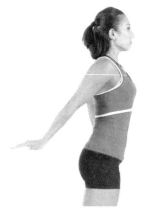

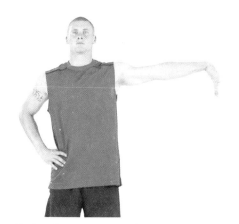

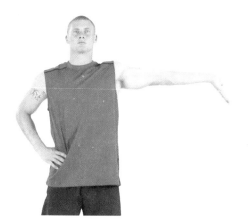

Static biceps stretch

Static wrist extensor stretch

Static wrist flexor stretch

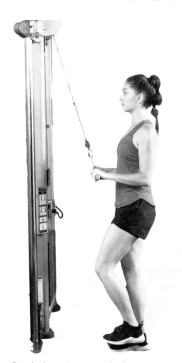

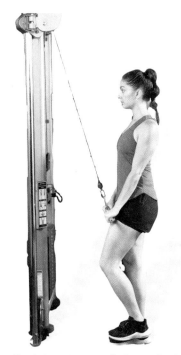

Single-leg triceps push down—start

Single-leg triceps push down—finish

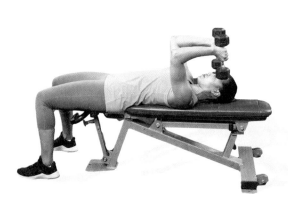

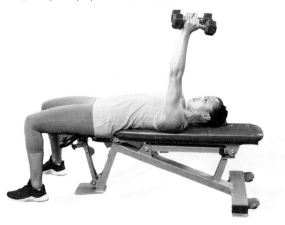

Supine dumbbell triceps extension—start

Supine dumbbell triceps extension—finish

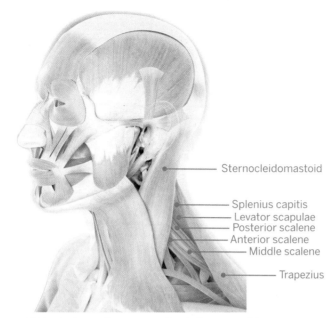

Figure 16-5 Neck muscles associated with the upper oblique subsystem

Sternocleidomastoid

Splenius capitis
Levator scapulae
Posterior scalene
Anterior scalene
Middle scalene

Trapezius

can lead to forward head migration and the rounding of the shoulders commonly seen in the upper crossed syndrome postural distortion (Page et al., 2010).

The cervical extensors can also become shortened and overactive in individuals with **forward head posture (FHP)** (Hallgren et al., 2017; Kim & Koo, 2016; Singla & Veqar, 2017). The suboccipital muscles, which are part of the cervical extensors, can become overactive and be a source of neck pain and headaches (Kalmanson et al., 2019; Park et al., 2017). The suboccipital muscles consist of four deep muscles located in the upper cervical spine below the occipital bone (Moore et al., 2013).

Altered Cervical Spine Posture and Movement

Individuals may assume different head and neck positions during various activities. FHP is one of the most common postural impairments seen by health and fitness professionals. It is common among desk workers, individuals who use smartphones, and adolescents who play video games for an extended period of time (Singla & Veqar, 2017). The following sections will discuss FHP as it pertains to static posture, muscle pattern activity, and movement.

Static Malalignments

FHP can be considered a malalignment of the head and neck where the head protrudes forward, forcing the lower cervical spine to flex and the upper cervical spine to extend to keep the head upright. FHP may cause abnormal stress to the cervical vertebrae, lengthen the anterior neck muscles, and shorten the posterior neck muscles (Singla & Veqar, 2017). These compensations alter the muscle balance in the upper body, which can affect regions below the head and neck. For example, during a static postural assessment, it is not uncommon to observe FHP with rounded shoulders and increased thoracic kyphosis (Singla & Veqar, 2017). These findings are common in Janda's upper crossed syndrome (**Figure 16-6**). The static assessment provides an organized approach to observing and classifying the different postural distortions or malalignments along

Forward head posture

Occurs when the head is protruding anterior to the shoulders in the sagittal plane; can lead to development of head and neck pain, movement restrictions, and compensations above and below the cervical spine.

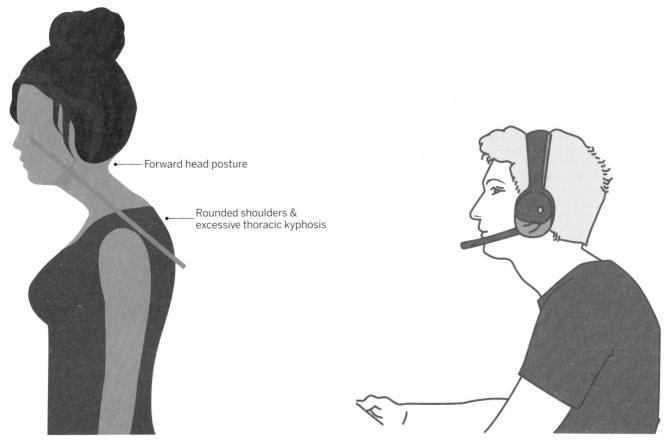

Figure 16-6　Upper crossed syndrome

Forward head posture

Rounded shoulders &
excessive thoracic kyphosis

Figure 16-7　Upper crossed syndrome with gaming

the body's kinetic chain. It also provides insight into possible compensatory muscle imbalances that may occur with a particular postural dysfunction.

CAUSES OF FORWARD HEAD POSTURE

Children and adolescents who maintain poor posture, such as when playing video games for extended periods of time, can bring their skeletal malalignments into adulthood (**Figure 16-7**) (Pop et al., 2018). If young adults continue to maintain poor posture, it can eventually lead to **spinal remodeling**, which increases the risk for degenerative changes to occur in the spine over the life span (Pop et al., 2018; Stone et al., 2015).

Similarly, adults can also develop pain and other musculoskeletal symptoms by maintaining poor posture when working at their desk or workstation for extended periods of time. For example, frequent computer users commonly experience pain in the cervical spine, shoulders, back, and wrist (Borhany et al., 2018). Sitting with abnormal head and neck posture while using computers on a regular basis is also associated with higher incidences of headaches (Mingels et al., 2016). Being aware of risk factors for developing neck pain while using a computer, such as sitting with abnormal neck posture, can help reduce the occurrence of this musculoskeletal disorder (Mani et al., 2016).

While the invention of cell phones has enhanced the ability to rapidly communicate, looking down at a phone for extended periods of time can accentuate FHP and contribute to the onset and prevalence of neck pain (Damasceno et al., 2018; Gustafsson et al., 2017). Spinal surgeons report an increase in young patients who are experiencing upper back and neck pain due to cell phone use (Cuéllar & Lanman, 2017). A new diagnosis, known as **text neck**, has been established to describe this condition (Cuéllar & Lanman, 2017).

Spinal remodeling

Abnormal reshaping of the spine's physiologic curvatures due to sustained abnormal posture.

Text neck

Neck and upper back pain caused by poor posture during excessive cell phone use.

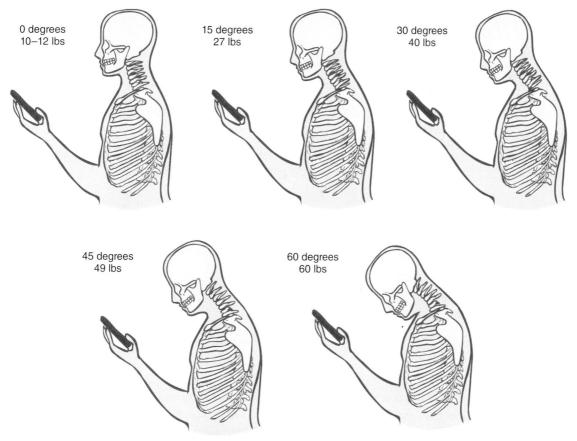

Figure 16-8 Posture when texting
Inspired by Dr. Kenneth K. Hansraj, https://realspinesurgery.com/text-neck/

The adult human head weighs approximately 10 to 12 pounds; however, when the neck flexes to look down, the relative stress placed on the neck increases to significantly higher than just the weight of the head (**Figure 16-8**). Every inch of forward displacement of the head requires a 10-fold increase of muscular effort to support posture (Cailliet, 1981).

Abnormal Movement Patterns

When FHP is observed during the static assessment, it is reasonable to consider that imbalances in the myofascial system can also occur that will affect movement. More specifically, muscles may be overactive/shortened or underactive/lengthened due to the malposition of the body region. With FHP, potential shortened/overactive muscles may include, but are not limited to, the sternocleidomastoid, levator scapulae, scalenes, upper trapezius, cervical extensors, and

 GETTING TECHNICAL

The Importance of Maintaining a Neutral Posture When Using Mobile Devices
When the neck is flexed to 15 degrees, the relative stress on the neck can be increased to approximately 30 pounds. A shift to 30 degrees of neck flexion can increase the relative stress to 40 pounds, 45 degrees can increase the relative stress to 50 pounds, and 60 degrees of neck flexion increases the relative neck stress to 60 pounds (Hansraj, 2014). Providing education for recommended posture (**Figure 16-9**) when using a mobile device can help prevent text neck from occurring.

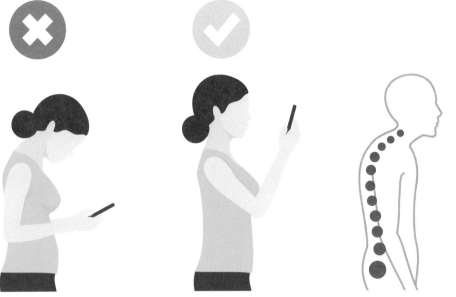

Figure 16-9 Recommended posture when texting

Figure 16-10 Advanced forward head posture

suboccipitals (Singla & Veqar, 2017). Lengthened/underactive muscles may include, but are not limited to, the deep cervical flexors (Gupta et al., 2013; Kim & Kwag, 2016; Mujawar & Sagar, 2019). With some extreme FHPs, the lower cervical extensors may be lengthened (Singla & Veqar, 2017). Other muscles may be also shortened or lengthened when the FHP is combined with rounded shoulders and thoracic kyphosis. These compensatory muscle imbalances affect regions below the head and neck during activity.

For healthy individuals with normal head and neck posture, approximately 50% of cervical spine rotation occurs between the first cervical vertebra (C1) and the second cervical vertebra (C2; Mercer & Bogduk, 2001). However, in clients with an FHP, rotation as well as side-bending of the neck is often reduced. During function, the cervical spine requires balance between left and right associated musculature to maintain optimal posture. When this does not occur, abnormal asymmetric shifting can also be seen when assessing statically. This may be related to an overactive and underactive right and left sternocleidomastoid, scalenes, levator scapulae, and upper trapezius (Falla et al., 2003, 2004, 2006).

Advanced stages of FHP (**Figure 16-10**) can cause compression in the upper cervical spine, which can significantly reduce the ability of C1 to rotate around C2. When this occurs, the middle and lower cervical spine segments try to make up for the restrictions above by attempting to rotate through greater ranges of motion than they normally would. This can result in cervical spine instability or **hypermobility** in the middle and lower cervical spine, which increases the risk for cervical spine degeneration and pain (Pop et al., 2018).

DYNAMIC MALALIGNMENT

During movement, the head, neck, shoulder girdle, and thoracic spine all work as an interdependent region of the body. In the presence of FHP, excessive strain can be placed in regions below the head. For example, FHP can cause excessive stress to the cervical and upper thoracic spines that contributes to pain and decreased range of motion (ROM) of those regions (Kim et al., 2018; Quek et al., 2013). In fact, FHP can cause expansion of the upper thorax and

---

Hypermobility

Increased movement and functionality of a joint beyond normal range of motion.

contraction of the lower thorax, resulting in decreased respiratory function (Koseki et al., 2019). FHP is also associated with tension headaches (Fernández-de-Las-Peñas et al., 2007), shoulder impingement (Alizadehkhaiyat et al., 2017), and carpal tunnel syndrome (De-la-Llave-Rincón et al., 2009). FHP may make individuals more prone to nerve entrapment disorders (e.g., carpal tunnel) along the upper kinetic chain (Ozudogru Celik et al., 2020). Individuals with FHP may also have poor proprioception or joint position sense in the cervical region (Yong et al., 2016). These issues related to FHP are most prevalent in adults or adolescents who participate in prolonged computer work and online gaming or use smartphones (Brink & Louw, 2015; Eitivipart et al., 2018; Szczygieł et al., 2017).

Cervical Spine Dysfunction and the Regional Interdependence Model

Optimal function of the cervical spine is dependent on the entire kinetic chain. In accordance with the Regional Interdependence (RI) model, dysfunction at the ankle, lumbo-pelvic-hip complex (LPHC), thoracic spine, or shoulder can negatively influence the region of the cervical spine. Similarly, dysfunction in the cervical spine can have a significant effect throughout the human movement system. Similar to how dysfunction at the LPHC can lead to knee or thoracic spine pain, dysfunction in the neck can cause issues both above and below the cervical region of the spine.

Hyoid Bone Positioning

Located in the upper anterior neck, the hyoid bone is considered a *floating bone*; it is not attached to any other bone, and its position is controlled by a sling of muscles (German et al., 2011). The hyoid bone serves as an important link between the cervical spine and the head as it plays a major role in the ability to chew, swallow, speak, and breathe properly (Deljo et al., 2012; Zheng et al., 2012). FHP can promote altered length-tension and force-couple relationships within the musculature attaching to this bone (Zheng et al., 2012).

Specifically, FHP increases tension in the musculature located directly above the hyoid bone (suprahyoids), which can cause the hyoid bone to elevate above its normal resting position (Zheng et al., 2012). This may contribute to the onset of anterior neck pain and jaw pain, as well contribute to other symptoms, such as difficulty swallowing food (An et al., 2015; Zheng et al., 2012). Restoring postural alignment of the head and neck has also been demonstrated to re-establish proper hyoid bone position (Pettit & Auvenshine, 2018).

 CRITICAL

If a client is reporting neck pain, headaches, jaw pain, breathing difficulty, or difficulty swallowing, the Corrective Exercise Specialist must stay within their scope of practice by referring the client to a healthcare professional who is licensed to diagnose and treat the condition.

To help illustrate the effects of FHP on muscle tightness in the anterior neck, go through a simple demonstration. With the head in a neutral position and eyes looking forward, swallow as if eating normally. Now, extend the neck backward to look upward and swallow again. Feel for the difference in muscle tightness between these two neck positions. Individuals with FHP may regularly experience similar muscular tightness in the anterior aspect of their neck.

Influence Above the Cervical Spine

Myofascial trigger points

Painful regions within a tight band of skeletal muscle that also give rise to referred pain.

FHP results in increased load bearing on the musculature and facet joints located in the upper cervical spine (Patwardhan et al., 2018). If FHP is chronically sustained, it may also lead to overactivity and shortening of the cervical extensors and suboccipital musculature (Page et al., 2010; Patwardhan et al., 2018). In addition, FHP is linked to reduced pain thresholds and predisposition to **myofascial trigger points** (Hong et al., 2019; Patwardhan et al., 2018).

Myofascial trigger points are painful regions within a tight band of skeletal muscle; they give rise to **referred pain** (Simons et al., 1999). Suboccipital trigger points can contribute to the onset of cervicogenic headaches (headaches originating from the neck; Barmherzig & Kingston, 2019). These trigger points can refer and radiate pain to the posterior and lateral portions of the head (**Figure 16-11**) (Barmherzig & Kingston, 2019).

However, not all individuals who have a headache that occurs with neck pain at the same time are diagnosed with **cervicogenic headaches**, as there are many different forms of headaches, including tension, migraine, and other types associated with various medical conditions (Blumenfeld & Siavoshi, 2018).

Referred pain

Pain perceived at a different location than the source.

Cervicogenic headaches

Headaches originating from the neck.

GETTING TECHNICAL

Cervicogenic Headaches
Cervicogenic headaches, which are common in individuals with FHP, can arise from myofascial trigger points from muscles in the head and neck region (Barmherzig & Kingston, 2019). As shown in Figure 16-11, the upper trapezius, sternocleidomastoid, and suboccipitals can radiate pain to the many regions around the head (Simons et al., 1999).

INFLUENCE ON THE TEMPOROMANDIBULAR JOINT (TMJ)

The temporomandibular joint (TMJ) is a modified hinge joint that allows the mandible (jawbone) to move upward, downward, anterior, and posterior, as well as side to side. From a biomechanical standpoint, the TMJ is highly complex because its function is not only influenced by muscles located throughout the head and neck, but also by a cartilaginous disc located within the joint (Zafar et al., 2000).

A link exists between head and neck posture and TMJ function (Zafar et al., 2000). FHP can contribute to the development of pain in the musculature surrounding the TMJ by altering length-tension relationships in the head and neck musculature (Chaves et al., 2014). This

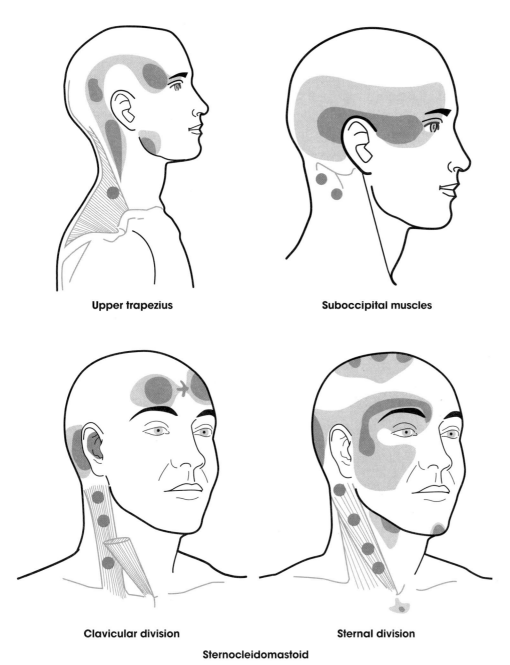

Upper trapezius

Suboccipital muscles

Clavicular division

Sternal division

Sternocleidomastoid

Figure 16-11 Myofascial trigger point referral patterns
Data from Simons, D. G., Travell, J. G., Simons, L. S. (1999). *Travell & Simons' myofascial pain and dysfunction: Upper half of body.* Philadelphia, PA: Lippincott, Williams, & Wilkins.

posture creates excessive tension in the muscles above the hyoid bone, which, in turn, places greater force demands on the muscles that close the jaw (mandibular elevators; An et al., 2015). Over time, these excessive force demands on the jaw muscles can lead to the development of myofascial trigger points and pain around the TMJ (Fernández-de-las-Peñas et al., 2010).

FHP can also influence the location where the upper and lower teeth come together, which can also affect TMJ function (Khan et al., 2013). Overactivity in the upper trapezius, sterno-cleidomastoid, levator scapulae, cervical extensors, and suboccipitals is also associated with TMJ disorders, because **cocontractions** occur in these muscles when teeth are clenched to-gether excessively (Giannakopoulos et al., 2013).

> **Cocontractions**
>
> The simultaneous contraction of muscles around a joint.

Influence Below the Cervical Spine

Many individuals with FHP also demonstrate rounded shoulders. These two postural observations comprise Janda's upper crossed syndrome. Because FHP is associated with overactivity of the upper trapezius and levator scapulae muscles, this can negatively affect **scapulohumeral rhythm**, leading to scapular dyskinesis. **Scapular dyskinesis** refers to when the scapula does not move in a normal fashion during humeral elevation and is associated with the development of shoulder pain and impingement. The thoracic spine, especially the upper region, contributes to neck mobility (Tsang et al., 2013). Abnormal scapulothoracic posture, such as an increased **thoracic kyphosis (TK)**, can promote **hyperextension** in the upper cervical spine, which contributes to neck pain and stiffness (Roussouly & Pinheiro-Franco, 2011). Increased TK is a common postural impairment observed in individuals with Janda's upper crossed syndrome (Olszewska et al., 2018). A forward head, rounded shoulders, and excessive TK predisposes to contracture (shortening) of the pectoral muscles, which also negatively affects overhead reaching ability (Olszewska et al., 2018).

 TRY THIS

Sit with a slouched posture and forward head and shoulders and then try to raise one arm over your head. Feel the tightness in the shoulder and note the limited mobility when performing this. Compare the difference when sitting in an upright posture with shoulders and scapulae slightly retracted (pulled back). Notice the ease of movement as well as how much higher the reach is.

THE INFLUENCE OF FHP ON THE RESPIRATORY SYSTEM

Sustained FHP can also negatively influence the respiratory system. Normal inspiration (breathing in) is initiated by contraction of the primary respiratory muscles, the diaphragm, and external intercostals (Kenney et al., 2015). However, in individuals with FHP, muscle activity and function of the diaphragm may decrease, which can reduce lung expansion during inspiration (Okuro et al., 2011). To make up for impaired muscle power of the diaphragm, individuals with FHP may compensate by utilizing accessory respiratory muscles such as the sternocleidomastoid for inspiration (inhalation; Okuro et al., 2011). Excessive sternocleidomastoid activity when breathing at rest can cause the client's shoulders to move up and down rather than remaining in their normal stationary position (Okuro et al., 2011). Correction of FHP has been demonstrated to improve respiratory function (Kim et al., 2015).

Assessment Results for the Cervical Spine

Like the other regions of the body, assessment of the cervical spine region (i.e., head and neck) can be accomplished using static postural assessments, transitional and dynamic movement assessments, and ROM (mobility) assessments. A summary of common findings indicating potential dysfunction at the cervical spine is provided in **Table 16-2**.

TABLE 16-2 Head and Neck Assessment Results

Assessment	Results
Static posture	Forward head in cervical extension Shoulders rounded forward
Transitional and loaded movement assessments	Arms fall forward Excessive cervical extension Scapular elevation
Dynamic movement assessments	Excessive cervical extension
Mobility Cervical flexion and extension, rotation, and lateral flexion	Limited cervical extension ROM Limited cervical flexion ROM Limited cervical lateral flexion ROM Limited cervical rotation ROM

Static Posture

Postural distortion patterns that highlight potential cervical spine dysfunction include Janda's upper crossed and layered crossed syndromes, and Kendall's flat-back, sway-back, and kyphosis-lordosis postures. All include a combination of the FHP and rounded shoulder position in their classifications (**Figure 16-12**) (Kendall et al., 2014; Page et al., 2010).

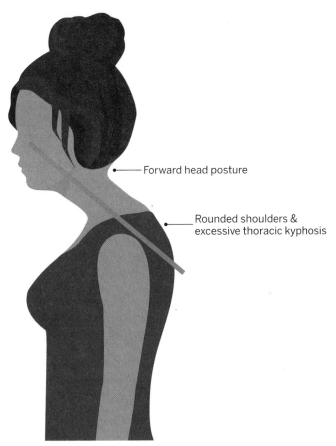

Forward head posture

Rounded shoulders & excessive thoracic kyphosis

Figure 16-12 Forward head posture and rounded shoulders

Transitional Movement Assessment

Based on the collective information obtained from the static postural assessment, the Corrective Exercise Specialist will have a high-level estimation of which muscles might be overactive/shortened and which ones are underactive/lengthened. Occasionally, clients might have relatively impairment-free static posture; however, when in motion, active muscle imbalances may come to light. With essentially all movement having some influence on the cervical spine, transitional movement assessments provide objective information from which to design effective corrective exercise programs.

OVERHEAD SQUAT ASSESSMENT

During the overhead squat assessment (OHSA), the cervical spine may extend excessively into FHP. This is typically caused by overactive cervical extensors causing the deep neck flexors to become underactive and lengthened. As previously mentioned, even if the overactivity of the cervical extensor muscles is not severe enough to produce FHP while standing still, performing the overhead squat pattern can highlight underlying muscle overactivity that causes the head to protrude while in motion.

When observing static posture, a forward head and rounded shoulders are typically seen together due to commonalities in activities of daily living. The arms fall forward and excessive cervical extension movement impairments are similarly observed during dynamic postural assessment. During the OHSA, the Corrective Exercise Specialist might see the ears move in line with the arms as they fall forward at the bottom of the squat movement.

LOADED MOVEMENT ASSESSMENT

Clients who demonstrate proper static and dynamic posture under body weight alone can be progressed to using loaded variants of primary movement patterns. This provides more challenge to the musculature and can help draw attention to any remaining imbalance at the joints. While the OHSA is likely to uncover the significant movement impairments, loaded pushing and pulling assessments may uncover other areas of dysfunction, provided the client is able to perform them.

Overactivity of the sternocleidomastoid, upper trapezius, and/or scalenes can cause FHP and influence the dynamic posture of the shoulders. On top of their normal isolated functions, they are also synergists for elevating the shoulders, and when overactive, they can become synergistically dominant. If the shoulders elevate during loaded pushing or pulling, that is a sign that neck muscles are working more than they should be. While elevating shoulders could very well be a consequence of underactive muscles of the trunk that help keep the shoulders retracted and depressed, that movement impairment can also be considered a cervical spine issue. For that reason, corrective protocols for FHP can also be beneficial for individuals whose shoulders elevate during pushing or pulling tasks, even if they do not present with overt static FHP.

Dynamic Movement Assessments

Because it shares similar biomechanics to loaded pushing movements, the Davies test is the dynamic assessment that best highlights dysfunction in the cervical spine region. Specifically, look for a client's head to drop below the shoulders either during the push-up starting position or when in motion. In either case, this is an example of FHP, and corrective protocols should be followed to help the client better hold their neck in an efficient position in line with the rest of the spine. This is an advanced technique, so the Corrective Exercise Specialist should make sure their clients have proper push-up and plank form, as well as adequate strength to remain in the "high plank" push-up position for prolonged periods of time.

GETTING TECHNICAL

Pelvo-Ocular Reflex
The **pelvo-ocular reflex** is the neuromotor response of the pelvic girdle and lower extremity (Lewit, 1985) that serves to orient the body in response to head position and anticipatory visual reference cues. It is theorized that head position affects pelvic position. As the head migrates forward, the pelvis reflexively rotates anteriorly to readjust the center of gravity (pelvo-ocular reflex). This rotation of the pelvis with concomitant forward head migration can lead to thoracolumbar pain (Lewit, 1985; Morningstar et al., 2005). This example illustrates how FHP can lead to dysfunction and pain in different (and distal) regions of the body.

Pelvo-ocular reflex

A postural reflex in which anterior rotation of the pelvis occurs as a result of forward head posture.

Mobility Assessments

If the client demonstrates static or dynamic postural impairments at the head and neck or shoulder kinetic chain checkpoints, the Corrective Exercise Specialist should perform mobility assessments for the cervical spine. Cervical flexion, extension, rotation, and lateral flexion can be performed to observe general cervical mobility and help specifically identify muscles with flexibility deficits that may be contributing to a client's FHP or elevating shoulders (Floyd, 2017), thus narrowing the focus of the corrective exercise program.

TRAINING TIP

The same muscles that contribute to FHP when overactive/shortened are also the ones that can create ROM deficits for cervical rotation and lateral flexion (i.e., the sternocleidomastoid, scalenes, and upper trapezius). If ROM is restricted when rotating or side bending in one direction over the other, follow the corrective protocol for FHP discussed next while preferentially stretching the muscles on the side of the neck opposite to the restriction. This will help restore bilateral balance and allow the client to keep their head and neck in a straight, neutral position.

Corrective Strategies for the Cervical Spine

The integrated assessment process will reveal movement compensation patterns that may warrant the implementation of corrective programming for the cervical spine, with the most common one being FHP. Once the static, movement, and mobility assessments have been performed and impairments have been identified, the corrective exercise strategy can be developed using the NASM Corrective Exercise Continuum. Most programs can be performed daily or multiple times per week (**Table 16-3**).

Phase	Modality	Muscle(s)/Exercise	Acute Training Variables
Inhibit	Self-myofascial rolling	Cervical extensors (suboccipitals) Levator scapulae Sternocleidomastoid Thoracic spine Upper trapezius	Hold areas of discomfort for 30 to 60 seconds Perform four to six repetitions of active joint movement
Lengthen	Static stretching	Levator scapulae Scalenes (included when stretching the upper trapezius and sternocleidomastoid) Sternocleidomastoid Upper trapezius	30-second hold
Activate	Isolated strengthening	Cobra progressions Deep cervical flexors (chin-tuck progressions) Scapular retraction progressions	10 to 15 reps with 4-second eccentric contraction, 2-second isometric contraction at end-range, and 1-second concentric contraction
Integrate	Integrated dynamic movement	Ball combo 1 Ball combo 2 Lunge to scaption Scaption progressions Squat to row	10 to 15 reps under control

Common Exercise Selections for the Cervical Spine

Exercises used for cervical spine corrective strategies look to improve commonly observed movement impairments such as forward head posture and scapular elevation. Oftentimes, these movement impairments are interrelated and occur together across the kinetic chain assessment process, and therefore may benefit from exercises that address more than one. For example, inhibition and lengthening of the upper trapezius may improve more than one impairment. As such, the Corrective Exercise Specialist may create a program that efficiently addresses multiple movement impairments. Incorporation of previously outlined corrective exercise strategies for the thoracic spine and shoulder, particularly for arms fall forward and scapular elevation, will often occur concurrently with those for the cervical spine.

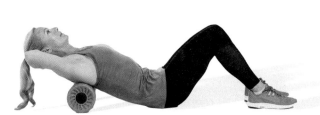

Thoracic spine

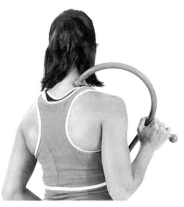

Levator scapulae (instrument assisted)
© Courtesy of National Academy of Sports Medicine

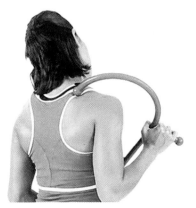

Upper trapezius (instrument assisted)
© Courtesy of National Academy of Sports Medicine

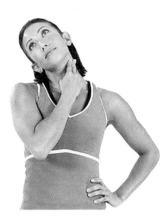

Sternocleidomastoid (self-applied pressure)
© Courtesy of National Academy of Sports Medicine

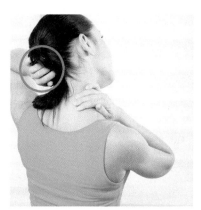

Cervical extensors (suboccipitals; self-applied pressure)
© In Green/Shutterstock

 CRITICAL

Inhibiting the Cervical Spine Region

There are several areas of the body where it is best to avoid using a foam roller for self-myofascial rolling due to risk of pain or potential injury in the structures below the skin. The cervical spine is a great example of a contraindicated region for foam roller use because of the sensitive nature of this region of the body. Appropriate regions to inhibit via myofascial rolling or instrument-assisted devices include the thoracic spine, levator scapulae, and upper trapezius. To ensure client safety, the Corrective Exercise Specialist should address inhibition of the cervical extensors (suboccipitals) and the sternocleidomastoid by using self-applied pressure techniques rather than rollers or instrument-assisted devices.

The upper trapezius and levator scapulae may have mild pressure applied using one of many hook- or cane-type tools with rounded ends. It is important to note that the levator scapulae lies partially under the upper trapezius and sternocleidomastoid on either end. Only the middle portion of the muscle is "superficial" on the lateral portion of the neck. However, to maintain safety, it is recommended that the levator scapulae be inhibited by applying pressure to the medial portion of the upper trapezius, where its trigger points are normally located. The suboccipital muscles may benefit from simply placing a thumb or finger on the base of the skull and applying mild pressure. The sternocleidomastoid can be accessed by placing one or two fingers on the belly of the muscle and applying light pressure on identified trigger points. Care should be taken to avoid applying pressure to the carotid artery.

LENGTHEN: STATIC STRETCHING

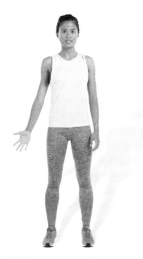
Neck static stretches—start

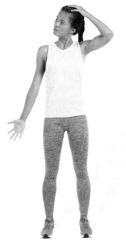
Sternocleidomastoid—finish

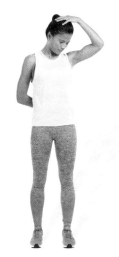
Levator scapulae—finish

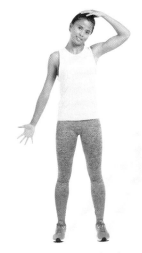
Upper trapezius—finish

NOTE: The three static stretches presented share the same starting position.

ACTIVATE: ISOLATED STRENGTHENING

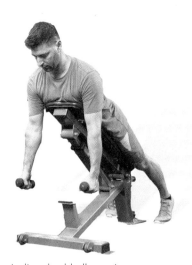
Incline dumbbell scaption—start

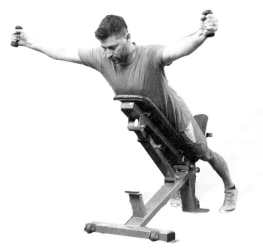
Incline dumbbell scaption—finish

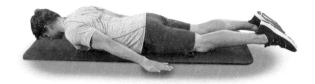
Prone floor scapular retraction

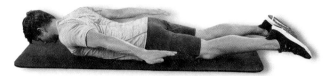
Prone floor scapular retraction—progression

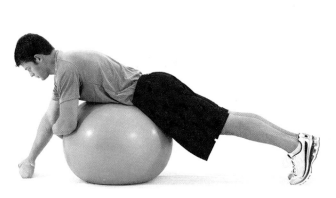

Single-arm ball dumbbell cobra—start

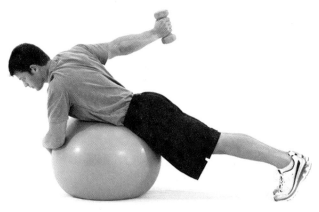

Single-arm ball dumbbell cobra—finish

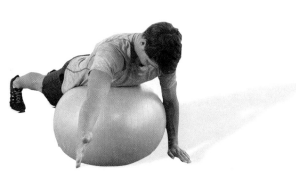

Single-arm ball quadruped scaption—start

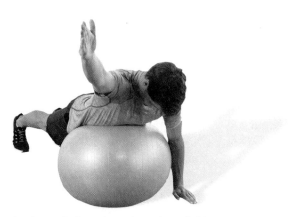

Single-arm ball quadruped scaption—finish

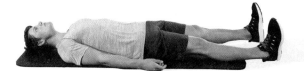

Supine chin tuck—start

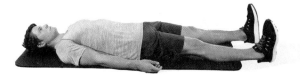

Supine chin tuck—finish

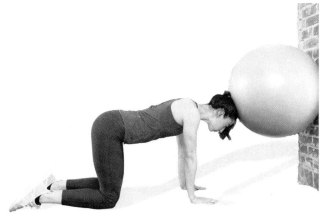

Quadruped chin tucks with stability ball—start

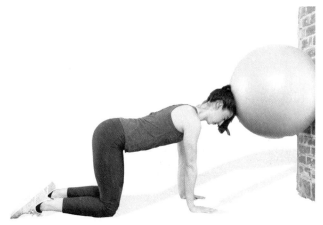

Quadruped chin tucks with stability ball—finish

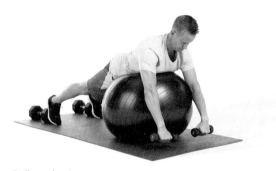

Ball combo 1—start

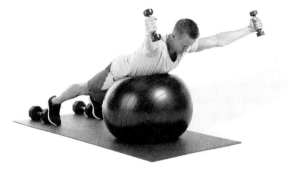

Ball combo 1—scaption

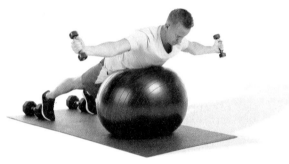

Ball combo 1—retraction

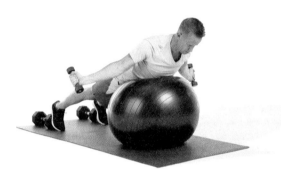

Ball combo 1—cobra (finish)

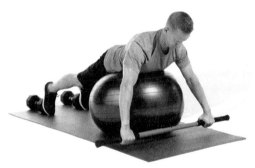

Ball combo 2 with dowel rod—start

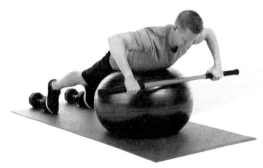

Ball combo 2 with dowel rod—row

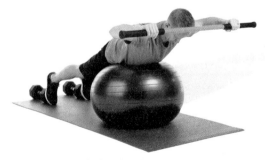

Ball combo 2 with dowel rod—rotate

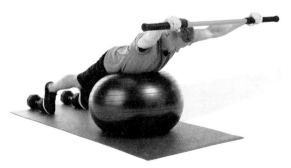

Ball combo 2 with dowel rod—press

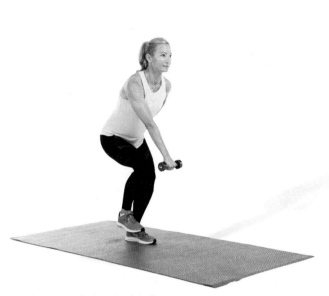

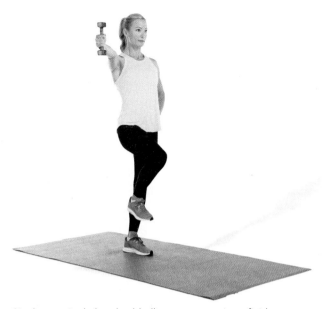

Single-arm single-leg dumbbell squat to scaption—start

Single-arm single-leg dumbbell squat to scaption—finish

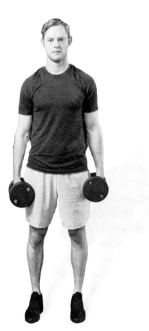

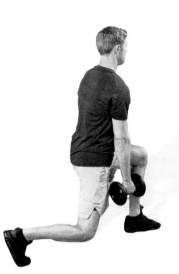

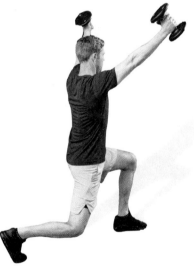

Lunge to scaption, transverse—start

Lunge to scaption, transverse—movement

Lunge to scaption, transverse—finish

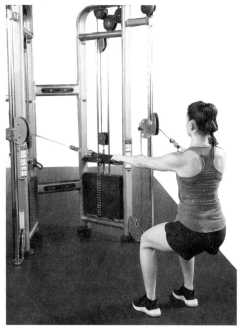
Squat to row—start

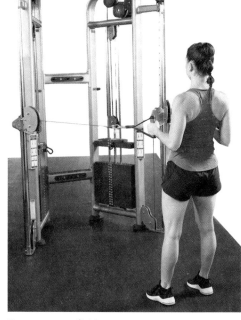
Squat to row—finish

Importance of Cervical Stability During Exercise

The deep neck flexors are primarily made up of the longus colli and longus capitis muscles. These muscles stabilize the cervical spine in all positions against the effects of gravity. They play a pivotal role in cervical spine conditions and are often overlooked as a source of locomotor system dysfunction. The anatomic action of the longus capitis and longus colli is to nod the chin. If muscle recruitment is impaired, the balance between the stabilizers on the front and the back of the neck will be disrupted. This will cause loss of proper alignment of the spinal segments and a posture that could lead to cervical pain (Falla et al., 2011). Thus, maintaining proper cervical alignment (chin tuck) during exercise is crucial to decrease the stress on the cervical spine and the risk of injury (Falla & Farina, 2007; Falla et al., 2003, 2004, 2006).

Forward Head Posture

The Corrective Exercise Specialist should be selective regarding the techniques recommended to each client. To improve client adherence, it is recommended that the Corrective Exercise Specialist employ as few exercises as are effective in each phase of the continuum. The following exercises are the ones most used for the compensation of FHP. In this compensation, the client may demonstrate a combination of a forward head with rounding of the shoulders statically and scapular elevation upon introducing motion and/or load. The broad objectives of the program are to improve ideal cervical spine and scapular positioning and stability. When applied systematically, the Corrective Exercise Continuum contributes to efficient neuromuscular control and proper alignment of the cervical spine during movement.

PHASE 1: INHIBIT

Key regions to inhibit via rollers, self-applied pressure, or instrument-assisted devices include the cervical extensor (suboccipital), upper trapezius, levator scapulae, and sternocleidomastoid muscles and the thoracic spine. To ensure client safety, it is recommended that the Corrective Exercise Specialist address inhibition of the cervical extensor (suboccipital) and sternocleidomastoid muscles utilizing self-applied pressure techniques.

PHASE 2: LENGTHEN

Key lengthening exercises with static stretches generally include the bilateral (right + left) upper trapezius, scalenes, levator scapulae, and sternocleidomastoid muscles (Bae et al., 2016). If mobility assessment reveals asymmetrical restriction, additional sets may be performed for the more restricted side.

TRAINING TIP

Given the attachments of the scalene muscles, they will also be lengthened when performing stretches for the upper trapezius and sternocleidomastoid muscles.

PHASE 3: ACTIVATE

Key activation exercises with isolated strengthening exercises include the deep cervical flexors, middle and lower trapezius, and rhomboids.

GETTING TECHNICAL

Activation of the Middle and Lower Trapezius
The trapezius muscle plays a pivotal role in maintaining proper mechanics and stability of the shoulder girdle. Since shoulder elevation is often associated with FHP, activation of the middle and lower trapezius is beneficial for addressing it. Kinney et al. (2008) studied the relationship between shoulder abduction angle and activation of the middle and lower trapezius. They found the greatest level of middle and lower trapezius activation occurred at 90 and 125 degrees of shoulder abduction. To the Corrective Exercise Specialist, this translates to the application of horizontal row and scaption progressions within the Corrective Exercise Continuum whenever lower and middle trapezius activation is targeted.

PHASE 4: INTEGRATE

An integration progression should be implemented first to emphasize scapular positioning and cervical spine stability. One integration exercise that could be implemented is ball combo 1 while maintaining cervical retraction. Although this exercise can also be considered an activation exercise for the shoulder complex, it can be used as an integration exercise for cervical spine impairments to integrate the use of the cervical spine musculature with the inferior shoulder musculature. Performing this movement on a stability ball also forces the exerciser to use these muscles in concert with the core and lower extremity musculature to provide stability. This movement can be progressed by incorporating other dynamic functional movements involving the lower extremity such as squat-to-scaption variations and lunging to scaption while maintaining proper cervical retraction. Squat-to-row variations can also be done to further challenge the client. See **Table 16-4** for a sample program.

TABLE 16-4 Sample Corrective Exercise Program for the Cervical Spine: Forward Head Posture

Phase	Modality	*Muscle(s)/Exercise	Acute Training Variables
Inhibit	Self-myofascial technique appropriate to the region	Cervical extensors (suboccipitals) Levator scapulae Sternocleidomastoid Upper trapezius	Hold areas of discomfort for 30 to 60 seconds Perform between four and six repetitions of active joint movement 90 to 120 seconds per muscle group
Lengthen	Static stretching	Levator scapulae Sternocleidomastoid Upper trapezius	30-second hold
Activate	Isolated strengthening	Incline dumbbell scaption Quadruped chin tucks with stability ball	10 to 15 reps with 4-second eccentric contraction, 2-second isometric contraction at end-range, and 1-second concentric contraction
Integrate	Integrated dynamic movement	Ball combo 1 Squat to row	10 to 15 reps under control

*NOTE: Inhibit/lengthen bilaterally (right + left).

 TRAINING TIP

The Corrective Exercise Specialist needs to consider that the suggested Corrective Exercise Continuum selections in this section detail common strategies for FHP. The strategies in this section highlight exercises for the major muscle groups involved in this movement impairment. The corrective suggestions provide a basic framework. Other muscles may be involved, such as those related to rounded shoulders, and should be considered with each individual client based on their assessment results.

Common Issues Associated with the Cervical Spine

Common local injuries or dysfunctions associated with the cervical spine include neck pain or stiffness, text neck, elevated hyoid bone, trapezius dysfunction, levator scapulae dysfunction, cervical joint dysfunction, cervical strains, deep flexor dysfunction, and cervical disc lesions. Common complaints above the cervical spine (that may stem from dysfunction in the cervical spine) are often seen with symptoms associated with the head. This includes TMJ disorders, headaches, dizziness, or lightheadedness (Sahrmann, 2001). Common injuries below the cervical spine toward the shoulder include shoulder pain, trapezius–levator scapulae dysfunction, acromioclavicular (AC) joint impingement, scapulothoracic dysfunction, and thoracic outlet dysfunction. At the thoracolumbar spine, low back pain and sacroiliac joint dysfunction may be seen with various compensations in posture (thoracic extension, anterior pelvic tilt, and sacroiliac joint translation) related to cervical spine dysfunction (**Table 16-5**).

TABLE 16-5 Common Injuries Associated with Cervical Spine Impairment

Local Injuries	Injuries Above the Cervical Spine	Injuries Below the Cervical Spine
Cervical disc lesions	Cervicogenic headaches	AC impingement
Cervical joint dysfunction	Dizziness/lightheadedness	Anterior pelvic tilt/low-back pain
Cervical strains	TMJ-related symptoms	Dysfunctional breathing
Deep flexor dysfunction		Sacroiliac joint dysfunction
Elevated hyoid bone		Scapulothoracic dysfunction
Levator scapulae dysfunction		Thoracic outlet syndrome
Pain/stiffness		Upper extremity pain/weakness
Text neck		
Trapezius dysfunction		

Each of the typical injuries can be problematic for any individual, and the reduction in pain or severity is often the focus of many rehabilitation programs conducted by licensed healthcare professionals. However, these injuries may at times be signs of a postural or movement dysfunction further down the kinetic chain. Although the origin of these injuries is multifactorial and complex, using exercise techniques to correct postural and movement dysfunctions throughout the kinetic chain may reduce a client's risk of developing the conditions described in the following sections.

Corrective exercise protocols are intended for healthy individuals who are looking to move, feel, and perform better, and the specific treatment of pain (especially in the spine) is well outside the Corrective Exercise Specialist's scope of practice. Always refer out to a medical professional when injury is suspected and ensure that clients are cleared for exercise by their doctor before beginning a corrective fitness program.

A Corrective Exercise Specialist's job is to evaluate movement and provide strategies for improving movement quality and injury resistance. Diagnosis or treatment of any of the following pathologies is outside of the scope of practice. The presence of any of the following pathologies requires consultation with or referral to a qualified medical professional.

 CRITICAL

This section is intended to provide general information about specific medical conditions for the cervical spine. The information provided should not be used to diagnose any medical condition. The fitness professional should refer to the appropriate medical professional if a client needs a diagnosis of a potential medical condition. This will ensure client safety and proper scope of practice.

Muscle Strain

Because the cervical spine is often an exposed region of the body during sports and athletics, it is at risk for injury during collision and contact sports (Mayer et al., 2012). The most common neck injury in athletes is muscle strain (Schroeder & Vaccaro, 2016). A muscle strain occurs when a tendon or muscle is overstretched and/or overworked, which results in disruption or tearing of the muscle tissue. Also commonly known as a pulled muscle, muscle strains may result in pain, spasm, swelling, and muscle weakness. In mild cases, this injury occurs only to the musculotendinous tissue itself; however, in severe cases, such as those caused by traumatic sport injuries, falls, or motor vehicle accidents, nerves may become damaged as well (Todd, 2011). Muscle strains in the cervical spine are not always caused by an acute traumatic force, as they can also be caused by sustained muscle contractions. Individuals who maintain poor or awkward neck posture for prolonged periods while working are also susceptible for developing a muscle strain in their neck. For example, using a laptop computer on the legs results in greater neck flexion, torque, and neck strain compared to using a standard computer on a desk (Berkhout et al., 2004).

Stenosis of the Cervical Spine

Spinal stenosis is a condition most commonly seen in older individuals; however, it can affect some middle-aged individuals who have a genetic predisposition for this condition. In this pathology, the spinal canal narrows, causing compression of the spinal cord. A reduction in disc height as well as thickening and reduced flexibility of spinal ligaments are often the main causes of this condition (Okada et al., 2009). Common symptoms of spinal stenosis include chronic, dull pain that remains deep in the neck; however, if this pathology also results in compression of nerve roots, individuals can also experience radiating pain, numbness, tingling sensations, or motor weakness in the upper extremities (Todd, 2011). In severe cases, if the spinal cord is under significant compression, spinal stenosis can cause chronic muscle spasms in the extremities, as well as gait abnormalities (Malone et al., 2015).

Degenerative Disc Disease

Intervertebral discs make up approximately 25% of the height of a healthy spine (Betts et al., 2013). During the natural aging process, spinal discs slowly lose their ability to retain fluid, resulting in gradual loss of disc height as well as reduction in shock-absorbing capability (Brzuszkiewicz-Kuźmicka et al., 2018). In advanced age, the discs dry out and become thinner. This contributes to the reduction of overall body height while aging. Not everyone experiences spinal discomfort as a result of aging; however, some individuals may experience pain, stiffness, and inflammation in the spine due to the effects of reduced disc height (Peng & DePalma, 2018).

Degenerative disc disease (DDD) can lead to excessive compression forces placed on the facet joints, which can cause pain and predisposition to arthritic degeneration (Kumaresan et al., 2001) (**Figure 16-3**). Excessive compression restricts the facet joints' ability to function properly. For example, some facets may lose their ability to slide over each other, which contributes to neck stiffness or instability in the cervical spine. In addition, some individuals with DDD may also develop bone spurs in and around the facets, which can cause significant neck pain, stiffness, and inflammation (Kumaresan et al., 2001). Although DDD in the cervical spine is more commonly observed in middle-aged to elderly populations, it can occur in younger individuals who maintain poor posture (including FHP) or who have sustained a traumatic neck injury that resulted in damage to an intervertebral disc (Boucher et al., 2008).

DDD may also lead to a herniated disc (also known as a bulged disc). When the gel-like substance that is normally contained in the center of the disc (nucleus pulposus) projects out of the disc, it can irritate or compress a nerve root that is located next to the spine. This often results in burning pain, numbness, or tingling that also radiates to the upper extremity. Weakness in upper extremity musculature is also a common symptom (Todd, 2011). Interestingly, if the projecting disc material does not make direct contact with a nerve, it may not produce pain symptoms because the spinal discs themselves do not contain nerve endings (Antoni & Croft, 2006). Up to 35% of individuals between 40 and 64 years of age may have a cervical disc herniation without symptoms (Antoni & Croft, 2006).

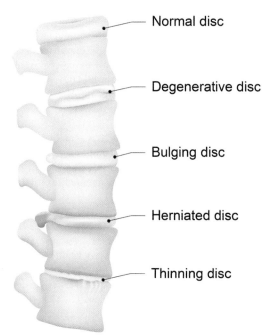

Normal disc

Degenerative disc

Bulging disc

Herniated disc

Thinning disc

Figure 16-13 Disc degeneration
© Designua/Shutterstock

SUMMARY

A chronic forward head posture and rounded shoulders (Janda's upper crossed syndrome) may develop in individuals who maintain an unsupported, abnormal, or awkward body position during recreational or work-related activities. Not only can forward head posture increase the risk for early onset of degenerative changes within the cervical spine, but it also negatively influences the position and function of structures above and below such as the hyoid bone, temporomandibular joint, and respiratory system. By addressing postural abnormalities associated with the cervical spine and encouraging cervical stability while exercising by utilizing the Corrective Exercise Continuum, the Corrective Exercise Specialist can help improve their client's function as well as their movement quality and durability.

As described by the RI model, pain or dysfunction in one region of the body can likely be caused by dysfunction in another region of the body. This can be especially true for cervical spine dysfunction, owing to the compensatory chain reaction that can occur resulting from human movement impairment. Although the cervical spine is a complex region of the body, having an understanding of functional anatomy, functional biomechanics, and the overall human movement system will greatly assist the Corrective Exercise Specialist with understanding potential causes for cervical spine dysfunction and key elements that must be addressed to help correct these dysfunctions via the Corrective Exercise Continuum.

REFERENCES

Alizadehkhaiyat, O., Roebuck, M. M., Makki, A. T., & Frostick, S. P. (2017). Postural alterations in patients with subacromial impingement syndrome. *International Journal of Sports Physical Therapy*, *12*(7), 1111–1120.

An, J. S., Jeon, D. M., Jung, W. S., Yang, I. H., Lim, W. H., & Ahn, S. J. (2015). Influence of temporomandibular joint disc displacement on craniocervical posture and hyoid bone position. *American Journal of Orthodontics and Dentofacial Orthopedics*, *147*(1), 72–79. https://doi.org/10.1016/j.ajodo.2014.09.015

Antoni, A. V. D., & Croft, A. C. (2006). Prevalence of herniated intervertebral discs of the cervical spine in asymptomatic subjects using MRI scans: A qualitative systematic review. *Journal of Chiropractic Education*, *20*(1), 58.

Bae, W. S., Lee, H. O., Shin, J. W., & Lee, K. C. (2016). The effect of middle and lower trapezius strength exercises and levator scapulae and upper trapezius stretching exercises in upper crossed syndrome. *Journal of Physical Therapy Science*, *28*(5), 1636–1639. https://doi.org/10.1589/jpts.28.1636

Barmherzig, R., & Kingston, W. (2019). Occipital neuralgia and cervicogenic headache: Diagnosis and management. *Current Neurology and Neuroscience Reports*, *19*(5), 20. https://doi,org/10.1007/s11910-019-0937-8

Berkhout, A. L., Hendriksson-Larsén, K., & Bongers, P. (2004). The effect of using a laptop station compared to using a standard laptop PC on the cervical spine torque, perceived strain and productivity. *Applied Ergonomics*, *35*(2), 147–152. https://doi.org/10.1016/j.apergo.2003.11.008

Betts, J. G., Young, K. A., Wise, J. A., Johnson, E., Poe, B., Kruse, D. H., Poe, B., Wise, J. A., Womble, M., Young, K. A., & DeSaix, P. (2013). *Anatomy and physiology*. OpenStax.

Blumenfeld, A., & Siavoshi, S. (2018). The challenges of cervicogenic headache. *Current Pain and Headache Reports*, *22*(7), 47. https://doi.org/10.1007/s11916-018-0699-z

Borhany, T., Shahid, E., Siddique, W. A., & Ali, H. (2018). Musculoskeletal problems in frequent computer and internet users. *Journal of Family Medicine and Primary Care*, *7*(2), 337–339. https://doi.org/10.4103/jfmpc.jfmpc_326_17

Boucher, P., Descarreaux, M., & Normand, M. C. (2008). Postural control in people with osteoarthritis of the cervical spine. *Journal of Manipulative & Physiological Therapeutics*, *31*(3), 184–190. https://doi.org/10.1016/j.jmpt.2008.02.008

Brink, Y., Louw, Q. A., Grimmer, K. A., & Jordaan, E. R. (2015). The relationship between sitting posture and seated-related upper quadrant musculoskeletal pain in computing South African adolescents: A prospective study. *Manual Therapy, 20*(6), 820–826.

Brzuszkiewicz-Kuźmicka, G., Szczegielniak, J., & Baczkowicz, D. (2018). Age-related changes in shock absorption capacity of the human spinal column. *Clinical Interventions in Aging*, *13*, 987–993. https://doi.org/10.2147/CIA.S156298

Cailliet, R. (1981). *Neck and arm pain*. F.A. Davis.

Chaves, T. C., Turci, A. M., Pinheiro, C. F., Sousa, L. M., & Grossi, D. B. (2014). Static body postural misalignment in individuals with temporomandibular disorders: A systematic review. *Brazilian Journal of Physical Therapy*, *18*(6), 481–501. https://doi.org/10.1590/bjpt-rbf.2014.0061

Cuéllar, J. M., & Lanman, T. H. (2017). "Text neck": An epidemic of the modern era of cell phones? *The Spine Journal*, *17*(6), 901–902. https://doi.org/10.1016/j.spinee.2017.03.009

Cunha, A. C., Burke, T. N., França, F. J., & Marques, A. P. (2008). Effect of global posture reeducation and of static stretching on pain, range of motion, and quality of life in women with chronic neck pain: A randomized clinical trial. *Clinics (Sao Paulo)*, *63*(6), 763–770.

Damasceno, G. M., Ferreira, A. S., Nogueira, L. A. C., Reis, F. J. J., Lara, R. W., & Meziat-Filho, N. (2018). Reliability of two pragmatic tools for assessing text neck. *Journal of Bodywork and Movement Therapies*, *22*(4), 963–967. https://doi.org/10.1016/j.jbmt.2018.01.007

De-la-Llave-Rincón, A. I., Fernández-de-las-Peñas, C., Palacios-Ceña, D., & Cleland, J. A. (2009). Increased forward head posture and restricted cervical range of motion in patients with carpal tunnel syndrome. *Journal of Orthopaedic & Sports Physical Therapy*, *39*(9), 658–664. https://doi.org/10.2519/jospt.2009.3058

Deljo, E., Filipovic, M., Babacic, R., & Grabus, J. (2012). Correlation analysis of the hyoid bone position in relation to the cranial base, mandible and cervical part of vertebra with particular reference to bimaxillary relations/teleroentgenogram analysis. *Acta Informatica Medica*, *20*(1), 25–31. https://doi.org/10.5455/aim.2012.20.25-31

Eitivipart, A. C., Viriyarojanakul, S., & Redhead, L. (2018). Musculoskeletal disorder and pain associated with smartphone use: A systematic review of biomechanical evidence. *Hong Kong Physiotherapy Journal*, *38*(2), 77–90.

Falla, D., & Farina, D. (2007). Neural and muscular factors associated with motor impairment in neck pain. *Current Rheumatology Reports*, *9*(6), 497–502.

Falla, D., Jull, G., Dall'Alba, P., Rainoldi, A., & Merletti, R. (2003). An electromyographic analysis of the deep cervical flexor muscles in performance of craniocervical flexion. *Physical Therapy, 83*(10), 899–906.

Falla, D., Jull, G., & Hodges, P. (2004). Patients with neck pain demonstrate reduced electromyographic activity of the deep cervical flexor muscles during performance of the craniocervical flexion test. *Spine*, *29*(19), 2108–2114.

Falla, D., Jull, G., O'Leary, S., & Dall'Alba, P. (2006). Further evaluation of an EMG technique for assessment of the deep cervical flexor muscles. *Experimental Brain Research*, *16*(6), 621–628.

Falla, D., O'Leary, S., Farina, D., & Jull, G. (2011). Association between intensity of pain and impairment in onset and activation of the deep cervical flexors in patients with persistent neck pain. *The Clinical Journal of Pain, 27*(4), 309–314.

Fernández-de-las-Peñas, C., Galán-del-Río, F., Alonso-Blanco, C., Jiménez-García, R., Arendt-Nielsen, L., & Svensson, P. (2010). Referred pain from muscle trigger points in the masticatory and neck-shoulder musculature in women with temporomandibular disorders. *The Journal of Pain, 11*(12), 1295–1304.

Fernández-de-Las-Peñas, C., Cuadrado, M. L., & Pareja, J. A. (2007). Myofascial trigger points, neck mobility, and forward head posture in episodic tension-type headache. *Headache, 47*(5), 662–672. https://doi,org/10.1111/j.1526-4610.2006.00632.x

Floyd, R. T. (2017). *Manual of structural kinesiology* (20th ed.). McGraw-Hill Education.

German, R. Z., Campbell-Malone, R., Crompton, A. W., Ding, P., Holman, S., Konow, N., & Thexton, A. J. (2011). The concept of hyoid posture. *Dysphagia, 26*(2), 97–98.

Giannakopoulos, N. N., Schindler, H. J., Rammelsberg, P., Eberhard, L., Schmitter, M., & Hellmann, D. (2013). Co-activation of jaw and neck muscles during submaximum clenching in the supine position. *Archives of Oral Biology, 58*(12), 1751–1760. https://doi.org/10.1016/j.archoralbio.2013.09.002

Gustafsson, E., Thomée, S., Grimby-Ekman, A., & Hagberg, M. (2017). Texting on mobile phones and musculoskeletal disorders in young adults: A five-year cohort study. *Applied Ergonomics, 58*, 208–214. https://doi.org/10.1016/j.apergo.2016.06.012

Gupta, B. D., Aggarwal, S., Gupta, B., Gupta, M., & Gupta, N. (2013). Effect of deep cervical flexor training vs. conventional isometric training on forward head posture, pain, neck disability index in dentists suffering from chronic neck pain. *Journal of Clinical and Diagnostic Research, 7*(10), 2261–2264. https://doi.org/10.7860/jcdr/2013/6072.3487

Häkkinen, A., Kautiainen, H., Hannonen, P., & Ylinen, J. (2008). Strength training and stretching versus stretching only in the treatment of patients with chronic neck pain: A randomized one-year follow-up study. *Clinical Rehabilitation, 22*(7), 592–600. https://doi.org/10.1177/0269215507087486

Häkkinen, A., Salo, P., Tarvainen, U., Wirén, K., & Ylinen, J. (2007). Effect of manual therapy and stretching on neck muscle strength and mobility in chronic neck pain. *Journal of Rehabilitation Medicine, 39*(7), 575–579.

Hallgren, R. C., Pierce, S. J., Sharma, D. B., & Rowan, J. J. (2017). Forward head posture and activation of rectus capitis posterior muscles. *Journal of the American Osteopathic Association, 117*(1), 24–31. https://doi.org/10.7556/jaoa.2017.004

Hansraj, K. K. (2014). Assessment of stresses in the cervical spine caused by posture and position of the head. *Surgical Technology International, 25*, 277–279.

Hong, S. W., Lee, J. K., & Kang, J. H. (2019). Relationship among cervical spine degeneration, head and neck postures, and myofascial pain in masticatory and cervical muscles in elderly with temporomandibular disorder. *Archives Gerontology and Geriatrics, 81*, 119–128. https://doi.org/10.1016/j.archger.2018.12.004

Hoy, D. G., Smith, E., Cross, M., Sanchez-Riera, L., Buchbinder, R., Blyth, F. M., Brooks, P., Woolf, A. D., Osborne, R. H., Fransen, M.,

Driscoll, T., Vos, T., Blore, J. D., Murray, C., Johns, N., Naghavi, M., Carnahan, E., & March, L. M. (2014). The global burden of musculoskeletal conditions for 2010: An overview of methods. *Annals of Rheumatic Diseases, 73*(6), 982–989. https://doi.org/10.1136/annrheumdis-2013-204344

Jull, G., Falla, D., Treleaven, J., Hodges, P., & Vicenzino, B. (2007). Retraining cervical joint position sense: The effect of two exercise regimes. *Journal of Orthopaedic Research, 25*(3), 404–412.

Kalmanson, O. A., Khayatzadeh, S., Germanwala, A., Scott-Young, M., Havey, R. M., Voronov, L. I., & Patwardhan, A. G. (2019). Anatomic considerations in headaches associated with cervical sagittal imbalance: A cadaveric biomechanical study. *Journal of Clinical Neuroscience, 65*, 140–144. https://doi.org/10.1016/j.jocn.2019.02.003

Kendall, F. P., McCreary, E. K., Provance, P. G., McIntyre Rodgers, M., & Romani, W. A. (2014). *Muscles: Testing and function with posture and pain* (5th ed.). Wolters Kluwer Health.

Kenney, W. L., Wilmore, J. H., & Costill, D. L. (2015). *Physiology of sport and exercise* (6th ed.). Human Kinetics.

Khan, M. T., Verma, S. K., Maheshwari, S., Zahid, S. N., & Chaudhary, P. K. (2013). Neuromuscular dentistry: Occlusal diseases and posture. *Journal of Oral Biology and Craniofacial Research, 3*(3), 146–150.

Kim, D. H., Kim, C. J., & Son, S. M. (2018). Neck pain in adults with forward head posture: Effects of craniovertebral angle and cervical range of motion. *Osong Public Health and Research Perspectives, 9*(6), 309–313.

Kim, J. Y., & Kwag, K. I. (2016). Clinical effects of deep cervical flexor muscle activation in patients with chronic neck pain. *Journal of Physical Therapy Science, 28*(1), 269–273. https://doi.org/10.1589/jpts.28.269

Kim, S. Y., Kim, N. S., & Kim, L. J. (2015). Effects of cervical sustained natural apophyseal glide on forward head posture and respiratory function. *Journal of Physical Therapy Science, 27*(6), 1851–1854.

Kim, S.-Y., & Koo, S.-J. (2016). Effect of duration of smartphone use on muscle fatigue and pain caused by forward head posture in adults. *Journal of Physical Therapy Science, 28*(6), 1669–1672. https://doi.org/10.1589/jpts.28.1669

Kinney, E., Wusthoff, J., Zyck, A., Hatzel, B., Vaughn, D., Strickler, T., & Glass, S. (2008). Activation of the trapezius muscle during varied forms of Kendall exercises. *Physical Therapy in Sport, 9*(1), 3–8. https://doi.org/10.1016/j.ptsp.2007.11.001

Koseki, T., Kakizaki, F., Hayashi, S., Nishida, N., & Itoh, M. (2019). Effect of forward head posture on thoracic shape and respiratory function. *Journal of Physical Therapy Science, 31*(1), 63–68. https://doi.org/10.1589/jpts.31.63

Kumaresan, S., Yoganandan, N., Pintar, F. A., Maiman, D. J., & Goel, V. K. (2001). Contribution of disc degeneration to osteophyte formation in the cervical spine: A biomechanical investigation. *Journal of Orthopaedic Research, 19*(5), 977–984. https://doi.org/10.1016/S0736-0266(01)00010-9

Lewit, K. (1985). Muscular and articular factors in movement restriction. *Manual Medicine, 1*, 83–85.

Malone, A., Meldrum, D., & Bolger, C. (2015). Three-dimensional gait analysis outcomes at 1 year following decompressive surgery for cervical spondylotic myelopathy. *European Spine Journal, 24*(1), 48–56. https://doi.org/10.1007/s00586-014-3267-1

Mani, K., Provident, I., & Eckel, E. (2016). Evidence-based ergonomics education: Promoting risk factor awareness among office computer workers. *Work, 55*(4), 913–922. https://doi.org/10.3233/WOR-162457

Mayer, J., Cho, S., Qureshi, S., & Hecht, A. (2012). Cervical spine injury in athletes. *Current Orthopaedic Practice, 23*(3), 181–187.

Mercer, S. R., & Bogduk, N. (2001). Joints of the cervical vertebral column. *Journal of Orthopaedic & Sports Physical Therapy, 31*(4), 174–182.

Mingels, S., Dankaerts, W., van Etten, L., Thijs, H., & Granitzer, M. (2016). Comparative analysis of head-tilt and forward head position during laptop use between females with postural induced headache and healthy controls. *Journal of Bodywork and Movement Therapies, 20*(3), 533–541. https://doi.org/10.1016/j.jbmt.2015.11.015

Moore, K. L., Dalley, A. F., & Agur, A. M. R. (2013). *Clinically oriented anatomy* (7th ed.). Lippincott, Williams, & Wilkins.

Morningstar, M. W., Pettibon, B. R., Schlappi, H., Schlappi, M., & Ireland, T. V. (2005). Reflex control of the spine and posture: A review of the literature from a chiropractic perspective. *Chiropractic & Osteopathy, 13*(16). https://doi.org/10.1186/1746-1340-13-16

Mujawar, J. C., & Sagar, J. H. (2019). Prevalence of upper cross syndrome in laundry workers. *Indian Journal of Occupational and Environmental Medicine, 23*(1), 54–56. https://doi.org/10.4103/ijoem.IJOEM_169_18

National Center for Health Statistics. (2006). Special feature: Pain. In *Chartbook on trends in the health of Americans.* Hyattsville, MD. http://www.cdc.gov/nchs/data/hus/hus06.pdf

Nikander, R., Mälkiä, E., Parkkari, J., Heinonen, A., Starck, H., & Ylinen, J. (2006). Dose-response relationship of specific training to reduce chronic neck pain and disability. *Medicine & Science in Sports & Exercise, 38*(12), 2068–2074.

Okada, E., Matsumoto, M., Ichihara, D., Chiba, K., Toyama, Y., Fujiwara, H., Momoshima, S., Nishiwaki, Y., Hashimoto, T., Ogawa, J., Watanabe, M., & Takahata, T. (2009). Aging of the cervical spine in healthy volunteers: A 10-year longitudinal magnetic resonance imaging study. *Spine, 34*(7), 706–712. https://doi:10.1097/BRS.0b013e31819c2003

Okuro, R. T., Morcillo, A. M., Ribeiro, M. A., Sakano, E., Conti, P. B., & Ribeiro, J. D. (2011). Mouth breathing and forward head posture: Effects on respiratory biomechanics and exercise capacity in children. *Jornal Brasileiro Pneumologia, 37*(4), 471–479. https://doi.org/10.1590/s1806-37132011000400009

Olszewska, E., Tabor, P., & Czarniecka, R. (2018). Magnitude of physiological curvatures of the spine and the incidence of contractures of selected muscle groups in students. *Biomedical Human Kinetics, 10*, 31–37. https://doi.org/10.1515/bhk-2018-0006

Ozudogru Celik, T., Duyur Cakit, B., Nacir, B., Genc, H., Cakit, M. O., & Karagoz, A. (2020). Neurodynamic evaluation and nerve conduction studies in patients with forward head posture. *Acta Neurologica Belgica, 120*, 621–628. https://doi.org/10.1007/s13760-018-0941-9

Page, P., Frank, C. C., & Lardner, R. (2010). *Assessment and treatment of muscle imbalance: The Janda approach.* Human Kinetics.

Park, S. K., Yang, D. J., Kim, J. H., Heo, J. W., Uhm, Y. H., & Yoon, J. H. (2017). Analysis of mechanical properties of cervical muscles in patients with cervicogenic headache. *Journal of Physical Therapy Science, 29*(2), 332–335. https://doi.org/10.1589/jpts.29.332

Patwardhan, A. G., Khayatzadeh, S., Havey, R. M., Voronov, L. I., Smith, Z. A., Kalmanson, O., Ghanayem, A. J., & Sears, W. (2018). Cervical sagittal balance: A biomechanical perspective can help clinical practice. *European Spine Journal, 27*(Suppl. 1), 25–38. https://doi.org/10.1007/s00586-017-5367-1

Peng, B., & DePalma, M. J. (2018). Cervical disc degeneration and neck pain. *Journal of Pain Research, 11*, 2853–2857. https://doi.org/10.2147/JPR.S180018

Pettit, N. J., & Auvenshine, R. C. (2018). Change of hyoid bone position in patients treated for and resolved of myofascial pain. *Cranio, 31*, 1–17.

Pop, M. S., Mihancea, P., & Debucean, D. (2018). Posture optimization—Is it the key to myofascial neck pain relief? *Archives of the Balkan Medical Union, 53*(4), 573–579.

Quek, J., Pua, Y. H., Clark, R. A., & Bryant, A. L. (2013). Effects of thoracic kyphosis and forward head posture on cervical range of motion in older adults. *Manual Therapy, 18*(1), 65–71. https://doi.org/10.1016/j.math.2012.07.005

Roussouly, P., & Pinheiro-Franco, J. L. (2011). Sagittal parameters of the spine: Biomechanical approach. *European Spine Journal, 20*(Suppl. 5), 578–585. https://doi.org/10.1007/s00586-011-1924-1

Sahrmann, S. A. (2001). *Diagnosis and treatment of movement impairment syndromes.* Mosby.

Schroeder, G. D., & Vaccaro, A. R. (2016). Cervical spine injuries in the athlete. *Journal of the American Academy of Orthopaedic Surgeons, 24*(9), e122–133. https://doi.org/10.5435/JAAOS-D-15-00716

Simons, D. G., Travell, J. G., Simons, L. S. (1999). *Travell & Simons' myofascial pain and dysfunction: Upper half of body.* Lippincott, Williams, & Wilkins.

Singla, D., & Veqar, Z. (2017). Association between forward head, rounded shoulders, and increased thoracic kyphosis: A review of the literature. *Journal of Chiropractic Medicine, 16*(3), 220–229. https://doi.org/10.1016/j.jcm.2017.03.004

Stone, M. A., Osei-Bordom, D. C., Inman, R. D., Sammon, C., Wolber, L. E., & Williams, F. M. (2015). Heritability of spinal curvature and its relationship to disc degeneration and bone mineral density in female adult twins. *European Spine Journal, 24*(11), 2387–2394. https://doi.org/10.1007/s00586-014-3477-6

Szczygieł, E., Weglarz, K., Piotrowski, K., Mazur, T., Metel, S., & Golec, J. (2015). Biomechanical influences on head posture and the respiratory movements of the chest. *Acta of Bioengineering and Biomechanics, 17*(2), 143.

Taimela, S., Takala, E. P., Asklöf, T. Seppälä, K. & Parviainen, S. (2000). Active treatment of chronic neck pain: A prospective randomized intervention. *Spine, 25*(8), 1021–1027.

Todd, A. G. (2011). Cervical spine: Degenerative conditions. *Current Reviews in Musculoskeletal Medicine, 4*(4), 168–174. https://doi.org/10.1007/s12178-011-9099-2

Tsang, S. M., Szeto, G. P., & Lee, R. Y. (2013). Normal kinematics of the neck: The interplay between cervical and thoracic spines. *Manual Therapy, 18*(5), 431–437.

Ylinen, J., Häkkinen, A., Nykänen, M., Kautiainen, H., & Takala, E. P. (2007). Neck muscle training in the treatment of chronic neck pain: A three-year follow-up study. *Europa Medicophysica, 43*(2), 161–169.

Ylinen, J., Häkkinen, A. H., Takala, E. P., Nykänen, M. J., Kautiainen, H. J., Mälkiä, E. A., Pohjolainen, T. H., Karppi, S.-L., & Airaksinen, O. V. (2006). Effects of neck muscle training in women with chronic neck pain: One-year follow-up study. *Journal of Strength & Conditioning Research, 20*(1), 6–13.

Ylinen, J., Kautiainen, H., Wirén, K., & Häkkinen, A. (2007). Stretching exercises vs. manual therapy in treatment of chronic neck pain: A randomized, controlled cross-over trial. *Journal of Rehabilitation Medicine, 39*(2), 126–132.

Ylinen, J., Takala, E. P., Nykänen, M., Häkkinen, A., Mälkiä, E., Pohjolainen, T., Karppi, S.-L., Kautiainen, H., & Airaksinen, O. (2003). Active neck muscle training in the treatment of chronic neck pain in women: A randomized controlled trial. *JAMA, 289*(19), 2509–2516.

Yong, M.-S., Lee, H.-Y., & Lee, M.-Y. (2016). Correlation between head posture and proprioceptive function in the cervical region. *Journal of Physical Therapy Science, 28*(3), 857–860. https://doi.org/10.1589/jpts.28.857

Zafar, H., Nordh, E., & Eriksson, P. O. (2000). Temporal coordination between mandibular and head-neck movements during jaw opening-closing tasks in man. *Archives of Oral Biology, 45*(8), 675–682.

Zheng, L., Jahn, J., & Vasavada, A. N. (2012). Sagittal plane kinematics of the adult hyoid bone. *Journal of Biomechanics, 45*(3), 531–536. https://doi.org/10.1016/j.jbiomech.2011.11.040

CHAPTER 17

Self-Care and Recovery

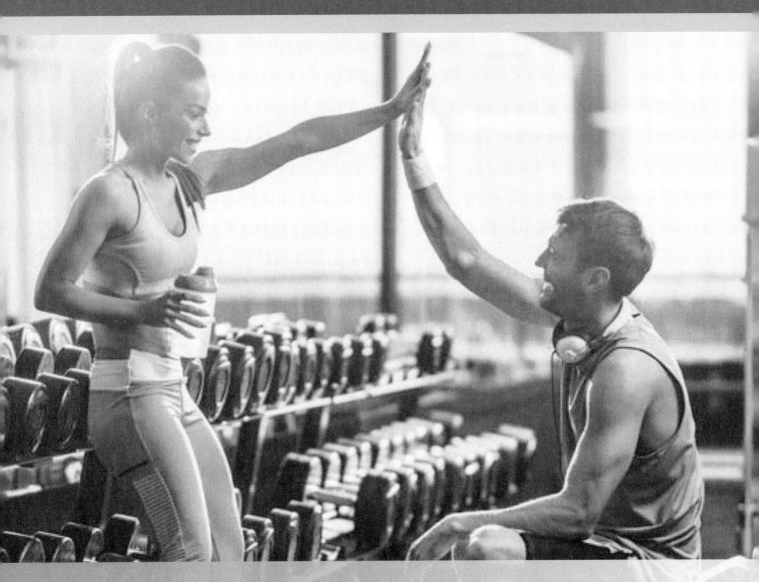

Learning Objectives

After reading this content, students should be able to demonstrate the following objectives:

- **Demonstrate** effective coaching and communication techniques to maximize adherence to and engagement in recovery techniques.
- **Identify** proven client restorative methods and recovery strategies.
- **Communicate** effective recovery strategies for a client's overall wellness.

© Skynesher/E+/Getty Images

Introduction

Acute muscle soreness, musculoskeletal discomfort, and fatigue are just a few of the physiological and psychological effects a client experiences when increasing novel demands on their body. These effects may have a profound influence on subsequent training and exercise. Health and fitness professionals have turned to recovery research to help mitigate these effects to ensure that clients are able to perform at an optimal level, quickly adapt to stressors, and maximize physical and mental preparedness for the next bout of activity. Additionally, this has prompted the general public to seek out more information about the science of recovery in fitness and athletic environments. **Recovery** is a term used to describe a systematic physiological and psychological post-exercise process in which the body and brain require replenishment and rejuvenation in order to prepare for upcoming training or competition. Whether a client has just completed an intense cardiovascular workout, a light weight training session, or competed in a championship game, recovery strategies are imperative at all levels in order to combat the stress placed on the body and brain and maintain optimal work capacity.

As the use of recovery strategies has grown, so, too, has the production of recovery tools and methods. Vibrating foam rollers, percussive massagers, sleep pods, compression boots, and wearable devices are just some of the several tools and methods flooding the market to provide a competitive advantage to their users. The presence of several tools may overcomplicate the process to achieve optimal recovery; thus, actual implementation must start with "the basics" and can be more simplistic in practice. The recovery process begins at the personal knowledge base and understanding of the professional and client, and progresses with carefully selected individual strategies. The Corrective Exercise Specialist will focus on recommending strategies and practices that are foundational to effective exercise recovery in the areas of sleep, nutrition, hydration, psychological relaxation, and movement (preparatory and restorative). These strategies can be grouped into three phases: **rest**, **refuel**, and **regenerate** (**Figure 17-1**).

Recovery

A systematic physiological and psychological process in which the body and brain require replenishment and rejuvenation in order to prepare for the next training or competition.

Rest

Aspect of recovery that focuses on improving daily sleep amount and quality, limiting stress, and increasing physical and psychological relaxation.

Refuel

Aspect of recovery that focuses on nutrition and hydration habits prior to, during, and after activity.

Regenerate

Aspect of recovery that focuses on movement-based self-care strategies to optimize movement quality and minimize compensation.

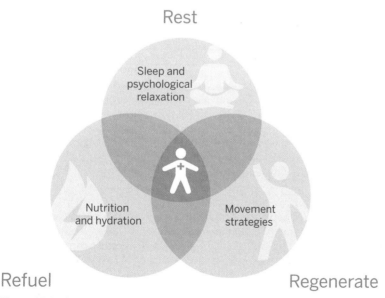

Figure 17-1 Recovery strategies

Exercise, Recovery, and Overall Wellness

Six dimensions of wellness

Interdependent categories used by the National Wellness Institute to illustrate the primary properties of an individual's holistic health and overall functioning.

Each recovery strategy is vital to the overall process. If any one of these strategies is not addressed, a client's performance could be compromised. It is important to note, however, that optimal recovery from training and competition is just one part of a larger focus on the overall health and wellness of the client.

Recovery is an essential component of the client's overall wellness because it contributes to both the psychological and physical components of well-being. Much like flawed performance programming, which focuses solely on uniplanar exercises or heavy strength training, health and fitness professionals who place physical gains above the total wellness of a client will find themselves on the wrong side of evidence-based practice. Corrective Exercise Specialists must take a holistic approach to optimal physical and emotional health. If any dimension of wellness is impaired by stress, self-esteem, fear, inactivity, insecurity, or disbelief, an individual's total wellness is affected.

 CHECK IT OUT

Dr. Bill Hettler (1976), cofounder of the National Wellness Institute (NWI), identified the **six dimensions of wellness**. The model comprises the six key elements of wellness: occupational, physical, social, intellectual, spiritual, and emotional. The implementation of the rest, refuel, and regenerate exercise recovery strategies will work to complement and enhance multiple wellness dimensions, such as the ones outlined here. Although the Corrective Exercise Specialist is not qualified to assess and attempt to provide strategies in all six dimensions, it is important to understand the effect that proper recovery strategies may have on one or more of the domains of overall wellness:

- **Occupational.** Occupational wellness focuses on a person's work and their attitude toward it. An individual will only be content with their occupation if that career aligns with their personal interests, moral and political beliefs, and values.
- **Physical.** The benefits of physical wellness have been well documented and include nutrition, hydration, and physical activity components. Individuals who consume a well-balanced diet, meet at least minimal physical activity requirements, and refrain from consuming toxic substances such as drugs, alcohol, and tobacco are more likely to have a healthy lifestyle and are less likely to sustain injury and illness.
- **Social.** Social interaction is a necessity for human existence. Positive, healthy relationships lead to a healthier lifestyle. Those who commit to not only improving their own social welfare but also the welfare of those around them will find an environment built on trust and harmony. Conversely, negative relationships, built on conflict, will have a drastic impact on social wellness.
- **Intellectual.** Education and creativity are the keys to development. Individuals who consistently challenge their own beliefs, are open to new ideas, encourage creative thinking, and who are strategic in problem solving and planning are less likely to report stress and conflict. Just like the need for continuous physical activity, human minds need constant positive stimulus to maintain intellectual wellness.
- **Spiritual.** Intolerance and a closed-minded perspective are two of the biggest detriments to spiritual wellness. Those who consistently question their own existence, values, and beliefs while at the same time are tolerant and open to other individuals' spiritual beliefs have a deep appreciation for the universe. A person should strive to have their actions align with their beliefs/values to achieve spiritual wellness.
- **Emotional.** Emotional wellness is the ability to identify and accept feelings and emotions. An individual who can freely express their feelings will find more meaningful relationships and will be able to handle conflict with maturity and clarity. Emotional wellness is a person's ability to accept other individuals' feelings while understanding and responding to their own feelings.

Reproduced from Hettler, B. (1976). *The six dimensions of wellness.* National Wellness Institute. https://nationalwellness.org/resources/six-dimensions-of-wellness/

The principles of corrective exercise and recovery are integral to the overall wellness of a client or athlete. Although health and fitness professionals are not qualified to provide strategies to improve every dimension of wellness (e.g., occupational or spiritual), their role is to optimize the physical wellness and performance of their clients through proper exercise and recovery programming. In this way, the related dimensions of wellness can be maximized, contributing to the client's overall health and well-being.

Recovery Planning

A parallel can be drawn between the recovery process and the Corrective Exercise Specialist's three-step process of identifying the problem, creating the solution, and then implementing the solution (**Figure 17-2**). By adapting the same steps to the creation of a recovery plan, the Corrective Exercise Specialist can outline an individualized and systematic recovery process for their client.

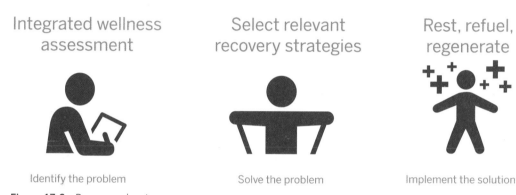

Integrated wellness assessment	Select relevant recovery strategies	Rest, refuel, regenerate
Identify the problem	Solve the problem	Implement the solution

Figure 17-2   Recovery planning process

The first step in the development of a recovery plan for athletes and clients at all levels begins with a recovery questionnaire. A recovery questionnaire can be used during client intake and even before each training session or athletic practice. This provides subjective data to the Corrective Exercise Specialist on a client's recovery-related habits. Some key information to obtain from a recovery assessment include daily sleep (e.g., self-reports of total daily sleep amounts, quality, and daytime sleepiness), relaxation, nutrition and hydration habits, stress, muscle soreness, mental readiness, and pre- and post-training self-care routines.

The second step in the development of a successful recovery plan is to create a targeted recovery strategy based on the client's reporting. This strategy should address both physiological and psychological rejuvenation in order to ensure that the client is ready for the next training session or competition. It is important the fitness professional and client select only those strategies that are most relevant and effective for their recovery plan. Working on a smaller number of actionable strategies creates a higher likelihood of adherence.

The final step in a recovery plan is implementation. The Corrective Exercise Specialist must be able to effectively communicate programs, recovery strategies, and goals in a manner that increases adherence and compliance. A variety of recovery and regeneration paradigms have been developed, but the process and the strategies presented here provide the necessary starting framework for the Corrective Exercise Specialist to optimize a client's overall recovery. Once the basics of the rest, refuel, and regenerate strategies are implemented, additional modalities may be utilized to optimize recovery for each individual.

Recovery Questionnaire

A systematic and strategic recovery plan begins with an assessment of a client's habits in the form of recovery questionnaires. Questions specifically targeting rest, refueling, and regeneration status provide a wealth of information to the Corrective Exercise Specialist. The fitness professional is encouraged to use the combination of questions that best suits their clientele's needs. Many of these questions are adapted from validated questionnaires used by clinicians to determine the level of influence these factors have on an individual's overall wellness and readiness to increase activity. These questions do not serve as formal diagnostic tools. They are used only to increase awareness around and track contributing factors to enhanced recovery and to allow the client to pinpoint helpful strategies. **Figure 17-3** offers a sample recovery questionnaire that can

Figure 17-3 Recovery questionnaire

be administered during client intake. During each training session, a subset of questions may be asked to assess workout or session readiness, as shown in **Figure 17-4**. **Table 17-1** offers example responses that would indicate the targeted behaviors in each recovery phase are optimized.

NASM

Session Readiness Questionnaire

Name ______________________________ Date ____________

REST

Sleep

- ☐ How many hours of sleep did you get last night? ____________
- ☐ How rested do you currently feel?

  Very Tired / Tired / Rested / Well Rested

Stress

- ☐ On a scale of 1 to 10, how stressed do you feel today?

  (1 = No Stress; 10 = Extremely Stressed)

  1 2 3 4 5 6 7 8 9 10

REFUEL

Nutrition

- ☐ Did you eat a nutritious pre-training meal/snack today? If yes, please describe.

  ____

Hydration

- ☐ Do you feel that you have consumed enough water prior to training?

  ____

REGENERATE

Pre-activity

- ☐ Did you engage in movement strategies to prepare for this workout (e.g., myofascial rolling, stretching, or dynamic warm-up)? If yes, please describe.

  ____

Figure 17-4 Session readiness questionnaire

TABLE 17-1 Recovery Questionnaire Targeted Responses

Rest		
Sleep	■ How many hours of sleep did you get last night? ■ Was your sleep disrupted more than usual? ■ How rested do you currently feel? Very Tired / Tired / Rested / Well Rested ■ Do you need to consume more than your usual dose of caffeine in order to stay awake and perform at your best?	■ Aim for 8+. ■ Minimize sleep disruption beyond their baseline. ■ Maximize the sense of feeling rested, which helps to gauge sleep quality. ■ Minimize reliance on stimulants and empty calories, which helps to gauge sleep quality.
Relaxation	■ How many cumulative minutes of psychological relaxation do you achieve per day? ■ How do you achieve this relaxation (e.g., reading, meditation, breathing exercises)?	■ Target 60+ minutes per day.

(continues)

TABLE 17-1 Recovery Questionnaire Targeted Responses (*continued*)

Stress	■ On a scale of 1–10 how stressed are you today? (1= No Stress; 10 = Extremely Stressed) 1 2 3 4 5 6 7 8 9 10	■ Reflects client's perceived stress level. ■ Track over time to assist the client in identifying behaviors and circumstances that correlate with stress levels.
Refuel		
Nutrition	■ Do you consume nutritious pre-training meals/snacks? If yes, please describe. ■ Do you consume nutritious post-training meals/snacks? If yes, please describe.	■ Target a balanced nutritional approach appropriate to performance goals.
Hydration	■ How many ounces of water have you consumed today?	■ Aim to replace fluid lost through sweat and retain hydration status prior to the next bout of training. ■ If less than 3% of body weight will be lost during competition or training, recommend fluid consumption as desired, or 500 mL (16.9 oz) before bed and within the hour prior to exercise.
Regenerate		
Pre-activity	■ How many days per week do you use myofascial rolling, trigger point massage, stretching, yoga, hot–cold modalities, targeted strengthening, or other movement strategies to prepare for a workout or competition?	■ Warm-up and movement preparation should follow the Corrective Exercise Continuum.
Post-activity	■ How many days per week do you use myofascial rolling, trigger point massage, stretching, yoga, hot–cold modalities, or other recovery strategies post-workout?	■ Cool-down and recovery or deloading workouts should follow the Corrective Exercise Continuum.

Rest

The first phase, rest, focuses on improving daily sleep amount and quality, limiting stress, and increasing physical and psychological relaxation. Sleep, stress, and relaxation have been shown to have a direct influence on next-day performance and the likelihood of injury (Halson & Juliff, 2017; Hamlin et al., 2019; Mah et al., 2011; Nedeltcheva et al., 2010; Pelka et al., 2017). Individuals should aim to achieve a minimum of 8 hours of sleep per night and 60 minutes of accumulated psychological relaxation per day and minimize the amount of perceived stress they experience. Psychological relaxation can take many forms depending on the individual and include breathing exercises, meditation, or reading.

Refuel

The next phase, refuel, addresses the principles of proper hydration and nutrition. It is recommended to consume adequate levels of carbohydrate, protein, and fat to prepare for and support activity and provide the substrates needed for tissue repair and recovery. In general, this equates to nutritious meals or snacks higher in carbohydrates, moderate in protein, and low in fat. Macronutrient distribution should be modified to adequately support activity goals and duration. Hydration levels should be restored to pre-activity levels using pre- and post-activity weight measurements, when realistic.

Regenerate

The final phase of recovery is regenerate. Musculoskeletal discomfort leads to a decrease in physical activity, an increase in muscular dysfunction, and potential injury. Regeneration is the cumulative process of deloading workouts and pre- and post-training routines to maintain optimal movement efficiency and recover from repetitive posture and movements. Corrective exercise is the pillar of regeneration and forms the basis of its strategies. Maximizing movement quality enhances neuromusculoskeletal efficiency, thereby reducing wasted motion and energy, sparing the kinetic chain's resources throughout activity. This enables the kinetic chain to recover from only necessary stimuli and activity. Components of the Corrective Exercise Continuum also function to reduce muscle tension and overactivity, contributing to post-workout recovery and the body's readiness for the next bout of work.

Recovery Strategies

The strategies provided serve as the basis for the rest, refuel, and regenerate framework. The fitness professional will be able to select and recommend specific methods to maximize their client's exercise recovery.

Recovery Tools and Methods

As the use of recovery strategies has grown, so has the production of recovery tools and methods. Recovery tools and methods have one of three underlying principles: physical manipulation, cognitive manipulation, and behavioral modification/goal-oriented behavior. These principles serve to increase range of motion (ROM), reduce muscle soreness, flush out lactate accumulation in the blood during high-intensity exercise, and/or reduce psychosocial stress.

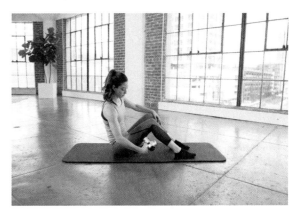

© Courtesy of National Academy of Sports Medicine

Physical manipulation recovery tools and methods include percussion instruments, foam rollers (vibrating and nonvibrating), and compression boots. Percussion instruments are newer physical manipulation tools aimed to optimize and enhance recovery. Their intent is to keep the myofascia compliant to maintain its flexibility and health with repeated training in order to prevent overuse injuries. However, because percussion tools are relatively recent, clinical research regarding application variables and overall efficacy in comparison to long-standing recovery tools and methods is limited and still evolving.

Research studies have found foam rollers to be sufficient for increasing ROM through selective muscle activation pre-workout and reducing muscle soreness post-workout (Healey et al., 2014; MacDonald et al., 2014). Respectable clinical research has also examined the use of compression boots as a recovery tool and method. The recovery-enhancing principle of compression boots is to flush out lactate accumulation in blood during high-intensity exercise through repeated vascular compression and subsequent release. In practice, compression boots have been found to have a clinically significant effect on recovery (Hanson et al., 2013) post-workout, but they are not meant to be performance-enhancing pre-workout (Martin et al., 2015).

Rapid advancements in neuroscience and further examination of brain–muscle connections have led to the implementation of several cognitive manipulation tools and methods for purposes of recovery. First, the stigma of an afternoon nap being linked to laziness has diminished in recent years (Alger et al., 2019) and has been replaced by high-performing executives and athletes recognizing the physiological and psychological benefits of a power nap as studied for decades in research laboratories (Alger et al., 2019). It has become commonplace for high-performance training centers of professional and collegiate athletic teams to offer sleeping pods that have the added utility of minimizing environmental noise and light while providing comfort for a power nap. Corporate health clubs now offer these services as well.

 GETTING TECHNICAL

Advancements in Recovery Technology

Sensory deprivation chambers have been added to high-performance training centers and elite health clubs and have become stand-alone businesses in recent years due to burgeoning research on the principles through which sensory deprivation chambers optimize and enhance performance and recovery. Research shows that sensory deprivation chambers can not only flush out lactate accumulation in blood post-exercise (Morgan et al., 2013), but can also more rapidly transition the brain into a state of active rest and restoration (Ben-Soussan et al., 2019). Sensory deprivation chambers are thought to offer the same cognitive-enhancing benefits for physical rest and restoration as ancient meditation and mindfulness practices used for centuries. An additional and burgeoning area of cognitive manipulation tools and methods are transcranial stimulation devices in order to coax the brain into a state of preparation pre-workout or into a state of rest and restoration post-workout. However, the clinical research is extremely limited regarding efficacy and determination of undue side effects with chronic use; therefore, use of transcranial stimulation technology ought to be approached with caution.

The past decade has also seen a significant boom in the use of wearables to measure daily fitness strain and nighttime recovery in order to predict next-day performance. The market is saturated with devices that monitor one or several elements of physiology and behavior passively and noninvasively (Piwek et al., 2016). Metrics include changes in the intensity of daily movement patterns, resting heart rate, variability in the speeding up and slowing down of heart rate (heart rate variability), and respiratory rate. At present, clinical centers are investigating the legitimacy of these wearables for replacing gold-standard yet cumbersome measures of sleep and cardiorespiratory health for disease prevention and diagnosis, but no formal consensus has been reached. At a minimum, wearables can be useful for behavioral modification and enforcing goal-oriented behaviors by holding the professional and client or athlete accountable for daily values of fitness strain and recovery reported by these devices.

The overall message is that not all recovery tools and methods are one size fits all. Selection of one or several recovery tools and methods requires a meaningful conversation between the Corrective Exercise Specialist and client to determine how one or two of these recovery tools and methods will help the client reach their primary and/or overall fitness goals. For example, an older client may be interested in the physical manipulation tools and methods in order to combat age-related decline in muscle function and overall flexibility, whereas a competitive athlete may opt for selecting one physical, cognitive, and wearable recovery tool and method for performance optimization and enhancement.

Sleep Strategies

Beyond integrating recent advancements in recovery tools and methods, one of the most undervalued, overlooked, and yet critical recovery strategies is achieving adequate amounts of restorative nighttime sleep. Restorative sleep is necessary and, when done right, sufficient for replenishing energy stores depleted from training. Restorative sleep also facilitates the release of anabolic hormones. A direct correlation exists between hours of deep, restorative sleep; nighttime anabolic hormone release; and optimization of next-day performance (Prinz, 1995; Ukraintseva et al., 2018; Van Cauter, 2000).

To achieve sufficient amounts of restorative sleep, the bedtime routine is a process beginning no less than an hour before bedtime. The process begins with adopting a strict regimen of bedtime and risetime that varies by no more than an hour. The intent is to "lock on" to daily rhythms of hormone release and physiological processes that are entrained, in part, through consistent cues in an individual's environment. Consistency in bedtime and risetime ensures that nighttime release of the sleep-promoting hormone melatonin is optimized. Melatonin release is also optimized by dim light. Outfitting a home with

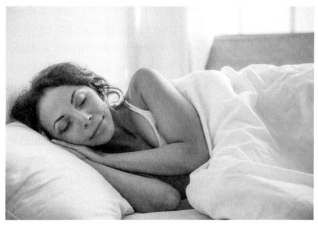
© George Rudy/Shutterstock

light dimmers and minimizing screen time are two of the most effective strategies. Taking a hot shower can also facilitate consolidated and restorative sleep through the act of vasodilation and increasing blood flow to skeletal muscle and tissues.

Finally, over-the-counter sleep supplements can be integrated on an as needed basis. Natural products such as magnesium, zinc, and cherry root are preferred, whereas "Z drugs" such as antihistamines and diphenhydramine should be used with caution. The addition of any supplemental sleep aids requires physician clearance. During sleep, light exposure should be at an absolute minimum and the room temperature should be no greater than 72 degrees Fahrenheit if reasonably possible. Overly thick, warm blankets can additionally disrupt the ability to achieve restorative sleep by means of interfering with the body's thermostat. Restorative sleep can also be achieved through the integration of meditation and mindfulness practices that have been shown to transition brain activity from higher to lower (sleep- and recovery-promoting) frequencies. Sleep strategies are an easy and cost-effective solution but require diligence and discipline for long-term benefits to recovery and next-day performance.

Nutrient-Timing Applications: Endurance and Strength-Based Activities

Carbohydrates and fat are the main substrates used by the body during endurance activity. The intensity and duration of the activity determines the contribution of each. Carbohydrates are the main substrate used during moderate- to high-intensity exercise, whereas fat is the predominant substrate used during lower-intensity exercise. In addition to intensity, as exercise duration continues (prolonged bouts of exercise), fuel substrates begin to shift, moving more from carbohydrates (glycogen) to fat stores.

Like endurance activity, resistance-based exercise relies primarily on carbohydrates as the primary fuel source, making liver and muscle glycogen stores important for performance (Robergs et al., 1991). It is important to keep muscles fueled and hydrated to optimize performance and support adequate recovery. The body takes time to digest foods, so total energy intake and composition should be considered in the meals leading up to exercise. During exercise greater than 60 minutes, glycogen depletion can be delayed when exogenous glucose is present.

ENDURANCE EXERCISE

The amount of carbohydrates an endurance athlete needs varies tremendously based on their size, training program, and sport (Ivy, 1991). Often, elite endurance athletes struggle to consume enough calories to balance the day-to-day energy demands. Glycogen stores are maximized with a higher carbohydrate diet and can be depleted with high-volume exercise such as consistent endurance activity (Kerksick et al., 2017). Carbohydrates are critical for an endurance athlete and a continuous supply (8 to 12 grams/kilogram of body weight/day) is optimal (Kerksick et al., 2017). Athletes who continuously eat a carbohydrate-rich versus a protein- or fat-rich diet have greater muscle glycogen stores to draw from during training and racing (Ivy, 1991).

It is well-established that adequate muscle glycogen stores help delay the onset of fatigue (Impey et al., 2018). Although the research around carbohydrate timing and intake is plentiful, at this time, research is inadequate to suggest timing of fat intake as it relates to exercise.

Endurance athletes should consume frequent meals and snacks throughout the day and avoid skipping meals. Good-quality carbohydrates, lean protein, and healthy fats should be the focus of all meals and snacks. Active individuals training for a race of some kind (e.g., 5K or 10K) and exercising consistently for over an hour should also ensure adequate carbohydrate intake to fuel exercise and speed recovery from training bouts (Eberle, 2014). **Table 17-2** suggests timing (and general content) of meals pre-, peri- (during), and post-workout.

TABLE 17-2 Fueling Strategies for Endurance Athletes

Timing	Composition	Hydration
Pre-exercise Meal		
3 to 4 hours before exercise	High-quality carbohydrates that digest easily (e.g., English muffin, pancakes, waffles, low-fiber cereal, or whole grain bread) Lean protein (e.g., eggs, turkey, ham, roast beef, chicken, or tuna) Low in fiber and fat	4 hours before activity, start hydration strategies. Example: Drink about 20 oz of water.
Pre-exercise Snack		
30 minutes to 1 hour before exercise	High in carbohydrates (e.g., chocolate milk, yogurt, fruit, and nut butter or sports drink with protein powder) Moderate in protein Low in fat and fiber	Continue hydrating. Example: Drink 15 to 20 oz of water.
Peri-exercise Meal		
Carbohydrate intake should begin shortly after onset of activity, but only if the exercise session is continuous and will last more than 60 minutes. Otherwise, no additional carbohydrate intake during exercise is required.	Products providing multiple transportable carbohydrates such as sports gels, blocks, sport beans, sports drinks, fruit, or high-carbohydrate bars with little to moderate protein	Continue hydrating, which is dependent on the athlete's sweat rate. Example: Drink 0.4 to 0.8 L per hour. Sports drinks should contain 6% to 8% carbohydrate solution. Replace electrolytes lost with sports drinks or foods high in sodium and potassium.

Timing	Composition	Hydration
Post-exercise Meal/Snack		
Critical only if another exercise bout is planned within 24 hours; however, no harm in replenishment within 2 hours after exercise.	Quality carbohydrate and lean protein Carbohydrates: 1 to 1.2 g/kg per hour for 4 to 6 hours post-exercise Protein: 0.2 to 0.5 g/kg post-exercise as a complement to carbohydrate intake above	Continue hydrating. Example: Drink 16 to 24 oz of water or sports drink for every pound lost during exercise (1.25 to 1.5 liters per kilogram of body weight lost during exercise).

Data from Aragon, A. A., & Schoenfeld, B. J. (2013). Nutrient timing revisited: Is there a post-exercise anabolic window? *Journal of the International Society of Sports Nutrition, 10*(1), 5. https://doi.org/10.1186/1550-2783-10-5; Kerksick, C. M., Arent, S., Schoenfeld, B. J., Stout, J. R., Campbell, B., Wilborn, C. D., Taylor, L., Kalman, D., Smith-Ryan, A. E., Kreider, R. B., Willoughby, D., Arciero, P. J., VanDusseldorp, T. A., Ormsbee, M. J., Wildman, R., Greenwood, M., Ziegenfuss, T. N., Aragon A. A., & Antonio, J. (2017). International society of sports nutrition position stand: Nutrient timing. *Journal of the International Society of Sports Nutrition, 14*, 33. https://doi.org/10.1186/s12970-017-0189-4

RESISTANCE EXERCISE

For a strength-training athlete, the main goals are to provide calories for daily activity and intense training and competition and to build and repair muscle mass. Focusing on eating and hydrating often and nutrition before, after, and possibly during exercise is key to training and performing at an optimal level and achieving specific fitness and athletic goals. Although traditional resistance exercise has less of an influence on muscle glycogen concentration than exhaustive endurance exercise, studies have demonstrated that resistance exercise can also significantly decrease muscle glycogen (Robergs et al., 1991).

It is well established that resistance exercise stimulates muscle protein synthesis (MPS), which is further stimulated and augmented by protein ingestion (Damas et al., 2015). MPS is an important factor for increasing the size of muscles, known as muscle hypertrophy.

Nutrient timing is simply one part of the equation of increasing muscle mass. In fact, muscle hypertrophy cannot occur without a properly designed and simultaneous resistance-training program. In reality, many factors play a role in achieving hypertrophy and strength gains, including hormone levels, stimulating lean muscle with a properly designed resistance-training program, and the consumption of the right fuel (total energy and protein). **Table 17-3** describes fueling strategies to support these goals.

TABLE 17-3 Fueling Strategies for Strength Athletes		
Timing	Composition	Hydration
Pre-exercise Meal		
2 to 4 hours before exercise	High quality carbohydrates (1 to 4 g/kg) 20 to 30 g lean protein Lower in fiber and fat	Start hydration strategies 4 hours before activity. Example: Drink about 20 oz of water.
Pre-exercise Snack		
30 minutes to 2 hours before exercise	High in carbohydrates Moderate in protein Low in fat and fiber	Continue hydrating. Example: Drink 15 to 20 oz of water.

(continues)

TABLE 17-3 Fueling Strategies for Strength Athletes (*continued*)

Timing	Composition	Hydration
Peri-exercise		
Carbohydrate intake (and possibly protein) should begin shortly after onset of activity only if the exercise session lasts more than 60 minutes	30 to 60 g of carbohydrates per hour spaced every 15 to 20 minutes for exercise lasting more than 60 minutes	Continue hydrating, which is dependent on the athlete's sweat rate. Example: Drink 0.4 to 0.8 L per hour. Sports drinks should contain a 6% to 8% carbohydrate solution. Replace electrolytes lost with sports drinks or foods high in sodium and potassium.
Post-exercise Meal/Snack		
Critical only if exercising again within 24 hours, but not harmful to try to consume quality carbohydrates and protein soon after exercise session comes to an end and at repeated intervals (about every 4 hours), particularly with protein.	Quality carbohydrates and lean protein. Carbohydrates: 1 to 1.2 g/kg for 4 to 6 hours post-exercise. Protein: 20 to 30 g consumed after exercise	Continue hydrating. Example: Drink 16 to 24 oz of water or sports drink for every pound lost during exercise (1.25 to 1.5 liters per kilogram of body weight lost during exercise).

Data from Aragon, A. A., & Schoenfeld, B. J. (2013). Nutrient timing revisited: Is there a post-exercise anabolic window? *Journal of the International Society of Sports Nutrition, 10*(1), 5. https://doi.org/10.1186/1550-2783-10-5; Kerksick, C. M., Arent, S., Schoenfeld, B. J., Stout, J. R., Campbell, B., Wilborn, C. D., Taylor, L., Kalman, D., Smith-Ryan, A. E., Kreider, R. B., Willoughby, D., Arciero, P. J., VanDusseldorp, T. A., Ormsbee, M. J., Wildman, R., Greenwood, M., Ziegenfuss, T. N., Aragon A. A., & Antonio, J. (2017). International society of sports nutrition position stand: Nutrient timing. *Journal of the International Society of Sports Nutrition, 14*, 33. https://doi.org/10.1186/s12970-017-0189-4; Burd, N., & Phillips, S. (2017). Protein and exercise. In C. Karpinski & C. Rosenbloom (Eds.), *Sports nutrition. A handbook for professional sports.* Academy of Nutrition and Dietetics.

 TRAINING TIP

The nutrition recommendations presented are designed to maximize high-level athletic training and competition, and may be overly complicated or unnecessary for a large majority of clients. The Corrective Exercise Specialist should maximize adherence by prioritizing and focusing on basic strategies. These should be simple to apply, such as drinking water as desired during activity or consuming a healthy snack 30 to 60 minutes prior to exercise that provides quick-digesting carbohydrates and some protein. In this way, clients will remain hydrated and fueled without feeling like it is yet another chore to complete so they can exercise. Remember, a program that is consistently performed is superior to the perfect program that is never done.

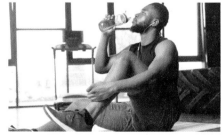
© LightField Studios/Shutterstock

HYDRATION

The objective of hydration relating to planned activity is to replace fluid lost through sweat and to maintain hydration status prior to the next bout of training. If less than 3% of body weight will be lost during competition or training, the client may simply be directed to consume fluid as desired. However, for clients or athletes requesting specific recommendations, 500 mL (16.9 oz) before bed and within the hour prior to exercise will satisfy the hydration needs for most exercisers.

Movement Strategies

Optimizing recovery can be pigeonholed as being a more passive component of health, wellness, and performance. As has already been mentioned, factors such as sleep, psychological relaxation, nutrition, and hydration are some of the key components in this process. Self-care and recovery-based movement strategies can also have an effect on the mental as well as physical aspects of regeneration.

Corrective exercise within fitness and performance-based programs, when formally integrated into a workout plan, will have its own segment in the earlier phases of the conditioning plan. This is to establish postural integrity and improve stabilization and muscle balance before increasing intensity and volume in the training phases to follow. This phase of improving overall movement efficiency does not have to end when subsequent training phases begin, but, rather, can have a weekly, if not daily, part in maintaining muscle balance and decreasing the stress of higher-intensity training through the use of pre- and post-training movement sequences. Corrective exercise programs prepare the body for work and help it recover from work.

Long-term exercise and recovery program design must consider the 168-hour week in a holistic manner. After considering the responsibilities of home, family, work/school, social commitments, workouts, and practice for sport/recreation, the pockets of "free" time may be slim. However, time needs to be carved out to address postural positions given the effects of prolonged sitting in front of the computer at work or school; the overuse patterns of sports-related movements such as side-dominant throwing, kicking, or running; or excessive use of mobile devices. Many clients are seated at least 8 to 9 hours per day with a commute–desk job–commute cycle. Some time must be dedicated to counter movements and postures to offer relief from the prolonged forward head with cervical extension; protracted shoulders; and hip, knee, and ankle flexed positions. Proper movement strategies can be a significant factor in offsetting postural distortion patterns.

TRAINING TIP

Encouraging clients to move more requires an understanding of what movement may mean to different people and contexts. Movement strategies can be delivered in a few key contexts to maximize adherence:

1. Formal assessment-based strategies
2. Strategies based on what "feels right"
3. Preformatted routines

(continues)

Formal Assessment-Based Strategies

Corrective exercise strategies at times may require formal 30- to 60-minute sessions contained within a 4- to 6-week plan of slow tempos and low intensity to elicit improved posture. However, improving posture can take place over a matter of 5 to 10 minutes daily with the right coordinated movement sequences. Depending on the environment, the client may choose self-myofascial techniques (SMTs) that do not involve getting on the floor with a roller. Self-applied pressure or a percussive device may be used to accomplish the goals of phase 1 of the Corrective Exercise Continuum in this case.

Sample assessment-based strategy for a desk worker—upper extremity:

- SMT or percussion tool for the anterior shoulder girdle
  - Performance tip: Exerciser may remain seated.
- Static pectorals stretch
  - Performance tip: Find closest wall or door jamb.
- Single-leg cobra
  - Performance tip: Use an open area that is at least arms-width across.

"Feels Right" Strategies

Reading a textbook or tablet requires directing the eyes and head position to the screen or book. This requires a forward head position that can instigate upper neck and shoulder tension. At the onset of tension, relief can come by way of the following sequence right at the time of need:

- SMT using hook-shaped tool with downward pressure into the upper trapezius
- Levator scapulae stretch
- Cervical flexion (chin tuck) with active holds

Preformatted Routines

If working with corporate groups or athletic teams, preformatted routines can be offered that are designed to address many of the muscle imbalances that much of the greater population collectively experience. Some sample programs can be offered with suggested opportunities for execution. Many can be completed in 5 to 10 minutes and with minimal equipment:

- Anterior hip routine
  - SMT hip flexor complex (TFL, rectus femoris)
  - Three-dimensional standing hip flexor stretch
  - Hip hinge pattern (e.g., Romanian deadlift using body weight)
- Shoulder routine
  - SMT latissimus dorsi
  - Static latissimus dorsi stretch using ball or fixed anchor (e.g., chair)
  - Standing scaption
- Foot and ankle routine
  - SMT calf complex
  - Dynamic calf stretch (leg swings side to side)
  - Anterior tibialis activation

EXAMPLE PROGRAMMING FOR SEASON-BASED SPORTS

Strength and conditioning programs at the collegiate and professional level will have progressive and stratified training plans that include phase-based training. If designed correctly, the training plan (i.e., training cycles) will consider recovery. When looking at the athletic needs of any sport, the adaptations of stability, strength, and power need to be integrated as well as progressed in sync with seasonal competition. Whether for the recreational or competitive athlete, careful long- and short-term planning are essential to maximizing recovery. In this way, recovery is "built in" to the athlete's periodization strategy. Generally, season-dependent progressions are coordinated cycles of training with desired adaptation goals:

- Preseason: Corrective exercise, stabilization, strength, and power
- In-season: Maintain strength and power; stabilization via self-care routines
- Off-season: Corrective exercise, self-care routines, and active rest

This concept is not specific or isolated to collegiate, club, or professional-based sports as some degree of variation can be implemented with the weekend warrior or recreational athlete. Despite the level of competition variation in volume, intensity and exercise selection is crucial for diversifying stresses on the body and maximizing recovery, thereby minimizing overuse patterns and injury. The following example is a sample layout of short- and long-term planning for a competitive golfer (**Figure 17-5**).

NASM — Sample Training Plan – Collegiate Golfer

Name ___Juliette Smith_____   Training Period ____In-season, January, Week 1__

MACROCYCLE

	Assessment & Corrective Exercise	Stabilization	Strength Endurance	Muscular Development	Maximal Strength	Power Endurance	Maximal Power
Pre-season (Fall, with pre-season play)	X	X	X			X	X
In-Season (Winter/ Spring)	X	X	X			X	X
Off-Season (Summer)	X	X	X		X	X	

IN-SEASON MONTHLY PLANNING

	Assessment & Corrective Exercise	Stabilization	Strength Endurance	Muscular Development	Maximal Strength	Power Endurance	Maximal Power
January	X	X	X			X	X
February			X			X	X
March	X	X	X			X	X

IN-SEASON MESOCYCLE – JANUARY

	Assessment & Corrective Exercise	Stabilization	Strength Endurance	Muscular Development	Maximal Strength	Power Endurance	Maximal Power
Week 1	X	X	X				
Week 2		X	X				
Week 3			X			X	
Week 4			X			X	X

MICROCYCLE – JANUARY – WEEK 1

	Monday	Tuesday	Wednesday	Thursday	Friday	Saturday	Sunday
Self-Care		X	X	X	X	X	X
Assessment & Corrective Exercise	Re-assessment						
Stabilization	X		X				
Strength Endurance					X		

Figure 17-5 Sample planning: competitive golfer

Athletes have many opportunities to incorporate strategies that improve or at least maintain muscle balance and postural endurance. Often, these self-care and corrective exercise strategies must be built into the strength and conditioning or workout schedule. They can also be integrated incrementally as a daily "mini" workout or built into the workout plan as a movement preparation and/or cool-down. However it is executed, planning recovery through movement will help maintain established stability as well as offset overuse due to high-volume, high-intensity load through exercise programming as well as practice and competitive play.

Communication Skills for Adherence

Much of the challenge around encouraging recovery behaviors lies in increasing adherence to "homework" away from the session. During the initial sessions, much time is spent discovering the status and needs of the client. As discussed, conversations on both mental and physical wellness are meant to calculate the current behaviors that have contributed to their current situation. This, combined with goal setting, lays the foundation for the different behaviors that need to be addressed for improved recovery through structured and measurable strategies.

Recovery Strategies and Lifestyle Compatibility

When implementing new or modified habits, client inclusion in the process helps with adherence. Having the client play an active role in what behaviors need to be addressed as well as the extent to which they are implemented can help with compliance. This means exploring current behaviors and how they came about, whether due to work schedule, family obligations, team practice, or conditioning sessions. With that in mind, the Corrective Exercise Specialist and client must develop a plan that considers the nonnegotiable (e.g., work schedule) and the negotiable (e.g., recreational and leisure time) as a way of making room for new behaviors or modifying current ones.

For example, a client reports spending 4 hours watching TV per day between morning and evening. Some of this time can be carved out for exercise, meal preparation, relaxation, meditation, and getting in the habit of going to bed earlier. As the fitness professional works with the client to develop a plan, the client has options they can opt into, such as the following:

- Watching TV during a bus ride so that it does not interfere with health-enhancing behaviors
- Watching programming that educates on exercise, meditation or relaxation, or cooking skills for more nutritious meals
- Being more selective in the programs watched to reduce screen time and create more time for movement and sleep

Another example is for someone who has been assessed as having overactive muscles and thus needs a flexibility or movement strategy for daily tension relief. Such a plan may incorporate the following options:

- Perform myofascial rolling before and after workouts, while watching TV or immediately after getting home from the evening commute.
- Invest in a percussion tool that can be taken on business trips and used in a hotel room or fitness center to improve circulation.
- Take breaks between calls or meetings with a preset stretching program that takes no more than 2 minutes to execute.

Clients can incorporate many different types of options, with the best ones being those that offer compatibility with the client's lifestyle with the least amount of perceived disruption. Another consideration is to look at actions that will give the biggest return on effort or even those that dovetail and improve other life-enhancing behaviors. For example, when sleep deprived, the client may lose energy toward the mid-afternoon. If an afternoon nap is not an option, they can reduce sleepiness through a walk for a cup of coffee at the local cafe. Individuals sensitive to caffeine should consider tea over coffee to avoid insomnia at night. In brief, by improving one behavior (such as prioritizing sleep in order to avoid excessive daytime sleepiness for a homework assignment) additional behaviors may be affected as well.

Improving Client Self-Care Adherence

Consistent practice and self-efficacy on the part of the client are crucial for long-term adoption of a self-care plan. The necessity of regular follow-up by the fitness professional cannot be understated when maximizing client or athlete adherence to their self-care and recovery programs. The client or athlete is tasked with a new behavior that has been agreed upon with the fitness professional and now the real-time environment must be tested for practicality and effectiveness.

The average fitness professional is not going to see a client more than a few times per week. This makes it necessary to hold the client accountable for the other hours of the week. When the self-care assignment has been presented and agreed upon, it is up to the Corrective Exercise Specialist to follow up for effectiveness.

As an example, the fitness professional and client agree that the priority for the week is getting 8 hours of sleep per night. After evaluating late nights watching movies combined with early morning commutes, the client is likely to spend an average of 5 hours in bed and, in general, sleeping less than 5 hours per night. As a result, the following behavioral modifications were advocated: stopping screen time after 9 p.m. (so as not to interfere with the natural nighttime release of melatonin) and reserving full-length movies for the weekends. When the client comes back for the next training session, one of two things occurs:

1. A verbal and nonverbal (i.e., handshake or high five) congratulations for successfully incorporating a positive change in quality of life, after which the next behavior for achieving adequate nighttime sleep will be addressed.
2. A re-evaluation or new strategy is provided to achieve the proper sleep amount and quality.

One key component is to keep the session positive and to find the small "wins" in effort and to celebrate and encourage any behavior that is close to the ultimate desired result. In this example, it may be determined that an additional accommodation needed is to watch TV and movies earlier in the evening in order to start a bedtime routine around 9 p.m.

Questions become the fitness professional's lifeline in the discovery of alternative solutions when initial attempts are not successful. All that has been learned up to this point for the client and professional is what has not worked in its current format. Here are some sample questions that can be used in order to find alternative solutions:

- "On a scale of 1 to 5, how challenging was this assignment, and what can we do to make it easier?"
- "This didn't work this time, but what can we do to remove some of the obstacles you encountered?"

- "Do you think there is anything we could have done differently to achieve the desired result?"
- "Is this a behavior that you feel can be done on a daily basis?"

Such questions have no right or wrong answers, because they are designed to guide the client's introspection and reflection on the actions they took (or did not take) over a certain time frame. From there, the question is also designed to spark conversation, continue the strategy creation process, and empower the client to think about how they can address other behaviors that need to be changed.

Transtheoretical Model for Fitness and Recovery Strategies

In addition to understanding human movement science, exercise science, and exercise program design, the fitness professional needs to understand the concept of the transtheoretical model (TTM) of behavior change (**Figure 17-6**) (Prochaska, 1979). The TTM is a concept that considers the stage at which someone is apt to create behavior change for desired behaviors or habits. The following are brief descriptions of the stages of the TTM:

- **Precontemplation:** The person does not know that they have a problem or that a new behavior is needed.
- **Contemplation:** The person understands that there is an issue that needs to be addressed and that the current behavioral path is detrimental to their goals or health.
- **Preparation:** Research and planning on lifestyle change is taking place.
- **Action:** Behaviors are being executed to reverse the problem.
- **Maintenance:** Consistent action is taking place for improved condition or lifestyle.
- **Termination:** An undesirable status is no longer a temptation and new counter behavior has taken hold.

Understanding the TTM is important for fitness professionals because it sets the foundation for communications with the client or a prospective client who may be researching options for fitness improvement. If a client does not realize that their progress may be stalled because

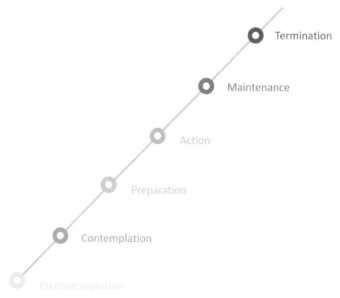

Figure 17-6 The transtheoretical model

of movement dysfunction observed during an overhead squat assessment, it could possibly be holding them back from making progress and strength gains. In this example, the client is in the precontemplation stage because they did not realize what a movement impairment is and how that would affect performance. Now that the education process has begun with further discussion with the fitness professional, the client is more aware of the effects of muscle imbalance and how it can detract from improvement in their fitness status. The client can now be considered in the contemplation stage as they are now aware of other factors that influence exercise and their results.

Preparation from this point can mean diving deeper into corrective exercise strategies and how to implement them into the exercise plan. Sample strategies may include 10- to 15-minute bouts of daily self-care. Once the strategies have been weighed and considered for optimal effectiveness, it is time for action. From here, with the possible assistance or aid of the fitness professional, exercise programming to address movement dysfunction is executed and underway.

After 6 months of consistent time in the action stage, the client is now in the maintenance stage. Here, they have been on a regularly scheduled program that addresses proper muscle balance with varied programming that improves movement quality and increases the likelihood of proper muscular function. Although the termination stage is possible for things like smoking cessation, where an individual who has truly quit will completely lack the desire to start again, it is never truly achieved with regard to exercise adherence. Due to the vast amount of unexpected events life undoubtedly has in store for every individual—changing jobs, moving to a new city, having a baby, falling ill, grieving a death in the family, getting injured, and so much more—even the most dedicated athletes tend to cycle back and forth between the preparation, action, and maintenance stages of the TTM.

Understanding where the client is in their comprehension of corrective exercise in relation to their readiness for change is crucial. What the client is ready to learn and accept will influence the level of discussion. For example, all too often, a Corrective Exercise Specialist will try to discuss corrective exercise protocols and what can be done to improve performance. If a client has no understanding of the benefits or sees no relevance to their current situation, they will have no concern, and therefore no motivation to execute the proposed plan. Conversely, if a trainer is still trying to educate on the benefits of corrective exercise but the client is ready to execute and move forward, then there may be a missed opportunity to involve the client in training sessions. The discussion and conversation need to match and mirror the TTM stage the client is currently in.

Talking About Corrective Exercise with Clients

Corrective exercise is a relatively new concept to exercise, having risen in popularity and awareness among fitness professionals over the last 15 to 20 years. Even after its development, with the goal of improving movement quality and injury resistance, there have been many variations in its implementation by industry professionals. It is because of this that clients may have different understandings of what corrective exercise is and who needs it. If it is determined that a client needs corrective exercise strategies, the fitness professional needs to be clear on what issues it is designed to solve, as well as how successful integration within an exercise and recovery plan will benefit the client.

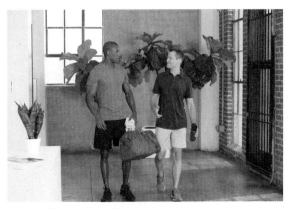

© Courtesy of National Academy of Sports Medicine

The discussion for corrective exercise begins with the explanation of the assessment process. The client needs to understand that before any comprehensive workout plan can be developed a baseline understanding of what the body needs to improve posture and minimize excess strain on the muscular system will be established. The information gained from the assessment will reveal muscle imbalances and give insight into what muscles are overactive and generally in a chronically shortened state and those muscles that are underactive and tend to be in a chronically lengthened state.

Tying movement back to the individual's "why" or motivation for achieving results is a vital part of increasing adherence to their self-care routines. As clients begin their workout plan with integration of corrective exercise programming, there must be reminders of why and how the program will help the client achieve their goals in the safest, quickest, and most effective manner possible. This is done by addressing movement efficiency and recruiting the proper muscles at the proper time. Using this format of conditioning at least in the beginning of the program decreases the chances that they will overtrain and it lays the groundwork or practice for what will be a regular self-care plan moving forward.

SUMMARY

Simply put, adequate recovery is just as important for optimizing health and wellness as the corrective exercise workouts themselves. Without proper recovery habits in place, overtraining can occur and lead to the development of additional movement impairments, increasing the chance that an individual will enter and potentially stay within the cumulative injury cycle. For maximal quality of life, exercise, recovery, and optimization of the six dimensions of wellness must work hand in hand.

The first step is to understand the components that make up recovery: the combination of adequate rest, refueling, and regeneration practices. Rest encompasses not only proper sleep habits, but also daily techniques to help reduce psychological stress. Refueling encompasses eating a healthy, balanced diet and maintaining proper hydration. Regeneration is the practice of optimizing movement patterns so that the body is ready to train at varied intensities and possibly for multiple adaptations.

To help clients properly recover, it is important to foster adherence to a self-care plan, considering all three phases of recovery in their everyday lives. Techniques to assist with this process include using recovery questionnaires to keep clients thinking about their life outside of training, implementing physical recovery tools after workouts, teaching basic guidelines for athlete-focused nutrition and hydration, providing tips on how to achieve proper sleep, and then communicating all that information in the most effective way possible. When recovery is planned and implemented as carefully as workouts, success in both a corrective exercise program and self-care will be achieved.

Alger, S. E., Brager, A. J., & Capaldi, V. F. (2019). Challenging the stigma of workplace napping. *Sleep, 42*(8). https://doi.org/10.1093/sleep/zsz097

Aragon, A. A., & Schoenfeld, B. J. (2013). Nutrient timing revisited: Is there a post-exercise anabolic window? *Journal of the International Society of Sports Nutrition, 10*(1), 5. https://doi.org/10.1186/1550-2783-10-5

Ben-Soussan, T. D., Mauro, F., Lasaponara, S., Glicksohn, J., Marson, F., & Berkovich-Ohana, A. (2019). Fully immersed: State absorption and electrophysiological effects of the OVO Whole-Body Perceptual Deprivation chamber. *Progress in Brian Research, 244*, 165–184. https://doi.org/10.1016/bs.pbr.2018.10.023

Burd, N., & Phillips, S. (2017). Protein and exercise. In C. Karpinski & C. Rosenbloom (Eds.), *Sports nutrition. A handbook for professional sports*. Academy of Nutrition and Dietetics.

Damas, F., Phillips, S., Vechin, F. C., & Ugrinowitsch, C. (2015). A review of resistance training-induced changes in skeletal muscle protein synthesis and their contribution to hypertrophy. *Journal of Sports Medicine, 45*(6), 801–807. https://doi.org/10.1007/s40279-015-0320-0

Eberle, S. G. (2014). *Endurance sports nutrition*. Human Kinetics.

Halson, S. L., & Juliff, L. E. (2017). Sleep, sport, and the brain. *Progress in Brain Research, 234*, 13–31. https://doi.org/10.1016/bs.pbr.2017.06.006

Hamlin, M. J., Wilkes, D., Elliot, C. A., Lizamore, C. A., & Kathiravel, Y. (2019). Monitoring training loads and perceived stress in young elite university athletes. *Frontiers in Physiology. 10*, 34. https://doi.org/10.3389/fphys.2019.00034

Hanson, E., Stetter, K., Li, R., & Thomas, A. (2013). An intermittent pneumatic compression device reduces blood lactate concentrations more effectively than passive recovery after Wingate testing. *Journal of Athletic Enhancement, 2*(3). https://doi.org/10.4172/2324-9080.1000115

Healey, K. C., Hatfield, D. L., Blanpied, P., Dorfman, L. R., & Riebe, D. (2014). The effects of myofascial release with foam rolling on performance. *Journal of Strength & Conditioning Research, 28*(1), 61–68. https://doi.org/10.1519/JSC.0b013e3182956569

Hettler, B. (1976). *The six dimensions of wellness*. National Wellness Institute. https://www.nationalwellness.org/page/Six_Dimensions

Impey, S. G., Hearris, M. A., Hammond, K. M., Bartlett, J. D., Louis, J., Close, G. L., & Morton, J. P. (2018). Fuel for the work required: A theoretical framework for carbohydrate periodization and the glycogen threshold hypothesis. *Sports Medicine, 48*(5), 1031–1048. https://doi.org/10.1007/s40279-018-0867-7

Ivy, J. L. (1991). Muscle glycogen synthesis before and after exercise. *Sports Medicine, 11*(1), 6–19.

Kerksick, C. M., Arent, S., Schoenfeld, B. J., Stout, J. R., Campbell, B., Wilborn, C. D., Taylor, L., Kalman, D., Smith-Ryan, A. E., Kreider, R. B., Willoughby, D., Arciero, P. J., VanDusseldorp, T. A., Ormsbee, M. J., Wildman, R., Greenwood, M., Ziegenfuss, T. N., Aragon A. A., & Antonio, J. (2017). International society of sports nutrition position stand: Nutrient timing. *Journal of the International Society of Sports Nutrition, 14*, 33. https://doi.org/10.1186/s12970-017-0189-4

MacDonald, G. Z., Button, D. C., Drinkwater, E. J., & Behm, D. G. (2014). Foam rolling as a recovery tool following an intense bout of physical activity. *Medicine & Science in Sports & Exercise, 46*(1), 131–142. https://doi.org/10.1249/MSS.0b013e3182a123db

Mah, C. D., Mah, K. E., Kezirian, E. J., & Dement, W. C. (2011). The effects of sleep extension on the athletic performance of collegiate basketball players. *Sleep, 34*(7), 943–950. https://doi.org/10.5665/SLEEP.1132

Martin, J. S., Friedenreich, Z. D., Borges, A. R., & Roberts, M. D. (2015). Preconditioning with peristaltic external pneumatic compression does not acutely improve Wingate performance nor does it alter blood lactate concentrations during passive recovery compared with sham. *Applied Physiology, Nutrition, and Metabolism, 40*(11), 1214–1231. https://doi.org/10.1139/apnm-2015-0247

Morgan, P. M., Salacinski, A. J., & Stults-Kolehmainen, M. A. (2013). The acute effects of flotation restricted environmental stimulation technique on recovery from maximal eccentric exercise. *Journal of Strength & Conditioning Research, 27*(12), 1367–1374. https://doi.org/10.1519/JSC.0b013e31828f277e

Nedeltcheva, A. V., Kilkus, J. M., Imperial, J., Schoeller, D. A., & Penev, P. D. (2010). Insufficient sleep undermines dietary efforts to reduce adiposity. *Annals of Internal Medicine. 153*(7), 435–441. https://doi.org/10.7326/0003-4819-153-7-201010050-00006

Pelka, M., Kolling, S., Ferrauti, A., Meyer, T. M., Pfeiffer, M., & Kellmann, M. (2017). Acute effects of psychological relaxation techniques between two physical tasks. *Journal of Sports Sciences, 35*(3), 216–223.

Piwek, L., Ellis, D. A., Andrews, S., & Joinson, A. (2016). The rise of consumer health wearables: Promises and barriers. *PLoS Medicine, 13*(2), e1001953. https://doi.org/10.1371/journal.pmed.1001953

Prinz, P. N., Moe, K. E., Dulberg, E. M., Larsen, L. H., Vitiello, M. V., Toivola, B., & Merriam, G. R. (1995). Higher plasma IGF-1 levels are associated with increased delta sleep in healthy older men. *The Journals of Gerontology. Series A, Biological Sciences and Medical Sciences, 50*(4), M222–M226. https://doi.org/10.1093/gerona/50a.4.m222

Prochaska, J. O. (1979). *Systems of psychotherapy: A transtheoretical analysis*. Dorsey Press.

Roberg, R. A., Pearson, D. R., Costill, D. L., Fink, W. J., Pascoe, D. D., Benedict, M. A., Lambert, C. P., & Zachweija, J. J. (1991). Muscle glycogenolysis during differing intensities of weight-resistance exercise. *Journal of Applied Physiology, 70*(4), 1700–1706.

Ukraintseva, Y. V., Liaukovich, K. M., Polishchuk, A. A., Martynova, O. V., Belov, D. A., Simenel, E. S., Meira e Cruz, M., & Nizhnik, A. N. (2018). Slow-wave sleep and androgens: Selective slow-wave sleep suppression affects testosterone and 17α-hydroxyprogesterone secretion. *Sleep Medicine, 48*, 117–126.

Van Cauter, E. (2000). Slow wave sleep and release of growth hormone. *JAMA, 284*(21), 2717–2718.

CHAPTER 18

Real-World Application of Corrective Exercise Strategies

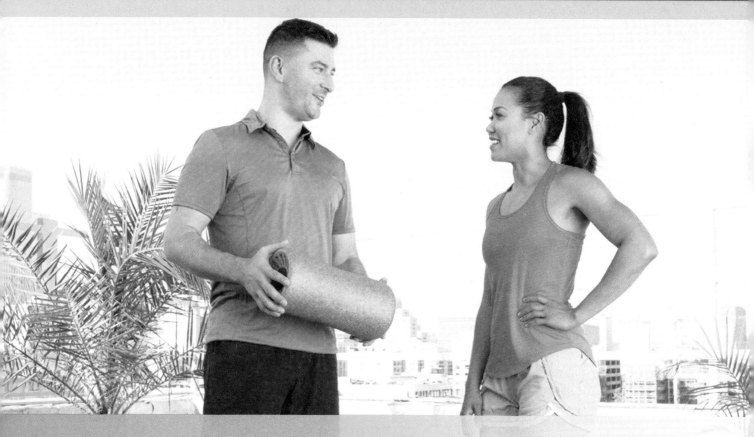

Learning Objectives

After reading this content, students should be able to demonstrate the following objectives:

- **Design** individualized corrective exercise programs based on assessment results.
- **Apply** a spectrum of corrective tools, protocols, and modalities aligned to client needs and goals.
- **Explain** the integration of corrective exercise for various scenarios and circumstances (e.g., warm-up, workout, group exercise, etc.).
- **Explain** the progression of corrective exercise programming from low- to high-threshold tasks.
- **Explain** common segmental integrations and their influence on corrective exercise programming.

Introduction

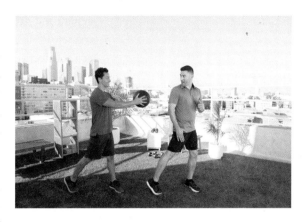

At this point in the text, it should be clear that the NASM Corrective Exercise Continuum is more than just a collection of individual assessments, techniques, and exercises, and instead presents a comprehensive assessment and programming *system* for enhancing and optimizing human movement, recovery, and durability. Greater than the sum of its individual components, the Corrective Exercise Continuum leverages evidence-based strategies and solutions rooted in concepts and principles of human movement science (functional anatomy, biomechanics, exercise science, neurophysiology, and neuroscience), affording the Corrective Exercise Specialist the opportunity to employ a variety of techniques, tools, and tactics in order to accomplish desired outcomes with their clients and athletes. While the Corrective Exercise Continuum is grounded in evidence and application, the ideal program extends beyond the complexities of the science; it must be client centric!

It is important to define some of these terms within the context of corrective exercise in order to establish a common framework and set of principles that can guide the application of corrective exercise:

- **System:** The four phases of the Corrective Exercise Continuum are an organized science- and evidence-based model in which individual components (inhibit, lengthen, activate, integrate) work together to improve human movement. It is the foundation for all corrective programs.

- **Solutions and strategies:** Solutions are answers to a problem. With respect to corrective exercise, the problem to be solved is the presence of observable movement impairments and compensation resulting from muscle imbalance. The solution is the high-level understanding of the client's needs using the four phases of the Corrective Exercise Continuum. Recommendations are created based on the probable overactive and underactive muscles associated with each movement impairment. The Corrective Exercise Specialist will identify which tissues to address within each phase of the continuum. For example, if scapular winging is present, scapular control, activation of the serratus anterior, reduction in pectoralis minor overactivity, and integrated motion of the scapulae and upper extremities all become priorities to be addressed in a program.

  A strategy is the translation of a solution into a goal-directed plan; in other words, it is how the Corrective Exercise Specialist transforms recommended solutions into corrective programs for their clients. This requires an understanding of not only the needs of one segment of the kinetic chain, but also how the segments interrelate, along with client preferences, adherence level, abilities, and needs.

- **Techniques:** Techniques are technical skills or specific methods used to accomplish particular outcomes. In corrective exercise, specific techniques are best suited to accomplish the intended outcome of each phase of the Corrective Exercise Continuum:
  - **Inhibit:** Myofascial techniques such as foam rolling and local muscle vibration
  - **Lengthen:** Static, neuromuscular, or dynamic stretching
  - **Activate:** Isolated strengthening exercises
  - **Integrate:** Integrated dynamic movements

- **Tools:** Not to be confused with techniques, tools are the specific equipment and/or modalities used to perform or augment recommended techniques. Often, health and fitness professionals are guilty of chasing "shiny objects," getting caught up in using only specific tools and modalities to address client needs, versus implementing a principles-focused system and using the best tool for the job. The beauty of a system is that it provides a framework for inclusivity of multiple tools, whereby a variety of tools and modalities can be effectively employed dependent on a professional's credentials, knowledge, skills, and abilities. Although not an exhaustive list, the following are just some example tools/modalities appropriate for each phase of the Corrective Exercise Continuum:

- **Inhibit:** Foam roller, roller ball, muscle vibration device, etc.
- **Lengthen:** Stretch strap, elastic resistance band, stretching stick
- **Activate:** Resistance cables, resistance machines, elastic resistance tubes/bands, dumbbells, kettlebells, stability balls, medicine balls
- **Integrate:** Body weight, resistance machines, dumbbells, kettlebells, stability balls, medicine balls

■ **Tactics:** Tactics are the art or skill of employing available means to accomplish an end; essentially, it is how one supports and encourages the client to actually *perform* their scheduled program.

The corrective exercise paradigm just described is represented by the CES Pyramid of Success (**Figure 18-1**).

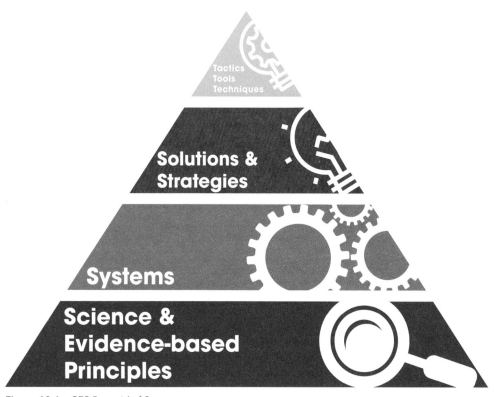

Figure 18-1   CES Pyramid of Success

Although an ideal program must certainly take into consideration the client's needs and assessment results, it must also be intentionally designed and implemented in a way that meets their goals and expectations and is executed correctly and consistently over time to elicit improvement. The perfectly designed program that is never done is not the best program; rather, it is the consistently performed program that achieves results.

Although the CES Assessment Flow and Corrective Exercise Continuum are straightforward processes, many questions arise regarding the application of these strategies in multiple environments and real-world client scenarios. The coming sections will focus on factors that influence program design and provide best practices and guidelines to assist the Corrective Exercise Specialist in maximizing the benefits of corrective exercise.

Factors Influencing Program Design, Adherence, and Success

Multiple factors influence how a corrective exercise program is designed and implemented that ultimately will affect client adherence and success. These include, but are not limited to:

- Client-related factors
- Training-related factors
- Environment-related factors

Taking each of these factors into consideration when developing a corrective exercise program will ensure that it complements and supports the exercise and training plan required to achieve the client's target goals and objectives. Any potential obstacles that could impede consistent execution of the program are identified and addressed, leading to enhanced effectiveness and improved outcomes.

Client-Related Factors

Client Needs/Assessment Results

- In what areas does the client need to improve based on their current functional status and assessment results?
- What functional and lifestyle needs exist that the program must take into consideration?

Client Goals

- What specific goals and outcomes has the client expressed they want to accomplish and achieve through exercise and training that their program must support?

Client Expectations

- What are the client's or athlete's expectations for their exercise or training program? Do they have preconceived thoughts, ideas, or beliefs about what they should be doing, such as the frequency and length of their program, based on what they want to achieve? Does corrective exercise align with their expectations?

Client Capabilities

- Does the client have any physical or functional limitations that could affect their ability to successfully perform certain exercises or techniques in their program?

Training-Related Factors

Program or Training Goals

- What are the objectives of the corrective exercise program?
  - Post-rehab/reconditioning/return-to-performance?
  - Health and wellness optimization?
  - Workout preparation/targeted warm-up?
  - Injury risk reduction/durability?
  - Performance readiness?
  - Recovery and regeneration?
- What are the objectives of the overall training program?
  - What neuromuscular and physiological adaptations are necessary to achieve the target objective(s)?
  - What specific competencies and qualities must be improved for adaptation to occur?
  - How will the corrective exercise program support and enhance this?

(continues)

Training Schedule

- How much time can the client commit to performing their program?
- When will the client be doing their corrective exercise program?
  - What time of day?
  - Before exercise/training, after, or both?
- Will the program ever be done stand-alone?

Frequency

- How many days per week is the client willing and/or able to do their program?
- How many days per week is recommended to achieve the program objective?
  - If there is lack of alignment between what the client is willing and/or able to do and what is recommended, how can that be rectified? What tactics can be employed, compromise can be reached, or creative solution found?

Environment-Related Factors

Location/Setting

- Where will the client or athlete(s) be performing their program primarily?
  - Gym or training facility
  - Work/office
  - Home
  - Athletic field or court
  - Hotel

- Will the program be performed with multiple clients/athletes at the same time?
  - Small group
  - Group exercise
  - Athletic team

Equipment

- Based on location/setting, what equipment is accessible?
  - If the client will be doing their program in multiple settings with varied levels of equipment access, alternative program options may be necessary.
  - Contingency plans, including substitute exercises, may be necessary if desired equipment is unavailable at time of need.

Provider Involvement

- Self-care/self-led programs
  - Self-care/self-led programs are those the client or athlete performs independently without direct supervision or coaching once they have been instructed or provided a plan of what to do.
  - Typically, self-care/self-led programs consist of techniques and exercises that are limited in complexity and easy for the client to perform to minimize any barriers or obstacles to completion.
- Provider-directed programs
  - Provider-directed programs are those performed under the supervision and guidance of the health and fitness professional.
  - As with self-care/self-led programs, provider-directed programs may consist of techniques and exercises that are lower in complexity and easy for the client to perform; however, because there is an opportunity for coaching and direction, provider-directed programs may progress in complexity and difficulty to promote overload, adaptation, and adherence.

Provider Involvement

- Provider-delivered programs
  - Provider-delivered programs are those directly administered by the health and fitness professional and consist of techniques and exercises that require direct application by the provider.
  - For providers qualified to do so, examples include, but are not limited to, local muscle vibration or percussion techniques and assisted stretching techniques.
  - For providers qualified to perform manual techniques, other techniques may include hands-on myofascial, joint mobilization, and muscle activation techniques.

Corrective Exercise for Any Goal

To increase adherence to, and therefore the effectiveness of, recommended corrective exercise routines, it is important that client and athlete communication is tailored to their desired outcomes. **Table 18-1** shows common goals and example language designed to reinforce the importance of corrective exercise. Options to incorporate corrective strategies for each client or athlete to maximize adherence are also included.

TABLE 18-1 Corrective Exercise for Desired Outcomes

Desired Outcome	Benefits of Corrective Exercise	Individual Suggestions for Adherence
Muscular development	"Creating and supporting the right movement patterns helps your spine, joints, and muscles become more efficient at handling load. The more load you can handle safely, the more work you can accomplish and muscle development you can experience. Corrective exercise also creates fewer movement compensations, which helps you target the right muscles at the right time. You also won't be 'wasting energy' because of inefficient movement, so recovery is more focused on helping you become stronger and more muscular over time."	Corrective strategies should be easy to apply and a natural part of the movement prep sequence. Focus on decreasing impairment in joints that will be working hard (e.g., shoulder joint mobility on chest day) and activating muscles that will contribute to the lifts executed. If compliance is an issue, pick fewer muscles to roll and stretch and activate only what is necessary. Select exercises and tools that are more desirable by the exerciser (e.g., muscle vibration device versus a cane tool). **Example corrective strategy for chest day:** ■ **Inhibit and lengthen:** Pectoralis minor, upper trapezius ■ **Activate:** Prone cobra ■ **Integrate:** Perform warm-up sets on the bench press
Weight loss	"Workouts should support your efforts to be stronger and healthier and give your body a reason to adapt to exercise. A proper warm-up is essential to getting more work done and fully benefitting from your workouts. I have individualized your flexibility and preparation routines to make sure your body is moving the best it can, so it gets the most from your workouts."	Exercise selection and sequencing should maximize adherence. The health and fitness professional has discretion regarding the number of exercises to recommend. In general, providing too many flexibility and movement preparation exercises may overwhelm a client. For many weight-loss clients, consistency is a priority, so focus on one to three selections for each of the Corrective Exercise Continuum phases.

(continues)

TABLE 18-1 Corrective Exercise for Desired Outcomes (*continued*)

Desired Outcome	Benefits of Corrective Exercise	Individual Suggestions for Adherence
		Example corrective strategy before a full-body resistance training session: ■ **Inhibit:** Myofascial technique of choice for gastrocnemius/soleus, hip flexor complex, latissimus dorsi ■ **Lengthen:** Static stretch gastrocnemius, hip flexor complex, latissimus dorsi ■ **Activate:** Floor bridge, prone cobra ■ **Integrate:** Step-up to overhead press
Health and wellness and/or movement longevity and independence	"Your workouts will focus on improving strength and cardiorespiratory health. Part of maximizing the health of your joints and muscles is maintaining the quality of your movement. The flexibility and strengthening routines that you will perform prior to and in between your workouts are a form of regular joint and muscle tissue maintenance, just like daily brushing and flossing maintain the health of your teeth."	Corrective exercise selection should prioritize ease of completion and convenience. Daily strategies and maintenance of the human movement system will be helpful in maximizing the health, fitness, and recovery of the client, with the primary goal of maintaining a baseline level of health and wellness. **Example corrective strategy before a cardio session:** ■ **Inhibit and lengthen:** Gastrocnemius/soleus, hip flexor complex, thoracic spine, upper trapezius ■ **Activate:** Floor bridge, quadruped arm/opposite-leg raise ■ **Integrate:** Step-up to overhead press
Athletic performance	"Moving with higher quality and efficiency positively affects performance on the field or court while minimizing risk of injury. Based on the assessments we did, which show us how your body prefers to move, we will create targeted flexibility and strengthening strategies to optimize your movement and body control."	Movement preparation for strength and conditioning, practice, and competition must include sequences that optimize flexibility, neuromuscular efficiency, movement quality, and performance specific to the upcoming activity. **Performance-related best practices:** ■ **Inhibit and lengthen:** Myofascial and stretching techniques of choice, focusing on individual areas that contribute to the athlete's movement impairments, muscles affecting the foot/ankle, lumbo-pelvic-hip complex, and shoulder generally require attention. ■ **Activate:** Focus on muscle groups requiring intramuscular coordination specific to the athlete's assessment results and sport (e.g., gluteus medius activation in jumping athletes). ■ **Integrate:** Use movements that are task and demand specific to the upcoming activity (e.g., hip swings, cutting maneuvers).

Prioritizing Corrective Exercise Programming

Common concerns expressed by many Corrective Exercise Specialists are the challenge of knowing where to start programming when a client exhibits various compensations during the assessment process, how to make the time to incorporate corrective exercise into a client's routine, and how to establish client buy-in of corrective exercises. There are multiple ways to prioritize a corrective exercise strategy; ultimately, it will be up to the Corrective Exercise Specialist's judgment to decide where a client will focus their time and effort. Establishing client and athlete buy-in and making time to prioritize corrective exercise can be challenging due to the perception that it will negatively affect results by taking time away from other aspects of the training program, when quite the opposite is true. Poor movement has been associated with decreased athletic performance (Yamamoto et al., 2016, p. 104); however, with appropriate guidance, coaching, and planning, performing just a 10- to 12-minute corrective/preventive program prior to training or physical activity in lieu of a more traditional warm-up can have a positive effect on fitness and performance measures (Peck et al., 2017)—the ends will justify the means! The following are some considerations to help guide that decision making. Note that a client many times falls into multiple frameworks, and that a strategy will often reveal itself in that overlap.

The fitness professional's objective is to program for all identified movement compensations, when possible. However, in the real world, not all clients are willing to perform several foam rolling, stretching, and activation exercises prior to a session or on their own in between bouts of training and exercise. To increase client and athlete program adherence, the exercise programs provided should include fewer and simpler-to-execute movements. Although all compensations will be addressed over the first months of training, the fitness professional must prioritize which compensations and regions of the body to tackle first. Based on the Regional Interdependence (RI) model, improving movement in one region of the body will likely have a positive influence on the movement quality of the individual overall (Bell et al., 2013). Remember, the best corrective exercise program for the client is the one they will actually do. The OPT® CES Programming Template is available in Appendix B.

Prioritize a Region

A region or kinetic chain checkpoint may emerge as an obvious place to focus corrective exercise programming. As the Corrective Exercise Specialist completes the assessment flow, a particular region may present multiple compensations and impairments. For example, the lumbo-pelvic-hip complex (LPHC) may display the most compensations across static, movement, and mobility assessments when compared to other kinetic chain checkpoints. As a result, the Corrective Exercise Specialist may focus programming on the LPHC.

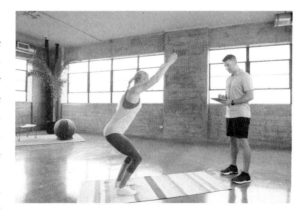

An additional way to prioritize a corrective exercise program is to focus on the region with the compensation that "sticks out" the most (i.e., the deviation that is the most prominent relative to others). This may be particularly useful if clients are limited on time or are able to execute only a few corrective exercises. For example, say that a client displays feet turn out that is more pronounced than their other compensations. After additional assessments, such as the heels-elevated overhead squat and the weight-bearing lunge test, the professional feels limited dorsiflexion is a primary contributor to additional compensations at the knee (e.g., valgus due to tibial external rotation)

and the LPHC (e.g., excessive forward lean). Therefore, improving the mobility at the foot and ankle complex may provide the most "bang for the buck" for this client and would be a great place to start their program.

Functional and Lifestyle Needs of the Client

The corrective exercise professional may also choose to prioritize exercise selection based on the functional and lifestyle needs of the client. Creating programs that match assessment results with client needs is a sweet spot that combines personal relevance with exercise science. This winning combination can improve adherence and commitment to a program.

For example, a client who is an avid cyclist has sought out a fitness and performance professional because they heard strength and conditioning is something they should do. This recreational athlete may not be excited at the prospect of training away from a bike but would like to improve their performance, resistance to injury, and recovery. With a client like this one it will be important to program according to their lifestyle and functional needs. Cyclists repeatedly maintain specific postures over long periods of time. Hips are flexed, head is forward, shoulders are often rounded. This will likely create muscular imbalances and overuse patterns, which may initiate the cumulative injury cycle if their movement is not optimized away from the bike.

It is highly likely that the assessment results of this client would reveal regions and compensations related to cycling. In any case, the corrective exercise professional will want to program corrective sequences based on the client's repetitive activity as well as their assessment results. Being able to connect exercises to this client's love for cycling will increase their program's relevance, and therefore adherence.

Needs of the Workout or Activity

One of the simplest ways to program corrective exercise and make it easy to understand for the client is to frame corrective exercise as a customized movement preparation or "warm-up" sequence based on the functional requirements and performance demands of a particular workout, training session, or activity. Mills et al. (2015) found that limitations in range of motion (ROM) can negatively affect prime mover performance while increasing recruitment of synergists. Therefore, to achieve maximum performance and optimal adaptation from a training session, the Corrective Exercise Specialist will want to ensure that the client addresses any limitations present that may affect the specific requirements associated with the movements they will have to perform.

For example, a client whose resistance training session is focused on vertical pushing (pressing)/pulling exercises for the upper body and hinge-dominant exercises for the lower body presents unique mobility and stability requirements that can be addressed with a corrective movement preparation program. Optimal thoracic extension, shoulder flexion, and hip extension ROM and hip, trunk, and scapulothoracic stability will be crucial to maximize execution and performance outcomes of the resistance training exercises in the session.

Example programming selections may include:

- **Inhibit (tool of choice):** Tensor fascia latae (TFL), quadriceps, thoracic spine, latissimus dorsi
- **Lengthen (static stretch):** Hip flexor complex, pectoralis minor, latissimus dorsi
- **Activate:** Ball bridge, quadruped opposite arm/leg raise
- **Integrate:** Single-leg Romanian deadlift (RDL) to proprioceptive neuromuscular facilitation (PNF), warm-up sets on first exercise

Conversely, a client who may be performing a horizontal pushing/pulling-focused upper body and knee-dominant lower body workout would be presented with similar yet slightly different movement requirements to the previous example. In this case some pre-workout priorities should include thoracic rotation; shoulder horizontal abduction and internal and external rotation; hip internal rotation; and ankle dorsiflexion ROM; as well as scapulothoracic, core, hip, and lower extremity stability/neuromuscular control.

Example programming selections may include:

- **Inhibit (tool of choice):** Gastrocnemius/soleus, adductor complex, pectoralis minor, thoracic spine
- **Lengthen (static stretch):** Gastrocnemius/soleus, adductor magnus, pectoralis major and minor
- **Activate:** Floor bridge, side plank, prone cobra
- **Integrate:** Squat to row, warm-up sets on first exercise

If the client in either example already possesses adequate mobility at the primary joints involved, lengthening techniques may be omitted, with more emphasis placed on light myofascial techniques to reduce any local tension in the upper and lower body (inhibit), targeted exercises to enhance activity of the stabilizers and prime movers that will be challenged during the workout (activate), and dynamic warm-up exercises that move their upper and lower body through their full available range of motion (integrate).

Progressing Corrective Exercise to Improve Adherence

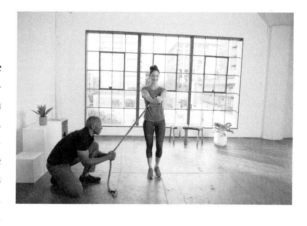

Integrating, implementing, and adhering to a corrective exercise program may seem overwhelming to both the professional and client, particularly if there are multiple regions to address based on assessment results and/or functional, lifestyle, and training needs. An incremental and progressive approach can be used when developing and scheduling corrective exercise programs. For example, the Corrective Exercise Specialist could first create multiple programs based on assessment data and client needs, and then prioritize them in order of relative importance based on their professional judgment, the client's needs, and other training program components. For the first 1 to 2 weeks, the corrective exercise professional would only provide the client with, and schedule, whichever program is determined to be the priority program and work with them to ensure that it is completed at least three to five times each week—ideally prior to any other physical activity, if applicable. Once the client is familiar with the exercises and has created the habit of performing corrective workouts, for the third week, the fitness professional could introduce the second program and have the client replace at least 2 days with the new program. This adds variety, as well as starts to address secondary compensations without completely abandoning focus on primary compensations. And finally, during weeks four, five, and beyond, the corrective exercise professional can introduce the remaining programs, if any, to address tertiary needs/compensations. With this approach, the client is not completely overwhelmed with multiple programs to learn and do, their compensations are prioritized and addressed accordingly, and by the end of 4 to 6 weeks they are regularly and consistently focusing on all areas of need.

Table 18-2 provides an example where the objective is to perform a corrective program(s) at least three to five times per week. Over time, the client is provided program options on five days or more per week, which gives them flexibility and autonomy to choose which days they

Self-efficacy

An individual's belief and confidence in their capacity to execute necessary behaviors to attain specific performance results.

perform the workouts. Providing options and involving the client challenges them to take responsibility in the process, promoting and reinforcing **self-efficacy**.

Additionally, if the client would benefit from a recovery and regeneration or deloading day, perform multiple sets of a single program, or simply combine all programs into one workout and perform an extended, total-body, corrective routine for the desired number of sets.

TABLE 18-2 Example Corrective Program Plan

Weeks	Days of Week	Program (Ordered by Priority)
1–2	Monday/Friday	Program 1: Focused on ankle, knee, and hip
3	Monday/Wednesday/Friday	Program 1
	Tuesday/Thursday/Saturday	Program 2: Focused on hip and core
4+	Monday/Thursday	Program 1
	Tuesday/Friday	Program 2
	Wednesday/Saturday	Program 3: Focused on shoulder and cervical spine
	Sunday	Client's choice

Programming When Compensations Are Present

Many clients and athletes will display movement compensations of some type. It is important to recognize that both positive and negative changes in movement quality are not permanent; that is, movement quality can both improve and regress as a result of the intensity, type, and duration of demands imposed on the kinetic chain. Understanding how to work within a client's level of ability and current state of movement quality while still achieving their desired outcomes is crucial. This section will explore considerations and strategies to incorporate and work with, not around, clients' movement impairments.

Throughout the corrective exercise program, it is important to reinforce its objectives at every opportunity with careful, intentional exercise selection. When at all possible, exercises included in a client's or athlete's overall fitness and performance training program (and how those exercises are performed) should support, not counteract, the assessment-based needs of the client. For example, if a client demonstrates excessive external rotation of the legs during their overhead squat assessment and limited hip internal rotation during their mobility assessment, it may be prudent to initially limit exercises that emphasize involvement of the hip and lower extremity external rotators, such as sumo deadlifts or plié-style squatting patterns, at least until the identified movement impairments are improved. Such exercises would likely exacerbate those impairments—effectively "undoing" all of the work and progress made in the preceding corrective program. This strategy does not preclude them from squatting motions in general, but rather only those that may worsen an already faulty movement pattern.

Reinforcing Proper Movement Patterns

Health and fitness professionals sometimes abandon certain movement patterns because their client lacks the requisite mobility or neuromuscular control to perform them with correct technique. At times, squatting, overhead, and hinging motions are avoided until the professional believes the client can handle them. This often presents a paradox because these are foundational movement patterns most or all exercisers should be able to successfully perform; however, they will never improve and master these patterns if not given the opportunity to work through them. Simply because someone compensates does not mean training a particular pattern must be abandoned.

Corrective exercise presents an opportunity to help the professional and client alike in achieving performance of fundamental movement patterns. The following are some strategies when training fundamental movement patterns in clients who compensate:

- Focus inhibition and lengthening techniques on areas that exhibit impairments specific to the desired pattern (e.g., self-myofascial roll and stretch hip flexors to allow for better recruitment of hip extensors in a hinge pattern).
- Even if it is considered partial, have the client move through the exercise's range of motion they can perform successfully instead of omitting the exercise completely.
- During the activation and integration phases of the continuum perform complementary movements that support and reinforce the primary pattern being trained (e.g., if an overhead press is challenging, include scaption exercises to reinforce correct shoulder flexion and abduction).

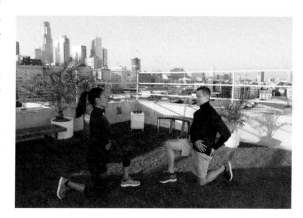

Using All Phases of the Corrective Exercise Continuum

The use of all phases of the Corrective Exercise Continuum *in the recommended sequence* is crucial to effective corrective exercise programs. It is common for corrective exercise professionals and clients alike to skip steps—especially exercises during the activate and integrate phases. Each phase accomplishes a specific objective for the human movement system (HMS), and when combined with the other phases, creates an ideal environment for proper movement to automatically, naturally, and organically integrate itself into the client's or athlete's training and everyday activities.

While movement compensations are multifactorial and could be caused solely by muscles that are relatively shortened and overactive (mobility), or muscles that are relatively underactive (stability), they are often caused by a combination of both, which is why *all four phases* in the Corrective Exercise Continuum are paramount to improving client movement (**Figure 18-2**) (Bell et al., 2013).

As highlighted previously, two critical steps to the movement retraining process are the third and fourth phases of the Corrective Exercise Continuum—activate and integrate. The first and second phases help to address overactive tissues, restore optimal length-tension relationships, and improve ROM. For clients to take full advantage of their improved ROM, their HMS must

Corrective Exercise
Continuum Objectives

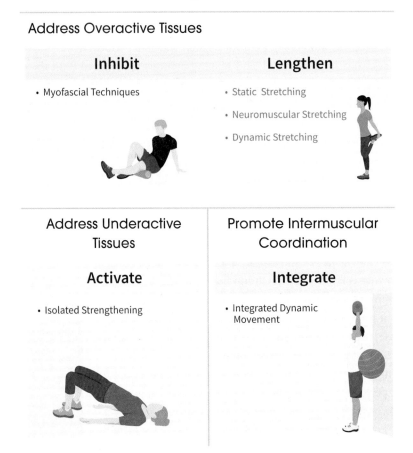

Address Overactive Tissues

Inhibit	Lengthen
• Myofascial Techniques	• Static Stretching • Neuromuscular Stretching • Dynamic Stretching

Address Underactive Tissues	Promote Intermuscular Coordination
Activate	**Integrate**
• Isolated Strengthening	• Integrated Dynamic Movement

Figure 18-2 Corrective Exercise Continuum objectives

relearn how to utilize and control this new-found mobility during functional activities. The third and fourth phases accomplish this task. Without these phases, clients will have what is referred to as **naive range of motion**, whereby the HMS possesses mobility that it has not learned to handle effectively or incorporate into existing or required functional movement patterns.

Gains in mobility will be short-lived if they are not reinforced in the third and fourth phases. Activation reestablishes local neuromuscular control around the joints that were just made more mobile and flexible and may even further enhance the effects of the first and second phases on ROM by taking advantage of and leveraging reciprocal inhibition. Contracting target muscle(s) during activation techniques will create further inhibition and relaxation to identified overactive muscles addressed during inhibitory and/or lengthening steps—reinforcing improvements in ROM and muscle balance around affected joints. However, although beneficial in their own right, many activation techniques are performed in isolation and in nonfunctional positions, which is where the integration phase becomes significant. Integration typically involves total-body, dynamic, multi-joint movements performed in multiple planes of motion. This requires the neuromuscular system to take the improvements in ROM, stability, strength, and control of the affected joints attained in the previous three phases and utilize them in positions where they can be progressively challenged functionally against gravity in multiple directions, environments, intensities, and speeds. Carefully planned progression replicates the demands that the body will have to contend with in exercise, life, or sport. Optimizing dynamic stability and neuromuscular control are the end goals.

Lastly, while the specific exercises selected for inclusion in a client or athlete program are critical to its effectiveness, *how* clients do their exercises is just as important as *why* they do them. Proper instruction, cueing, coaching, and feedback on movement technique (e.g., "land softly," "keep your knees over your toes," "bend your knees and hips") during phases 3 and 4 are integral to precise exercise performance and ultimately the transfer of benefits from a corrective exercise program to life, sport, or occupational tasks (Frost et al., 2015; Padua et al., 2018). To ensure maximum effectiveness, no compensations should be allowed, and techniques should not be sacrificed for increased load or intensity; strength and power adaptations can be made a focus as the program progresses and technique can be maintained.

CHECK IT OUT

Setting Expectations

Although the benefits and improvements in movement quality from corrective exercise *may* be realized in as few as 10 sessions over the course of a few weeks (Bell et al., 2013), the speed of improvement is influenced by many factors. Often, the mobility improvements seen from corrective exercise take time to become the "new normal" for the client or athlete. The improvements in mobility and neuromuscular control brought about by the Corrective Exercise Continuum are most likely temporary at first. Although it is unclear regarding the duration of those improvements, it is reasonable to assume that they are fairly short-lived, given that clients return to dysfunctional movement patterns in between training bouts (daily commutes, postures at work/school, etc.). Research on the topic suggests a 3-month injury prevention program that included flexibility and strengthening exercises based on individual movement quality assessment performed 3 to 4 days per week did not produce lasting improvements in movement quality. Instead, a 9-month application of the identical program produced lasting improvements (Padua et al., 2012).

It is important for the Corrective Exercise Specialist to understand that enhancements in movement quality brought about by corrective exercise protocols are temporary within the workout and during early phases of training. This underscores the importance of *regular and consistent* application of corrective exercise not only before and/or after the workout, but over the long-term planning of their client's training and in between sessions with assigned homework and/or deloading workouts. Corrective techniques should become the backbone of body maintenance and recovery techniques; think of them as the "brushing and flossing" for the HMS.

Corrective Exercise Progressions

It is common for health, fitness, and performance professionals to view corrective exercises as only low-intensity, low-demand activities. However, corrective exercise programs must be progressed in their level of challenge as with any training program along the **principle of overload**. As mentioned previously, not only is exercise progression very important to enhance dynamic stability for the transfer to life, sport, and/or occupation-specific tasks, but also to maintain client engagement—eliminating boredom and plateaus and enhancing adherence. Improvements achieved by the Corrective Exercise Continuum must be put to use in activities that match the desired outcomes of the client's or athlete's needs. The HMS must be challenged in the appropriate speeds, loads, and directions to meet the training demands of the client or athlete. For example, a recreational basketball player's corrective exercise plan should eventually be progressed to include integrated movements such as jumps, hops, agility drills, etc. Consider manipulating the items listed in **Table 18-3** when progressing corrective exercises for clients, particularly for the integration phase of the program.

However, the exercises, movements, and progressions in a program do not need to be overly complex in order to be effective and for positive adaptations in dynamic neuromuscular control to occur (Sasaki et al., 2019). Consider the program used by Bell et al. (2013) to improve medial knee displacement (MKD)/knee valgus. The program was developed using the exact

> **Principle of overload**
>
> Implies that there must be a training stimulus provided that exceeds the current capabilities of the kinetic chain to elicit the optimal physical, physiological, and performance adaptations.

TABLE 18-3 CES Progressions and Variables

Variables	Progression Options
Muscle action spectrum	Eccentric, isometric, concentric
Plane of motion	Sagittal, frontal, transverse
Proprioceptive demand	Stable to less stable surface
Contraction speed spectrum	Tempo selection: Slow, medium, fast, explosive
Complexity	Movement demands progress from simple to complex
Frequency, sets, repetitions	Low to high volume

procedures outlined by the NASM Corrective Exercise Continuum—focusing on joints both proximal and distal to the knee—and consisting of only bodyweight and elastic band–resisted exercises. Over the course of 10 sessions, exercises were progressed by increasing sets, repetitions, or level of resistance band, or changing to a new exercise entirely (for the bodyweight integration techniques).

In addition to successful execution of current exercises guiding the decision to progress a program, involve the client or athlete in the process as well by eliciting feedback. Once a client indicates that an exercise is becoming easier, incorporate a progression, if applicable, the next time they perform their program. Regularly communicate with clients about the exercises in their program to ensure they are continually being challenged by proper levels of resistance, volume, intensity, and complexity.

Incorporating Corrective Exercise in Different Scenarios

Corrective exercise strategies have the objective of optimizing client movement not only for the immediate workout ahead, but also for maximizing the long-term health and performance of the kinetic chain. Although the phases of the Corrective Exercise Continuum will not differ, the way they are applied can vary depending on the training-related, client-related, and environment-related factors presented earlier in this chapter. To optimize corrective exercise outcomes (acutely and chronically), it is generally advisable to perform movement-focused programming *at least* three to five times per week; however, this is highly dependent on the prevalence, magnitude, and severity of movement compensations; the amount and types of activity (or inactivity); the intensity of the activities performed; and the recovery behaviors of the individual—some clients or athletes may need greater frequency/exposure (e.g., up to seven times per week) and others less. Frequency and consistency are paramount to successful outcomes from corrective programs; shorter, targeted programs done consistently well and frequently will be a more effective strategy than longer, more comprehensive—but perhaps unrealistic—programs that are never done.

Corrective Exercise as the Warm-Up

The most common application of corrective exercise will be in the pre-workout or pre-activity warm-up. Many professionals also refer to this as the "movement prep" portion of a workout. The highest priority is individualization to the client's needs based on their movement assessment results in order to maximize performance of the upcoming workout and minimize the risk of injury. Based on the assessment process, the corrective exercise professional will know which muscle groups to inhibit, lengthen, activate, and integrate.

Depending on how much time for movement prep is available, the professional will select exercises that prioritize the targeted muscle groups most beneficial to the client's workout. As previously mentioned, other influences such as client lifestyle and functional needs and subjective reporting on factors such as stress and soreness will also affect exercise selection. Myofascial (inhibitory) and stretching (lengthening) techniques are applied to one to three overactive/shortened muscle groups each. For example, if the upcoming workout focuses on the lower body, these techniques may focus on the gastrocnemius/soleus, hip flexor, and/or adductor complexes.

To optimize neuromuscular control of the lower extremity and trunk, activation exercises would likely target the anterior tibialis, gluteus medius, gluteus maximus, and core stabilizers (Sasaki et al., 2019). Integration exercises can feel more like "working out" to the client and can take many forms. Practicing proper movement patterns for the main portion of the workout is one way to maximize integration. For example, if a client performs squats or deadlifts in the main portion of the workout, integration exercises could take the form of a bodyweight deadlift, step-up, or squat. This presents the opportunity to reinforce proper activation and timing of the muscles the client is about to work. Both activation and integration exercises will serve as a neuromuscular primer for the patterns that will be loaded later in the workout, essentially creating a potentiating effect that would cause enhanced muscle force production with less effort and improving movement quality (Parr et al., 2017).

The time spent on corrective exercise as movement prep can vary but does not usually require more than 10 to 15 minutes to be effective (Padua et al., 2018; Peck et al., 2017; Sasaki et al., 2019).

Corrective Exercise Post-Workout

While corrective exercise is often thought of as a pre-workout process, restoring ROM and movement quality with corrective exercise post-workout can be just as important to a client's overall needs and goals, as well as recovery from their training program. Components such as inhibitory and lengthening techniques can also be performed—and offer substantial benefits—after training as part of a cool-down, reducing sympathetic nervous system activity/tone and blood pressure (Lastova et al., 2018), as well as effects associated with delayed-onset muscle soreness (DOMS), enhancing recovery from exercise, and setting up the body for enhanced performance in subsequent training sessions (Pearcey et al., 2015). Emphasis can be placed on improving primary compensations identified during the client's assessment or on the tissues targeted and challenged during the workout or training session.

Corrective Exercise as the Entire Workout

Corrective exercise may also be applied as a full workout, often 30 to 60 minutes in duration. In this case, the priority is to take a long-term view in restoring the optimal function and efficiency of the client's kinetic chain based on their individual assessment results and needs.

Though not exhaustive, a list of common use cases for implementing corrective exercise as an entire workout include:

- **Post-rehabilitation/return to play or performance:** A client has completed treatment and has been cleared by their healthcare provider to return to exercise, using corrective programming to recondition and bridge the gap from rehab to fitness and/or performance.
- **Deconditioned clients:** Movement patterns and work capacity must be established before any higher demands can be placed on the kinetic chain to minimize the risk of overuse or acute musculoskeletal injury.
- **Separate recovery/deload/restorative workouts:** Many clients can benefit from occasional (or regularly scheduled) corrective exercise workouts as a form of active recovery placed within their mesocycle or microcycle planning to address subjective muscle soreness and maintain kinetic chain health and performance in the midst of high-intensity, high-demand training and/or competition.

For example, White (2018) investigated the use of an integrated corrective exercise workout and its effects on recovery and fatigue-induced ROM deficits after a bout of high-intensity exercise. Athletes who performed a 30-minute workout (following the NASM Corrective Exercise Continuum) 24 hours after high-intensity exercise minimized ROM deficits in knee extension (i.e., maintained hamstrings extensibility). The workout included inhibition and lengthening techniques for muscle groups that may restrict knee extension (e.g., lateral hamstrings, gastrocnemius), followed by activation and integration exercises that emphasized the gluteals. That is, the workout design reinforced activity of hip extension prime movers (e.g., gluteals), thereby reducing synergistic dominance of the hamstrings, effectively deloading and sparing them additional stress.

The inclusion of corrective exercise–based recovery workouts may reduce the negative effects of high-intensity training related to decreases in soft tissue extensibility and joint ROM, thereby preparing and optimizing the HMS for the next bout of training or activity.

Corrective Exercise in Group Settings

Small group training and group exercise environments can sometimes be challenging to apply corrective exercise strategies because of the professional-to-client ratio. These exercising populations can still benefit from corrective exercise and optimized movement like any other. Although not an exhaustive list, the fitness professional may consider the following when designing and delivering corrective exercise programs in group settings:

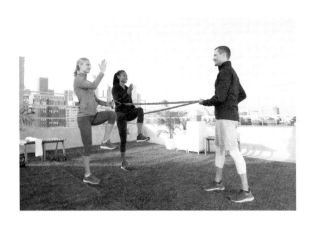

- **Assume common dysfunctions.** Deliver corrective exercise warm-ups based on the likely presence of muscle imbalances within the group. For example, an indoor cycling class is likely to have overactive shoulder protractors, gastrocnemius/soleus, and hip flexors, given the maintained/prolonged position on the bike.
- **Prepare participants for the specific demands of the class routine or session.** Deliver corrective exercise warm-ups based on planned movement patterns and exercises, as addressed earlier in the chapter.
- **Perform individual movement assessments and assign homework.** Take time to perform individual assessments and give corrective programs to exercisers to complete on their own, and even before a class starts. A best practice is to assign pairs of participants to keep each other accountable for their homework. For hybrid/crossover fitness professionals who instruct group classes as

well as provide personal training, not only is this a great value-add, but it also is a great opportunity to prospect for new training clients. Providing individual assessments and homework highlights the value of one-on-one instruction/training, which could generate interest in one's services and lead to new-client acquisition.

Corrective Exercise in Athletic Team and Sport Environments

Incorporating corrective exercise programming for an athletic team has similarities to the group exercise setting discussed; however, there are some distinct differences. Contrary to group exercise settings, members of an athletic team roster remain relatively constant for a period of time, which may facilitate greater structure, individualization, and consistency within corrective programming. Challenges often presented with implementing corrective exercise in a team or sport environment include establishing buy-in and support from key stakeholders such as coaches, administrators/staff, parents, and even the athletes themselves, as well as logistical barriers such as working within contact/time limitations often present at the various levels of sport (Padua et al., 2014).

As mentioned earlier, establishing stakeholder buy-in and prioritizing corrective exercise can be difficult due to the perception that it will be counterproductive by taking time away from other more sport-specific activities. It will be critical to educate stakeholders at all levels on the importance of incorporating corrective, multicomponent programming as a regular part of team/athlete preparation and development. Due to factors such as overuse and pattern overload, many athletes lack optimal movement quality. Not only is poor movement quality associated with decreased performance (Yamamoto et al., 2016 , p. 104), it is also associated with alterations in muscle strength, ROM, and neuromuscular control; greater mechanical load exposure and systemic stress, potentially decreasing recovery and biomechanical resilience (Frank et al., 2019); as well as increased risk of injury (Eckard et al., 2018; Padua et al., 2018).

 GETTING TECHNICAL

Successful Injury Rate Reduction in Athletic Populations
Although training programs designed to reduce injury risk may vary, certain common features have been shown to be successful in reducing injury rates and improving neuromuscular function and physical performance. Adapted from Padua et al. (2018), the following are general guidelines, recommendations, and suggested best practices regarding the development, adoption, and implementation of multicomponent training programs:

- Multicomponent preventive training programs that include feedback regarding technique and at least three of the following exercise categories—strength, plyometrics, agility, balance, and flexibility—are recommended to reduce noncontact and indirect-contact ACL injuries during physical activity and should be performed at least two to three times per week throughout the preseason and in-season.
- Multicomponent training programs are advocated to improve lower extremity biomechanics, muscle activation, balance, strength, power, and functional performance measures as well as decrease landing impact forces.
- Exercises should be performed at progressive intensity levels that are challenging and allow for excellent movement quality and technique.
- To maintain the benefits of reduced injury rates and improved neuromuscular function and performance over time, multicomponent training programs (preseason, in-season, and off-season) should be performed each year and not discontinued after a single season.
- Multicomponent training programs are effective when implemented as a dynamic warm-up or as part of a comprehensive strength and conditioning program and should be regularly supervised by individuals who are skilled in identifying faulty movement patterns to ensure excellent movement quality and provide feedback on exercise technique.

(continues)

- To facilitate the adoption and adherence of multicomponent training programs, education of athletes, coaches, parents, and administrators on the value of such programs is paramount. Things to highlight include the prevalence of lower extremity injuries in sports; costs (physically, psychologically, and financially) associated with ACL injury; that these programs not only are effective in reducing injury but also can improve physical performance and can be seamlessly incorporated into preseason, in-season, and off-season training practices without taking time away from skill development; and if time constraints are a concern, some evidence indicates that multicomponent training programs can be performed in 10 to 15 minutes as part of a dynamic warm-up before the start of practices and games.
- All individuals involved in sports and physical activity are advised to participate in a multicomponent training program focusing on injury resistance and movement quality; however, those who are active in particular sports or display certain traits should be targeted for preventive training because they either are at a relatively higher risk of ACL injury or have a greater potential for benefit. For example, athletes and children participating in higher-risk sports that involve landing, jumping, and cutting tasks (e.g., basketball, soccer, football, team handball, etc.), especially women, should be targeted for injury risk reduction training. And, because a history of ACL injury is one of the strongest predictors of future ACL injury, individuals with such a history, especially younger individuals who return to sport-related activities, should be targeted for injury risk reduction training.

Data from Padua, D. A., DiStefano, L. J., Hewett, T. E., Garrett, W. E., Marshall, S. W., Golden, G. M., Shultz, S. J., & Sigward, S. M. (2018). National Athletic Trainers' Association position statement: Prevention of anterior cruciate ligament injury. *Journal of Athletic Training, 53*(1), 5–19. https://doi.org/10.4085/1062-6050-99-16

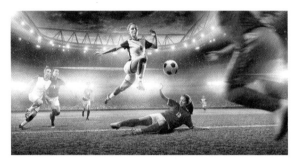
© Alex Kravtsov/Shutterstock

Success in sports is typically measured in terms of wins and losses. While many would state physical and athletic abilities are the primary determinants of a team's success, it has been shown that teams who keep a higher percentage of players on the court or field and off the injured list through the majority of the season win more than those that don't (Hägglund et al., 2013; Podlog et al., 2015; Williams et al., 2016), suggesting that the ability most associated with team performance and success is *availability*. To be fair, teams must still have a decent pool of talent, good coaching, conditioning, execution, and so on; however, if a team cannot capitalize on that because its best players are hurt, and therefore unavailable to play, it can be argued that training to avoid injury should be a priority and training to maximize performance should be secondary (Kucera et al., 2005).

This underscores and reinforces the importance and relevance of implementing corrective exercise programming strategies as part of athlete development. With the right leadership, planning, communication, and support, many opportunities exist to incorporate strategies and programs to both enhance athlete movement quality and reduce the risk of injury.

When designing and delivering corrective exercise programs within an athletic team environment, the Corrective Exercise Specialist should consider the following:

- If applicable, have athletes incorporate corrective exercises as part of an integrated warm-up or movement preparation sequence prior to strength and conditioning; individualized programs can be performed if schedule, facility design, and resources allow. Alternatively, a templated program performed by all, based on the lifts scheduled for the day, can be used. This is similar to what might be done in a group personal training or group exercise setting.
- Specific corrective, multicomponent preventive programming may be incorporated as part of team-based dynamic warm-ups prior to training, practice, or competition; 10 to 15 minutes seems to be both realistic and effective at improving neuromuscular control of the lower extremity and trunk (Pfile et al., 2013; Sasaki et al., 2019), reducing injury, and enhancing performance measures (Peck et al., 2017).

- Prepare different strategies based on where athletes have to perform and what equipment is available. Consider constraints and requirements if the program has to be implemented offsite or on the road at competitive venues, practice facilities, or on the court/field of play, as compared to programs done on-site at "home" facilities that are familiar and equipment availability is known.
- Assume common impairments based on movement, sport, and even positional demands. Deliver corrective exercise warm-ups based on the presence of likely muscle imbalances accordingly. For example, if working with a baseball team, while there will likely be many similarities among all players, there may be distinct differences between the programs for pitchers versus position players. Depending on sport type and level, consider the differences in program requirements that may exist between starters, utility players, and role players.
- Perform individual movement assessments and provide homework. Take time to perform individual assessments and give corrective exercise programs to athletes to complete on their own prior to, or even after, training, practice, or competition as well as on days off. If providing programs individualized to each athlete is not realistic, group athletes based on common impairments and schedules to foster responsibility, camaraderie, and accountability. To aid in assigning athletes to the appropriate programming groups, calculate the frequency/occurrence of each individual compensation among the roster and classify individuals based on compensation rate or prevalence at the different kinetic chain checkpoints or regions of the body. For example, groups can be classified and programs designed based on select compensations at the foot and ankle complex/lower leg, knee, LPHC, shoulder/upper extremity, and combinations thereof. Similarly, a threshold could be established (say, if a particular compensation occurred in more than 50% of the athletes) and programs designed based on each compensation that exceeded the designated threshold.

TRAINING TIP

Integrating Dynamic Stretching into Corrective Exercise for Athletes

Note that static, neuromuscular, and dynamic stretching are presented as effective flexibility techniques to be used in the lengthen phase of the Corrective Exercise Continuum. The Corrective Exercise Specialist is encouraged to use the technique that works best for the specific goals of each client.

Dynamic stretching is beneficial as part of a corrective exercise program for those focused on athletic performance in particular. Static stretching followed by dynamic stretching has been shown to improve flexibility without impairing performance (Wong et al., 2011). In Wong et al. (2011), subjects performed static stretching of the plantar flexors, quadriceps, and hamstrings followed by a dynamic stretching routine that included knee lifts, butt kicks, and straight-leg skipping. Thus, the inclusion of dynamic exercises into a corrective exercise program may help to re-engage and excite the nervous system before athletic performance.

If using a corrective exercise program as part of an integrated warm-up prior to an athletic event or sports performance training, include dynamic stretching within the integration phase. It is recommended that the individual perform at least one basic integrated movement before moving to dynamic stretches. This is important to ensure that a high-quality movement pattern is utilized prior to the often quicker and momentum-based exercises of dynamic stretching. An example program for an athlete with an excessive forward trunk lean may include:

- Self-myofascial rolling (SMR): Gastrocnemius/soleus, hip flexors
- Static stretching: Gastrocnemius, kneeling hip flexor
- Isolated strengthening: Heel walking (tibialis anterior), floor bridge (gluteus maximus)
- Integration: Goblet squat, lunge to rotation (dynamic), leg swings (dynamic), A-skips (dynamic)

Keep in mind that the four phases of the program should be specific to the movement impairment demonstrated by the athlete, whereas the dynamic flexibility exercises chosen may be specific to the demands of competition or practice.

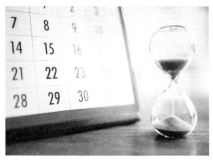
© Brian A Jackson18/Shutterstock

Corrective Exercise with Time or Schedule Constraints

A common barrier to performing corrective exercise may be a perceived lack of time. For many clients—especially those new to regular exercise—taking the time to perform a corrective program in addition to their regular exercise and training program is very daunting. A most important consideration when developing corrective exercise programs (and exercise programs overall) is to ensure client adherence. Meeting the client where they are, and determining what they are *willing* to do is extremely important. Health and fitness professionals have a responsibility to their clients to create an environment that helps them adhere to an exercise routine. They should instill confidence and competence while fostering client autonomy and self-efficacy to complete their program on terms that work for them.

If the primary objection or obstacle is the inability for the client to commit a 15- to 20-minute block of time to completing their entire corrective program at once, suggest breaking it into smaller chunks or "mini programs" that the client can perform at scheduled intervals or structured break times throughout the day, making it more manageable and realistic to complete. This may also be welcomed by the client as an opportunity for some self-care and to break up the monotony of their day.

With that said, because the effects are often more immediate and tangible, it is very common for clients to develop an affinity for the inhibitory and lengthening techniques in their program while neglecting the activation and integration techniques. Breaking the program up into smaller chunks may exacerbate this tendency. Remember that to maximally affect movement compensations, all four phases of the Corrective Exercise Continuum should be completed in succession and in their entirety—regardless of program length. This should be continually reinforced with clients. Additionally, the design of the program must be supported by their environment to maximize adherence. For example, if the program calls for a cable-based activation exercise, but the client will be at work in their office without access to a cable machine, the desired workout is already facing obstacles.

To encourage adherence, avoid overwhelming the client, and establish patterns of success, **Table 18-4** provides an example of how to break up a program addressing multiple areas of need

TABLE 18-4 Example 5-Minute Corrective Strategies		
Strategy 1	**Strategy 2**	**Strategy 3**
Inhibit (tool of choice): ■ Gastrocnemius/soleus 1 × 30 seconds	Inhibit (tool of choice): ■ Adductors complex 1 × 30 seconds	Inhibit (tool of choice): ■ Thoracic spine 1 × 30 seconds
Lengthen (static stretch): ■ Soleus 1 × 30 seconds	Lengthen (static stretch): ■ Adductor magnus 1 × 30 seconds	Lengthen (static stretch): ■ Child's pose using desk 1 × 30 seconds
Activate (isolated strength): ■ Heel walking (anterior tibialis) 1 × 20	Activate (isolated strength): ■ Wall slides (gluteus medius) 1 × 20	Activate (isolated strength): ■ Standing cobra 1 × 20
Integrate (total-body pattern): ■ Multiplanar single-leg balance reach 1 × 10	Integrate (total-body pattern): ■ Side lunge to balance 1 × 10	Integrate (total-body pattern): ■ Squat to scaption 1 × 10

into more manageable strategies—each taking 5 minutes or less—for a client with time constraints and who displays movement impairment of excessive forward trunk lean, knee valgus, and arms fall forward.

If a client displays only one compensation versus multiple, or the Corrective Exercise Specialist wants to prioritize a particular compensation over others based on need/severity or training schedule (e.g., upper body resistance training workout later in the day), then simply repeat a single strategy multiple times per day (in this example strategy 3) to maximize exposure and effect.

Corrective Exercise for Return to Performance

Corrective exercise can be a fantastic complement to a rehabilitation or post-rehabilitation return-to-performance program. Due to a variety of factors, rehabilitation programs may not be able to address reconditioning multiple components of the kinetic chain. However, it is understood from the RI model that multiple segments of the kinetic chain may have significant influence on the original site of injury. For example, as a client returns from ACL reconstruction, early phases of rehabilitation will focus on restoring knee ROM, as well as quadriceps, hamstrings, and general lower extremity strength. However, deficits in ankle dorsiflexion, hip rotation, and hip abduction ROM; and proximal stability, strength, and neuromuscular control of the LPHC all influence biomechanical risk factors associated with increased loading to the ACL. Therefore, to potentially accelerate recovery and optimize outcomes by mitigating stress to the ACL from these factors, it is imperative to take a more holistic approach to the overall program by incorporating concurrent corrective exercise strategies to restore and maintain mobility of the ankle and hip, as well as proximal stability, strength, and neuromuscular control of the LPHC. Taking this approach may help to minimize risk of injury/re-injury and also build client or athlete confidence as they prepare to return to full physical or sport-related activities. This is accomplished by executing the CES Assessment Flow and programming along the Corrective Exercise Continuum.

Corrective Exercise Without Equipment

Without tools or equipment, bodyweight movement patterns are all that may be available to promote movement quality and recovery. Effective combinations of movements are more than sufficient to serve as corrective exercise for the client or athlete in these situations. Although inhibition tools may not be available, targeted flexibility and strengthening movements will still contribute to improving ROM, control, and stability at select joints. Utilizing integration movements that focus on more than one region can be effective in reinforcing overall movement quality. To maximize client response and program benefits, more sets can be performed if time permits. **Table 18-5** provides sample 5- to 10-minute mobility routine themes and areas of focus.

TABLE 18-5 Sample Mobility Routine Themes	
Hip and shoulder region combination	▪ Static stretch: Standing hip flexor with overhead reach 1 × 30 seconds ▪ Hip swings 1 × 10 per leg ▪ Single-leg balance with multiplanar arm reach 1 × 10 per leg ▪ Multiplanar lunge with arm reach 1 × 10 per leg ▪ Single-leg windmill 1 × 10 per leg

(continues)

TABLE 18-5   Sample Mobility Routine Themes (*continued*)

Lower body alignment and control	▪ Static stretch: Gastrocnemius 1 × 30 seconds ▪ Static stretch: TFL 1 × 30 seconds ▪ Activate: Heel walking (i.e., walk while dorsiflexed) 1 × 20 ▪ Activate: Calf raise with toes in (medial gastrocnemius) 1 × 10 ▪ Activate: Side-lying leg raise or wall slides 1 × 10 per leg ▪ Multiplanar lunge to balance 1 × 10 per leg
LPHC alignment and control	▪ Static stretch: Kneeling hip flexor 1 × 30 seconds ▪ Static stretch: Adductors 1 × 30 seconds ▪ Dynamic stretch: Hamstring 1 × 30 seconds ▪ Activate: Quadruped opposite arm/leg raise 1 × 20 ▪ Single-leg RDL to shoulder scaption/retraction/cobra 1 × 5 per leg
Upper body alignment and control	▪ Static stretch: Levator scapulae 1 × 30 seconds ▪ Static stretch: Scalenes 1 × 30 seconds ▪ Static stretch: Pectorals 1 × 30 seconds ▪ Single-leg standing cobra × 10 per leg ▪ Single-leg squat to scaption × 10 repetitions per leg
Head and neck alignment and control	▪ Static stretch: Levator scapulae 1 × 30 seconds ▪ Static stretch: Scalenes 1 × 30 seconds ▪ Static stretch: Sternocleidomastoid 1 × 30 seconds ▪ Chin tucks against wall or chair headrest 1 × 20 ▪ Standing scaption/retraction/cobra 1 × 10

SUMMARY

Everyone—regardless of their level or type of activity—must move well to perform at the frequencies and intensities required to elicit improvements in health, fitness, and performance while minimizing risk of pain and injury. Many considerations and factors influence corrective exercise program design for clients and athletes. Corrective exercise may be delivered in a multitude of training schemes and applications such as movement preparation, post-workout recovery, deloading workouts, or post-rehabilitation. Ultimately, the corrective exercise professional will have the task of considering the client's assessment results, environment, preferences, outcomes, and level of adherence when creating programs. It is critical to effectively use all four phases of the Corrective Exercise Continuum and progress its programs to meet the functional capacity and needs of the end-user.

Corrective programs do not need to be complex to be effective and often require only 10 to 15 minutes to complete. Indeed, simpler programs may actually maximize adherence. Consistency and frequency are crucial to success. The ideal frequency of corrective exercise workouts is three to five times per week; however, some clients may require up to seven. Like any exercise program, corrective exercise should progress following the principle of overload to reduce boredom, maintain challenge, and increase engagement.

REFERENCES

Bell, D. R., Oates, D. C., Clark, M. A., & Padua, D. A. (2013). Two- and 3-dimensional knee valgus are reduced after an exercise intervention in young adults with demonstrable valgus during squatting. *Journal of Athletic Training, 48*(4), 442–449. https://doi.org/10.4085/1062-6050-48.3.16

Eckard, T., Padua, D., Mauntel, T., Frank, B., Pietrosimone, L., Begalle, R., Goto, S., Clark, M., & Kucera, K. (2018). Association between double-leg squat and single-leg squat performance and injury incidence among incoming NCAA Division I athletes: A prospective cohort study. *Physical Therapy in Sport: Official Journal of the Association of Chartered Physiotherapists in Sports Medicine, 34*, 192–200. https://doi.org/10.1016/j.ptsp.2018.10.009

Frank, B. S., Hackney, A. C., Battaglini, C. L., Blackburn, T., Marshall, S. W., Clark, M., & Padua, D. A. (2019). Movement profile influences systemic stress and biomechanical resilience to high training load exposure. *Journal of Science and Medicine in Sport, 22*(1), 35–41. https://doi.org/10.1016/j.jsams.2018.05.017

Frost, D. M., Beach, T. A., Callaghan, J. P., & McGill, S. M. (2015). Exercise-based performance enhancement and injury prevention for firefighters: Contrasting the fitness- and movement-related adaptations to two training methodologies. *Journal of Strength and Conditioning Research, 29*(9), 2441–2459. https://doi.org/10.1519/JSC.0000000000000923

Hägglund, M., Waldén, M., Magnusson, H., Kristenson, K., Bengtsson, H., & Ekstrand, J. (2013). Injuries affect team performance negatively in professional football: An 11-year follow-up of the UEFA Champions League injury study. *British Journal of Sports Medicine, 47*(12), 738–742. https://doi.org/10.1136/bjsports-2013-092215

Kucera, K. L., Marshall, S. W., Kirkendall, D. T., Marchak, P. M., & Garrett, W. E., Jr. (2005). Injury history as a risk factor for incident injury in youth soccer. *British Journal of Sports Medicine, 39*(7), 462. https://doi.org/10.1136/bjsm.2004.013672

Lastova, K., Nordvall, M., Walters-Edwards, M., Allnutt, A., & Wong, A. (2018). Cardiac autonomic and blood pressure responses to an acute foam rolling session. *Journal of Strength and Conditioning Research, 32*(10), 2825–2830. https://doi.org/10.1519/JSC.0000000000002562

Mills, M., Frank, B., Goto, S., Blackburn, T., Cates, S., Clark, M., Aguilar, A., Fava, N., & Padua, D. (2015). Effect of restricted hip flexor muscle length on hip extensor muscle activity and lower extremity biomechanics in college-aged female soccer players. *International Journal of Sports Physical Therapy, 10*(7), 946–954. https://spts.org/member-benefits-detail/enjoy-member-benefits/journals/ijspt

Padua, D. A., DiStefano, L. J., Marshall, S. W., Beutler, A. I., de la Motte, S. J., & DiStefano, M. J. (2012). Retention of movement pattern changes after a lower extremity injury prevention program is affected by program duration. *American Journal of Sports Medicine, 40*(2), 300–306.

Padua, D. A., DiStefano, L. J., Hewett, T. E., Garrett, W. E., Marshall, S. W., Golden, G. M., Shultz, S. J., & Sigward, S. M. (2018). National Athletic Trainers' Association position statement: Prevention of anterior cruciate ligament injury. *Journal of Athletic Training, 53*(1), 5–19. https://doi.org/10.4085/1062-6050-99-16

Padua, D. A., Frank, B., Donaldson, A., de la Motte, S., Cameron, K. L., Beutler, A. I., DiStefano, L. J., & Marshall, S. W. (2014). Seven steps for developing and implementing a preventive training program: Lessons learned from JUMP-ACL and beyond. *Clinics in Sports Medicine, 33*(4), 615–632. https://doi.org/10.1016/j.csm.2014.06.012

Parr, M., Price, P. D., & Cleather, D. J. (2017). Effect of a gluteal activation warm-up on explosive exercise performance. *BMJ Open Sport & Exercise Medicine, 3*(1), e000245. https://doi.org/10.1136/bmjsem-2017-000245

Pearcey, G. E. P., Bradbury-Squires, D. J., Kawamoto, J-E., Drinkwater, E. J., Behm, D. G., & Button, D. C. (2015). *Foam rolling for delayed-onset muscle soreness and recovery of dynamic performance measures.* National Athletic Trainers' Association.

Peck, K. Y., DiStefano, L. J., Marshall, S. W., Padua, D. A., Beutler, A. I., de la Motte, S. J., Frank, B. S., Martinez, J. C., & Cameron, K. L. (2017). Effect of a lower extremity preventive training program on physical performance scores in military recruits. *Journal of Strength and Conditioning Research, 31*(11), 3146–3157. https://doi.org/10.1519/JSC.0000000000001792

Pfile, K. R., Hart, J. M., Herman, D. C., Hertel, J., Kerrigan, D. C., & Ingersoll, C. D. (2013). Different exercise training interventions and drop-landing biomechanics in high school female athletes. *Journal of Athletic Training, 48*(4), 450–462. https://doi.org/10.4085/1062-6050-48.4.06

Podlog, L., Buhler, C. F., Pollack, H., Hopkins, P. N., & Burgess, P. R. (2015). Time trends for injuries and illness, and their relation to performance in the National Basketball Association. *Journal of Science and Medicine in Sport, 18*(3), 278–282. https://doi.org/10.1016/j.jsams.2014.05.005

Sasaki, S., Tsuda, E., Yamamoto, Y., Maeda, S., Kimura, Y., Fujita, Y., & Ishibashi, Y. (2019). Core-muscle training and neuromuscular control of the lower limb and trunk. *Journal of Athletic Training, 54*(9), 959–969. https://doi.org/10.4085/1062-6050-113-17

White, J. (2018). *Can an integrated corrective exercise intervention mitigate range of motion changes post high intensity exercise in female athletes?* [Master's Thesis, University of North Carolina at Chapel Hill Graduate School]. https://doi.org/10.17615/9cvr-np80

Williams, S., Trewartha, G., Kemp, S. P., Brooks, J. H., Fuller, C. W., Taylor, A. E., Cross, M. J., & Stokes, K. A. (2016). Time loss injuries compromise team success in Elite Rugby Union: A 7-year prospective study. *British Journal of Sports Medicine, 50*(11), 651–656. https://doi.org/10.1136/bjsports-2015-094798

Wong, D. P., Chaouachi, A., Lau, P. W. C., & Behm, D. G. (2011). Short durations of static stretching when combined with dynamic stretching do not impair repeated sprints and agility. *Journal of Sports Science & Medicine, 10*(2), 408–416.

Yamamoto, A. K., Frank, B. S., Stanley, L. E., Prentice, W. E., Aguilar, A. A., & Padua, D. A. (2016). Landing error scoring system scores are associated with field-based measures of athletic performance. *Journal of Athletic Training, 61*(6)(Suppl.), 104. https://doi.org/10.4085/1062-6050-51.6.s1

CES Assessment Flow

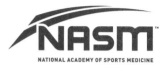

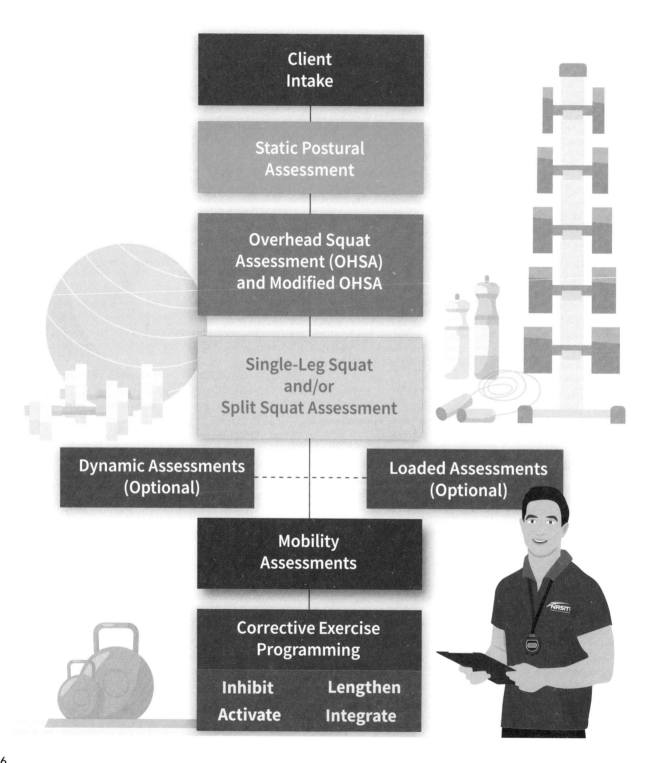

Client Intake

Static Postural Assessment

Overhead Squat Assessment (OHSA) and Modified OHSA

Single-Leg Squat and/or Split Squat Assessment

Dynamic Assessments (Optional)

Loaded Assessments (Optional)

Mobility Assessments

Corrective Exercise Programming

Inhibit   Lengthen

Activate   Integrate

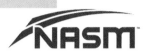

Static Postural Assessment

Name_____ Date_____

OBSERVATIONAL FINDINGS

CHECKPOINT	STATIC POSITION	POTENTIAL OVERACTIVE/ SHORTENED MUSCLES	POTENTIAL UNDERACTIVE/ LENGTHENED MUSCLES
Foot and Ankle	☐ Feet: straight/parallel ☐ Feet: externally rotated ☐ Arch: neutral ☐ Arch: flattened (pes planus) ☐ Arch: raised (pes cavus) ☐ Lower leg is vertical ☐ Lower leg posteriorly displaced (plantar flexed)		
Knee	☐ In line w/2nd & 3rd toes ☐ Valgus (knock-kneed) ☐ Varus (bowlegged) ☐ Neutral (straight) ☐ Flexed ☐ Hyperextended		
LPHC	☐ Pelvis: level ☐ Pelvis: anterior tilt　☐ L-spine: normal curve ☐ Pelvis: posterior tilt　☐ L-spine: exc. lordosis ☐ Hips: neutral　☐ L-spine: red. lordosis ☐ Hips: extended　☐ L-spine: lateral shift ☐ Hips: flexed		
Shoulders and Thoracic Spine	☐ Shoulders: level ☐ Shoulders: elevated ☐ Shoulders: in line w/hips & ears ☐ Shoulders: rounded forward ☐ T-spine: normal curve ☐ T-spine: exc. kyphosis		
Head and Cervical Spine	☐ Head: neutral (not tilted or rotated) ☐ Head: forward in cervical extension ☐ C-spine: normal curve		
Pes Planus Distortion	☐ Yes ☐ No		

Additional Notes

_____

_____

_____

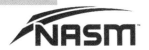

Transitional Movement Assessments

Name_____   Date_____

OVERHEAD SQUAT OBSERVATIONAL FINDINGS

CHECKPOINT	VIEWPOINT	MOVEMENT IMPAIRMENT	RESULT
Foot and Ankle	Anterior	• Feet turn out	• Right • Left • Both
	Lateral	• Heel rise	• Right • Left • Both
	Posterior	• Excessive pronation	• Right • Left • Both
Knee	Anterior	• Valgus	• Right • Left • Both
		• Varus	• Right • Left • Both
	Lateral	• Knee dominance	• Right • Left • Both
LPHC	Anterior or Posterior	• Asymmetric weight shift	Direction: • Right • Left
	Lateral	• Excessive anterior pelvic tilt	• YES • NO
		• Excessive posterior pelvic tilt	• YES • NO
		• Excessive forward trunk lean	• YES • NO
Shoulders and Thoracic Spine	Anterior or Posterior	• Scapular elevation	• Right • Left • Both
	Lateral	• Arms fall forward	• Right • Left • Both
Head and Cervical Spine	Lateral	• Excessive cervical extension/forward head	• YES • NO

Mark *Right* or *Left* or *Both* based on which limb a movement impairment was observed at. For asymmetric weight shift, mark the direction in which the shift occurred.

MODIFICATIONS

Heels Elevated	Squat performance improves?	• YES • NO
Hands on Hips	Squat performance improves?	• YES • NO

Additional Notes

_____

_____

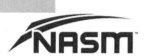

SINGLE-LEG and/or SPLIT SQUAT OBSERVATIONAL FINDINGS

CHECKPOINT	VIEWPOINT	MOVEMENT IMPAIRMENT	RESULT
Foot and Ankle	**Lateral**	• Heel Rise	• Right • Left • Both
	Posterior	• Excessive pronation	• Right • Left • Both
Knee	**Anterior**	• Valgus	• Right • Left • Both
		• Varus	• Right • Left • Both
	Lateral	• Knee dominance	• Right • Left • Both
LPHC	**Anterior**	• Asymmetric weight shift	*Direction:* • Right • Left
		• Inward trunk rotation	• Right • Left • Both
		• Outward trunk rotation	• Right • Left • Both
	Lateral	• Excessive anterior pelvic tilt	• YES • NO
		• Excessive posterior pelvic tilt	• YES • NO
		• Excessive forward trunk lean	• YES • NO

Right/Left/Both refers to the stance or forward leg when the impairment occurs. Mark *Right* or *Left* or *Both* based on which limb a movement impairment was observed at. For asymmetric weight shift, mark the direction to which the shift occurs.

Additional Notes

_____

_____

_____

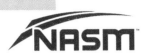

Loaded Movement Assessments

Name _____ Date _____

LOADED SQUAT OBSERVATIONAL FINDINGS

CHECKPOINT	VIEWPOINT	MOVEMENT IMPAIRMENT	RESULT
	Anterior	• Feet turn out	• Right • Left • Both
Foot and Ankle	Lateral	• Heel rise	• Right • Left • Both
	Posterior	• Excessive pronation	• Right • Left • Both
Knee	Anterior	• Valgus	• Right • Left • Both
		• Varus	• Right • Left • Both
	Lateral	• Knee dominance	• Right • Left • Both
LPHC	Anterior or Posterior	• Asymmetric weight shift	Direction: • Right • Left
	Lateral	• Excessive anterior pelvic tilt	• YES • NO
		• Excessive posterior pelvic tilt	• YES • NO
		• Excessive forward trunk lean	• YES • NO

Mark *Right* or *Left* or *Both* based on which limb a movement impairment was observed at. For asymmetric weight shift, mark the direction in which the shift occurred.

Additional Notes

_____

_____

_____

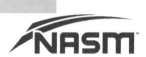

LOADED PUSH and/or PULL OBSERVATIONAL FINDINGS

CHECKPOINT	VIEWPOINT	MOVEMENT IMPAIRMENT	RESULT
LPHC	Lateral	• Excessive anterior pelvic tilt	• YES • NO
		• Excessive posterior pelvic tilt	• YES • NO
		• Trunk rotation	• YES • NO
Shoulders and Thoracic Spine	Lateral	• Scapular elevation	• YES • NO
		• Scapular winging (push assessment only)	• YES • NO
Head and Cervical Spine	Lateral	• Excessive cervical extension/forward head	• YES • NO

To observe *scapular winging* during the push assessment, view the client from a slight angle.

STANDING OVERHEAD DUMBBELL PRESS OBSERVATIONAL FINDINGS

CHECKPOINT	VIEWPOINT	MOVEMENT IMPAIRMENT	RESULT
LPHC	Lateral	• Excessive anterior pelvic tilt	• YES • NO
		• Excessive posterior pelvic tilt	• YES • NO
Shoulders and Thoracic Spine	Lateral	• Scapular elevation	• Right • Left • Both
		• Arms fall forward	• Right • Left • Both
Head and Cervical Spine	Lateral	• Excessive cervical extension/forward head	• YES • NO

Additional Notes

_____

_____

_____

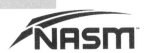

Dynamic Movement Assessments

Name _____   Date _____

GAIT ASSESSMENT OBSERVATIONAL FINDINGS

CHECKPOINT	VIEWPOINT	MOVEMENT IMPAIRMENT	RESULT
Foot and Ankle	Anterior	• Feet turn out	• Right • Left • Both
	Posterior	• Excessive pronation	• Right • Left • Both
Knee	Anterior	• Valgus	• Right • Left • Both
		• Varus	• Right • Left • Both
LPHC	Anterior	• Asymmetric weight shift	*Direction*: • Right • Left
	Lateral	• Excessive anterior pelvic tilt	• YES • NO
		• Excessive posterior pelvic tilt	• YES • NO

Mark **Right** or **Left** or **Both** based on which limb a movement impairment was observed at. For asymmetric weight shift, mark the direction in which the shift occurred.

Additional Notes

_____

_____

_____

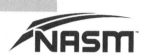

DEPTH JUMP OBSERVATIONAL FINDINGS

CHECKPOINT	VIEWPOINT	MOVEMENT IMPAIRMENT	RESULT
Foot and Ankle	Anterior	• Excessive pronation	• Right • Left • Both
		• Feet turn out	• Right • Left • Both
		• Asymmetric contact/landing	• Rt. first • Lt. first • NO
Knee	Anterior	• Valgus	• Right • Left • Both
		• Varus	• Right • Left • Both
	Lateral	• Knee dominance	• Right • Left • Both
		• Stiff landing	• YES • NO
LPHC	Anterior	• Asymmetric weight shift	Direction: • Right • Left
	Lateral	• Excessive anterior pelvic tilt	• YES • NO
		• Excessive posterior pelvic tilt	• YES • NO
		• Excessive forward trunk lean	• YES • NO

Mark *Right* or *Left* or *Both* based on which limb a movement impairment was observed at. For asymmetric weight shift, mark the direction in which the shift occurred.

Additional Notes

_____

_____

_____

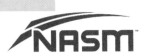

DAVIES TEST OBSERVATIONAL FINDINGS

CHECKPOINT	MOVEMENT IMPAIRMENT	RESULT
	• Excessive anterior pelvic tilt	• YES • NO
LPHC	• Excessive posterior pelvic tilt	• YES • NO
	• Excessive trunk movement	• YES • NO
Shoulders and Thoracic Spine	• Scapular elevation	• YES • NO
	• Scapular winging	• YES • NO
Head and Cervical Spine	• Excessive cervical extension/forward head	• YES • NO

TRIAL NUMBER	TIME	REPETITIONS (TOUCHES)
1	15 seconds	
2	15 seconds	
3	15 seconds	

Additional Notes

_____

_____

_____

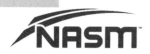

Mobility Assessments

Name _____ Date _____

OBSERVATIONAL FINDINGS

MOBILITY ASSESSMENT	MOBILITY RESTRICTED?	IF YES – OVERACTIVE/SHORTENED MUSCLES
	Yes No	
	Yes No	
	Yes No	
	Yes No	
	Yes No	
	Yes No	
	Yes No	
	Yes No	
	Yes No	

Choose appropriate mobility assessments based on the movement impairments observed during the OHSA, Modified OHSA, and any additional transitional, loaded, and dynamic movement assessments. The suggested mobility assessments listed on the assessment solutions table are a starting point that should be narrowed down. The Corrective Exercise Specialist may also choose mobility assessments for the purpose of reassessment at their discretion.

Additional Notes

_____

_____

_____

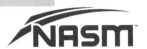

Session Readiness Questionnaire

Name _____ Date _____

REST

Sleep

☐ How many hours of sleep did you get last night? _____

☐ How rested do you currently feel?

    Very Tired / Tired / Rested / Well Rested

Stress

☐ On a scale of 1 to 10, how stressed do you feel today?

    (1 = No Stress; 10 = Extremely Stressed)
    1   2   3   4   5   6   7   8   9   10

REFUEL

Nutrition

☐ Did you eat a nutritious pre-training meal/snack today? If yes, please describe.

_____

Hydration

☐ Do you feel that you have consumed enough water prior to training?

_____

REGENERATE

Pre-activity

☐ Did you engage in movement strategies to prepare for this workout (e.g., myofascial rolling, stretching, or dynamic warm-up)? If yes, please describe.

_____

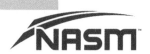

Recovery Questionnaire

Name _____ Date _____

REST

Sleep

☐ How many hours of sleep did you get last night? _____

Was your sleep disrupted more than usual?

_____

☐ How rested do you currently feel?

Very Tired / Tired / Rested / Well Rested

☐ Do you need to consume more than your usual dose of caffeine in order to stay awake and perform at your best?

_____

Relaxation

☐ How many cumulative minutes of psychological relaxation do you achieve per day?

_____

☐ How do you achieve this relaxation (e.g., reading, meditation, breathing exercises)?

_____

Stress

☐ On a scale of 1 to 10, how stressed do you feel today?

(1 = No Stress; 10 = Extremely Stressed)

1   2   3   4   5   6   7   8   9   10

REFUEL

Nutrition

☐ Do you consume nutritious pre-training meals/snacks? If yes, please describe.

_____

☐ Do you consume nutritious post-training meals/snacks? If yes, please describe.

_____

Hydration

☐ How many ounces of water have you consumed today? _____

REGENERATE

Pre-activity

☐ How many days per week do you use myofascial rolling, trigger point massage, stretching, yoga, hot-cold modalities, targeted strengthening, or other movement strategies to prepare for a workout or competition?

_____

Post-activity

☐ How many days per week do you use myofascial rolling, trigger point massage, stretching, yoga, hot-cold modalities, or other recovery strategies post-workout?

_____

SOLUTIONS TABLE

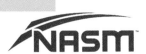

Movement Assessment Solutions Table

CHECKPOINT	VIEW	MOVEMENT IMPAIRMENT	POTENTIAL CONTRIBUTORS	SUGGESTED MOBILITY ASSESSMENTS*
Foot and Ankle	Anterior	Feet turn out	**Overactive/shortened** • Biceps femoris (short head) • Gastrocnemius (lateral) • Soleus **Underactive/lengthened** • Anterior tibialis • Gastrocnemius (medial) • Gluteus maximus • Gluteus medius • Hamstrings complex (medial) • Posterior tibialis	• Active knee extension • Ankle dorsiflexion • Hip abduction and external rotation • Modified Thomas test • Seated hip internal and external rotation
	Lateral	Heel rise	**Overactive/shortened** • Quadriceps complex • Soleus **Underactive/lengthened** • Anterior tibialis • Gluteus maximus	• Active knee flexion • Ankle dorsiflexion
	Posterior	Excessive pronation	**Overactive/shortened** • Fibularis (peroneal) complex • Gastrocnemius (lateral) • TFL **Underactive/lengthened** • Anterior tibialis • Gastrocnemius (medial) • Gluteus maximus • Gluteus medius • Intrinsic foot muscles • Posterior tibialis	• Ankle dorsiflexion • Modified Thomas test • Seated hip internal and external rotation
Knee	Anterior	Valgus (inward)	**Overactive/shortened** • Adductor complex • Biceps femoris (short head) • Gastrocnemius • Soleus • TFL • Vastus lateralis **Underactive/lengthened** • Anterior tibialis • Gluteus maximus • Gluteus medius • Hamstrings complex (medial) • Posterior tibialis • Vastus medialis oblique (VMO)	• Active knee extension • Ankle dorsiflexion • Hip abduction and external rotation • Modified Thomas test • Seated hip internal and external rotation

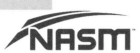

Knee (continued)				
		Varus (outward)	**Overactive/shortened** • Adductor magnus (posterior fibers) • Anterior tibialis • Biceps femoris (long head) • Piriformis • Posterior tibialis • TFL **Underactive/lengthened** • Adductor complex • Gluteus maximus • Hamstrings complex (medial)	• Active knee extension • Lumbar flexion • Modified Thomas test • Passive hip internal rotation • Seated hip internal and external rotation
	Lateral	Knee dominance	**Overactive/shortened^** • Adductor magnus • Piriformis • Quadriceps complex • Soleus **Underactive/lengthened** • Core stabilizers • Gluteus maximus	• Active knee flexion • Ankle dorsiflexion • Hip abduction and external rotation • Modified Thomas test • Passive hip internal rotation

LPHC	Anterior or Posterior	Asymmetric weight shift	**Overactive/shortened**
			• Same side as shift
			  ○ Adductor complex
			  ○ TFL
			• Opposite side of shift
			  ○ Biceps femoris
			  ○ Gastrocnemius/soleus
			  ○ Piriformis
			
			Underactive/lengthened
			• Core stabilizers
			• Same side as shift
			  ○ Gluteus medius
			• Opposite side of shift
			  ○ Adductor complex
				• Active knee extension
				• Ankle dorsiflexion
				• Hip abduction and external rotation
				• Modified Thomas test
				• Seated hip internal and external rotation

		Excessive trunk movement during testing (Davies test)	**Overactive/shortened:** • N/A **Underactive/lengthened:** • Local core stabilizers	N/A

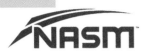

LPHC (continued)

		Overactive/shortened	

Lateral — Excessive anterior pelvic tilt (increased lumbar extension)

Overactive/shortened
- Adductor complex (anterior fibers)
- Latissimus dorsi
- Psoas
- Rectus femoris
- Spinal extensor complex (erector spinae, quadratus lumborum)
- TFL

Underactive/lengthened
- External obliques
- Gluteus maximus
- Hamstrings complex
- Local core stabilizers
- Rectus abdominis

- Active knee flexion
- Hip abduction and external rotation
- Lumbar flexion and extension
- Modified Thomas test
- Shoulder flexion

Lateral — Excessive posterior pelvic tilt (increased lumbar flexion)

Overactive/shortened
- Adductor magnus
- External obliques
- Hamstrings complex
- Piriformis
- Rectus abdominis

Underactive/lengthened
- Gluteus maximus
- Latissimus dorsi
- Local core stabilizers
- Psoas
- Rectus femoris
- Spinal extensor complex (erector spinae, quadratus lumborum)
- TFL

- Active knee extension
- Hip abduction and external rotation
- Lumbar flexion and extension
- Seated hip internal and external rotation

Excessive forward trunk lean

Overactive/shortened
- Adductor complex (anterior fibers)
- External obliques (if observed w/ lumbar flexion)
- Gastrocnemius
- Psoas
- Rectus abdominis (if observed w/ lumbar flexion)
- Rectus femoris
- Soleus
- TFL

- Active knee flexion
- Ankle dorsiflexion
- Modified Thomas test

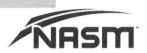

**LPHC
(continued)**

<table>
<tr><td rowspan="2">Anterior</td><td>Inward trunk rotation (single-leg and split squat)</td><td>**Overactive/shortened**
• Adductor complex
• TFL

Underactive/lengthened
• Gluteus maximus
• Gluteus medius
• Local core stabilizers</td><td>• Hip abduction and external rotation
• Modified Thomas test
• Seated hip internal and external rotation</td></tr>
<tr><td>Outward trunk rotation (single-leg and split squat)</td><td>**Overactive/shortened**
• Adductor magnus (posterior fibers)
• Hamstrings complex (lateral)
• Piriformis

Underactive/lengthened
• Adductor complex (anterior fibers)
• Gluteus maximus
• Gluteus medius
• Local core stabilizers</td><td>• Hip abduction and external rotation
• Modified Thomas test
• Seated hip internal and external rotation</td></tr>
</table>

Underactive/lengthened
- Anterior tibialis
- Gluteus maximus
- Hamstrings complex
- Local core stabilizers
- Spinal extensor complex (erector spinae, quadratus lumborum)

<table>
<tr><td rowspan="2">**Shoulders and Thoracic Spine**</td><td>Anterior or Posterior</td><td>Scapular elevation</td><td>**Overactive/shortened**
• Levator scapulae
• Pectoralis minor
• Upper trapezius

Underactive/lengthened
• Lower trapezius
• Serratus anterior</td><td>• Cervical flexion and extension
• Cervical lateral flexion
• Cervical rotation
• Seated thoracic rotation
• Shoulder retraction
• Thoracic extension</td></tr>
<tr><td>Lateral</td><td>Scapular winging (Davies test and push assessment)</td><td>**Overactive/shortened**
• Latissimus dorsi
• Pectoralis minor
• Upper trapezius

Underactive/lengthened
• Lower trapezius
• Middle trapezius
• Serratus anterior</td><td>• Seated thoracic rotation
• Shoulder flexion
• Shoulder retraction
• Thoracic extension</td></tr>
</table>

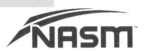

			Overactive/shortened	
Shoulders and Thoracic Spine (continued)		Arms fall forward	• Latissimus dorsi • Pectoralis major • Pectoralis minor • Teres major **Underactive/lengthened** • Infraspinatus • Lower trapezius • Middle trapezius • Posterior deltoids • Rhomboids • Teres minor	• Cervical flexion and extension • Cervical rotation • Cervical lateral flexion • Shoulder extension • Shoulder flexion • Shoulder internal and external rotation • Shoulder retraction • Seated thoracic rotation • Thoracic extension
Head and Cervical Spine	Lateral	Excessive cervical extension (forward head)	**Overactive/shortened** • Cervical extensors (suboccipital) • Levator scapulae • Sternocleidomastoid • Upper trapezius **Underactive/lengthened** • Deep cervical flexors • Lower trapezius • Middle trapezius • Rhomboids	• Cervical flexion and extension • Cervical lateral flexion • Cervical rotation

*It is not necessary to perform all of the listed mobility assessments associated with each movement impairment. The mobility assessments provided are a starting point that is narrowed down based on the results of the OHSA, Modified OHSA, and other movement assessments. It is likely that only a few mobility assessments will be needed.

^Movement competency, pain avoidance, or balance strategies should be ruled out prior to assuming over- and underactive muscles as contributing factors to knee dominance.

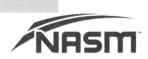

OPT® CES Programming Template

Client Name: _____

CLIENT GOAL:					
PHASE (include week #):					
DATE:					
Exercise Selection	**Sets**	**Reps**	**Tempo**	**Rest**	**Notes**
FLEXIBILITY – Inhibit with self-myofascial rolling or other technique and Lengthen w/ stretching technique					
ACTIVATION – isolated strengthening, trunk postural control (core), balance (hip/knee/ankle integration)					
INTEGRATION & SKILL DEVELOPMENT – integrated dynamic movement, SAQ, plyometrics, goal-specific prep					
RESISTANCE TRAINING – specific to phase and goal					
CLIENT'S CHOICE – single joint, additional core training, accessory movements, metabolic conditioning					
COOL DOWN – myofascial technique and static stretch					

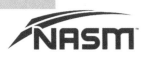

Sample Training Plan – Collegiate Golfer

Name ___Juliette Smith_____ Training Period ____In-season, January, Week 1___

MACROCYCLE

	Assessment & Corrective Exercise	Stabilization	Strength Endurance	Muscular Development	Maximal Strength	Power Endurance	Maximal Power
Pre-season (Fall, with pre-season play)	X	X	X			X	X
In-Season (Winter/ Spring)	X	X	X			X	X
Off-Season (Summer)	X	X	X		X	X	

IN-SEASON MONTHLY PLANNING

	Assessment & Corrective Exercise	Stabilization	Strength Endurance	Muscular Development	Maximal Strength	Power Endurance	Maximal Power
January	X	X	X			X	X
February			X			X	X
March	X	X	X			X	X

IN-SEASON MESOCYCLE – JANUARY

	Assessment & Corrective Exercise	Stabilization	Strength Endurance	Muscular Development	Maximal Strength	Power Endurance	Maximal Power
Week 1	X	X	X				
Week 2		X	X				
Week 3			X			X	
Week 4			X			X	X

MICROCYCLE – JANUARY – WEEK 1

	Monday	Tuesday	Wednesday	Thursday	Friday	Saturday	Sunday
Self-Care		X	X	X	X	X	X
Assessment & Corrective Exercise	Re-assessment						
Stabilization	X		X				
Strength Endurance					X		

GLOSSARY

A

Abduction A body segment is moving away from the midline of the body.

Activation techniques Corrective exercise techniques used to reeducate or increase activation of underactive muscle tissues.

Active motion The amount of motion obtained solely through voluntary contraction.

Ad libidum Latin phrase that translates to "as desired"; refers to eating or drinking as you are normally driven to (i.e., not purposely overeating or undereating).

Adduction A body segment is moving toward the midline of the body.

Afferent Sensory neurons that carry signals from sensory stimuli toward the central nervous system.

Agonist The prime mover muscle for a given movement pattern or joint action.

Altered length-tension relationships Occur when the resting length of a muscle is too short or too long to generate optimal force.

Altered reciprocal inhibition Process whereby an overactive/shortened muscle causes decreased neural drive, and therefore less-than-optimal recruitment of its functional antagonist.

Ankle sprain An injury to the ankle ligaments in which small tears occur in the ligaments.

Ankylosing spondylitis A form of arthritis that primarily affects the spine, although other joints can become involved; causes inflammation of the spinal joints (vertebrae) that can lead to severe chronic pain and discomfort.

Antagonist A muscle that acts in direct opposition to the prime mover.

Anterior cruciate ligament (ACL) injury One of the main knee ligaments; stabilizes the knee by stabilizing the anterior translation of the tibia relative to the femur. Injuries often take the form of overstretching or tearing due to sudden lower extremity movements such as stops, changes of direction, rotation, etc.

Autogenic inhibition The process by which neural impulses that sense tension are greater than the impulses that cause muscles to contract, providing an inhibitory effect to the muscle spindles.

B

Ballistic stretching Stretching that involves higher-velocity movements with bouncing actions at the end of the range of motion.

Biopsychosocial model of pain Treatment paradigm for chronic musculoskeletal pain that accounts for the role of biological, psychological, and social factors in an individual's experience of pain.

Breathing pattern dysfunction (BPD) A collection of suboptimal breathing patterns that can cause overactivity of accessory breathing muscles.

C

Cervical lordosis The curvature of the cervical spine.

Cervicogenic headaches Headaches originating from the neck.

Chronic ankle instability Repetitive episodes of giving way at the ankle, coupled with feelings of instability.

Cocontractions The simultaneous contraction of muscles around a joint.

Compensatory movement A nonideal movement strategy employed by the kinetic chain to fulfill the desired movement pattern.

Concentric muscle action Occurs when a muscle generates force while shortening to accelerate an external load.

Corrective exercise The systematic process of identifying a neuromusculoskeletal dysfunction, developing a plan of action, and implementing an integrated corrective strategy.

Corrective Exercise Continuum The systematic programming process used to address neuromusculoskeletal dysfunction using inhibitory, lengthening, activation, and integration techniques.

Cross-bridge mechanism The collective physiological processes that cause actin and myosin filaments to slide across each other, functionally shortening the muscle as it develops tension.

Cumulative injury cycle A cycle whereby an injury will induce inflammation, muscle spasm, adhesion, altered neuromuscular control, and muscle imbalances.

Cupping A form of myofascial therapy commonly practiced in Asian and Middle Eastern cultures that has recently become more popular in the United States.

D

Davis's law Law that states that soft tissue will model along the lines of stress.

De Quervain's tenosynovitis An inflammation or a tendinosis of the sheath or tunnel that surrounds two tendons that control movement of the thumb.

Deep neck flexors Muscle group that includes the longus colli, longus capitis, rectus capitis anterior, and lateralis.

Degenerative disc disease Thinning of the intervertebral discs as a result of the aging process, which can predispose pain, stiffness, bone spurs, and disc herniation.

Disfacilitation Occurs when a receptor decreases its firing frequency or neural discharge, resulting in a weaker signal. Example: Muscle spindles decrease their discharge frequency after prolonged static stretching.

Dynamic malalignments Deviations from optimal posture during functional movements.

Dynamic movement assessments Assessments that involve movement with a change in the base of support.

Dynamic posture How an individual is able to maintain an erect posture while performing functional tasks or in motion.

Dynamic stabilization Ability of the human movement system to control and minimize unwanted joint motions during movement.

Dynamic stretching The active extension of a muscle, using a muscle's force production and the body's momentum, to take a joint through the full available range of motion.

E

Eccentric muscle action Occurs when a muscle generates force while lengthening to decelerate an external load.

Efferent Motor neurons that carry signals from the central nervous system toward muscles to create movement.

Extensor mechanism Composed of the patellofemoral articulation, patellar tendon, quadriceps tendon, and tibial tubercle working together to produce concentric, eccentric, and isometric actions at the knee.

External (augmented) feedback Information provided by some external source, for example, a health and fitness professional, video, mirror, or heart rate monitor.

Extrinsic muscles Foot muscles that originate in the lower leg and insert in the foot as tendons.

F

Facet joints A set of synovial, plane joints located between and behind adjacent vertebrae.

Feedback The utilization of sensory information and sensorimotor integration to aid in the development of permanent neural representations of motor patterns for efficient movement.

Firing rate The frequency at which a motor unit is activated.

Flexibility The present state or ability of a joint to move through a range of motion.

Force transmission Muscle forces applied to the skeleton via pathways other than muscular origin and insertion.

Force-couple relationship The synergistic action of muscles to produce movement around a joint.

Forearm pronation Internal rotation of the forearm and hand so that the palm faces downward.

Forearm supination External rotation of the forearm and hand so that the palm faces upward.

Forward head posture Occurs when the head is protruding anterior to the shoulders in the sagittal plane; can lead to development of head and neck pain, movement restrictions, and compensations above and below the cervical spine.

Functional efficiency The ability of the neuromuscular system to recruit correct muscle synergies, at the right time, with the appropriate amount of force to perform functional tasks with the least amount of energy and stress on the human movement system (HMS).

G

Gamma loop The reflex arc consisting of small anterior horn nerve cells and their small fibers that project to the intrafusal bundle and produce its contraction, which initiates the afferent impulses that pass through the posterior root to the anterior horn cells, inducing, in turn, reflex contraction of the entire muscle.

Global muscular system Muscles responsible predominantly for movement and consisting of more superficial musculature that originates from the pelvis to the rib cage, the lower extremities, or both.

Golgi tendon organs (GTOs) Receptors sensitive to change in tension of the muscle and the rate of that change.

H

Hyperextension Extension of a limb or joint greater than the normal range of motion.

Hyperkyphosis A spinal disorder in which an excessive outward curve of the spine results in an abnormal rounding of the upper back.

Hypermobility Increased movement and functionality of a joint beyond normal range of motion.

Hypomobility Decrease in normal movement and functionality of a joint, which affects range of motion.

I

Iliotibial (IT) band syndrome Often associated with runner's knee; usually an overuse injury where the iliotibial band rubs on the femur, resulting in lateral knee pain.

Inelastic Possessing the inability to stretch.

Inhibitory techniques Corrective exercise techniques used to reduce tension or decrease activity of overactive neuromyofascial tissues in the body.

Instrument-assisted soft tissue mobilization (IASTM) Specifically designed instruments to provide a mobilizing effect to scar tissue and myofascial adhesions.

Integrated muscle function The joint motion(s) created when a muscle contracts eccentrically or isometrically.

Integration techniques Corrective exercise techniques used to retrain the collective synergistic function of all muscles through functionally progressive movements.

Intermuscular coordination The ability of different muscles in the body to work together to allow coordination of global and refined movements.

Internal (sensory) feedback The process by which sensory information is used by the body via length-tension relationships, force-couple relationships, and arthrokinematics to monitor movement and the environment.

Intramuscular coordination The ability of the neuromuscular system to allow optimal levels of motor unit recruitment and synchronization within a muscle.

Intrinsic muscles Refers to muscles located deep within a structure.

Isolated muscle function The joint motion created when a muscle contracts concentrically.

Isometric muscle action Occurs when a muscle generates force equal to an external load to hold it in place.

K

Kinematic adjustments Small alterations in movement pattern execution made in response to repetitive or novel performance conditions.

Kinetic chain The combination and interrelation of the nervous, muscular, and skeletal systems.

Kinetic chain checkpoints Key points on the body to observe and assess an individual's static

and dynamic posture; feet/ankles, knees, LPHC, shoulders, and head/neck.

Knowledge of performance Provides information about the quality of the movement.

Knowledge of results Used after the completion of a movement to inform individuals about the outcome of their performance.

Kyphosis Natural curvature of the thoracic spine toward the back of the body.

L

Leg dominance Limb-to-limb asymmetries in neuromusculoskeletal control or muscle recruitment.

Length-tension relationship The resting length of a muscle and the tension the muscle can produce at this resting length.

Lengthening techniques Corrective exercise techniques used to increase the extensibility, length, and range of motion of neuromyofascial tissues in the body.

Ligament dominance Decreased lower extremity frontal plane stability, usually evidenced by valgus and varus positioning, causing connective tissues to be the limiting factor of end range of motion control.

Loaded movement assessment Observing a client's posture under an additional source of resistance.

Local musculature system Muscles that connect directly to the spine and are predominantly involved in LPHC stabilization.

Lordosis Natural curvature of the lumbar or cervical spine toward the front of the body.

Lower crossed syndrome A postural distortion pattern characterized by an anterior tilt to the pelvis and lower extremity muscle imbalances.

M

Medial tibial stress syndrome (MTSS) Pain in the front of the tibia caused by an overload to the tibia and the associated musculature.

Mobility The entire available range of motion at a joint and the body's neuromuscular control of that motion.

Mobility restriction The inability to move a joint through what should be its full range of motion.

Motor behavior The human movement system's response to internal and external environmental stimuli.

Motor control The study of posture and movements with the involved structures and mechanisms used by the central nervous system to assimilate and integrate sensory information with previous experiences.

Motor development The change in motor behavior over time throughout a person's life span.

Motor learning The utilization of these processes through practice and experience leading to a relatively permanent change in a person's capacity to produce skilled movements.

Motor unit activation The progressive activation of a muscle by successive recruitment of contractile units (motor units) to accomplish increasing gradations of contractile strength.

Movement compensation When the body moves in a suboptimal way in response to kinetic chain dysfunction.

Movement impairment State in which the structural integrity of the human movement system is compromised because one or more segments of the kinetic chain are out of alignment.

Movement patterns Common combinations of joint motions the human body uses to move in all three planes of motion.

Muscle action spectrum The range of muscle contractions used to accelerate, decelerate, and stabilize forces.

Muscle imbalance Alteration of muscle length surrounding a joint.

Muscle innervation A muscle's point of connection to the nervous system.

Muscle insertion Where the end point of a muscle connects back to the skeleton.

Muscle origin The beginning attachment point of a muscle.

Muscle spasms Involuntary contraction of muscles surrounding a joint that immobilizes it in response to an injury.

Muscle spindles Receptors sensitive to change in length of the muscle and the rate of that change.

Muscle strain An injury to a muscle (tear in tendon) in which the muscle fibers tear as a result of overstretching; usually these are graded from I to III, with I being mild pulls and III being complete tears.

Muscular sling A group of muscles that, when contracted, provide stability.

Myofascia A strong, thin, fibrous connective tissue matrix that is woven throughout the body and surrounds muscles, bones, blood vessels, and nerves. The term *neuromyofascia* is also used.

Myofascial adhesions Knots in muscle tissue that can result in altered neuromuscular control.

Myofascial balls Spherical tools used for myofascial rolling that come in different sizes and densities; often called *massage balls*.

Myofascial flossing Method intended to increase flexibility by wrapping an elastic band around a region of the body and performing movements.

Myofascial rolling A compression intervention where an external object (e.g., foam roller) compresses the myofascia.

Myofascial trigger points Painful regions within a tight band of skeletal muscle that also give rise to referred pain.

N

Naive range of motion Range of motion improvements that are gained without being properly integrated into the existing proficiencies of the human movement system.

Neural drive The rate and volume of activation signals a muscle receives from the central nervous system.

Neuromuscular efficiency The ability of the neuromuscular system to allow agonists, antagonists, synergists, and stabilizers to work synergistically to produce, reduce, and dynamically stabilize the human movement system in all three planes of motion.

Neuromuscular stretching (NMS) A flexibility technique that incorporates varied combinations of isometric contraction and static stretching of the target muscle to create increases in range of motion. Also called proprioceptive neuromuscular facilitation (PNF).

Neutralizers Muscles that limit or cease an undesirable action of the mobile attachment site of the muscle.

Nociceptors Pain receptors that send pain information to the central nervous system through type III and IV afferents.

Nuclear chain and nuclear bag Fibers located in the muscle spindles that detect the amount of stretch and the rate and extent of stretch of the muscle. This information is relayed to the central nervous system by type I and II afferents.

O

Osteoarthritis The most common form of arthritis, affecting millions of people worldwide; occurs when the protective cartilage that cushions the ends of the bones wears down over time.

Osteoporosis Literally "porous bone"; a disease in which the density and quality of bone is reduced.

Overactive/shortened Occurs when elevated neural drive causes a muscle to be held in a chronic state of contraction.

P

Passive motion The amount of motion observed without any assistance from an external force.

Patellar tendinopathy Often associated with jumper's knee; commonly an overuse injury affecting the patellar tendon, resulting in anterior knee pain.

Patellofemoral pain syndrome A musculoskeletal condition in which a client experiences pain behind and around the patella with running, squatting, jumping, or other physical activity.

Pattern overload Occurs when a segment of the body is repeatedly moved or chronically held in the same way, leading to a state of muscle overactivity.

Pelvo-ocular reflex A postural reflex in which anterior rotation of the pelvis occurs as a result of forward head posture.

Perceptions The integration of sensory information with past experiences or memories.

Pes cavus A high medial arch during weight-bearing.

Pes planus A flattened medial arch during weight-bearing.

Pes planus distortion syndrome A postural distortion pattern characterized by flat feet, knee valgus, and an anterior pelvic tilt.

Physical Activity Readiness Questionnaire for Everyone (PAR-Q+) Series of questions designed to determine if a person is ready to undertake more strenuous physical activity.

Plantar fasciitis Irritation and swelling of the thick tissue on the bottom of the foot. The most common complaint is pain in the bottom of the heel.

Postural distortion Malalignments of bodily segments that place undue stress on the joints; for example, poor posture at one or more of the kinetic chain checkpoints.

Postural sway A measure of postural stability and control, often while standing. Refers to the amount of reflexive movement made by an individual around their center of gravity to remain balanced.

Posture The independent and interdependent alignment (static posture) and function (transitional and dynamic posture) of all components of the human movement system at any given moment, controlled by the central nervous system.

Primary movement patterns Common patterns of functional movement used by all humans.

Principle of overload Implies that there must be a training stimulus provided that exceeds the current capabilities of the kinetic chain to elicit the optimal physical, physiological, and performance adaptations.

Pronation A triplanar movement that is associated with force reduction.

Pronation distortion syndrome A movement impairment characterized by foot pronation and lower extremity muscle imbalances.

Pronation of the foot A multiplanar, synchronized joint motion that occurs with eccentric muscle function; the combination of subtalar eversion, dorsiflexion, and abduction.

Proprioception The cumulative neural input from sensory afferents to the central nervous system.

Q

Quadriceps dominance Decreased strength or recruitment of the posterior chain musculature relative to anterior chain musculature.

R

Range of motion (ROM) The amount of motion available at a specific joint.

Reciprocal inhibition When an agonist contracts, its functional antagonist relaxes to allow movement to occur at a joint.

Recovery A systematic physiological and psychological process in which the body and brain require replenishment and rejuvenation in order to prepare for the next training or competition.

Recurrent inhibition A feedback circuit that can decrease the excitability of motor neurons via interneurons called Renshaw cells.

Referred pain Pain perceived at a different location than the source.

Refuel Aspect of recovery that focuses on nutrition and hydration habits prior to, during, and after activity.

Regenerate Aspect of recovery that focuses on movement-based self-care strategies to optimize movement quality and minimize compensation.

Regional interdependence (RI) model Assessment and intervention model used by clinicians based on the concept that the site of a patient's primary complaint or symptoms is affected by dysfunction in remote musculoskeletal regions.

Relative flexibility The body's ability to find the path of least resistance to accomplish a task, even if that path creates dynamic malalignments.

Renshaw cells Interneurons that prevent excessive output of the central nervous system's contraction reflex response to sudden changes in muscle length.

Rest Aspect of recovery that focuses on improving daily sleep amount and quality, limiting stress, and increasing physical and psychological relaxation.

Resting length A muscle's state when the body is standing still; not contracting or stretching.

S

Sarcomere The functional unit of a muscle made up of overlapping actin and myosin filaments.

Scapular dyskinesis Occurs when the scapula does not move in a normal fashion during humeral elevation.

Scapulohumeral rhythm The interaction between the scapula and the humerus; important for shoulder function.

Scheuermann's disease A developmental disorder of the spine that causes abnormal growth of usually the thoracic (upper back) vertebrae, but it can also be found in the lumbar vertebrae.

Scoliosis Sideways curvature of the spine that occurs most often during the growth spurt just before puberty.

Scope of practice The procedures and actions professionals are permitted to administer in accordance with state and national law.

Screw-home mechanism External tibial rotation on the femur in open-chain exercises and femoral internal rotation in closed-chain exercises, resulting in the knee "locking-out."

Self-efficacy An individual's belief and confidence in their capacity to execute necessary behaviors to attain specific performance results.

Self-myofascial techniques The category of flexibility techniques used to reduce tension in muscle fibers. Primarily used for overactive tissue.

Sensations A process by which sensory information is received by the receptor and transferred either to the spinal cord for reflexive motor behavior, to higher cortical areas for processing, or both.

Sensorimotor integration The ability of the central nervous system to gather and interpret sensory information to execute the proper motor response.

Sensory information The data that the central nervous system receives from sensory receptors to determine such things as the body's position in space and limb orientation as well as information about the environment, temperature, texture, etc.

Shoulder girdle The bones and joints that connect the upper extremity to the axial skeleton. Composed of the scapulae, clavicles, and manubrium (broad upper portion) of the sternum.

Shoulder impingement Occurs when the space between the bone on top of the shoulder (acromion) and the tendons of the rotator cuff rub against each other during arm elevation.

Six dimensions of wellness Interdependent categories used by the National Wellness Institute to illustrate the primary properties of an individual's holistic health and overall functioning.

Spinal remodeling Abnormal reshaping of the spine's physiologic curvatures due to sustained abnormal posture.

Spinal stenosis Narrowing of the spinal canal resulting in compression of the spinal cord.

Stabilizers Muscles that support or stabilize the body while the prime movers and the synergists perform the movement patterns.

Static malalignments Deviations from ideal posture that can be seen when standing still.

Static posture The starting point from which an individual moves.

Static stretching The process of passively taking a muscle to the point of tension and holding the stretch for a minimum of 30 seconds.

Stretch-shortening cycle An active stretch (eccentric contraction) of a muscle followed by an immediate shortening (concentric contraction) of that same muscle.

Stretching An active process to elongate muscles and connective tissues in order to increase the present state of flexibility.

Structural efficiency The alignment of each segment of the human movement system, which allows posture to be balanced in relation to a person's center of gravity.

Subtalar eversion Occurs when the bottom of the heel (inferior calcaneus) swings laterally.

Subtalar inversion Occurs when the bottom of the heel (inferior calcaneus) swings medially.

Supination A triplanar motion that is associated with force production.

Supination of the foot A multiplanar, synchronized joint motion that occurs with concentric muscle function; the combination of subtalar inversion, plantar flexion, and adduction.

Synchronization The synergistic activation of multiple motor units.

Synergists Muscles that assist prime movers during functional movement patterns.

Synergistic dominance The process by which a synergist compensates for an inhibited prime mover to maintain force production.

T

Tendinopathy A broad term encompassing pain, swelling, and impaired performance occurring in and around tendons in response to overuse; commonly associated with the Achilles tendon.

Text neck Neck and upper back pain caused by poor posture during excessive cell phone use.

Thixotropic effects Reduced tissue viscoelasticity due to tissues being shaken, agitated, sheared, or stressed.

Thoracic kyphosis (TK) The outward curvature of the thoracic spine that provides the rounded appearance of the upper back.

Tissue creep An initial rapid increase in strain followed by a slower increase in strain at a constant stress.

Torque A force that produces rotation; most commonly measured in Newton-meters (Nm).

Transitional movement assessments Assessments that involve movement without a change in the base of support.

U

Underactive/lengthened Occurs when inhibited neural drive allows a muscle's functional antagonist to pull it into a chronically elongated state.

Upper crossed syndrome A postural distortion syndrome characterized by a forward head and rounded shoulders with upper extremity muscle imbalances.

V

Viscoelastic The collective properties related to fluid flow, heat dissipation, and elasticity of tissue.

Viscoelasticity See *Viscoelastic*.

INDEX

Note: Page numbers followed by "*f*" and "*t*" indicate figures and tables respectively.

C

capitis division
  longissimus, 27, 27f
  spinalis, 28, 28f
  transversospinalis, 30, 30f
carpal tunnel syndrome, 445–446
center of gravity, 233
cervical extension, excessive, 221f
cervical lordosis, 450
cervical spine (CS), 142f, 450
  assessment results, 460–463, 461t
  corrective exercise program, 464t, 472t
  curvature, 450
  dynamic malalignments, 456–457
  dynamic movement assessments,
      462–463
  functional anatomy
    bones and joints, 450–452, 451f
    muscles, 452–453, 452t
    neck region, 451f
  issues associated with, 472–475
    degenerative disc disease, 474–475
    muscle strain, 473–474
    stenosis of cervical spine, 474
  and Regional Interdependence model,
      457–460
  static malalignments, 453–454
  structure, 451f
  systematic corrective exercise strategies,
      463–472
  transitional movement assessment, 462
cervical vertebrae, 450
cervicis division
  iliocostalis, 26, 26f
  longissimus, 27, 27f
  spinalis, 28, 28f
  transversospinalis, 29, 29f
cervicogenic headaches, 458
CES Assessment Flow. See Corrective
    Exercise Specialist Assessment Flow
chronic ankle instability, 317
client communication, 165–166
client consent, 179
client intake and assessment, 164–180, 534f
  client communication, 165–166
  client consent, 179
  client intake screen, 168–178, 169f, 534f
  codes of professional conduct, 179
  ethical and legal considerations, 178–180,
      180t
  general lifestyle information, 171–174
    hobbies, 174
    lifestyle, 172–174
    occupation, 171–172
    recreation, 174
  goal setting, 177–178

medical history, 174–177
    cumulative injury cycle, 177f
    past injuries, 175–176, 175t
    past surgeries, 176–177
  readiness for activity, 168–170
  record keeping, 179
  scope of practice, 178–179
closed-packed position, 394
cocontractions, 459
codes of professional conduct, 179
communication skills, recovery and,
    496–500
compensatory movement, 166
concentric muscle actions, 14–15
contraindications for myofascial rolling,
    78–79, 79t
contralateral gluteus maximus, 55
corrective exercise, 3. See also Corrective
    Exercise Continuum; corrective
    exercise strategies
  client care and performance, 6–7
  defined, 3
  diagnosis and treatment, 8–9
  goals, 7–8
  philosophy of, 3
  populations, 8
  professional responsibilities, 7
  professional scope, 5–6
  professional settings, 8
  rationale for, 3
  Regional Interdependence model, 5
  specialist, 5–8
  techniques and skills, 8
Corrective Exercise Continuum, 3–5, 4f, 67f,
    89, 89f, 124f, 146, 146f, 533
  activation techniques, 124f
  for elbow and wrist, 436
  inhibitory techniques, 67f
  integration techniques, 146f
  lengthening techniques, 89f
  phase of, 124
Corrective Exercise Specialist Assessment
    Flow, 167, 167f, 185f, 191f, 229f, 235f,
    240f, 249f, 265f, 526–533
corrective exercise strategies
  application of, 502–524
    in athletic team and sport
      environments, 519–521
    client adherence and success, factors
      influencing, 505–507
    compensations and, 512–513
    for desired outcomes, 507–508t
    entire workout and, 517–518
    functional and lifestyle needs, 510
    goals and, 507
    in group settings, 518–519
    to improve adherence, 511–512

    incorporation to different scenarios,
        516–524
    movement patterns, reinforcing
        proper, 513
    phases, usage of, 513–515, 514f
    post-workout and, 517
    prioritizing of programming, 509–512
    program plan, 512t
    progressions, 515–516
    region, prioritizing, 509–510
    for return to performance, 523
    terminologies, 503–504
    with time and schedule constraints,
        522–523, 522t
    warm-up and, 517
    without equipment, 523–524
    workout or activity, needs of, 510–511
  for cervical spine, 463–472, 464t
  for desired outcomes, 507–508t
  for elbow and wrist, 436–442, 437t
  for foot and ankle, 303–313
  for knee, 330–343, 331t
  for LPHC, 361–377
  for shoulder impairments, 408–417
cross-bridge mechanism, 44
CS. See cervical spine
cumulative injury cycle, 58, 59f, 68–70, 177f
  myofascial rolling and, 68–70, 68f
cupping, myofascial rolling, 76, 76f
cutting maneuvers, 340
  integrated techniques and, 155f

D

Davies test
  movement, 256
  observation, 256–257
  observational findings template, 257f, 546f
  position, 255–256, 256f
  procedure, 255–256
Davis's law, 69
deep longitudinal subsystem (DLS),
    54–55, 54f
degenerative disc disease, 474–475
depth jump assessment, 252–254, 253f
  observational findings template, 254f, 545f
de Quervain tenosynovitis, 445
diaphragm, 25, 25f
disfacilitation, 92
distal bones, 322f
DLS. See deep longitudinal subsystem
dynamic functional movements,
    468–470f
dynamic malalignments
  cervical spine, 456–457
  elbow, 433
  foot and ankle, 296–297

scapulothoracic joint, 395, 395f, 396f
Scheuermann's disease, 418
scoliosis, 399, 400f
scope of practice, 6, 178–179
screw-home mechanism, 321
self-efficacy, 512
self-myofascial rolling. *See* myofascial
    rolling
self-myofascial techniques (SMT). *See also*
    myofascial rolling
  application guidelines for, 71–73
    density, 72
    diameter, 73
    pressure, 71–72
    texture, 73
  defined, 67
  tools, 73–77
semimembranosus, 17, 17f
semitendinosus, 17, 17f
sensations, 41
sensorimotor integration, 43
sensory feedback. *See* internal feedback
sensory information, 40
sensory receptors, 70
serratus anterior, 30, 30f
  isolated strengthening exercises, 137f
shin splints. *See* medial tibial stress
    syndrome
short foot, 129f
shortened muscle, 45
shoulder, 392f
  arms fall forward, 414–415
  assessment, 403–404t
    overhead press, 248t
  assessment process, 403
  assessment results, 403–404t, 403–408
  common issues associated with, 417–421
  corrective exercise strategies, 408–417
  dynamic malalignments, 401
  dynamic movement assessments, 407
  force-couples of, 396f
  frozen, 421
  functional anatomy
    bones and joints, 391–396
    dynamic stabilizers, 394
    glenohumeral joint, 393–394, 394f
    scapula, 392–393
    scapulothoracic joint, 395, 395f, 396f
    sternoclavicular joint, 395
  impingement, 418, 419, 419f
  injuries, 417
  instability, 421
  isolated strengthening exercises,
    137–139f
  muscles, 396–398
  overhead squat movement, 405–406
  pain, 399

scapular winging, 416, 417t
  shoulder elevation, 415
  static malalignments, 399
  transitional movement assessments,
    405–407
shoulder elevation, 415, 416t
  during pulling assessment, 406f
shoulder girdle, unique anatomy, 392, 393f
shoulder impingement syndrome (SIS),
    418–419
single-arm row to arrow position, integrated
    dynamic movement exercises, 157f
single-leg balance with multiplanar reach,
    integrated dynamic movement
    exercises, 158f
single-leg functional movements, 56
single-leg hop exercise, 340
single-leg horizontal jump test, integrated
    techniques and, 155f
single-leg Romanian deadlift to PNF
    pattern, 160f, 413f
single-leg squat assessment, 301
  knee, 329, 329f
  knee assessment, 329
  LPHC movement, 360f
  movement, 234
  observation, 234
  position, 234f
  procedure, 234
single-leg squatting, 338f
single-leg squat to overhead press,
    integrated dynamic movement
    exercises, 160f
six dimensions of wellness, 482
skeletal muscles, functional anatomy, 14
sleep strategies, recovery and, 488–489
SMT. *See* self-myofascial techniques
soleus, 15, 15f
  myofascial rolling, 332f, 363f
  neuromuscular stretches, 334f, 364f
  static stretches, 333f, 364f
spinalis
  capitis division, 28, 28f
  cervicus division, 28, 28f
  thoracis division, 28, 28f
spinal remodeling, 454
squat, 301
squat to row, integrated dynamic movement
    exercises, 158f
stabilization, dynamic, 52
stabilizers, 14
standing cable external rotation, isolated
    strengthening exercises, 136f
standing elbow extension, isolated
    strengthening exercises, 141f
standing elbow flexion, isolated
    strengthening exercises, 140f

standing gluteus maximus, isolated
    strengthening exercises, 132f
standing gluteus medius, isolated
    strengthening exercises, 133f
standing hip flexor, isolated strengthening
    exercises, 133f
standing overhead dumbbell press
  assessment, 248t
  movement, 247, 247f
  observation, 247–248
  observational findings template, 248f, 543f
  position, 246–247, 247f
  procedure, 246–248
standing pull assessment, 244–246, 245f
  observational findings template, 246f, 543f
standing push assessment, 243–244, 243f
  observational findings template, 244f, 543f
standing quadriceps, isolated strengthening
    exercises, 130f
static adductor magnus stretch, 111f
static ball latissimus dorsi stretch, 112f
static ball pectoral stretch, 112f
static biceps stretch, 438f
static erector spinae stretch, 112f
static gastrocnemius stretch, 110f
static kneeling hip flexor stretch, 114f
static kneeling TFL stretch, 115f
static levator scapulae stretch, 113f
static long head of biceps stretch, 113f
static malalignments
  cervical spine, 453–454
  elbow, 432
  foot and ankle, 296–297
  human movement science and, 59–60
  knee, 325
  LPHC, 354
  shoulder, 399
  thoracic spine, 399
  wrist, 432
static piriformis stretch, 112f
static posterior shoulder stretch, 112f
static postural assessment, 185–186, 461
  altered movement patterns, 189
  assessment observations form, 192f, 539f
  CES Assessment Flow, 191f
  distortional patterns, 191f
  habitual movement patterns, 189
  Janda's postural distortion syndromes,
    197–201, 207–208t
  Kendall's posture types, 202–205, 208t
  muscle imbalance, 186–190
  pes planus distortion syndrome, 206–207
  systematic approach, 190–193
  use, 209
static posture, 166, 185, 185f, 357, 404, 461
static seated ball adductor stretch, 111f
static soleus stretch, 110f